Ascorbic Acid:
Chemistry, Metabolism, and Uses

Ascorbic Acid:
Chemistry, Metabolism, and Uses

Paul A. Seib, EDITOR
Kansas State University

Bert M. Tolbert, EDITOR
University of Colorado

Based on a symposium

sponsored by the Division of

Carbohydrate Chemistry

at the Second Chemical Congress

of the North American Continent

(180th ACS National Meeting),

Las Vegas, Nevada,

August 26–27, 1980.

ADVANCES IN CHEMISTRY SERIES **200**

AMERICAN CHEMICAL SOCIETY
WASHINGTON, D. C.   1982

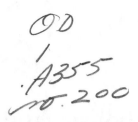

Library of Congress Cataloging in Publication Data

Ascorbic acid.

(Advances in chemistry series, ISSN 0065–2393; 200)

Includes bibliographies and index.

1. Vitamin C—Congresses.
I. Seib, Paul A., 1936–   . II. Tolbert, Bert M., 1921–   . III. American Chemical Society. Division of Carboydrate Chemistry. IV. Chemical Congress of the North American Continent (2nd: 1980: Las Vegas, Nev.). V. American Chemical Society. National Meeting (180th: 1980: Las Vegas, Nev.). VI. Series.

QD1.A355 no. 200 [QP772.A8]   540s   82–13795
ISBN 0–8412–0632–5 [574.19′26]   ADCSAJ 200
                                   1–604   1982

Copyright © 1982

American Chemical Society

Advances in Chemistry Series

M. Joan Comstock, *Series Editor*

FOREWORD

ADVANCES IN CHEMISTRY SERIES was founded in 1949 by the American Chemical Society as an outlet for symposia and collections of data in special areas of topical interest that could not be accommodated in the Society's journals. It provides a medium for symposia that would otherwise be fragmented, their papers distributed among several journals or not published at all. Papers are reviewed critically according to ACS editorial standards and receive the careful attention and processing characteristic of ACS publications. Volumes in the ADVANCES IN CHEMISTRY SERIES maintain the integrity of the symposia on which they are based; however, verbatim reproductions of previously published papers are not accepted. Papers may include reports of research as well as reviews since symposia may embrace both types of presentation.

CONTENTS

PREFACE

THE BRILLIANT SUCCESS OF ASCORBIC ACID RESEARCH in the 1930s led to the commercial production of inexpensive ascorbic acid in large quantities. The wide distribution of ascorbic acid, and its incorporation into many food products, so completely solved the problem of scurvy in both general and special populations that pressure for a more complete scientific understanding of this vitamin was sharply reduced. As a result many questions concerning ascorbic acid's chemistry, biochemistry, physiological roles and kinetics, and its nutritional requirements were deferred for more pressing scientific problems.

In spite of a relaxed position for ascorbic acid studies, our technical knowledge regarding this vitamin has greatly increased during the second half of the 20th century. Much remains to be done. The results described in this book will contribute to that development by summarizing current work in many areas.

The metabolism of ascorbic acid has yet to be clarified. Only one of the major water-soluble urinary metabolites of ascorbic acid has been isolated and characterized; the others and the matabolic pathways involved are yet to be defined. When these pathways and their intermediates are understood, there will be good possibilities for significant nutritional and medical innovation.

The physiological roles of ascorbic acid have not yet been described in a manner that is scientifically satisfactory. The presence of ascorbic acid in all eucaryote organisms suggests fundamental roles that are not understood. The absence of ascorbic acid in procaryote organisms suggests an unknown fundamental difference between these two classes of organisms in which ascorbic acid plays an essential role.

Perhaps more than any other nutritional factor, ascorbic acid has been the focus of the questions, "How much ascorbic acid is required in humans for optimum health and well-being?" and "What factors can change this requirement?" There seem to be no simple answers to these questions, but good progress has been made in fundamentals related to this problem, such as measurement of pool sizes and turnover in humans as a function of environmental variables. The lack of such physiological data for children, women, and pregnant women needs to be corrected.

Ascorbic acid has been implicated in a great variety of biological phenomena, such as the immune reactions, the cytochrome P_{450} system, cell division, neurological function, atherosclerosis, and free radical reactions in biological fluids. Unfortunately none of these different proposals have led to well defined and accepted uses of ascorbic acid. Even the demonstrated requirement for ascorbic acid in the formation of connective tissues is not sufficient to mandate post-operational supplementation of a diet with ascorbic acid. To prove beneficial effects from supplemental dietary ascorbic acid has been extremely difficult.

Large quantities of ascorbic acid are used by the pharmaceutical and food industries. Ascorbic acid is added to food as a nutrient or as a processing acid in brewing, wine making, bread making, meat curing, and freezing of fruits. Losses of the vitamin in processing, storing and cooking of foods are substantial. There is still a need for a stable form of vitamin C to use in foods.

Recently, C. F. Klopfenstein, E. Varriano-Marston and R. C. Hoseney (*Nutrition Reports International* 1981, 24: 1017–1028) found that a diet of 50% grain sorghum gave poor growth in guinea pigs receiving 2 mg of ascorbic acid/day. When the level of ascorbic acid was increased to 40 mg/day, the pigs grew normally. Wheat, millet, and oats did not depress the growth of pigs. The impact of these findings in human nutrition is not clear.

Much progress has been made in recent years in the chemistry of ascorbic acid. At least six new syntheses of L-ascorbic acid have been devised since 1971. One of those methods was used to prepare specifically labeled L-ascorbic acid to investigate its biosynthesis in plants. Proton magnetic resonance at 600.2 MHz has shown that the side chain of L-ascorbic acid and its sodium salt in aqueous solution adopt the same conformation as crystalline L-ascorbic acid. The conformation of crystalline sodium L-ascorbate, on the other hand, is different.

Assay methods for ascorbic acid have steadily improved. High performance liquid chromatography can now be used to separate and quantitate ascorbic, dehydroascorbic, and 2-ketogulonic acids. Improved analytical techniques are needed to identify and quantitate the oxidation products of ascorbic acid.

New derivatives of L-ascorbic acid have been synthesized including saccharoascorbic acid, 5-ketoascorbic acid, 2-phosphoric-ascorbic acid, 6-bromo-6-deoxyascorbic acid, 6-chloro-6-deoxyascorbic acid, the 5,6-dehydro-5,6-dideoxy derivative, the 4,5-dehydro-5-deoxy derivative, the 5,6-dideoxy derivative, and numerous nitrogen derivatives.

Dehydroascorbic acid is now readily prepared in pure form by the Ohmori–Takagi method in which ascorbic acid is dissolved in ethanol and oxygenated in the presence of charcoal. The structure of dehydro-L-ascorbic acid is solvent dependent. In water, dehydro-L-ascorbic acid exists almost exclusively in the bicyclic hydrated monomer in which 6-OH bonds to C3 through a hemiketal linkage. In *N,N*-dimethylformamide and acetonitrile, dehydroascorbic acid forms a mixture containing a symmetrical and asymmetrical dimer. Monodehydroascorbic acid is present in tissue as a relatively stable free radical. That radical anion has been postulated as an intermediate in the oxidation of ascorbic acid by metal ions. The stability of the radical anion and its disproportionation into dehydroascorbic acid and ascorbic acid helps explain the antioxidant role that ascorbate plays in biological systems and in foods.

There continues to be a fascination in the challenge of the scientific problems related to ascorbic acid. The authors of the chapters in this book have probably felt an intellectual curiosity about this commonplace substance: Why is it so unique? What does it do? The excitement and challenge will lead us on and intrigue the next generation of scientists working in this field.

It is our pleasure to thank Myron Brin, Frank Loewus, Dietrich Hornig, and Jack Bauernfeind for helpful discussions in planning the symposium and this book. We are grateful to the chairmen of the various sessions: Frank Loewus, Linus Pauling, and Benjamin Borenstein. The work of Suzanne B. Roethel and Robin Giroux of the ACS Books Department to assemble the manuscripts is gratefully acknowledged.

PAUL A. SEIB
Kansas State University
Manhattan, KS 66506

BERT M. TOLBERT
University of Colorado
Boulder, CO 80309

June 28, 1982

Synthesis of L-Ascorbic Acid

THOMAS C. CRAWFORD

Central Research, Chemical Process Research, Pfizer Inc., Groton, CT 06340

The methods by which L-ascorbic acid has been synthesized are readily divided into three major categories. The first involves coupling a C_1 fragment and a C_5 fragment, and the second involves coupling a C_2 fragment and a C_4 fragment. The third involves the conversion of a C_6 chain into the correct oxidation state and stereochemical configuration. All of these approaches will be reviewed with special regard given to those syntheses that are suitable for the preparation of analogues of L-ascorbic acid, the preparation of radiolabeled derivatives of L-ascorbic acid, and the current commercial synthesis of L-ascorbic acid.

Following the isolation of crystalline "hexuronic acid" from the adrenal cortex of the ox and from orange juice in 1928 (*1*) and the determination in 1933 (*2*) that the structure of this material was 1 (with other proton tautomers shown in Scheme 1), efforts were begun to synthesize this novel vitamin. In a very short time several syntheses were successfully accomplished that confirmed that the structure of L-ascorbic acid or vitamin C was indeed that proposed (*2*). Complete details of the crystal structure of 1 have since been obtained by both x-ray (*3, 4*) and neutron diffraction (*5*) analysis and are approximated by structure 1a.

Efforts directed toward the synthesis of L-ascorbic acid have been governed by the following factors:

1. The need to synthesize material to confirm the structure and provide larger quantities of material for further study.
2. The desire to synthesize analogues of L-ascorbic acid.
3. The desire to prepare radiolabeled material for use in the study of L-ascorbic acid metabolism in plants, fish, animals, and humans.
4. The need to develop a commercially viable, low cost synthesis. This is illustrated by the fact that in 1934 1 kg of L-ascorbic acid sold for $7000 (*6*).

0065-2393/82/0200–0001$10.00/0
© 1982 American Chemical Society

L-ASCORBIC ACID

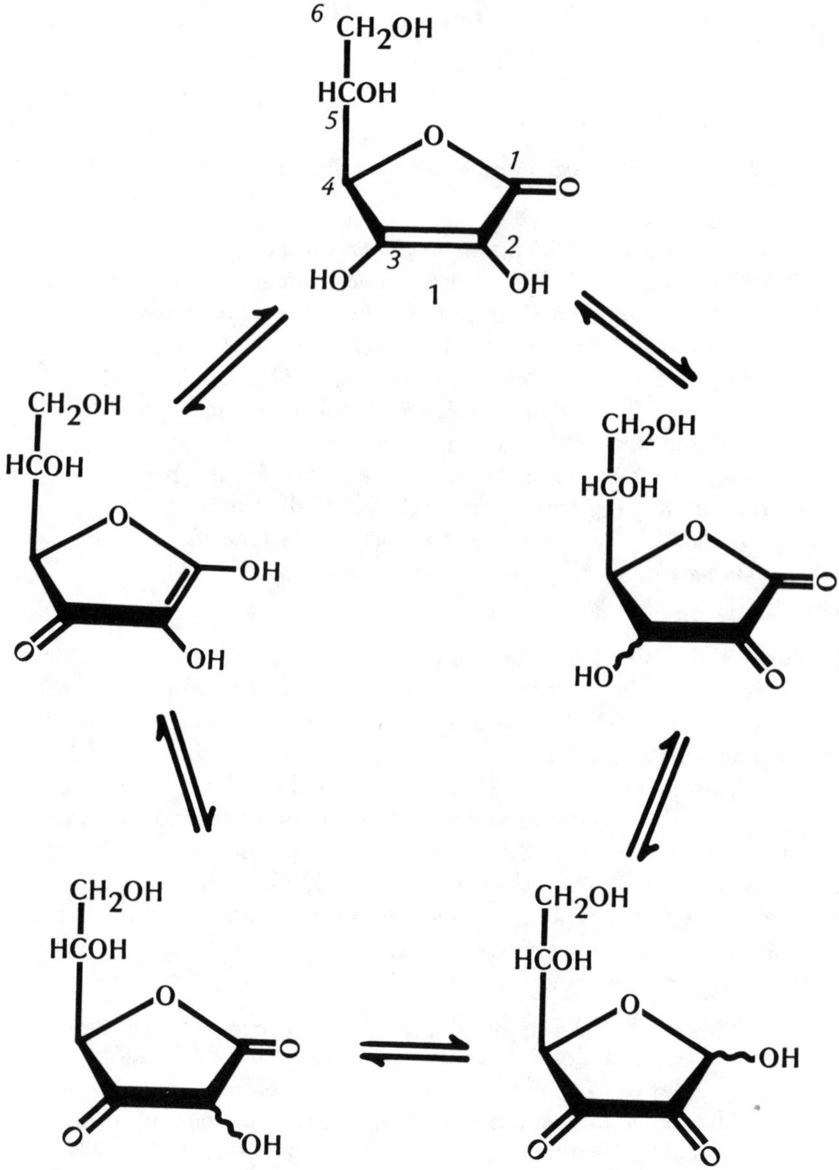

Scheme 1.

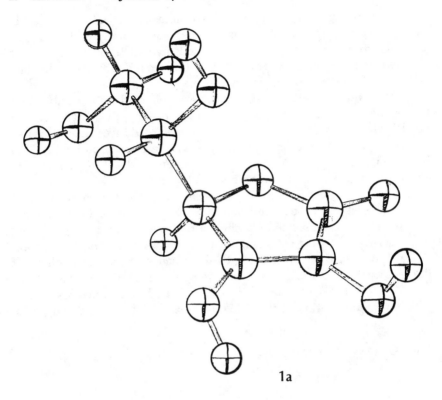

1a

The design of syntheses of L-ascorbic acid must take into consideration the following points:

1. The synthesis must be chiral since only the L-enantiomer is biologically active.
2. The final step in the synthesis must be carried out under nonoxidative conditions because of the very facile oxidation of L-ascorbic acid to dehydro-L-ascorbic acid followed by further degradation.
3. L-Ascorbic acid must be stable to the conditions used to generate it (i.e., no vigorous acid or base treatment in the final step because degradation of L-ascorbic acid can result).
4. For commercial use, the synthesis must be economical.

This chapter provides an overview of the various available syntheses of L-ascorbic acid. The key synthetic discoveries that have resulted in the preparation of L-ascorbic acid analogues, the preparation of radio-labeled derivatives of L-ascorbic acid, and the production of commercial quantities of L-ascorbic acid are highlighted. For a comprehensive review of all these approaches, *see* Reference 7.

All syntheses of L-ascorbic acid are actually partial syntheses because the chirality at C5 and C4 is obtained via naturally derived sugars
and not by total synthesis. Various methods by which the six carbons of
ascorbic acid have been assembled with the appropriate oxidation state
and stereochemistry are shown in Scheme 2.

One approach to the synthesis of L-ascorbic acid is by combining a
C_5 fragment and a C_1 fragment (in effect making the carbon–carbon
bond between C1 and C2 in **1**). Intermediates derived from L-xylose
and L-arabinose have been used in these syntheses. L-Ascorbic acid has
been synthesized by combining a C_2 fragment and a C_4 fragment (in
effect making the carbon–carbon bond between C2 and C3 in **1**) starting
with L-threose. No syntheses of L-ascorbic acid have been reported in
which the carbon–carbon bond between C3 and C4 or between C4 and
C5 (*see* **1**) has been formed (in effect a C_3 fragment plus a C_3 fragment
or a C_4 fragment plus a C_2 fragment representing C5 and C6, respectively). Most methods for making these carbon–carbon bonds will result
in the formation of a mixture of enantiomers and/or diastereomers.

Most syntheses of L-ascorbic acid start with preformed C_6 sugars,
which by manipulation of the oxidation state at C1, C2, C5, and/or C6

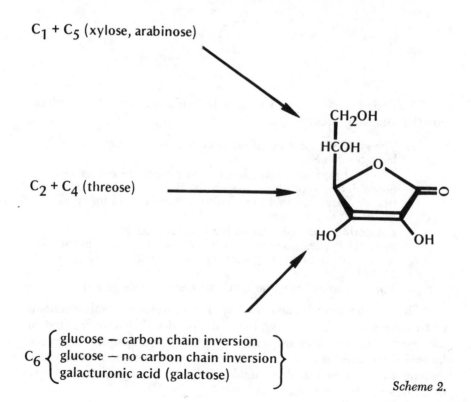

$C_1 + C_5$ (xylose, arabinose)

$C_2 + C_4$ (threose)

C_6 { glucose — carbon chain inversion
glucose — no carbon chain inversion
galacturonic acid (galactose) }

Scheme 2.

and by manipulation of the stereochemistry at C2 or C5 have been converted into L-ascorbic acid by a variety of reaction sequences. The most common C_6 sugar starting material is D-glucose, which has been converted into intermediates formally derived from L-gulose, L-galactose, L-idose, or L-talose.

A survey of the reported syntheses of L-ascorbic acid reveals that derivatives related to 2-keto acid (**2**) (Scheme 3) are the most frequently used intermediate to L-ascorbic acid. 3-Keto acid (**3**), ketolactone (**4**) (in protected form), and 6-aldehydo-L-ascorbic acid (**5**) are less frequently used. The use of each of these intermediates (**2–5**) will be illustrated in the following discussion of the different syntheses of L-ascorbic acid.

Ascorbic Acid via C_1 and C_5 Fragments

The first synthesis of L-ascorbic acid (**1**) was reported in 1933, before the correct structure had been determined. In early 1933, Micheel and Kraft (*8*) suggested that carboxylic acid (**6**) was the structure for L-ascorbic acid. A short time later the synthesis of D-ascorbic acid shown in Scheme 4 starting with D-xylosone was reported (*9–12*). This synthesis gave material identical with natural L-ascorbic acid, except for the specific rotation, and was used (*9–12*) as evidence to support structure **6** as the structure for L-ascorbic acid. Shortly after these initial reports (*9–12*), the same sequence of reactions was reported (*13–15*) and, having the advantage of knowing the correct structure of L-ascorbic acid, the sequence of reactions leading from L-xylosone to L-ascorbic acid was correctly depicted as that shown in Scheme 5; the synthesis proceeds via 3-keto acid derivative **3a**. It is ironic that one of the more difficult and important problems of those times—the synthesis of L-ascorbic acid— was accomplished before the correct structure of **1** was known.

This C_1 homologation of osones proved to be valuable in the preparation of L-ascorbic acid analogues (*16*) as well as in the preparation of radiolabeled L-ascorbic acid (*17–20*). This synthesis was greatly improved when aldoses were discovered to be directly oxidized to osones with cupric acetate (Equation 1) (*21*). Subsequently, the conditions were modified so that D-xylose could be oxidized to D-xylosone in 50–55% yield with cupric acetate in methanol. The intermediacy of the imino ether was proved by the isolation of **7** when D-glucosone was treated with potassium cyanide (*16*). The initial cyanohydrin adduct (**3a**) easily undergoes cyclization to the imino ether intermediate (aqueous solution for 10 min at room temperature, Scheme 5). This feature will be compared with the conditions required for the lactonization of other intermediates.

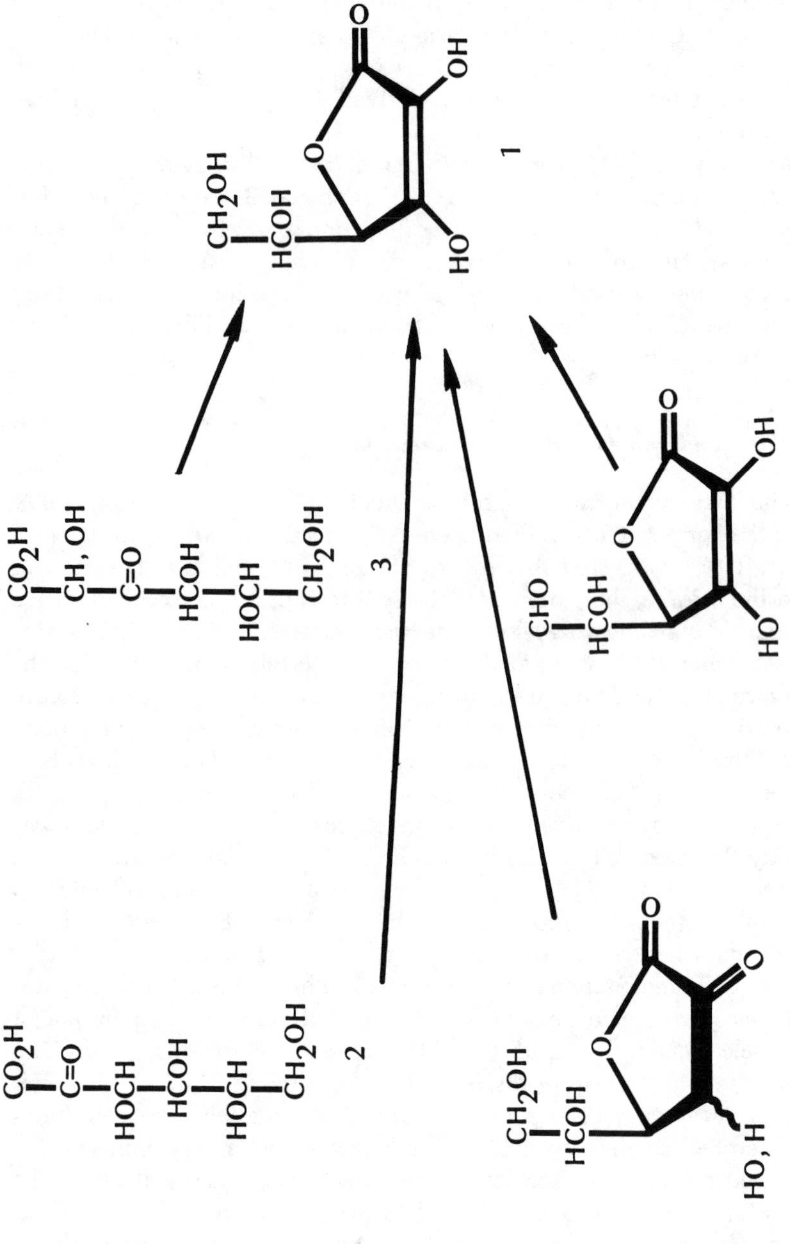

Scheme 3.

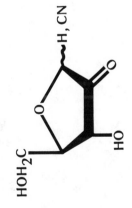

Scheme 4.

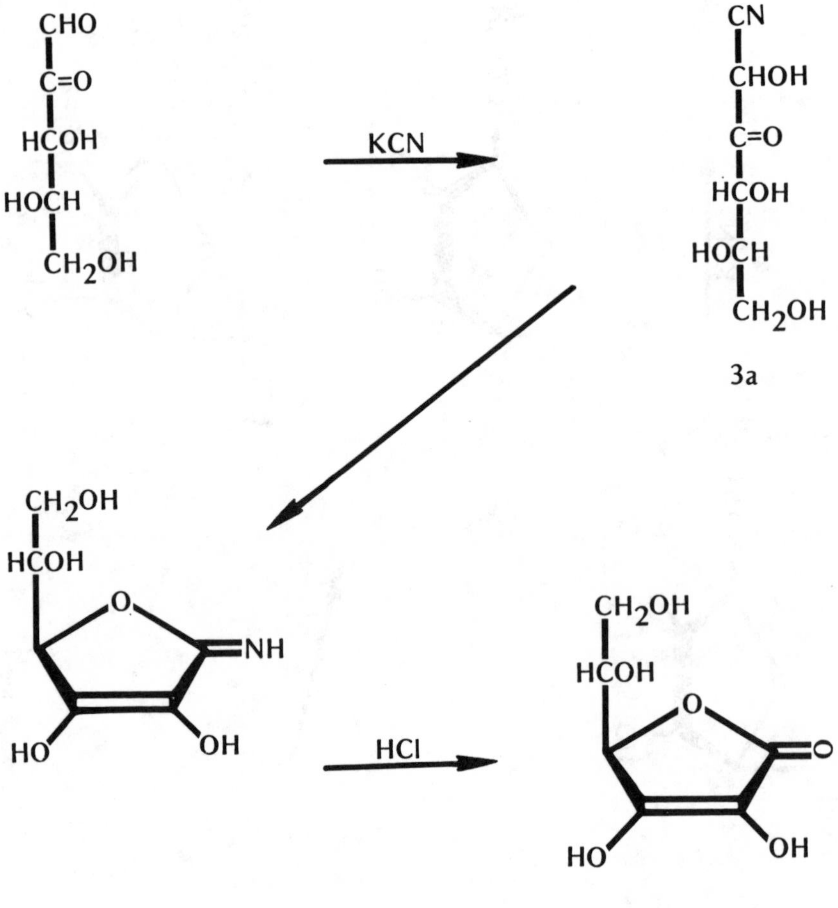

Scheme 5.

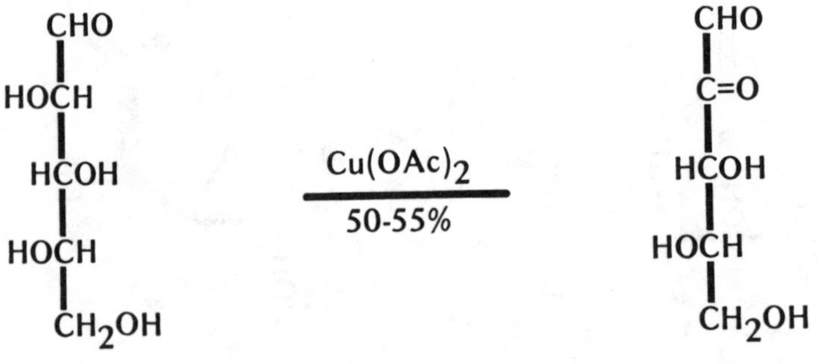

$$\text{structure 7}$$

7

A second synthesis in which a C_1 fragment was coupled with a C_5 fragment was reported in which acid chloride (8) was converted to the acyl nitrile (9) by use of silver cyanide (23) (Scheme 6). Hydrolysis and esterification produced ethyl 3,4,5,6-tetra-O-acetyl-DL-*xylo*-2-hexulosonate. The conditions required for the conversion of this material to DL-ascorbic acid will be discussed later. No yields were reported for this reaction sequence. This synthesis has not been used for the preparation of analogues or radiolabeled derivatives of L-ascorbic acid as has the osone–cyanide synthesis first reported (9–12). In contrast to the osone–cyanide synthesis (Scheme 5) in which a 3-ketogulonic acid derivative is produced, the acid chloride–silver cyanide synthesis (Scheme 6) results in the formation of a 2-ketogulonic acid derivative (2a) as an intermediate in the ascorbic acid synthesis.

A third synthesis utilizing a C_1 and C_5 coupling procedure to produce L-ascorbic acid was recently reported (24) (Scheme 7). L-Arabinose (10) was reduced to L-arabinitol and protected with formaldehyde to provide 1,3:2,4-di-O-methylene-L-arabinitol (11) along with a number of other products. Compound 11 with the free hydroxyl group at C5 and all other hydroxyl groups protected is suitably protected for conversion into L-ascorbic acid by oxidation to the aldehyde, carbon-chain extension with potassium cyanide, then conversion to L-ascorbic acid. This synthesis uses L-arabinose as the source of chirality by carbon-chain inversion. Thus C2 and C3 in arabinose, which have the same stereochemistry as C4 and C5 in L-ascorbic acid, become C4 and C5 in 1 by reducing C1 of arabinose, selectively (but inefficiently) protecting C1–C4, oxidizing, and extending the chain at C5.

Ascorbic Acid via C_2 and C_4 Fragments

L-Ascorbic acid was prepared by using L-threose as the chiral C_4 unit and extending to the required six carbons with the correct oxidation

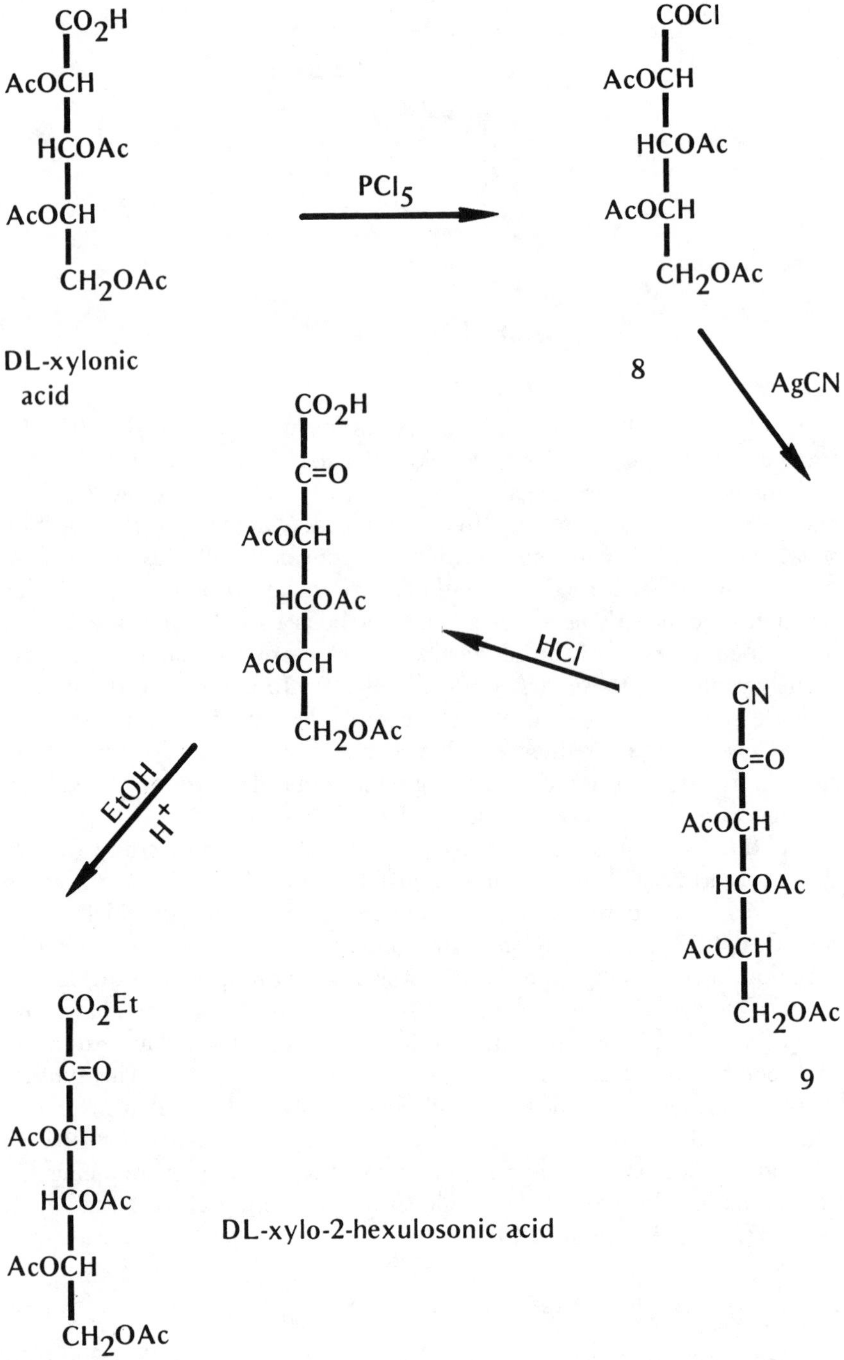
CO2H
AcOCH
HCOAc
AcOCH
CH2OAc
DL-xylonic acid
PCl5
COCl
AcOCH
HCOAc
AcOCH
CH2OAc
8
AgCN
CN
C=O
AcOCH
HCOAc
AcOCH
CH2OAc
9
HCl
CO2H
C=O
AcOCH
HCOAc
AcOCH
CH2OAc
EtOH
H+
CO2Et
C=O
AcOCH
HCOAc
AcOCH
CH2OAc
DL-xylo-2-hexulosonic acid

Scheme 6.

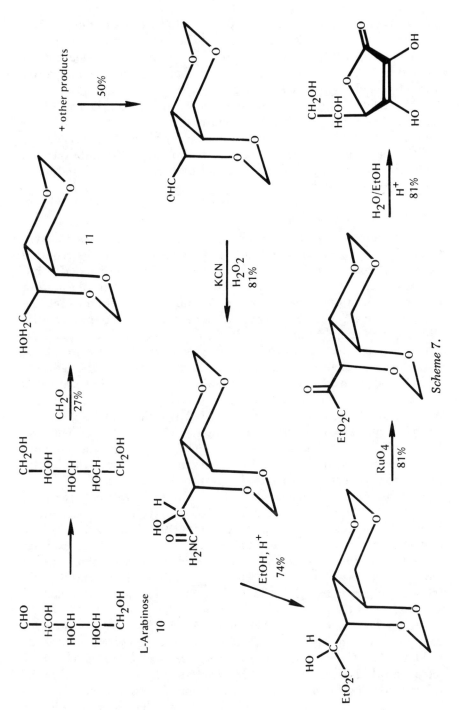

Scheme 7.

state by condensing L-threose (12) with ethyl glyoxylate in the presence of sodium cyanide (25, 26) (Scheme 8). The condensation proceeds via anion 13. When this synthesis is carried out in methanol using sodium methoxide as the base (25) and 12a as the starting L-threose derivative, L-ascorbic acid is produced in 75–80% yield.

In a related synthesis (Scheme 9) diethyl oxopropanedioate (15) is condensed with the protected cyanohydrin of L-threose (14), producing L-ascorbic acid (27). This condensation presumably proceeds via the addition of anion 16 to 15 followed by hydrolysis and decarboxylation. Both of these synthetic approaches could be used in the preparation of L-ascorbic acid analogues.

Ascorbic Acid via C_6 Sugars

The most important sugar used as a starting material for the synthesis of L-ascorbic acid is D-glucose (17), which contains the requisite six carbon atoms, some or all of the appropriate chiral centers (depending on synthetic approach), and an attractively low cost. D-Glucose can be converted into L-ascorbic acid by two different procedures (Scheme 10). In the first procedure, C1 of glucose becomes C1 of L-ascorbic acid. This approach requires that C1 and C2 be oxidized and the stereochemistry at C5 be inverted. In the second procedure, the carbon chain of D-glucose is inverted. In this approach C1 of glucose must be reduced, and C5 and C6 oxidized, with the chirality at C4 and C5 of L-ascorbic acid coming from that at C3 and C2, respectively, in D-glucose. Studies on the biosynthesis of L-ascorbic acid (28) have shown that D-glucose is converted into 1 by two different pathways, one in which C1 of D-glucose becomes C1 of L-ascorbic acid and one in which C1 of D-glucose becomes C6 of L-ascorbic acid. Synthetic approaches to L-ascorbic acid that belong to the latter category (carbon-chain inversion) will be discussed first.

Glucose to L-Ascorbic Acid. CARBON-CHAIN INVERSION. The most important synthesis in this class is the second synthesis developed by Reichstein and Grüssner (29) and reported in 1934 (Scheme 11). D-Glucose was reduced to D-glucitol (18), which was fermentatively oxidized to L-sorbose (19). On treatment with acetone and acid, a mixture of monoprotected (20) and diprotected (21) derivatives of L-sorbose was formed and separated. 2,3:4,6-Di-O-isopropylidene-L-xylo-2-hexulofuranose (21) was then oxidized to the corresponding acid (22). When 22 was heated in water, L-xylo-2-hexulosonic acid (2-keto-L-gulonic acid, 23) was obtained; on heating at 100°C 23 was converted in 13–20% yield into L-ascorbic acid. Alternatively, 23 was esterified to afford methyl L-xylo-2-hexulosonate (methyl-2-keto-L-gulonate, 24), which, after treatment with sodium methoxide in methanol followed by acidification, produced L-ascorbic acid in 73% yield from 22. This first short, efficient synthesis of L-ascorbic acid had an overall yield of 15–18%.

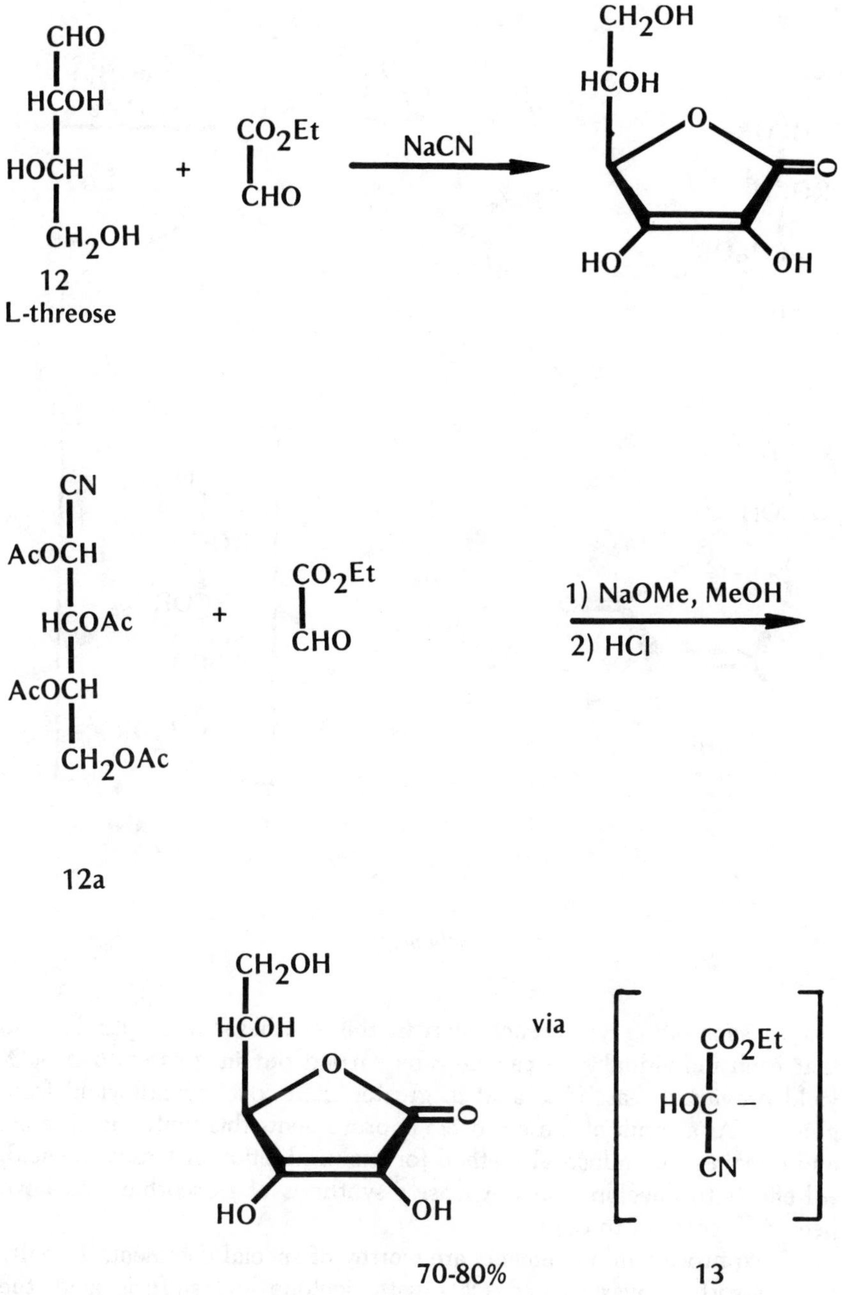
CHO
HCOH
HOCH
CH_2OH
12
L-threose
CO_2Et
CHO
NaCN
CH_2OH
HCOH
O
HO
OH
CN
AcOCH
HCOAc
AcOCH
CH_2OAc
12a
CO_2Et
CHO
1) NaOMe, MeOH
2) HCl
CH_2OH
HCOH
O
HO
OH
70-80%
via
CO_2Et
HOC −
CN
13

Scheme 8.

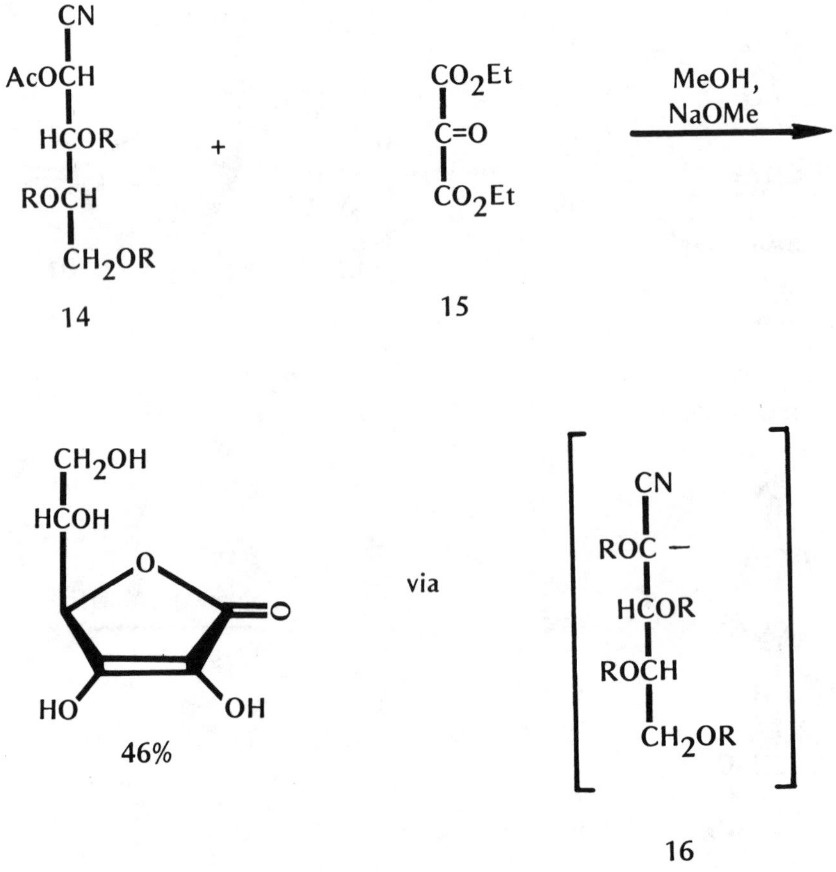

Scheme 9.

In succeeding years each step in this synthesis was optimized so that each individual step can now be carried out in greater than 90% yield providing L-ascorbic acid in greater than 50% overall yield from glucose. As a result of these process improvements this synthesis became, and remains, the industrial method for the production of L-ascorbic acid. All efforts to develop a less expensive synthesis of L-ascorbic acid have been unsuccessful to date.

Two process improvements are worthy of special comment. Initially when L-sorbose was treated (29) with acetone and sulfuric acid, the monoacetonide (20) and the diacetonide (21) were formed. In subsequent work researchers found that when the temperature of the reaction

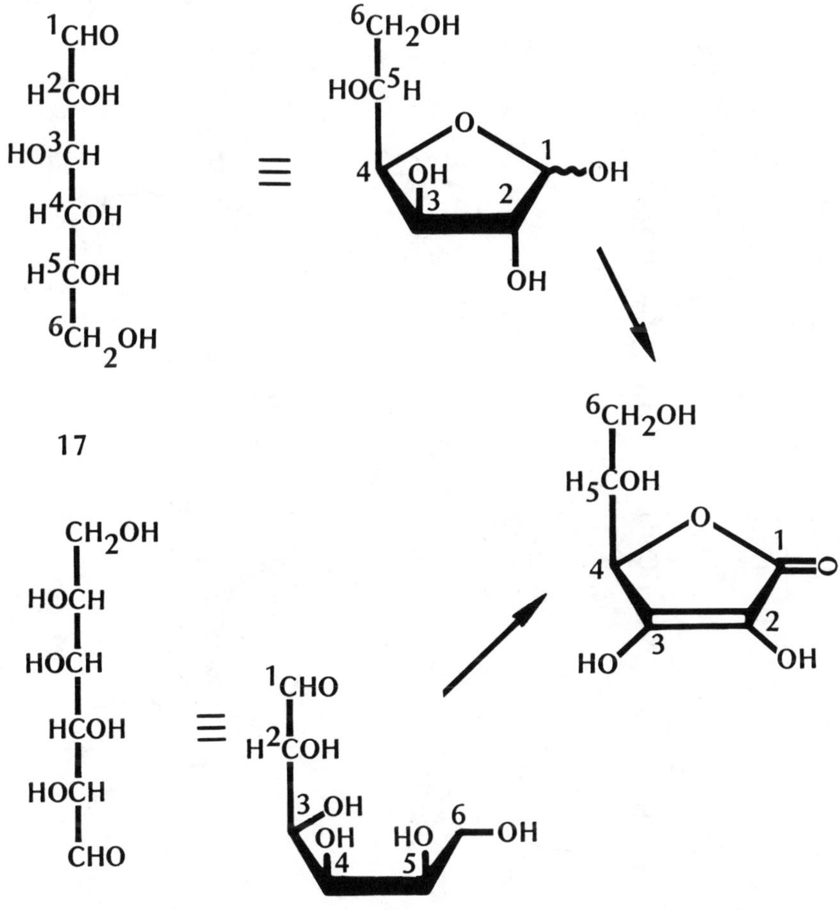

Scheme 10.

was reduced from room temperature to -8–$0°C$, the yield of **21** increased to greater than 85% (*30–32*). A second major improvement resulted when workers found that **22**, **23**, or **24** could be converted to L-ascorbic acid via acid catalysis under essentially nonaqueous conditions in greater than 90% yield (*33–35*). Although high yields can be obtained, the conditions required for this conversion are considerably more vigorous [toluene, $65°C$, 5 h (*34*) or chloroform–ethanol, $65°C$, 45–50 h (*33*), both with concentrated hydrochloric acid] than those required for the conversion of cyanohydrin adduct (**31**) to L-ascorbic acid (aqueous solution at room temperature for 10 min) as noted previously.

Scheme 11.

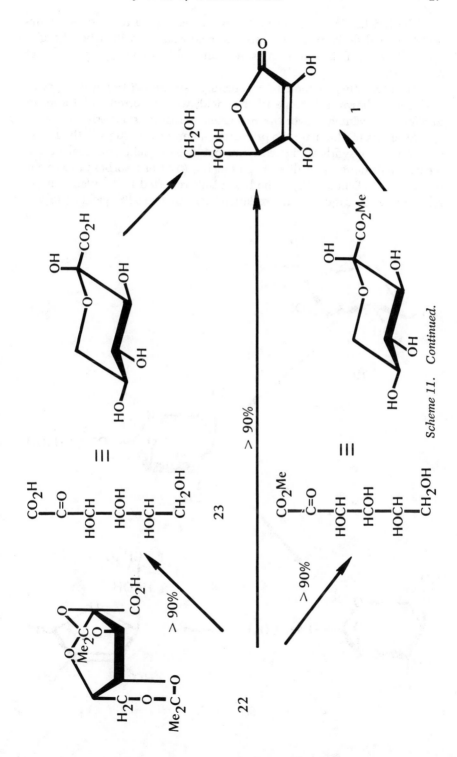

Scheme 11.   Continued.

The Reichstein–Grüssner synthesis has been used to prepare a number of labeled derivatives of L-ascorbic acid, starting with labeled D-glucose (36–40). This synthesis is not amenable to the preparation of analogues.

An alternative method for protecting L-sorbose (19) was reported (41) and is shown in Scheme 12. No yields were reported and it appears to offer no advantages over the Reichstein–Grüssner synthesis.

Attempts to eliminate the protection–deprotection steps in the Reichstein–Grüssner synthesis by carrying out a high-yield chemical or fermentative oxidation step directly on glucitol (18) or L-sorbose (19) were unsuccessful (Scheme 13). The best result reported is the platinum (or related metals) catalyzed air oxidation of 19 to 23 (62% yield) (42).

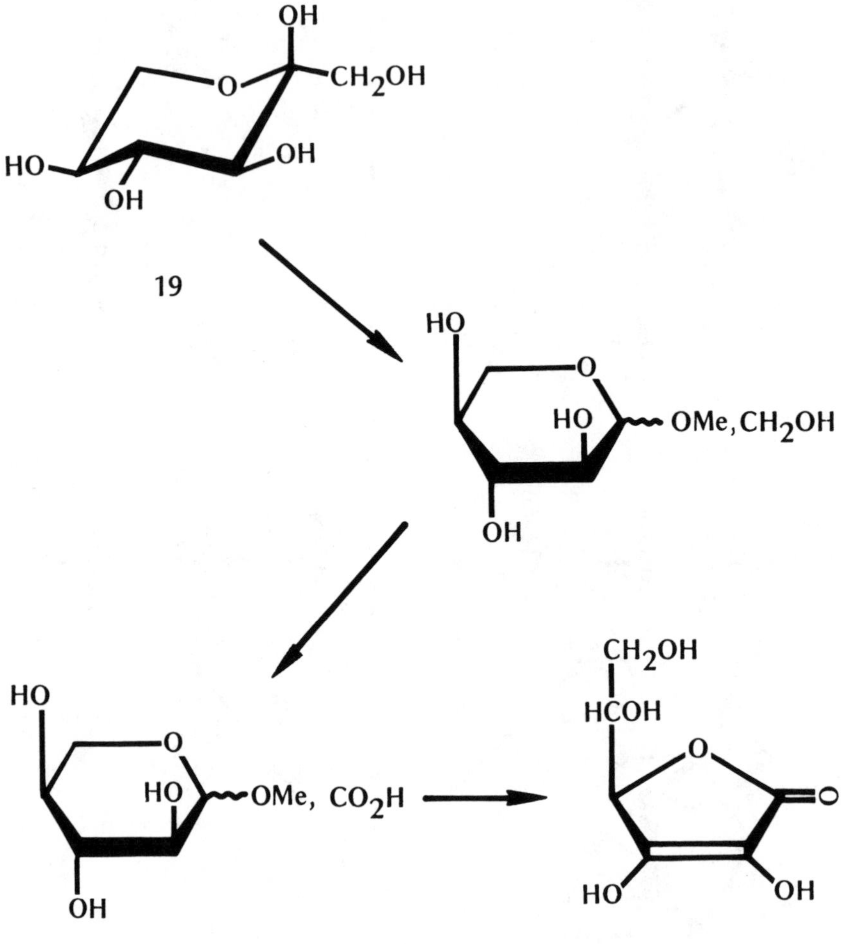

Scheme 12.

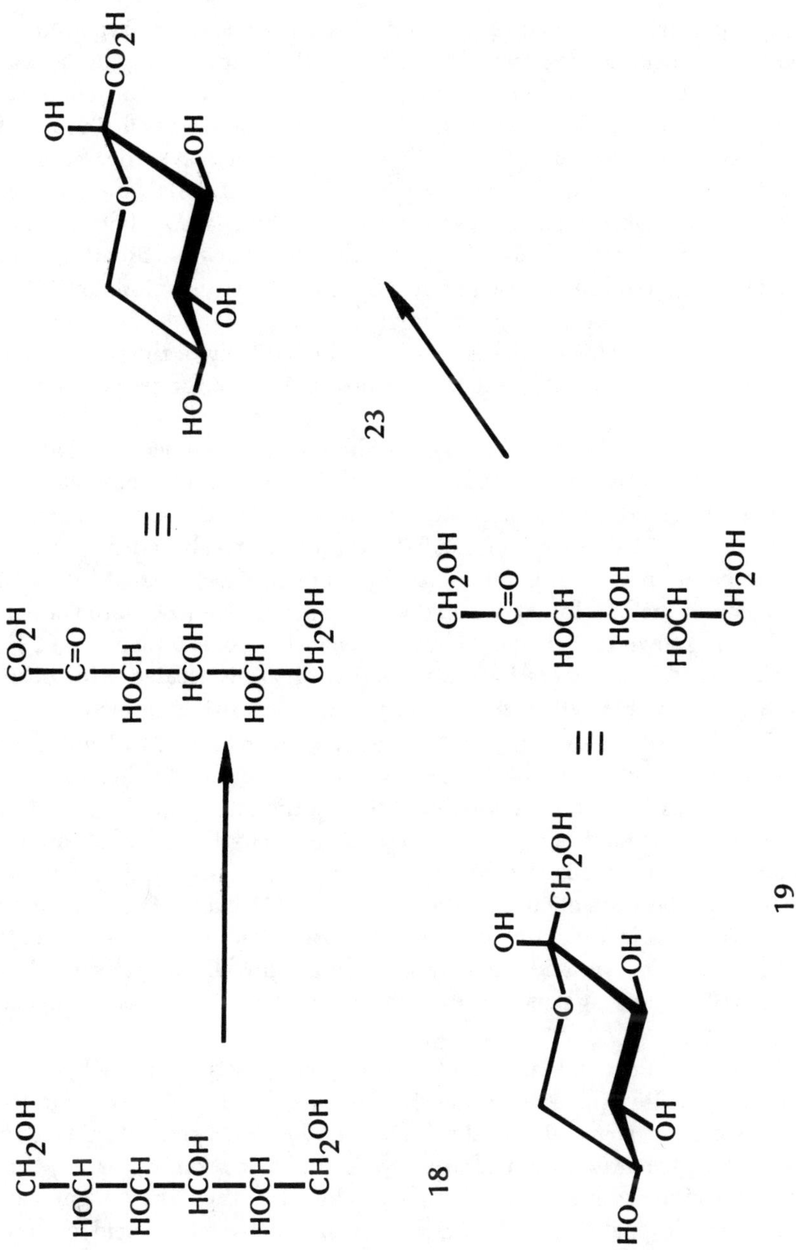

Scheme 13.

An alternative method of preparing L-ascorbic acid was reported by Bakke and Theander (Scheme 14) (43). In this synthesis D-glucose was first oxidized at C6, then at C5, and then reduced at C1. This contrasts with the Reichstein–Grüssner synthesis in which glucose was first reduced at C1, then oxidized at C5, and then at C6 to achieve the requisite inverted carbon chain. The key intermediate in the Bakke–Theander synthesis, ketolactone (25) was prepared earlier (44, 45) but was not converted to 1. Hydrolysis of 25 afforded 6-aldehydo-L-ascorbic acid (26, aldehydo-L-*threo*-hex-4-enurono-6,3-lactone) as an unisolated intermediate. Compound 26 was not previously synthesized. The reduction of 26 afforded 1. This synthesis of 1 is used effectively in the preparation of labeled derivatives of 1 (46). It is not useful for the preparation of analogues.

Another synthesis of L-ascorbic acid became obvious once the Bakke–Theander synthesis was reported (Scheme 15) (47). D-Glucuronolactone (27) is protected with acetone to afford 28, which can be oxidized to ketolactone (25), the key intermediate in the Bakke–Theander synthesis. The preparation of 25 was reported by a number of workers (44, 45, 48).

Another method for converting D-glucuronolactone (27) into L-ascorbic acid is shown in Scheme 16 (49). When L-gulono-1,4-lactone (29), which is readily available by the reduction of 27, is treated with benzaldehyde, 3,5-O-benzylidene-L-gulono-1,4-lactone (30) is formed.

Lactone 30 on oxidation at C2 gives ketolactone (31), which on hydrolysis in acetic acid–water afforded L-ascorbic acid (Scheme 16). This synthesis and the Bakke–Theander synthesis are among the few syntheses that do not have as the last step the lactonization of an appropriate 2- or 3-keto sugar acid or derivative. The approach shown in Scheme 16, the protection of either the C2 or C3 hydroxyl group in an appropriate 1,4-lactone followed by the oxidation of the unprotected hydroxyl to a ketone and then by hydrolysis, can be generally used to convert L-gulono-, L-galactono, and L-talono-1,4-lactone to L-ascorbic acid (50).

When L-gulono-1,4-lactone (29) was treated with benzaldehyde diethyl acetal, ethyl 3,5:4,6-di-O-benzylidene-L-gulonate (32) was formed (49) in greater than 90% yield (Scheme 17). This derivative can be converted efficiently into L-ascorbic acid by oxidation (> 90%) followed by hydrolysis of the resulting product to ethyl 2-keto-L-gulonate (L-*xylo*-hexulosonate) (86%) and lactonization by either acid or base (90%) to L-ascorbic acid.

Either this synthesis or that shown in Scheme 16 is suitable for the preparation of C6 deuterated or tritated derivatives of L-ascorbic acid reducing 27 with deuterium or tritium enriched gas or with labeled sodium borohydride (51).

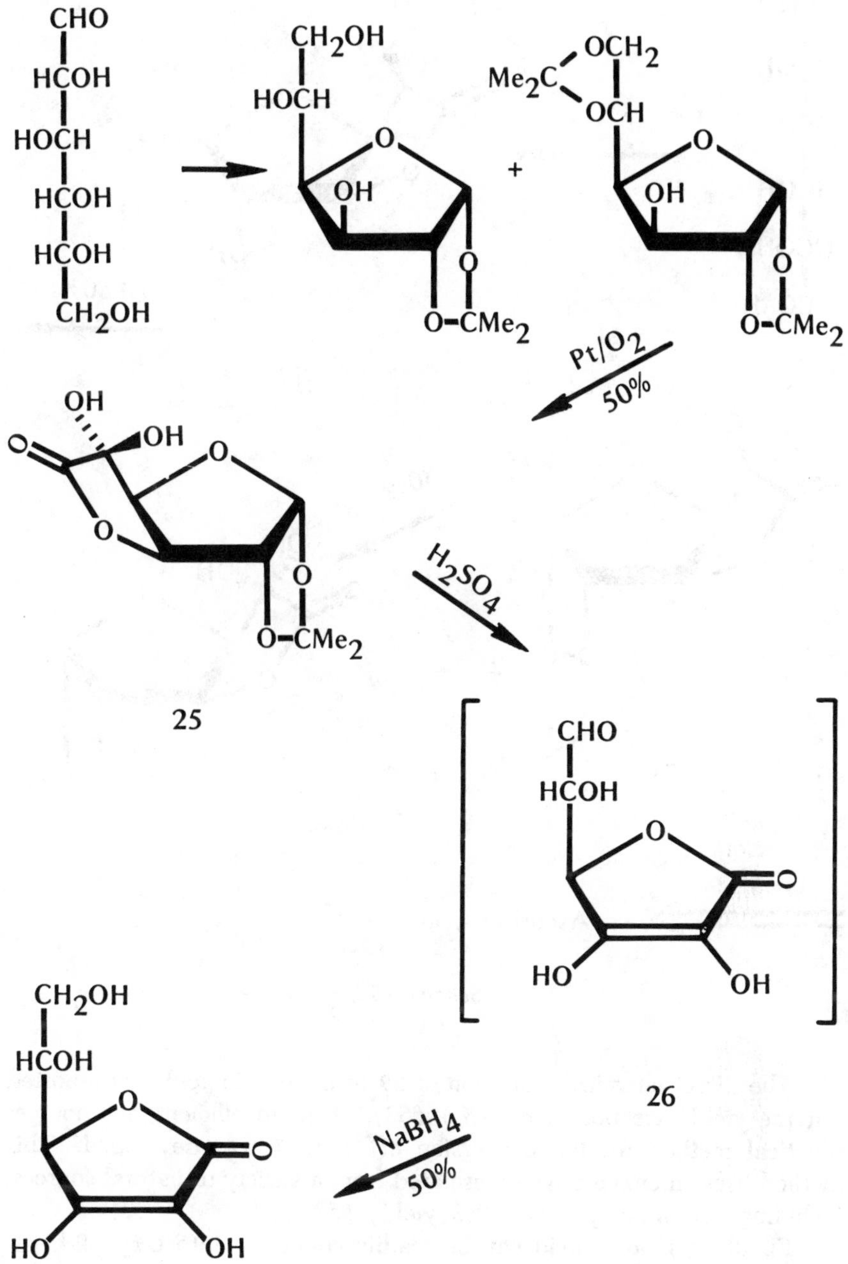

Scheme 14.

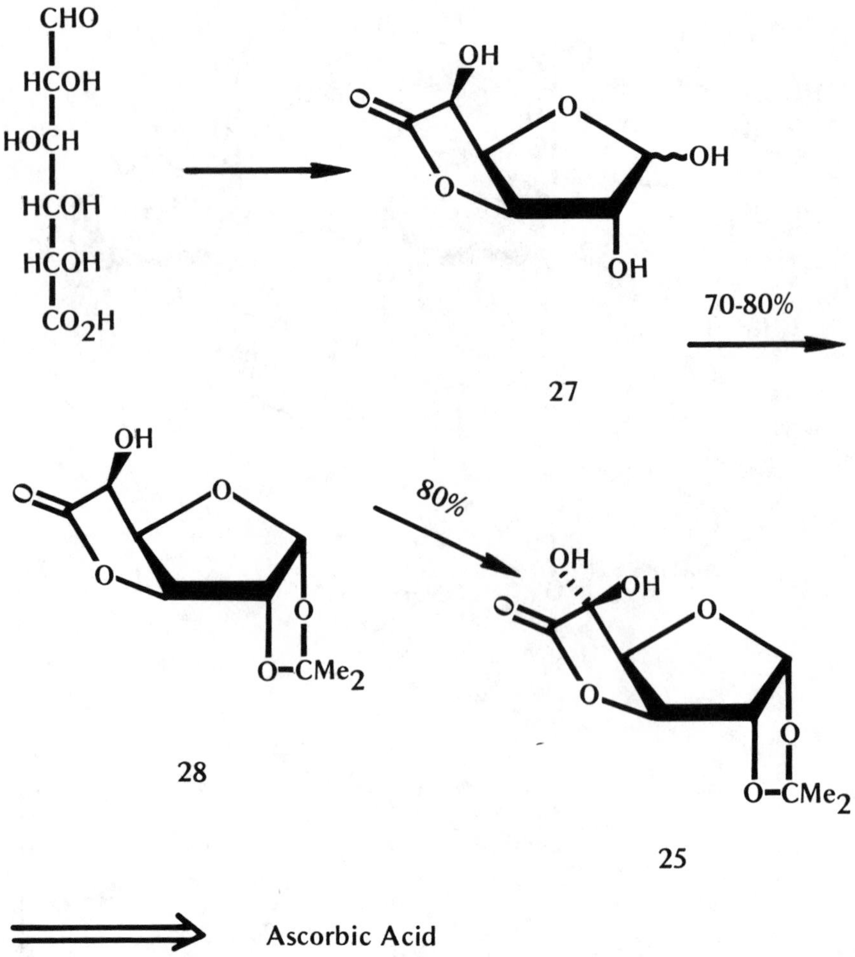

Scheme 15.

The direct chemical oxidation of 29 to L-ascorbic acid was reported but the yields are poor (< 10%) (52). A more efficient but not yet practical method for the conversion of 29 to 1 was developed. This method uses an enzyme system isolated from a variety of natural sources, including germinating peas (40% yield) (53).

Finally, L-gulonic acid can be readily converted into L-*xylo*-2-hexulosonate using a number of microorganisms (54, 55), including *Acetobacter suboxydans* and *Xanthomonas translucens* (Scheme 18).

A second synthesis that involves the oxidation of glucose at C6, reduction at C1, and then oxidation at C5 (glucose numbering) is shown

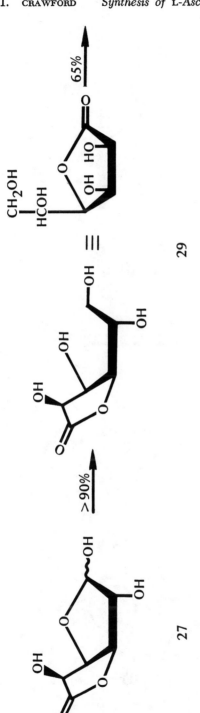

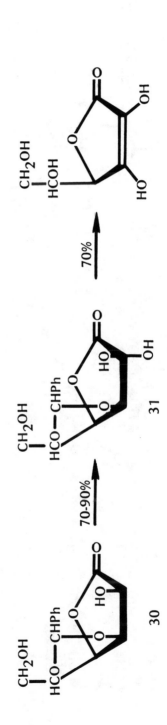

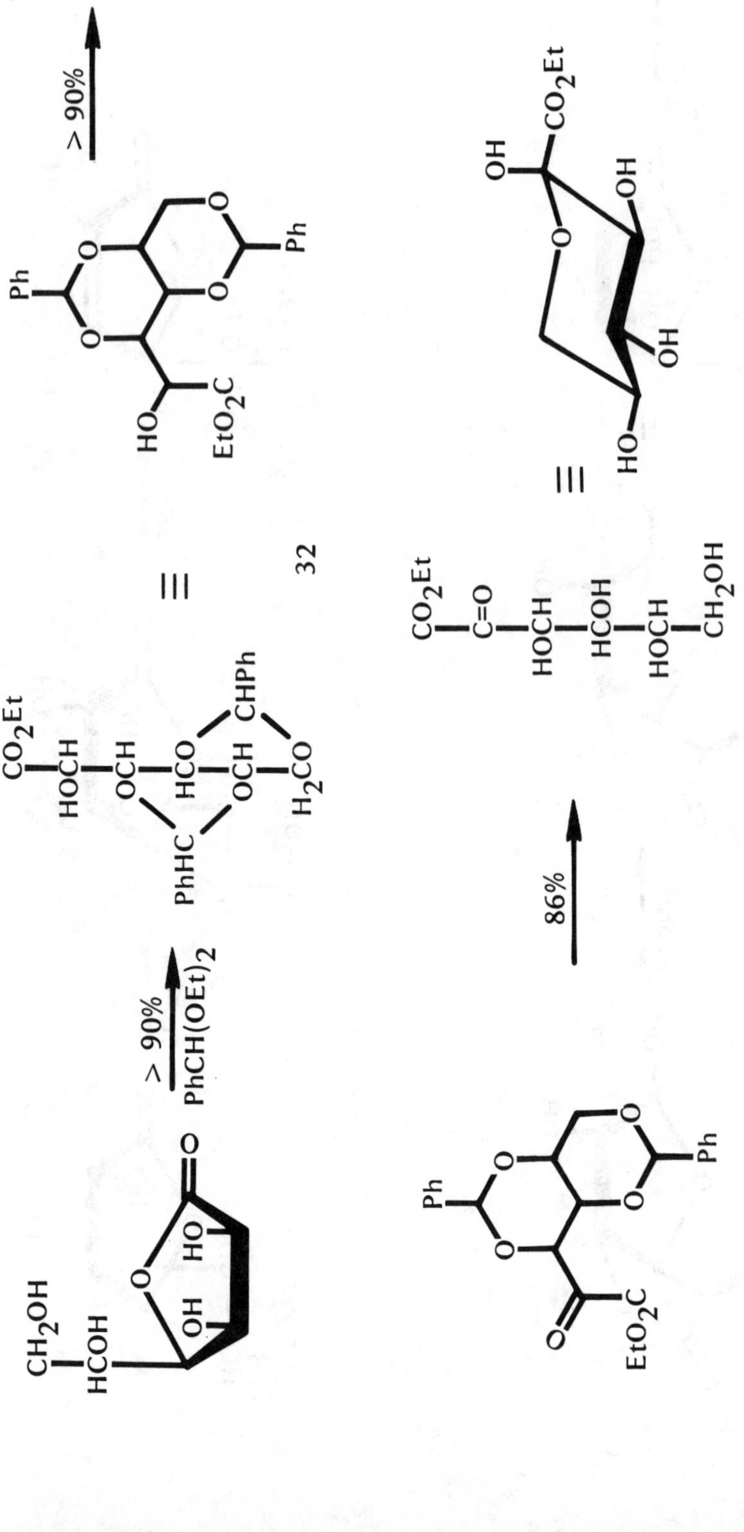

Scheme 17.

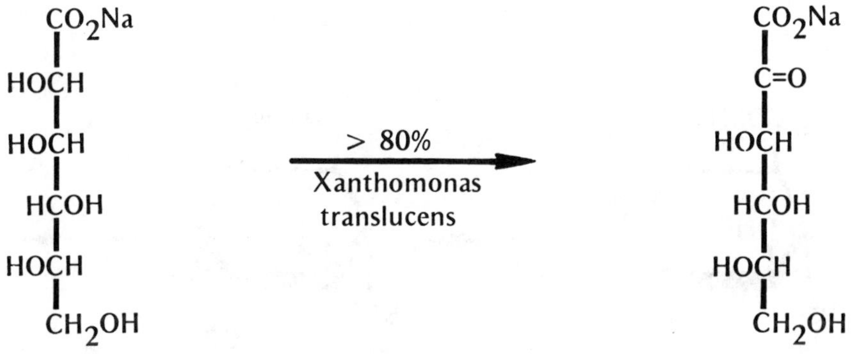

$$
\begin{array}{ccc}
\text{CO}_2\text{Na} & & \text{CO}_2\text{Na} \\
| & & | \\
\text{HOCH} & & \text{C=O} \\
| & & | \\
\text{HOCH} & \xrightarrow[\text{translucens}]{\substack{> 80\% \\ \text{Xanthomonas}}} & \text{HOCH} \\
| & & | \\
\text{HCOH} & & \text{HCOH} \\
| & & | \\
\text{HOCH} & & \text{HOCH} \\
| & & | \\
\text{CH}_2\text{OH} & & \text{CH}_2\text{OH}
\end{array}
$$

Scheme 18.

in Scheme 19 (*56–58*). This multistep synthesis involves the conversion of D-glucuronic acid into **33** (a derivative of gulonic acid) followed by oxidation to **34** and hydrolysis to methyl L-*xylo*-2-hexulosonate (**36**) via **35**.

No CARBON-CHAIN INVERSION. This section will discuss the methods by which D-glucose has been converted to L-ascorbic acid without carbon-chain inversion. These syntheses of L-ascorbic acid from D-glucose without carbon-chain inversion involve the oxidation of D-glucose at C1 and C2, and the inversion of chirality at C5.

The first synthesis reported in this class is shown in Scheme 20. D-Glucose can be efficiently (> 90%) oxidized fermentatively to calcium D-*xylo*-5-hexulosonate (**37**) using *Acetobacter suboxydans* (*59*). The reduction of **37** has been studied by several researchers. The best results were obtained using palladium boride and hydrogen and afforded a mixture of calcium idonate (**38**) and calcium gluconate (**39**) in the ratio of 73:27 (*60*). Other catalytic hydrogenation conditions resulted in a lower yield of **38**, but reduction with sodium borohydride afforded a 1:1 mixture of **38** and **39** (*61*). The mixture of **38** and **39** can be efficiently converted to pure L-*xylo*-2-hexulosonic acid (**23**) by fermentative oxidation of **38** to **23** and fermentative destruction of **39** using various organisms, including *Pseudomonas fluorescens* (*62, 63*). The yield of **23** based on starting idonic acid is greater than 90%. Based on D-*xylo*-5-hexulosonic acid, the yield of **23** is 50–60%. Acid **23** can be converted to L-ascorbic acid as previously described. Thus in this synthesis, C1 is oxidized, the stereochemistry at C5 is inverted via oxidation to the ketone and reduction, and then C2 is oxidized. This synthesis is not suitable for the preparation of analogues, but could be used for preparing C5-labeled derivatives of L-ascorbic acid.

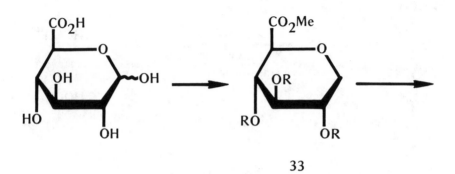

33

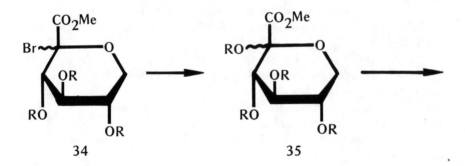

34   35

36

Scheme 19.

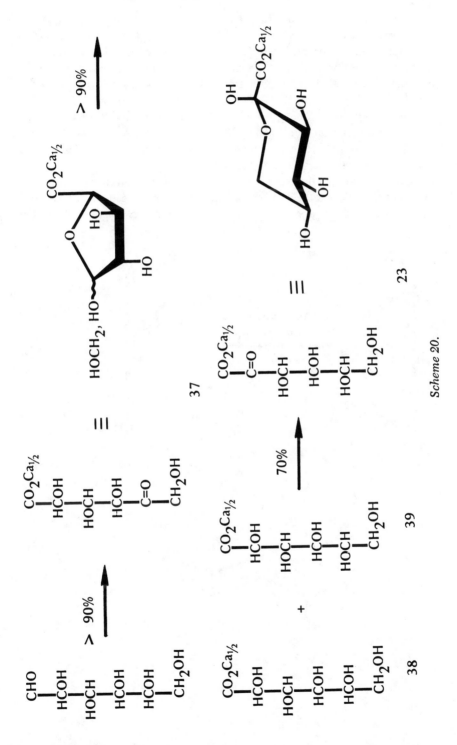

Scheme 20.

A second synthesis in which the carbon chain of D-glucose (17) is not inverted was reported (64). In 1953, glucose (17) was converted to D-threo-2,5-hexodiulosonic acid (2,5-diketo-D-gluconic acid, 40) by fermentative oxidation with *Acetobacter melanogenum* (Equation 2). Subsequently, more efficient fermentations of D-glucose to 40 using *Pseudomonas albosesame* (65, 66), *Acetobacter fragum* (67), and A. *cerines* (68) were reported. The gross chemical structure of this material was proved by Katznelson et al. (64). It was not until the work of Andrews and coworkers that 40 was shown to exist in aqueous solution in the hydrated pyranose form (40a) (69, 70).

D-*threo*-2,5-Hexodiulosonic acid (40) is a pivotal intermediate in this ascorbic acid synthesis because the oxidation of glucose at C1 and C2 has already been accomplished and the inversion of stereochemistry

$$\text{(2)}$$

17   40

40a

at C5 is half completed by oxidation of the C5 hydroxyl group to a ketone. All that remains is the demanding regiospecific and stereospecific reduction of the C5 ketone to the equatorial hydroxyl group (Scheme 21) to afford L-*xylo*-2-hexulosonic acid (23), which can be converted to L-ascorbic acid in high yield. For a summary of the methods by which this reduction was attempted, *see* Scheme 21.

The fermentative reduction of 40 using several microorganisms was reported. Most organisms produce 23 in low yield and, in some cases, as a mixture of C5 hydroxyl epimers (71, 72). The most promising fermentative reduction reported uses a *Corynebacterium* species and produces approximately 50% yield of 23 from 40 at 7.8% broth concentration (Scheme 21) (73, 74).

The regioselective catalytic hydrogenation of 40 afforded a mixture of D-*arabino*-2-hexulosonic acid (41) and L-*xylo*-2-hexulosonic acid (23) with 41 predominating (75, 76). This result is in complete accord with the proposed solution structure for 40 (40a) because catalytic hydrogenation of cyclohexanones affords predominantly axial hydroxyl groups.

With the catalytic hydrogenation results in hand and knowing the solution structure of 40, Andrews et al. (76) correctly predicted that the reduction of 40 with sodium borohydride would result in the formation of the desired L-isomer (23) as the major product. An 89% yield of an 86:14 mixture of 23:41 was obtained; the development of an efficient L-ascorbic acid synthesis (Scheme 22) followed. D-Glucose is converted to 40 in greater than 90% yield with either *Acetobacter fragum* (66) or *A. cerinus* (67). Reduction affords the above-mentioned mixture of 23 and 41 in 89% yield. This mixture can be converted to pure 23 by the selective fermentative destruction of 41 (77) using *Psuedomonas fluorescens*. Sodium L-*xylo*-2-hexulosonate is then isolated and converted to methyl L-*xylo*-2-hexulosonate (24) with methanol and acid, at the same time removing residual boric acid as trimethyl borate (78). As previously noted, 24 can be converted in high yield to 1. The mixture of 23 and 41 can also be converted to a mixture of methyl ester that on crystallization affords pure 24 (76). L-(5-^{2}H)Ascorbic acid has been prepared using this procedure (76). The reduction of 40 can be carried out more efficiently using dimethylamineborane, which affords a 92:8 mixture of 23:41 in 95% yield (79).

In a related synthesis methyl D-*arabino*-2-hexulosonate (42) was converted, via a series of selectively protected intermediates, into 43, a protected derivative of D-*threo*-2,5-hexodiulosonic acid (Scheme 23). Stereoselective reduction of 43 with sodium borohydride afforded 44, which was converted to L-ascorbic acid. The overall yield was 36%. This synthesis was also used to prepare L-(5-^{2}H)ascorbic acid.

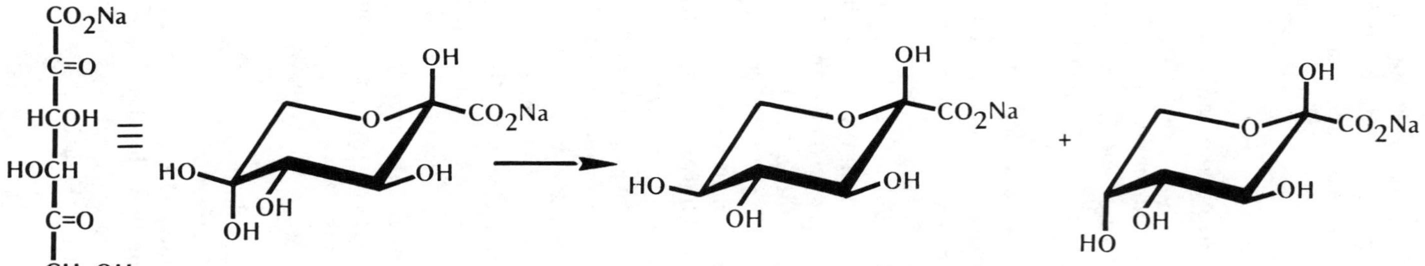

CO2Na
C=O
HCOH
HOCH
C=O
CH2OH
HO
OH
OH
O
OH
CO2Na
OH
HO
OH
O
OH
CO2Na
OH
+
HO
OH
O
OH
CO2Na
OH

40 23 41

			Yield	
Fermentative Reduction				
Brevibacterium	both isomers produced		17%	Sonoyama and coworkers (1975)
Corynebacterium	possibly a single isomer		50%	Sonoyama and coworkers (1977)
Chemical Reduction				
RaNi	minor	major		Wakisaka (1964)
RaNi	20%	80%	82%	Andrews, Bacon, Crawford, Breitenbach (1979)
$NaBH_4$	86 %	14%	89%	Andrews, Bacon, Crawford, Breitenbach (1979)
Me_2NHBH_3	92 %	8 %	95%	Andrews (1980)

Scheme 21.

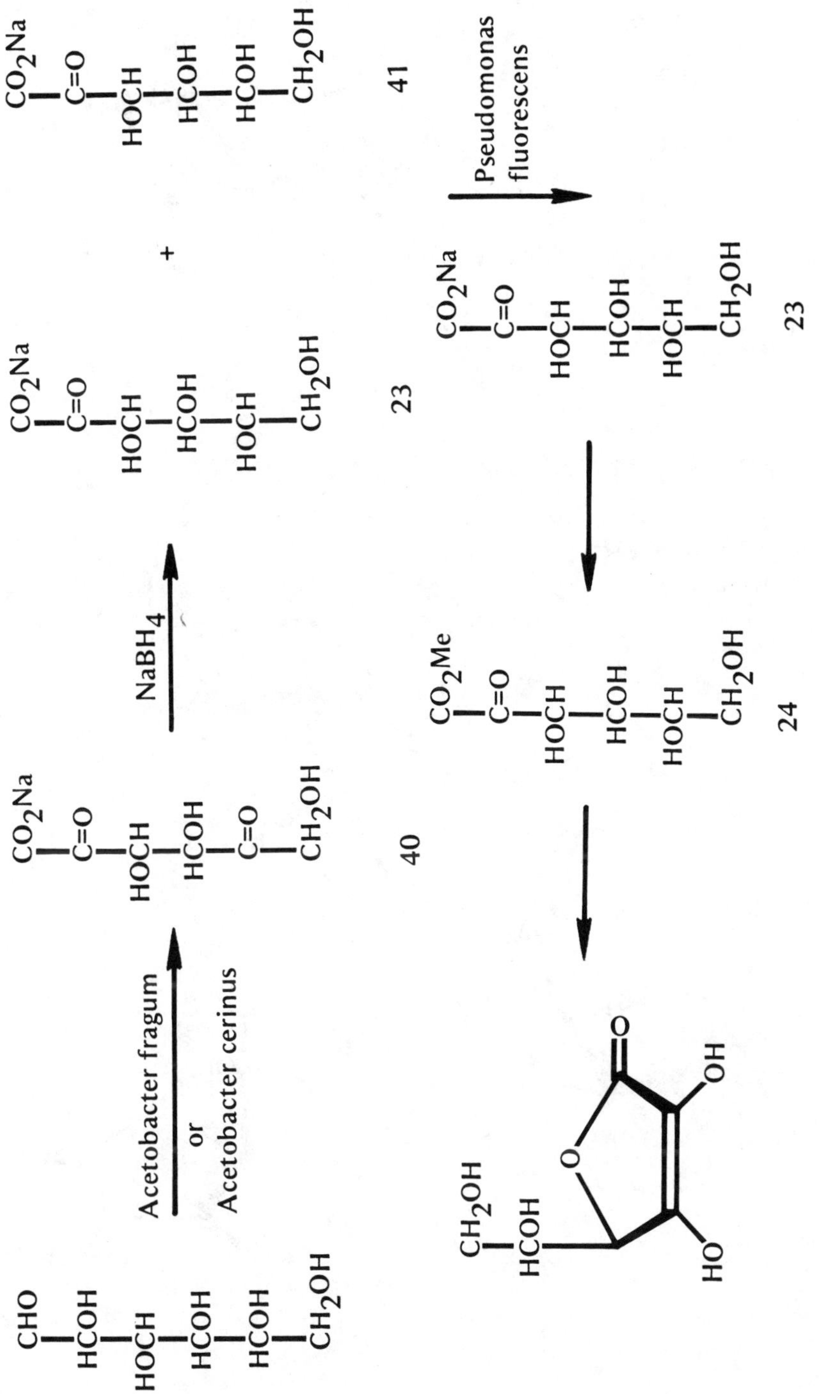

Scheme 22.

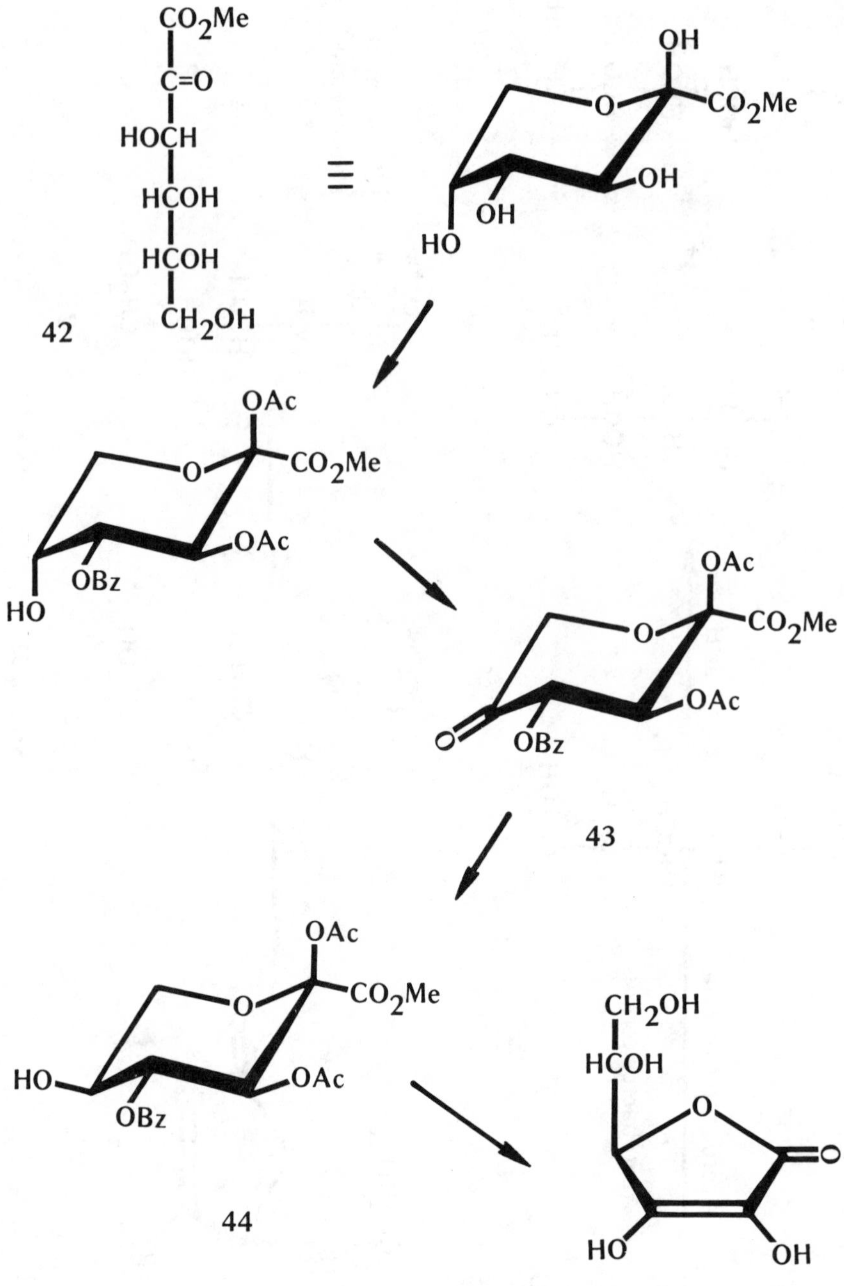
CO2Me
C=O
HOCH
HCOH
HCOH
CH2OH
42
≡
OH
CO2Me
OH
OH
HO
OAc
CO2Me
OAc
OBz
HO
OAc
CO2Me
OAc
OBz
43
OAc
CO2Me
HO
OAc
OBz
44
CH2OH
HCOH
HO
OH

Scheme 23.

Ascorbic Acid via C_6 Sugars Other Than Glucose

During the work directed toward the synthesis of L-ascorbic acid from D-glucose, a number of C_6 sugar acids was synthesized, including L-idonic and L-gulonic acids in particular. One other sugar acid, L-galactonic acid, which is not readily derived from D-glucose, was used to prepare L-ascorbic acid (82, Scheme 24). Pectin, which can be obtained from beet pulp or orange or grapefruit peel, can be converted to D-galacturonic acid (45) via enzymatic hydrolysis. Catalytic reduction of 45 over Raney nickel afforded L-galactonic acid (46) in 93% yield. Acid 46 was then oxidized to L-*lyxo*-2-hexulosonic acid (47) in 25–30% yield. Keto acid 47 was converted to 1 via esterification (90% yield) and base-catalyzed cyclization (71% yield). No fermentative oxidation of L-galactonic acid to 47 was reported. A high-yield fermentative oxidation probably could be developed. (Note added in proof: A recent U.S. patent describes an inefficient fermentation oxidation of L-galactonic acid to 47.)

No other C_6 sugar acids have proved important in the synthesis of L-ascorbic acid. In Scheme 25 the first method by which L-(4-^{3}H)ascor-

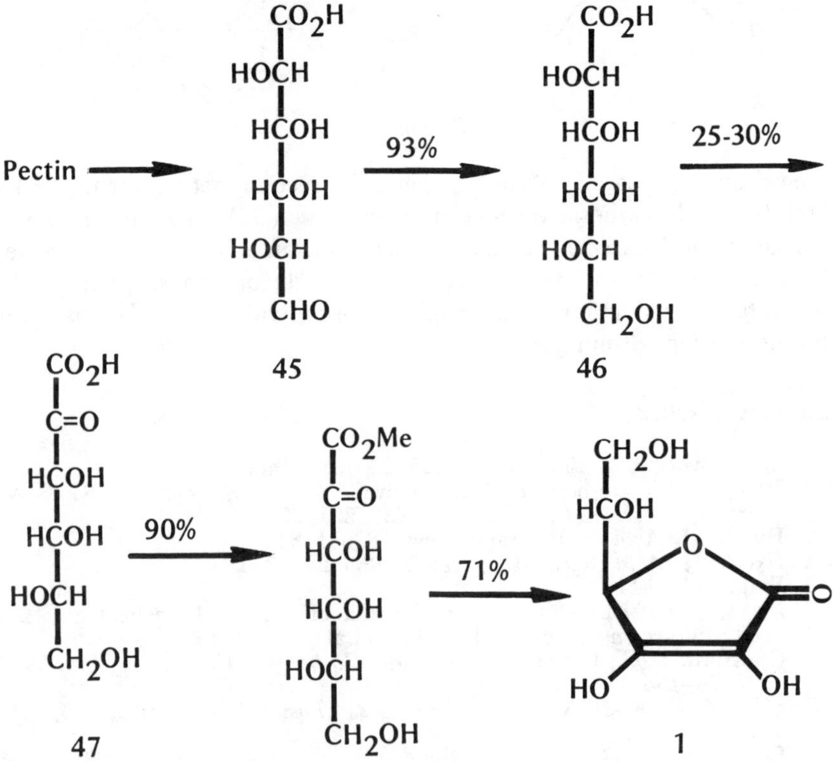

Scheme 24.

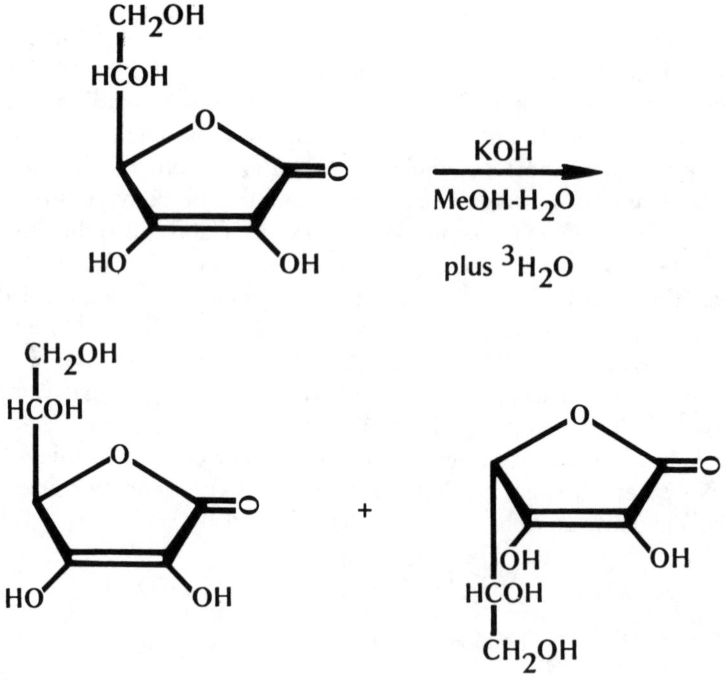

Scheme 25.

bic acid was prepared (83, 84) is shown. A second method for L-(4-³H)-ascorbic acid synthesis was recently reported (85). This material was prepared via the ascorbic acid synthesis shown in Scheme 14 (the Bakke–Theander synthesis), starting with D-(3-³H)glucopyranose prepared by the catalytic reduction of 1,2:5,6-di-O-isopropylidene-α-D-*ribo*-hex-3-ulo-furanose using tritium gas.

Literature Cited

1. Szent-Györgyi, A. *Biochem. J.* **1928,** *22,* 1387–1409.
2. Hirst, E. L.; Herbert, R. W.; Percival, E. G. V.; Reynolds, R. J. W.; Smith, F. *Chem. Ind. (London)* **1933,** 221–222.
3. Hvoslef, J. *Acta Chem. Scand.* **1964,** *18,* 841–842.
4. Hvoslef, J. *Acta Crystallogr., Sect. B* **1968,** *24,* 23–35.
5. Ibid., 1431–1440.
6. Burns, J. J. "Kirk-Othmer Encyclopedia of Chemical Technology," 2nd ed.; Interscience: New York, 1963; Vol. 2, pp. 747–762.
7. Crawford, T. C.; Crawford, S. A. *Adv. Carbohydr. Chem. Biochem.* **1980,** *37,* 79–155.
8. Micheel, F.; Kraft, K. *Hoppe-Seyler's Z. Physiol. Chem.* **1933,** *215,* 215–224.
9. Reichstein, T.; Grüssner, A.; Oppenauer, R. *Helv. Chim. Acta* **1933,** *16,* 561–565.
10. Reichstein, T.; Grüssner, A.; Oppenauer, R. *Nature (London)* **1933,** *132,* 280.

11. Reichstein, T.; Grüssner, A.; Oppenauer, R. *Helv. Chim. Acta* **1934**, *17*, 510–520.
12. Ibid., **1933**, *16*, 1019–1033.
13. Haworth, W. N. *Chem. Ind. (London)* **1933**, *52*, 482–485.
14. Haworth, W. N.; Hirst, E. L. *Chem. Ind. (London)* **1933**, *52*, 645–646.
15. Ault, R. G.; Baird, D. K.; Carrington, H. C.; Haworth, W. N.; Herbert, R. W.; Hirst, E. L.; Percival, E. G.; Smith, F.; Stacey, M. *J. Chem. Soc.* **1933**, 1419–1423.
16. Haworth, W. N.; Hirst, E. L. *Helv. Chim. Acta* **1934**, *17*, 520–523.
17. Burns, J. J.; King, C. G. *Science* **1950**, *111*, 257–258.
18. Salomon, L. L.; Burns, J. J.; King, C. G. *J. Am. Chem. Soc.* **1952**, *74*, 5161–5162.
19. von Schuching, S. L.; Frye, G. H. *Biochem. J.* **1966**, *98*, 652–654.
20. Rudoff, S., Univ. Microfilms, 58-2712; *Diss. Abstr.* **1959**, *19*, 1551–1552.
21. Stone, I. U.S. Patent 2 206 374, 1940; *Chem. Abstr.* **1940**, *34*, 7545.
22. Hamilton, J. K.; Smith, F. *J. Am. Chem. Soc.* **1952**, *74*, 5162–5163.
23. Major, R. T.; Cook, E. W. U.S. Patent 2 368 557, 1945; *Chem. Abstr.* **1946**, *40*, 354.
24. Othman, A. A.; Al-Timari, U. S. *Tetrahedron* **1980**, *36*, 753–758.
25. Helferich, B.; Peters, O. *Ber. Dtsch. Chem. Ges.* **1937**, *70*, 465–468.
26. Stedehouder, P. L. *Recl. Trav. Chim. Pays-Bas* **1952**, *71*, 831–836.
27. Helferich, B. U.S. Patent 2 207 680, 1940; *Chem. Abstr.* **1940**, *34*, 8184.
28. Loewus, F. *Annu. Rev. Plant Physiol.* **1971**, *22*, 337–364.
29. Reichstein, T,; Grüssner, A. *Helv. Chim. Acta* **1934**, *17*, 311–328.
30. Kristallinskaya, R. G. *Proc. Sci. Inst. Vitam. Res., Moscow* **1941**, *3*, 78–84; *Chem. Abstr.* **1942**, *36*, 3007.
31. Slobodin, Y. M. *J. Gen. Chem. USSR* **1947**, *17*, 485–488.
32. Strukov, I. T.; Kopylova, N. A. *Farmatsiya* **1947**, *10*, 8–12; *Chem. Abstr.* **1950**, *44*, 8327b.
33. Reichstein, T. British Patent 466 548, 1937; *Chem. Abstr.* **1937**, *31*, 8124.
34. Bassford, H. H.; Harmon, W. S.; Mahoney, J. F. U.S. Patent 2 462 251, 1949; *Chem. Abstr.* **1970**, *72*, 133,146k.
35. Politechnika Slaska, British Patent 1 222 322, 1971; Bogaczek, R.; Bogaczek, Fr. Demandé Pat. 2 001 090, 1969; *Chem. Abstr.* **1970**, *72*, 133,146k.
36. Flueck, N.; Wuersch, J. *J. Carbohydr. Nucleosides, Nucleotides* **1976**, *3*, 273–279.
37. Bothner-By, A. A.; Gibbs, M.; Anderson, R. C. *Science* **1950**, *112*, 363.
38. Dayton, P. B. *J. Org. Chem.* **1956**, *21*, 1535–1536.
39. Shnaidman, L. O.; Siling, M. I.; Kushchinskaya, I. N.; Eremina, T. N.; Shevyreva, O. N.; Shishkov, U. R.; Kosolapova, N. A.; Kazakevich, L. C.; Timafeeva, T. P. *Tr., Latv. Inst. Eksp. Klin. Med. Akad. Med. Nauk SSSR* **1962**, *27*, 1–14; *Chem. Abstr.*, **1963**, *58*, 4508a.
40. Karr, D. B.; Baker, E. M.; Tolbert, B. M. *J. Labelled Compd.* **1970**, *6*, 155–165.
41. Hinkley, D. F.; Hoinowski, A. M. U.S. Patent 3 721 663, 1973; *Chem. Abstr.* **1973**, *78*, 160,063m.
42. Heyns, K. *Justus Liebings Ann. Chem.* **1947**, *558*, 177–187.
43. Bakke, J.; Theander, O. *J. Chem. Soc. D* **1971**, 175–176.
44. Mackie, W.; Perlin, A. S. *Can. J. Chem.* **1965**, *43*, 2921–2924.
45. Heyns, K.; Alpers, E.; Weyer, J. *Chem. Ber.* **1968**, *101*, 4209–4213.
46. Williams, M.; Loewus, F. A. *Carbohydr. Res.* **1978**, *63*, 149–155.
47. Kitahara, T.; Ogawa, T.; Naganuma, T.; Matsui, M. *Agric. Biol. Chem.* **1974**, *38*, 2189–2190.
48. Dax, K.; Weidmann, H. *Carbohydr. Res.* **1972**, *25*, 363–370.
49. Crawford, T. C.; Breitenback, R. *J. Chem. Soc., Chem. Commun.* **1979**, 388–389.
50. Crawford, T. C. U.S. Patent 4 111 958, 1978.
51. Taylor, R. L.; Conrad, H. E. *Biochemistry* **1972**, *11*, 1383–1388.

52. Berends, W.; Konings, J. *Recl. Trav. Chim. Pays-Bas* **1955**, *74*, 1365–1370.
53. Isherwood, F. A.; Mapson, L. W., British Patent 763 055, 1956; *Chem. Abstr.* **1957**, *31*, 8387b.
54. Gray, B. E. U.S. Patent 2 421 612, 1947; *Chem. Abstr.* **1947**, *41*, 5683h.
55. Kita, D. U.S. Patent 4 155 812, 1979.
56. Ferrier, R. J.; Furneaux, R. H. *J. Chem. Soc., Chem. Commun.* **1977**, 332–333.
57. Ferrier, R. J.; Furneaux, R. H. *Carbohydr. Res.* **1976**, *52*, 63–68.
58. Ferrier, R. J.; Furneaux, R. N. *J. Chem. Soc., Perkin Trans. 1* **1978**, 1996–2000.
59. Stubbs, J. J.; Lockwood, L. B.; Roe, E. T.; Tabenkin, B.; Ward, G. E. *Ind. Eng. Chem.* **1940**, *32*, 1626–1631.
60. Chen, C.; Yamamoto, H.; Kwan, T. *Chem. Pharm. Bull.* **1969**, *17*, 1287–1289.
61. Hamilton, J. K.; Smith, F. *J. Am. Chem. Soc.* **1954**, *76*, 3543–3544.
62. Hori, I.; Nakatani, T. *Hakko Kogaku Zasshi* **1954**, *32*, 33–36.
63. Alieva, R. M. *Tr. Petergof. Biol. Inst. Leningr. Gos. Univ.* **1966**, 100–103; *Chem. Abstr.* **1966**, *65*, 19,025c.
64. Katznelson, H.; Tanenbaum, S. W.; Tatum, E. L. *J. Biol. Chem.* **1953**, *204*, 43–59.
65. Wakisaka, Y. *Agric. Biol. Chem.* **1964**, *28*, 369–374.
66. Wakisaka, Y. Japanese Patent 14 493, 1964; *Chem. Abstr.* **1964**, *61*, 16,742f.
67. Oga, S.; Sato, K.; Imada, K.; Asano, K. Japanese Patent 72 38 193, 1972; *Chem. Abstr.* **1973**, *78*, 82,947m.
68. Kita, D. Belgian Patent 872 095, 1979.
69. Andrews, G. C.; Bacon, B. E.; Bordner, J.; Hennessee, G. L. A. *Carbohydr. Res.* **1979**, *77*, 25–36.
70. Crawford, T. C.; Andrews, G. C.; Fauble, H.; Chmurny, G. N. *J. Am. Chem. Soc.* **1980**, *102*, 2220–2225.
71. Sonoyama, T.; Tani, H.; Kageyama, B.; Kobayashi, K.; Honjo, T.; Yagi, S. U.S. Patent 3 959 076, 1976; *Chem. Abstr.* **1976**, *85*, 121,786z.
72. Sonoyama, T.; Tani, H.; Kageyama, B.; Kobayashi, K.; Honjo, T.; Yagi, S. U.S. Patent 3 963 574, 1976; *Chem. Abstr.* **1976**, *85*, 44,945w.
73. Ikawa, K.; Tokuyama, K.; Kiyokawa, M.; Kimoto, M.; Yamane, S.; Tabato, T.; Sonoyama, T.; Honjo, T. Japanese Patent 7 766 684, 1977; *Chem. Abstr.* **1977**, *7*, 182,601y.
74. Ikawa, K.; Tokuyama, K.; Kiyokawa, M.; Kimoto, M.; Yamane, S.; Tobato, T.; Sonoyama, T.; Honjo, T. Japanese Patent 77 66 685, 1977; *Chem. Abstr.* **1977**, *87*, 182,600x.
75. Wakisaka, Y. *Agric. Biol. Chem.* **1964**, *28*, 819–827.
76. Andrews, G.; Bacon, B.; Crawford, T.; Breitenback, R. *J. Chem. Soc., Chem. Commun.* **1979**, 740–741.
77. Kita, D. European Patent 0 007 751, 1979.
78. Crawford, T. U.S. Patent 4 180 511, 1979.
79. Andrews, G. C. U.S. Patent 4 212 988, 1980.
80. Ogawa, T.; Taguchi, K.; Takasaka, N.; Mikata, M.; Matsui, M. *Carbohydr. Res.* **1976**, *51*, C1–C4.
81. Matsui, M.; Ogawa, T.; Taguchi, K.; Mikata, M., Japanese Patent 77 00 255, 1977; *Chem. Abstr.* **1977**, *87*, 53,526d.
82. Isbell, H. S. *J. Res. Natl. Bur. Stand.* **1944**, *33*, 45–61.
83. Bell, E. M.; Baker, E. M.; Tolbert, B. M. *J. Labelled Compd.* **1966**, *2*, 148–154.
84. Brenner, G. S.; Hinkley, D. F.; Perkins, L. M.; Weber, S. *J. Org. Chem.* **1964**, *29*, 2389–2392.
85. Williams, M.; Saito, K.; Loewus, F. A. *Phytochemistry* **1979**, *18*, 953–956.

RECEIVED for review February 9, 1981. ACCEPTED April 8, 1981.

Crystallography of the Ascorbates

JAN HVOSLEF

University of Oslo, Department of Chemistry, Blindern, Oslo 3, Norway

A review of the various ascorbates is given in terms of the results from crystal structure determinations. The acid itself and the simple, monovalent salts consist of roughly planar γ-lactone rings with side-chains in a more or less staggered conformation. The acidity of the compound is associated with the proton at O3 because of the conjugated O1=C1—C2=C3—O3 system in the ring. By esterification the location of the ester group can be at either C2 or C3, but the C2 position is presumably the stabler site. By oxidation of the vitamin dehydroascorbic acid is produced in different isomeric forms, depending on the solvent, on the time, and on a possible substituent in the lactone ring. The usual crystalline compound is a dimer comprising five fused rings, whereas monomeric derivatives are bicyclic, except in cases where the substituents induce sp² hybridization at C3.

In the mid 1930s x-ray crystallographers (1) attempted to assist chemists (2) in the elucidation of the chemistry of vitamin C. The trial was destined to be unsuccessful, but could nevertheless support the brilliant chemical works that eventually lead to a correct chemical formula and to the synthesis of the vitamin (3). This relatively small and simple molecule, comprising only 20 atoms, has intrinsic properties that diversify its chemical behavior and mask its constitution. Features such as acidity without a carboxyl group, an unusually stable γ-lactone ring, reducing power, and two chiral carbon atoms form a combination with enigmatic biological functions that still puzzle chemists and biologists in the 1980s.

With the advent of modern methods in crystallography the detailed geometries of ascorbates became accessible, and to date a number of crystal structures are known (Table I). The motivation for these investigations was originally not any doubt about the gross structures of the ascorbates arrived at by chemical means; the x-ray results also generally

0065-2393/82/0200–0037$06.25/0

Table I. Crystallographic Data on

Compound	Formula	Reference
L-Ascorbic acid	$C_6H_8O_6$	(6–8)
Sodium L-ascorbate	$Na^+C_6H_7O_6^-$	(10)
Calcium L-ascorbate dihydrate	$Ca^{2+}(C_6H_7O_6)_2^- \cdot 2H_2O$	(12–14)
Thallium (I)-L-ascorbate	$Tl^+C_6H_7O_6^-$	(11)
L-Serine-L-ascorbic acid	$C_3H_7NO_3 \cdot C_6H_8O_6$	(9)
L-Arginine L-ascorbate	$C_6H_5N_4O_2^+ \cdot C_6H_7O_6^-$	(15)
Barium 2-O-sulfonato-L-ascorbate dihydrate	$Ba^{2+}(C_6H_6O_9S)^{2-} \cdot 2\,H_2O$	(18)
3-O[(bismorpholino) phosphinyl]-5,6-O-isopropylidene-L-ascorbate	$C_{17}H_{27}N_2O_9P$	(21)
Dehydroascorbic acid dimer	$C_{12}H_{12}O_{12}$	(4)
p-Bromophenylhydrazine of monomeric dehydro-L-ascorbic acid	$C_{12}H_{11}O_5N_2Br$	(25)
Methyl glycoside of 2-C-benzyl-3-keto-L-lyxo-hexulosonic acid lactone	$C_{14}H_{16}O_6$	(24)
D-Isoascorbic acid	$C_6H_8O_6$	(26)
Sodium D-isoascorbate-monohydrate	$Na^+C_6H_7O_6^- \cdot H_2O$	(27)

[a] The technique used is indicated by: F, film; D, diffractometer; or N, neutron diffraction spectrometer.

confirmed the predicted chemical formulae and bonding properties. Surprises came, however, when the vitamin's oxidation product, dehydroascorbic acid, was examined by x-ray and NMR methods (4, 5). Virtually all textbooks are shown to be misleading in their assessment of the structure of this compound. This should actually not be surprising, for the formula commonly used is unacceptable for various reasons. Many details of the oxidation are still left to be sorted out, but they present difficult tasks because of the complicated reaction mechanism.

L-Ascorbic Acid and Some Derivatives

Space Group	Unit Cell Dimensions	Average e.s.d. in Bond Lengths [Method (Å) and Angles (°)][a]		
$P2_1$	$a = 17.299, b = 6.353, c = 6.411$ Å; $\beta = 102.18°$	0.003 Å	0.2°	F, N
$P2_12_12_1$	$a = 19.051, b = 4.490, c = 8.516$ Å	0.006	0.4	F
$P2_1$	$a = 8.335, b = 15.787, c = 6.360$ Å; $\beta = 107.48°$	0.004	0.2	D
$P2_12_12_1$	$a = 10.883, b = 18.598, c = 8.066$ Å	0.040	—	D
$P2_12_12_1$	$a = 5.335, b = 8.769, c = 25.782$ Å	0.005	0.3	D
$P2_1$	$a = 5.060, b = 9.977, c = 15.330,$ $\beta = 97.5°$	0.006	0.4	D
$P1$	$a = 5.201, b = 6.951, c = 8.732$ Å $\alpha = 99.54°, \beta = 93.92°, \gamma = 109.12°$	0.004	0.2°	D
$P2_1$	$a = 9.487, b = 13.570, c = 8.355$ Å	—	—	D
$C2$	$a = 15.728, b = 5.530, c = 9.453$ Å; $\beta = 130.56°$	0.006	0.5	F
$P2_12_12_1$	$a = 18.020, b = 12.859, c = 5.754$ Å	0.008	0.6	D
$P2_12_12_1$	$a = 6.339, b = 9.739, c = 22.484$ Å	0.004	0.3	D
$P2_1$	$a = 5.165, b = 14.504, c = 4.724$ Å; $\beta = 99.50°$	0.005	0.3	D
$P2_12_12_1$	$a = 8.307, b = 9.049, c = 11.181$	0.007	0.4	D

X-ray analyses have also proved useful in unraveling other complex structural problems in this field, and we shall review some work done on ascorbates by diffraction methods.

Ascorbic Acid and Its Salts

Ascorbic Acid. Vitamin C (L-ascorbic acid) was the first ascorbate to be studied in detail by diffraction methods (*6, 7, 8*). It crystallizes in the monoclinic space group $P2_1$ with four molecules in the unit cell as shown in Figure 1. There are two molecules, A and B, in the asymmetric unit, but they are related in pairs by pseudo screw axes along [010] in the positions ($x = 1/4$, $z = 5/8$) and ($x = 3/4$, $z = 3/8$). In the crystals the independent molecules are slightly different, mainly because of a small difference in the orientation of the almost identical side-chains. The distinction is defined by a $+/-7.9°$ twist about the C4—C5 bond to each side of an ideally staggered conformation where O5 is situated above the ring and where O6 is $+8.3°$ from *anti* to O5. The interatomic distances and angles, however, are almost identical in the independent molecules, which have the average values shown in Figure 2.

The C—C and C—O bond lengths show some interesting variations, and explain in a striking way the observed chemical properties. The localization of the protolytic proton to O3 was obvious from the bonding properties of the conjugated O1=C1—C2=C3—O3—H system, and it has later been confirmed by the structure of a number of salts. Whereas the ene—diolic group is entirely planar, the lactone group shows minor variations from planarity. These deviations are presumably caused by packing effects being different in the two independent molecules. However, the whole ring system can be adequately described as planar because the best planes through the lactone and the ene—diol group in each molecule are at only $0.6°$ to each other.

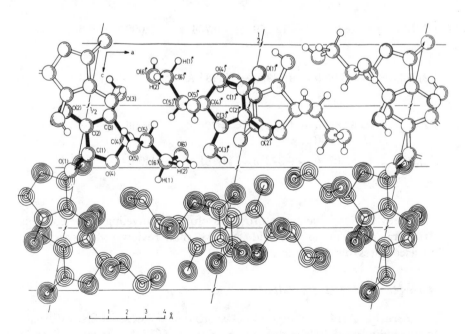

Figure 1. View of the structure of L-*ascorbic acid along [010] and the corresponding three-dimensional electron density. (Reproduced, with permission, from Ref. 7.)*

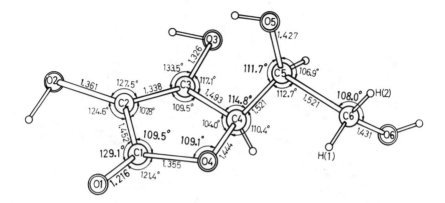

Figure 2. Average values of bonding distances and angles in L-ascorbic acid. (Reproduced, with permission, from Ref. 7.)

All the oxygen atoms, except O4, are engaged in hydrogen bonds, and the interactions involving the ene–diol oxygen atoms are particularly strong and about 0.15 Å shorter than the usual alcoholic interactions. The hydrogen bond system for each of the two independent molecules is shown in Figure 3, and it is noteworthy that the pattern is similar for A and B although the environments are different and the donor–acceptor sequence is reversed, except for O3.

The ascorbic acid molecule has also been studied in the crystalline complex with L-serine [CH₂(OH)CH(NH₂)COOH], recently reported by Sudhakar, Bhat, and Vijayan (9). The crystals are orthorhombic with $Z = 4$, and the molecules are mainly held together by hydrogen bonds. The individual components are both neutral, and the molecular dimensions in the ascorbic acid molecule are not significantly different from those in the pure acid. The side-chain conformation varies by rotation of O6 about the C5–C6 bond to a near *gauche* arrangement, thus bringing it close to the situation in sodium ascorbate (10). The hydrogen bond system is, of course, different, and it is interesting to note that the carboxyl group of L-serine is tied to the ene–diol group of L-ascorbic acid (Figure 4) through rather short hydrogen bonds (2.542 and 2.642 Å).

Salts of Ascorbic Acid. In salt formation the ionization of L-ascorbic acid is closely associated with the behavior of the ene–diol group and the conjugated O1=C1—C2=C3—O3 system. All the salts we know so far are formed by dissociation of the proton at O3 only, and are hence monovalent. Bivalent anions predicted from studies of solutions have not been isolated and characterized.

Common to the investigated ascorbate anions are the significant lengthening of the double, shortening of the single bonds in the conju-

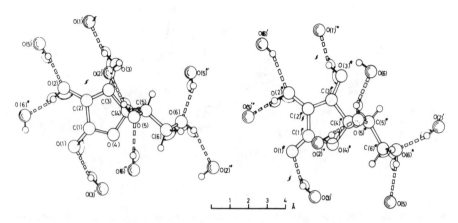

Figure 3.   Environment and hydrogen bonding for molecules A and B. Oxygen atoms in neighboring molecules are indicated by triple circles. (Reproduced, with permission, from Ref. 7.)

gated system, and changes in the angular distribution, especially at C2 and C3.

Selected values of bond lengths and angles in the ascorbate anion are given in Table II and are compared with those of the free acid.

Taking the bonding properties of the lactone group into account also, the observations support the view that the anion may be thought of as a resonance hybrid of **I, II,** and **III,** but with a dominating contribution from **I.**

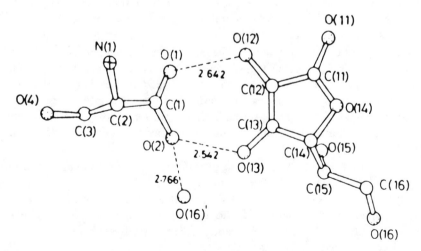

Figure 4.   The hydrogen-bonded interaction between the ene–diol group of ascorbic acid and the carboxylate group of serine. The primed atom belongs to a neighboring molecule. (Reproduced, with permission, from Ref. 9.)

Table II. Selected Bond Distances (Å) and Angles (°) in Ascorbate Anions[a]

	L-Ascorbic Acid (7)	D-Isoascorbic Acid (26)	Na L-Ascorbate (10)	Na Iso-ascorbate (27)	Ca L-Ascorbate (14) (A)	Ca L-Ascorbate (14) (B)	Arginine L-Ascorbate (15)	Ba 2-O-Sulfonato-L-ascorbate (18)
C1=O1	1.216	1.200	1.233	1.222	1.231	1.229	1.218	1.218 (Å)
C2—O2	1.361	1.340	1.384	1.364	1.375	1.366	1.364	1.389
C3—O3	1.326	1.329	1.287	1.301	1.275	1.288	1.275	1.265
C1—O4	1.355	1.365	1.358	1.381	1.365	1.374	1.361	1.376
C4—O4	1.444	1.437	1.448	1.465	1.453	1.451	1.440	1.455
C5—O5	1.427	1.416	1.410	1.420	1.436	1.431	1.424	1.421
C6—O6	1.431	1.428	1.423	1.441	1.422	1.425	1.401	1.422
C2=C3	1.338	1.331	1.373	1.362	1.371	1.370	1.364	1.367
C1—C2	1.452	1.446	1.416	1.418	1.417	1.421	1.423	1.422
C3—C4	1.493	1.493	1.516	1.516	1.516	1.518	1.499	1.515
C4—C5	1.521	1.531	1.536	1.521	1.533	1.528	1.510	1.523
C5—C6	1.521	1.520	1.503	1.513	1.514	1.508	1.497	1.524
C1—C2—C3	107.8	107.1	109.5	109.8	109.8	109.4	109.2	111.2 (°)
C2—C3—C4	109.5	110.1	105.8	107.5	106.2	106.9	106.9	105.7
C1—C2—O2	124.6	124.5	121.6	124.4	120.1	121.1	125.9	122.2
C2—C3—O3	133.5	132.8	131.3	130.7	130.9	131.9	130.8	131.4
O3—C3—C4	117.1	116.3	122.9	121.7	122.8	121.7	122.1	122.8
C4—C5—C6	112.7	112.5	110.1	110.9	114.6	115.6	111.9	111.2
C3—C4—C5	114.8	114.0	116.1	115.3	112.4	119.6	113.6	112.4

[a] The mean values of the L-ascorbic acid molecules and of D-isoascorbic acid are given for comparison. The values for Ca L-ascorbate dihydrate are weighed means of Refs. *12* and *13*.

I   II   III

The effect of an impaired sp^2 hybridization at C2 and C3 is conformational lability in the γ-lactone ring. As a result, the proximity of a metallic cation causes this ring to deviate from planarity; it also increases O2—C2=C3—O3 dihedral angles. Typical is the effect on salts like Na ascorbate (10), Tl(I)-ascorbate (11) and Ca ascorbate dihydrate (13, 14) where the angle between the mean planes defined by the lactone group (O4,C4,C1,O1,C2) and the ene–diol group (C2,O2,C3,O3) occasionally is as high as 8°. A somewhat smaller angle (5°) is observed in L-arginine ascorbate (15) where the influence of a metallic cation is avoided.

Whereas the conformational differences in the rings are moderate, the side-chains are found to be more susceptible to the influence of packing, metal coordination, and hydrogen bonding. In most cases the ascorbate ions have O5 in a roughly staggered position, but with appreciable tolerance. O6 has either a near *anti* or near *gauche* orientation as illustrated in Figure 5.

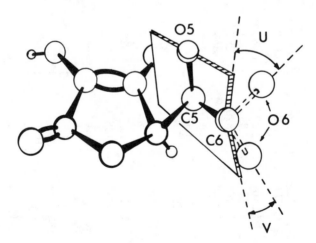

Figure 5. Dihedral angles (parentheses) U (gauche) and V (anti) for O5–C5–C6–O6 in ascorbates.

The gauche orientation occurs in: ascorbic acid in serine complex (66°), sodium ascorbate (70°), thallium ascorbate A (71.7°), arginine ascorbate (56°), barium 2-O-sulfonato-L-ascorbate dihydrate (73.3°). The anti orientation occurs in: ascorbic acid (8.3°), thallium ascorbate B (1°), p-bromophenylhydrazine of dehydroascorbic acid (1.2°).

In certain cases, exceptions to these rules are observed. In one of the two independent anions (**B**) of Ca ascorbate dihydrate, O5 (Figure 6) adopts a rare, unfavorable (peri) interaction (*16*) with O3. In addition, O6 is rotated about C5–C6 to permit the three oxygen atoms O3, O5 and O6 to form an interesting tridentate complex with Ca^{2+}. Mole-

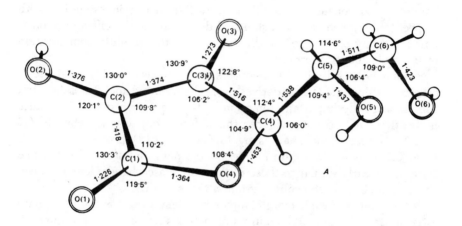

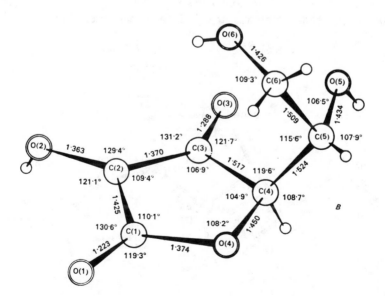

Figure 6.   Perspective drawing of the independent ascorbate anions A and B. Distances and angles for the nonhydrogen atoms are included in the drawing. (Reproduced, with permission, from Ref. 13.)

cule **A** can be derived from **B** by rotating the side-chain by $-117°$ around C4–C5, and the octahedral coordination around Ca^{2+} is completed by O5 and O6 from *A*, two water molecules, and O1 from a symmetry equivalent of *B*.

The structure of Ca ascorbate dihydrate was simultaneously determined by two independent groups (*12, 13*), and their data and results were subsequently compared and analyzed by Abrahams et al. (*14*). Some general conclusions could be drawn from this investigation with respect to the given values of standard deviations, to the effect of anomalous scattering on atomic coordinates, and to the absolute configuration of the molecule in question.

Among the salts in the ascorbate series is also Ba 2-*O*-sulfonato-L-ascorbate dihydrate that is derived from the ascorbic acid 2-sulfate ester. This biologically important compound (*17*) was much debated because it was difficult to decide whether the sulfate group was attached to C2 or C3. The structural analysis by McClelland (*18*) proved the site to be at C2 as shown in Figure 7. The bond lengths, angles, and resonance forms are clearly similar to those of the simple ascorbate anions irrespective of the effect of the sulfate group attached to C2.

A similar and even more complex problem arose for the phosphate ester of ascorbic acid, and again x-ray methods proved useful in unraveling the dilemma of where to assign the phosphate group. The position assigned by the original authors (*19*) was at C3, but Lee et al. (*20*) and others contended that was at C2. In a recent, interesting paper by

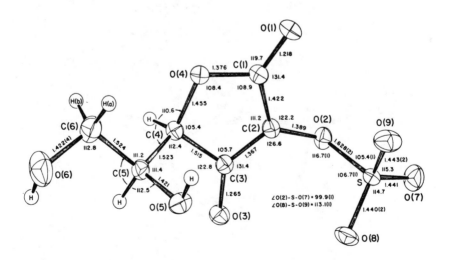

Figure 7.   Configuration, bond lengths (A), and bond angles (°) of the 2-O-sulfonato-L-ascorbate anion. (Reproduced, with permission, from Ref. 18.)

Jernow et al. (*21*) a brief crystallographic analysis demonstrates that a derivative of this ester, the (3-*O*-(bismorpholino)phosphinyl) 5,6-iso-propylidene-L-ascorbate, indeed has its phosphate group attached to C3. The molecular structure is shown in Figure 8, but unfortunately no details of the structure are given under the circumstances; only the gross structure was required. No information is therefore available with respect to the state of conjugation, but it is expected to be different from that in the simple salts and in the 2-*O*-esters. Upon acid hydrolysis of the compound, the authors claim that an unstable 3-*O*-phosphate is initially formed, but that it rapidly isomerizes to the stabler 2-*O*-phosphate. It is concluded that the tris(cyclohexyl)ammonium salt of the ascorbic acid phosphate, first prepared by Cutolo and Lorizza (*19*) and assigned the 3-*O*-phosphate, is in fact the 2-*O*-phosphate as proposed by Lee et al. (*20*).

All the compounds mentioned above have common features with respect to molecular and crystal structures, and the results arrived at by different authors are hearteningly unanimous. For the hydrogen bond system, for example, it is established that the distances associated with the ene–diolic hydroxyls are signficantly shorter than the others (Table III). A value well below 2.6 Å for a O2—H · · · O3 interaction is usual, and if O3 is an acceptor even an alcoholic hydroxyl group produces a strong interaction. This atom has an unusually high capacity for hydrogen bonding.

The orientation and conformations of the side-chain have only minor

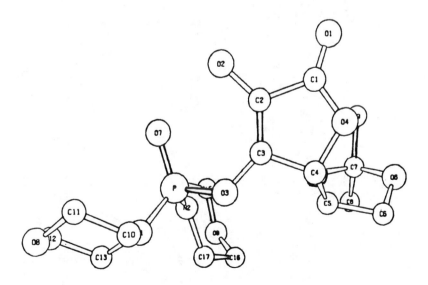

Figure 8.   Drawing showing the conformation of the ascorbate 3-O-phosphinate. (Reproduced, with permission, from Ref. 21.)

Table III. Examples of Hydrogen Bond Distances (Å) in Ascorbates[a]

Donor	Ascorbic Acid (7)	Ascorbic Acid in Serine Complex (9)	Isoascorbic Acid (26)	Na Ascorbate (10)	Na Isoascorbate (27)	Ca Ascorbate Dihydrate (13)	Arginine Ascorbate (15)	Ba 2-O-Sulfonato ascorbate (18)
O2—H	O6': 2.612	O1(S): 2.642	O6: 2.584	O3: 2.546	W: 2.699	O3': 2.549	O1(A): 2.676	
O2—H'	O5': 2.645					O3: 2.571		
O3—H	O1: 2.656	O2(S): 2.542	O1: 2.643					
O3—H'	O1': 2.666							
O5—H	O2: 2.786	O6: 2.709	O2: 2.827	O2: 2.709	O3: 2.801	O4': 2.862	O4: 2.921	O3: 2.693
O5—H'	O6: 2.707					O4: 2.742 O2: 2.793	O1: 2.913	
O6—H	O2': 2.935	O2: 2.766	O5: 2.777	O1: 2.820	O3: 2.993	O2: 2.715	O3: 2.622	W: 2.899
O6—H'	O5: 2.769					O1: 2.786		
O—H in water					O3: 2.828 O3: 2.785	O5': 2.972 O2': 2.921 O3: 2.707 O1: 2.782		

[a] If two independent molecules A and B are involved B is indicated by: S, serine; A, arginine; W, water.

influence on the bond lengths in the ring, but have some effect on its planarity. This is reflected in the angular distribution around C4 and C5, particularly in Ca-ascorbate dihydrate where deviations up to 7.2° are observed.

Dehydroascorbic Acid and Derivatives

Oxidation of L-ascorbic acid produces a variety of chemical species depending on the nature of the solvent, the time, and the strength of the oxidation agent. By careful, mild oxidation two hydrogen atoms are given off in successive steps. In the first step, an unstable radical "semi-dehydroascorbic acid" is formed. In the second, the biologically active dehydroascorbic acid results.

The commercially available isomer of dehydroascorbic acid is a crystalline, symmetric dimer comprising a system of five fused rings (*4, 22*), **IV,** and not the traditional "textbook compound" with the formula **V.** The latter has not been isolated and characterized, and is presumably not present in significant amount when the vitamin is oxidized. If the oxidation of L-ascorbic acid takes place in inert solvents such as dimethyl-formamide or dimethyl sulfoxide, it has been shown by Hvoslef and Pedersen (*5*), using NMR methods, that at low temperatures a dimer identical to the crystalline compound is formed. When the temperature

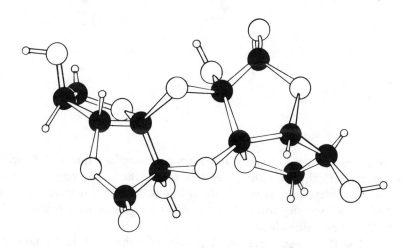

IV

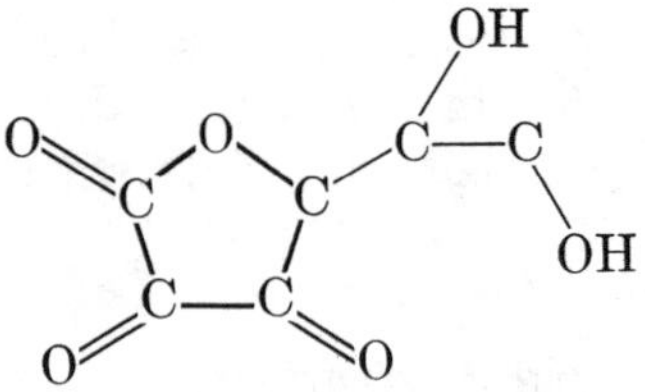

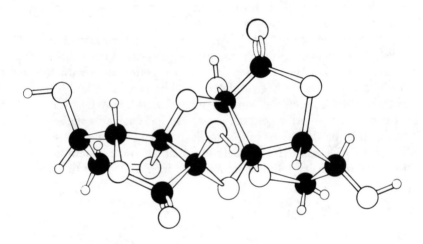

V

VI

rises, this dimer gradually transforms to another dimer, **VI**, which is unsymmetrical, but closely related to the first. However, in water a hydrated bicyclic monomer is the prime result. This is unstable in water, and with time the furanose ring opens to give a monocyclic molecule with an open side-chain.

The Dehydroascorbic Acid Dimer. Of the possible versions of pure dehydroascorbic acid, only the symmetric dimer has been obtained in crystalline state and investigated by diffraction methods. However, derivatives of monomers are known and will be discussed below.

Monoclinic crystals of the symmetric dimer can be precipitated by successive addition of formic acid and solid oxalic acid (23) to a dimethylformamide solution of the usual mixture of symmetric and asymmetric dimers. The solubility of the former is strongly decreased by these reagents, but leaves the latter in solution.

The space group C2 imposes twofold symmetry on the dimeric molecule with the dimensions shown in Figure 9. The two halves are joined by the O3 atoms originally associated by the ene–diol group, and establish a central dioxan ring in the twisted boat conformation. The fourth valence at C3 closes the side-chain to form an irregular furanose moiety with C6 0.55 Å from the best plane through the other atoms. Looking at the lactone ring one observes that the lactone group (C4,O4, C1,O1,C2) is almost planar, but that C3 deviates by 0.192 Å, which is moderate for furanose or furanoid lactone rings. The geometry of this moderately strained ring system is normal for a compound with covalent bonds. One may, however, notice that the C2–O2 bond is very short (1.352 Å) and that the two C–O bond lengths in the dioxan ring are unequal. On reaction with water the dioxan ring is split at the longer C2–O3 bond, and two bicyclic, hydrated monomers are formed (5). It is not unlikely that the short C2–O2 bond is responsible for the acidity of the compound.

The really interesting aspect of this structure is that it is dimeric. This fact obviously has relevance to the complicated reaction mechanism associated with the oxidation of the vitamin in inert solvents. Whether the dimer is formed as a short-lived intermediate by oxidation in water is still an open question. Attempts to determine the crystal structure of the asymmetric dimer are now being made in our laboratory.

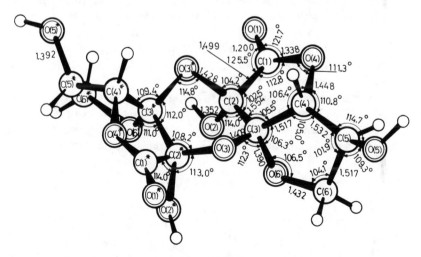

Figure 9.   Bonding distances and angles in dehydroascorbic acid. (Reproduced, with permission, from Ref. 4.)

Derivatives of Dehydroascorbic Monomers. Monomeric dehydro-ascorbic acid presumably is formed only in solvents that prevent the formation of dimers, for example, water and alcohols. The unstable evasive nature of the compound impedes its crystallization, and intractable syrups are often the result. However, derivatives of the monomer could be obtained with satisfactory crystalline quality for a regular x-ray study.

The question of whether a bi- or monocyclic molecule is present in these crystals was of major interest, but we have also sought possible factors that would cause an open side-chain in the monomer.

In the methyl glycoside of 2-C-benzyl-3-keto-L-lyxo-hexulosonic acid lactone (Figure 10) a bicyclic ascorbate isomer was found (24). The sugar moiety bears great resemblance to the asymmetric unit of the crystalline dimeric dehydroascorbic acid. Both five-membered rings have irregular envelope conformations with the common C3 atom deviating from the best planes through the four other atoms in the rings. The unique role of C3 is presumably caused by repulsion between the benzyl and methoxy groups, whereby an eclipsed conformation for O3 and C8 is avoided by a $+38.8°$ twist about the C2–C3 bond. The free OH group at C2 has the same orientation relative to the lactone ring as it has in the dimer, but the C–O bond is somewhat longer. Besides this, the bond lengths and angles are generally similar to those in the dimer, except for the conformational angles in the furanose moiety.

On the other hand, a monocyclic derivative was obtained when a solution of dehydroascorbic acid and p-bromophenylhydrazine in dimethylacetamide was allowed to stand overnight at room temperature (25). The compound was precipitated with water and recrystallized from absolute alcohol; its molecular structure is shown in Figure 11. The lactone ring is of the envelope type with C4 deviating by 0.126 Å from the plane defined by C1, O1, C2, and O4. The side-chain is very nearly staggered and with O5 and C6 anti.

A significant feature of this compound is the property of the C7–N2–N1–C2–C3 moiety with its planar, extended chain of atoms and its bond lengths and angles typical of sp^2 hybridization. The resonance structures that could describe the π-electron delocalization are:

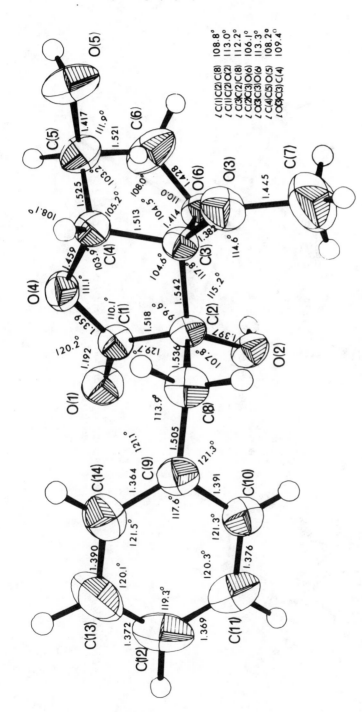

Figure 10. ORTEP plot of the methyl glycoside of the 2-C-benzyl-3-keto-L-lyxo-hexulosonic acid lactone molecule. (Reproduced, with permission, from Ref. 24.)

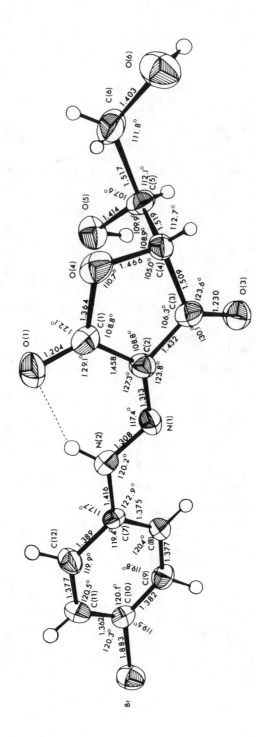

Figure 11. ORTEP plot of the p-bromophenylhydrazone of dehydroascorbic acid. (Reproduced, with permission, from Ref. 25.)

Obviously these are preferred to a system with a bicyclic ring as indicated by

The conclusion follows that any substituent at C2 that induces π-electron delocalization into the region will open the furanoid ring. The reason is simply that sp^2 hybridization at C3 precludes the necessary fourth valence for ring formation. It has recently been shown that solutions contain two isomers in equilibrium with 180° difference in orientation of the hydrazine group. The N–H group hence can establish hydrogen bonds to either O1 or O3 (*26*).

Ascorbate Isomers

Of substances closely related to vitamin C are isomers with inverted substituents at C4 and C5. The so called D-isoascorbic acid is a stereo-isomer with inversion of the OH group at C5 only. An x-ray investigation by Azarnia, Berman, and Rosenstein (*27*) revealed that in this compound the distances and angles are quite similar to those found in L-ascorbic acid (Table II). The plane relationship is also congruous, but the properties of the side-chain are, of course, different as a result of the inversion at C5. C4–C5–C6–O6 form a roughly planar zigzag chain where C6 adopts a position approximately corresponding to that of O5 in L-ascorbic acid. The dihedral C3–C4–C5–C6 angle is +78° vs. +58° for the C3–C4–C5–O5 angle in the vitamin. Relative to O5, O6 is in the *gauche* conformation that takes it farthest away from the ring; O6 is tied to O2 in a neighboring molecule by a short hydrogen bond (2.584 Å). Also, the hydrogen bond system duplicates one of the schemes found in the L-ascorbic acid.

Kanters, Roelofsen, and Alblas (*28*) have compared D-isoascorbic acid and L-ascorbic acid with respect to their behavior on ionization. They observed that almost the same changes in bond lengths and angles occur in the two compounds, exemplified by their sodium salts (Table II). Even the distortions in the rings are similar (Kanters et al.'s adversary conclusion was based upon a misprint in Table I of Ref. *10*). This is illustrated by the almost identical angles between the best planes through the lactone and ene–diol groups (1.4° vs. 0.6°). The side-chain conformation is nearly retained from the acid, but it is more staggered (by +31°) by a rotation about C4–C5.

Whereas most bond lengths and angles agree well with those of other ascorbate anions (Table II), the hydrogen bond interaction associated with O3 is unique: it accepts no less than four bonds ranging from 2.785 to 2.993 Å. Two of these are from water molecules. This unusually large number of bonds explains the fact that no short hydrogen bonds, which are usually encountered in the ene–diol group, are present in these crystals.

The fate of D-isoascorbic acid on oxidation has not yet been studied by diffraction methods, but NMR results (29) show that in inert solvents an asymmetric dimer is preferentially formed. In water, however, a mixture of two anomeric pyranose rings results, and the simple, reversible D-isoascorbic acid/dehydroisoascorbic acid equilibrium is lost. This may possibly be one of the factors that reduces the biological activity of D-isoascorbic acid. The latter has an effect that is only 5% of that of vitamin C (30).

Literature Cited

1. Cox, E. G.; Goodwin, T. H. *J. Chem. Soc.* **1936,** 769.
2. Herbert, R. W.; Hirst, E. L.; Percival, E. G. V.; Reynolds, R. J. W.; Smith, F. *J. Chem. Soc.* **1933,** 1275.
3. Haworth, W. N.; Hirst, E. L.; Jones, J. K. N.; Smith, F. *J. Chem. Soc.* **1934,** 1192.
4. Hvoslef, J. *Acta Crystallogr., Sect. B* **1972,** *28,* 916.
5. Hvoslef, J.; Pedersen, B. *Acta Chem. Scand., Ser. B* **1979,** *33,* 503.
6. Hvoslef, J. *Acta Chem. Scand.* **1964,** *18,* 841.
7. Hvoslef, J. *Acta Crystallogr., Sect. B* **1968,** *24,* 23.
8. Ibid., 1431.
9. Sudhakar, V.; Bhat, T. N.; Vijayan, M. *Crystallogr., Sect. B* **1980,** *36,* 125.
10. Hvoslef, J. *Acta Crystallogr., Sect. B* **1969,** *25,* 2214.
11. Hughes, D. L. *J. Chem. Soc., Dalton Trans.* **1973,** 2209.
12. Hearn, R. A.; Bugg, C. E. *Acta Crystallogr., Sect. B* **1974,** *30,* 2705.
13. Hvoslef, J.; Kjellevold, K. E. *Acta Crystallogr., Sect. B* **1974,** *30,* 2711.
14. Abrahams, S. C.; Bernstein, J. L.; Bugg, C. E.; Hvoslef, J. *Acta Crystallogr., Sect. B* **1978,** *34,* 2981.
15. Sudhakar, V.; Vijayan, M. *Acta Crystallogr., Sect. B* **1980,** *36,* 120.
16. Jeffrey, G. A.; Kim, H. S. *Carbohydr. Res.* **1970,** *14,* 207.
17. Tolbert, B. M.; Isherwood, D. J.; Atchely, R. W.; Baker, E. M. *Fed. Proc., Fed. Am. Soc. Exp. Biol.* **1971,** *30,* 529.
18. McClelland, B. W. *Acta Crystallogr., Sect. B* **1974,** *30,* 178.
19. Cutolo, E.; Lorizza, A. *Gazz. Chim. Ital.* **1961,** *91,* 964.
20. Lee, C. H.; Seib, P.; Hoseney, R. C.; Liang, Y. T.; Deyoe, C. W. *Cereal Chem.* **1975,** *20,* 456.
21. Jernow, J.; Blount, J.; Oliveto, E.; Perotta, A.; Rosen, P.; Toome, V. *Tetrahedron,* **1979,** *35,* 1483.
22. Albers, H.; Müller, E.; Dietz, H. *Hoppe–Seyler's Z. Physiol. Chem.* **1963,** *334,* 243.
23. Müller-Mulot, W. *Hoppe–Seyler's Z. Physiol. Chem.* **1970,** *351,* 50.
24. Hvoslef, J.; Nordenson, S. *Acta Crystallogr., Sect. B* **1976,** *32,* 1665.
25. Ibid., 448.

26. Pedersen, B. *Acta Chem. Scand., Ser. B* **1980,** *34,* 429.
27. Azarnia, N.; Berman, H.; Rosenstein, R. D. *Acta Crystallogr., Sect. B* **1971,** *27,* 2157.
28. Kanters, J. A.; Roelofsen, G.; Alblas, B. P. *Acta Crystallogr., Sect. B* **1977,** *33,* 1906.
29. Hvoslef, J.; Pedersen, B. *Carbohydr. Res.* **1981,** *92,* 9.
30. Brubacher, G.; Vuilleumier, J. P. *Wiss. Veröff. Dtsch. Ges. Ernähr.* **1965,** *14,* 61.

RECEIVED for review January 22, 1981. ACCEPTED April 8, 1981.

Recent Advances in the Derivatization of L-Ascorbic Acid

GLENN C. ANDREWS and THOMAS CRAWFORD

Central Research, Chemical Process Research, Pfizer Inc.
Groton, CT 06340

A survey of work since 1975 on the derivatization of ascorbic acid is reviewed from the perspective of the organic chemistry of ascorbic acid. Recent advances in the control of regioselectivity of alkylative derivatization of ascorbic acid have been made possible by the utilization of di- and trianions of ascorbic acid. Their use has allowed the facile synthesis of inorganic esters of ascorbic acid. New synthesis of acetal and ketal, side-chain oxidized, and deoxy derivatives are reviewed. The total synthesis of a new side-chain oxidized ascorbic acid derivative, 5-ketoascorbic acid, is reported.

There has been a great deal of recent work on the chemistry of L-ascorbic acid and ascorbic acid derivatives since the subject was last reviewed by Tolbert et al. in 1975 (*1*). Much of this work has been generated in three major areas of interest: the biosynthesis and catabolism of ascorbic acid; the commercial need for safe, food grade antioxidants; and investigations into the biological role of ascorbic acid in vivo. The recent literature has generated a wealth of new data on the chemistry of ascorbic acid and has given us a better understanding of how this functionally complex molecule can be modified and manipulated. Since the purpose of this chapter is to review the recent literature from the perspective of the organic chemistry of ascorbic acid, it is convenient to correlate the literature with respect to the reactivity of ascorbic acid to alkylation and acylation under basic and acidic conditions, its acetal and ketal derivatives, and finally with respect to the chemistry of its oxidation and reduction.

0065-2393/82/0200–0059$06.25/0

The Alkylation and Acylation of L-Ascorbic Acid
Under Basic Conditions

The reactivity of ascorbic acid toward electrophiles under basic conditions is a function of the acidity and steric environments of the four hydroxyl groups at the C2, C3, C5, and C6 positions (Figure 1). The first ionization of the molecule takes place at the C3 hydroxyl ($pK_a = 4.25$) (2). While readily ionized, the extensive delocalization of electron density into the enonolactone ring results in low reactivity to all but reactive alkylating and acylating agents such as diazomethane (1,3), benzyl chloride (4), trimethylchlorosilane (5), and acid chlorides (1). Furthermore, the unstable nature of the resulting vinyl ether or ester derivatives has resulted in few reports of selective O3 derivatization (1). Under more basic conditions, the ionization of the C2 hydroxyl occurs ($pK_a = 11.79$) (2) with the formation of the di-anion, 3. NMR investigations of the mono- and di-anions of ascorbic acid suggest retention of the lactone ring and the formulation of these species as 2 and 3, respectively (6,7,8). The di-anion of ascorbic acid reacts with electrophiles preferentially at the less stable O2 position (1,9,10), and allows the selective functionalization of this position in the presence of free hydroxyls at C3, C5, and C6. Selective O2 alkylation has also been observed with biological methylating agents in vivo. Catabolism of ascorbic acid in the guinea pig forms O2 methylascorbic acid as a minor product (11).

Under highly basic conditions, ascorbic acid may exhibit chemistry derived from ionization of the C4 hydrogen, presumably with the formation of a tri-anion, 4. Brenner et al. (12) reported the epimerization and racemization of ascorbic acid at high pH and elevated temperature.

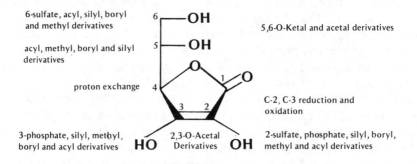

Figure 1.

Bell et al. (*13*), using similar conditions, prepared L-(4-³H)ascorbic acid via tritium oxide exchange.

If a leaving group resides at the C5 position of ascorbic acid, elimination can occur via ionization of the C4 hydrogen with the formation of a 4,5-dehydro derivative. This has been observed in the case of ascorbic acid derivative **5**, which on treatment with 1,5-diazabicyclo[4.3.0]non-5-ene (DBN) or potassium hydride affords the 5-deoxy-4,5-dehydro-derivative **6** as a mixture of olefinic isomers (*14*). The formation of 4,5-dehydroascorbic acid 2-*O*-sulfate, **8**, via the reaction of 6-*O*-valeroyl L-ascorbic acid, 7, with pyridine–SO₃ was reported to afford a single isomer (*15*). Interstingly, the C5 hydroxy epimer of compound **7**, (6-*O*-valeroyl-D-erythorbic acid) was also reported to afford a single 5,6-dehydro derivative isomeric with compound **8**, suggesting stereoselective elimination had occurred. Unfortunately, the configuration of the resulting olefins is unknown.

If both the C2 and C3 hydroxy groups are protected, alkylation or acylation occurs at the sterically most accessible C6 hydroxyl (*1*). Alkylation at the C5 position occurs only after derivatization of the other three functions. No O5 monosubstituted derivatives of ascorbic acid have been reported.

These generalizations are illustrated by the recent synthesis of L-ascorbic acid glucosides **11** and **12** (*16*). The monosodium salt of ascorbic acid in *N,N*-dimethylformamide (DMF) affords exclusively the O3 monoalkylated derivative **9** on alkylation with 2,3,4,6-tetra-O-α-D-glucopyranosyl bromide. To obtain the O2 glucosylated derivative **10**, under the same conditions, required the protection of the C3 hydroxyl as a methyl ether. Several workers have reported the biosynthesis of ascorbic acid glucosides in bacteria (*17*); however, the structure and position of glucosylation in these compounds has not been unambiguously determined.

Carbon vs. Oxygen Alkylation of Ascorbic Acid

The mono-anion of ascorbic acid is an ambident anion that can display nucleophilicity at the C2 as well as O3 positions. This ambident character was first observed by Jackson and Jones (*4*) in the synthesis of 3-O-benzylascorbic acid by alkylation of sodium ascorbate with benzyl chloride. In strongly cation solvating solvents, such as dimethyl sulfoxide (DMSO), exclusive O3 alkylation was observed. In water, a mixture of the expected O3 alkylated **13** and C2 benzylated product **14** was produced.

More recently, Brimacombe et al. (*18*) have also shown C2 alkylation of an ascorbic acid derivative in their attempted use of ascorbic acid as a synthon for the synthesis of spirodilactones. Dealkylation of 2-O-(*E*)-cinnamoyl-5,6-O-isopropylidene-3-O-methylascorbic acid, **15**, with lithium iodide in DMSO afforded the C2 alkylated isomer, **16**. It would appear that under conditions of reversible dealkylation at oxygen, C2 alkylation acts as a sink for the equilibrating mixture.

Inorganic Esters of Ascorbic Acid

The observation of L-ascorbic acid 2-O-sulfate, **18**, in a number of animal species, including humans, has provoked extensive research into the chemistry and biochemistry of this inorganic ester of ascorbic acid (*1, 19, 20*). Ascorbic acid 2-O-sulfate has been implicated as a biological sulfating agent and proposed as an anticholesteremic agent (*21–24*).

While early workers suggested the O3 sulfate structure for **18** based on chemical reactivity (*1*), x-ray analysis (*26*) and NMR data (*6*) have shown the stable monosulfate to be the O2 structure.

Several syntheses of ascorbic acid 2-O-sulfate have appeared that require the protection of the C5 and C6 hydroxyl groups and the O-sulfation of this protected derivative with SO_3 under basic conditions (*20, 26–29*). Deblocking the 5,6-O-protected 2-sulfate, **17**, with acid and purification using ion exchange chromatography affords the desired

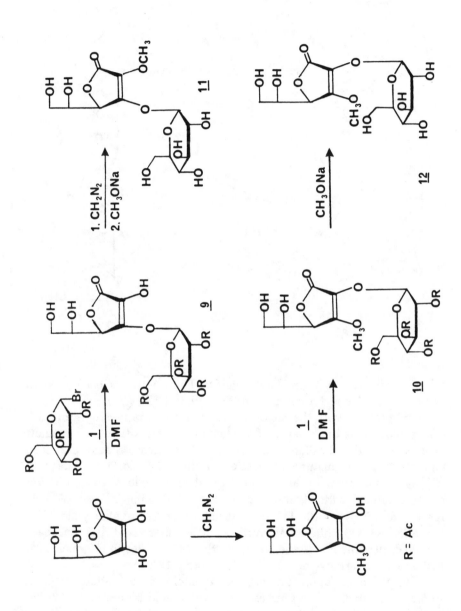

sulfate derivative **18** in moderate yields. This route has been used to prepare sulfur-labeled ascorbic acid 2-O-sulfate-(^{35}S) (27).

One problem with the use of the ketal or acetal protecting group for O5,6 protection is the removal of the ketal or acetal without concomitant hydrolysis of the 2-sulfate. Sulfation of free ascorbic acid has been reported to afford mixtures or sulfated products (23, 26, 30). Seib et al. (26) offered a rational solution to the problem of regioselective sulfation of ascorbic acid with his observation that the di-anion of ascorbic acid reacts exclusively at the O2 position affording **18** in high yield. The formation of O3 sulfated derivatives of ascorbic acid has not been observed, possibly due to the lability of the 3-O-sulfates to intermolecular hydrolysis or rearrangement to the more stable **18** (2).

The phosphorylation of ascorbic acid under basic conditions has been studied extensively. The synthesis of ascorbic acid 2-phosphate, **22**, has been reported by Seib et al. (9) via treatment of 5,6-O-isopropylidene ascorbic acid, with phosphorus oxychloride under highly basic conditions (pH 12). Hydrolysis of the ketal protecting group of the 2-phosphate intermediate **20** affords the 2-O-phosphate **22**, whose structure has been confirmed by NMR spectroscopy (7,9) and by spectroscopic and chemical means (2). Interestingly, the site of phosphorylation is dependent on the conditions of the phosphorylation. Jernow et al. (2) reported the O3 phosphorylation of 5,6-O-isopropylidene ascorbic acid using either thallium hydroxide or pyridine as base. The resulting 5,6-O-isopropylidene 3-O-phosphate derivative, 21, was found to rearrange to the more stable 2-O-phosphate 22 on hydrolysis of the protecting ketal. Seib et al. (9) also studied the phosphorylation of ascorbic acid under mildly basic conditions. Alkylation with phosphorus oxychloride in pyridine/acetone was shown to afford, after hydrolysis of the protecting group, a mixture of four products including 22 and the bis-2-O-phosphorylated dimer, 19.

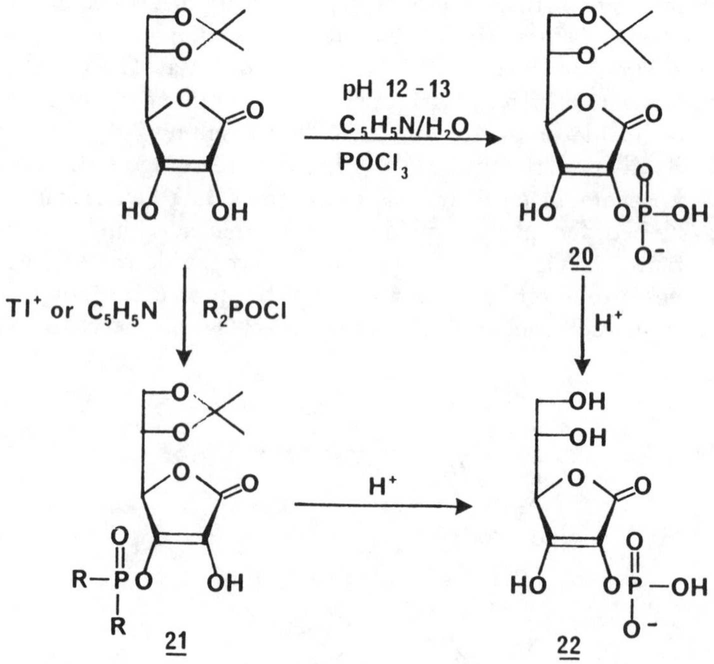
pH 12 - 13
C_5H_5N/H_2O
$POCl_3$
20
Tl^+ or C_5H_5N
R_2POCl
H^+
H^+
21
22

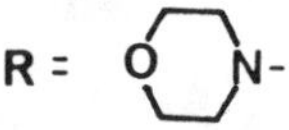
R =
N-

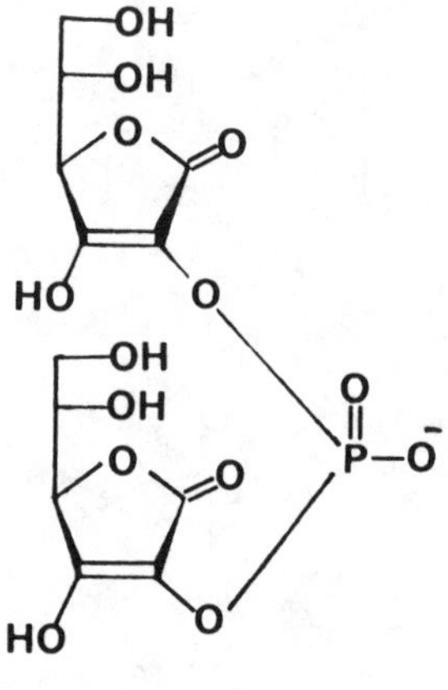

19

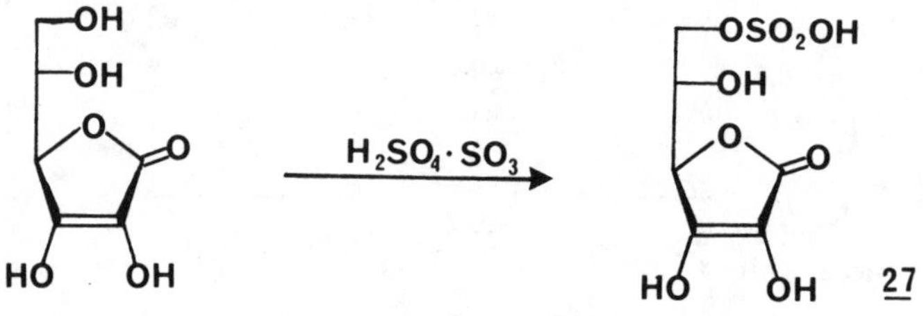
$H_2SO_4 \cdot SO_3$
OSO_2OH
27

Acid Catalyzed Derivatization of Ascorbic Acid:
Acetal and Ketal Derivatives

One of the most studied classes of ascorbic acid derivatives is that of 5,6-O-ketals, **23**, and acetals, **24** (*1*). These compounds are significant not only from their use in synthesis as protecting groups for the 5,6-hydroxyl functions, but also from their commercial importance as lipophilicity modifiers for ascorbic acid. Fodor and coworkers (*31,32*) have presented evidence that 2,3-O-acetals of ascorbic acid, **25**, are also formed with reactive aldehydes under kinetic conditions (*32*). Glyoxal is reported to afford the novel ene–diol bis acetal **26** (*33*).

The observation of 2,3-O-acetals of ascorbic acid opens up the possibility of direct oxidative modification of the ascorbic acid side-chain.

In recent work, Kamogawa et al. (*34*) reported the synthesis of 5,6-acetals of ascorbic acid with vinyl substituted benzaldehyde derivatives that, after polymerization, afford polymeric antioxidants capable of releasing ascorbic acid under mildly acidic conditions.

Acid Catalyzed Esterification of Ascorbic Acid

The acid catalyzed esterification of ascorbic acid is a thermodynamic process usually resulting in the formation of mixtures of products with a preponderance of O6 substitution. There is extensive patent literature on the formation of 6-ester derivatives of ascorbic acid both in aprotic (acetone, DMF, DMSO) (*1, 34, 35, 36*) and protic (sulfuric acid, hydrogen fluoride) (*37, 38*) solvents. The fatty acid ester derivatives of ascorbic acid have commercial importance due to the enhancement of lipophilicity that derivatization confers on ascorbic acid. These ester derivatives are used as antioxidants in edible oils, emulsifying agents, antiscaling agents, inhibitors of nitrosamine formation, and in bread making as dough modifiers (*39*). Under more stringent conditions, 5,6-diester derivatives are formed (*36*).

Cousins et al. (*38*) have reported the formation of ascorbic acid 6-O-sulfate, **27**, from the esterification of ascorbic acid with sulfur trioxide in sulfuric acid. The 6-sulfate derivatives have been proposed for use as anti-cholesteremics and as inhibitors of nitrosamine formation.

A relatively unstudied area of acid catalyzed derivatization is in the formation of boryl and boronate esters of ascorbic acid. The reaction of ascorbic acid with triethylborane using organic acid catalysis affords the 2,3,5,6-tetra-O-diethylborylated derivative (*40*). The boryl group is readily removed with methanol or acetylacetone in high yields. A borate derivative of ascorbic acid and boric acid has been claimed but not characterized (*41*).

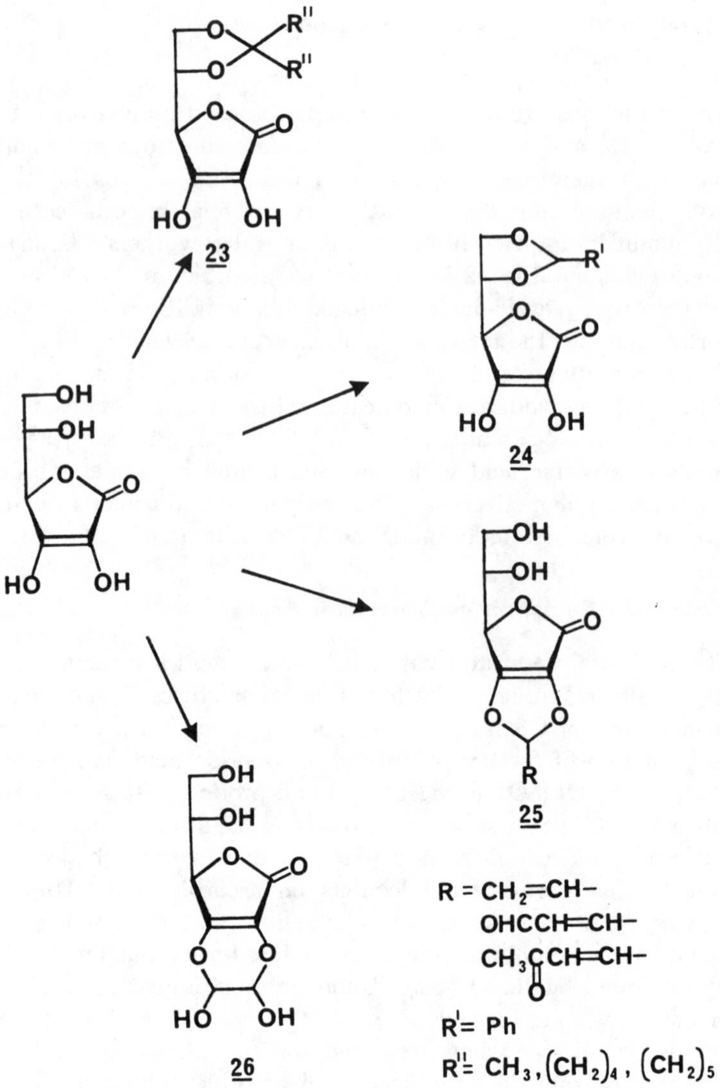
23
24
25
26
R = CH2=CH–
OHCCH=CH–
CH3CCH=CH–
O
R' = Ph
R'' = CH3, (CH2)4, (CH2)5

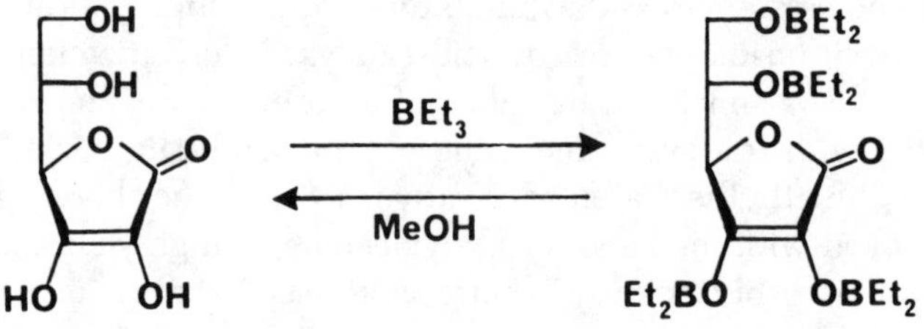
BEt3
MeOH

Oxidized Derivatives of Ascorbic Acid: Dehydroascorbic Acid

Oxidation of the reductone functionality of ascorbic acid is certainly its single most important reaction and results in the formation of its most biologically important derivative, dehydroascorbic acid, **28**. As chemistry and biochemistry of dehydroascorbic acid will be covered in a separate section of this volume, only a few of its reactions will be covered here.

An improved synthesis of dehydroascorbic acid has been reported (*42*). The oxidation of ascorbic acid in absolute methanol with oxygen over activated charcoal catalyst is reported to afford **28** in 95% yield. Dehydroascorbic acid has been characterized in solution as the monomer, **28** (*43*), and as the dimer (*44, 45*) and its tetra acetyl derivative **29** (*46*). Several studies of mono- and di-hydrazone (*48–53*) and osazone (*54*) derivatives of dehydroascorbic acid have been reported. Hydrazone derivatives of dehydroascorbic acid have been used in the reductive synthesis of 2,3-diaza-2,3-dideoxy- and 2-aza-2-deoxyascorbic acid derivatives **30**, **31**, and **32** (*55, 56*). Recently the reaction product of dehydro-L-ascorbic acid and L-phenylalanine in aqueous solution has been isolated and identified as tris(2-deoxy-2-L-ascorbyl)amine, **33**, based on spectral and chemical data and its symmetry properties (*57*).

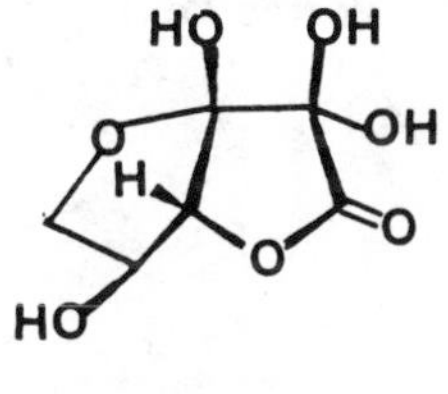

28

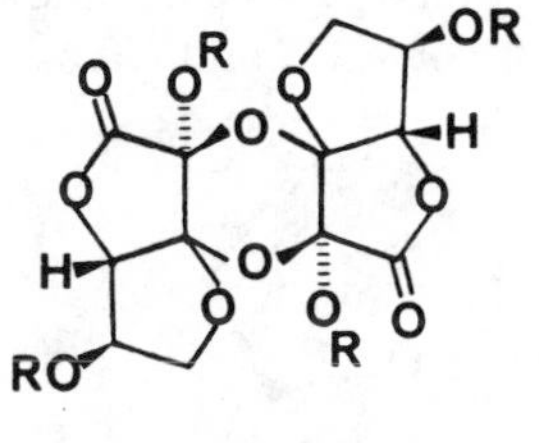

29 R = H
        R = Ac

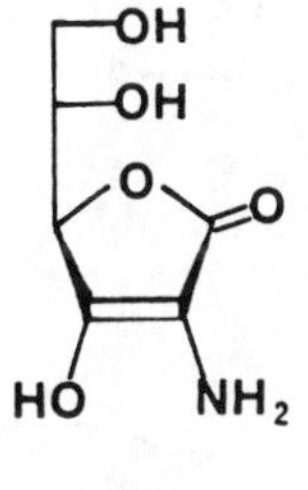

32 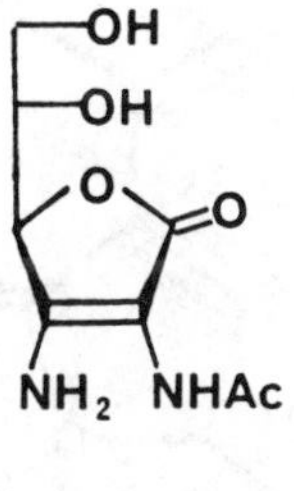   **30** 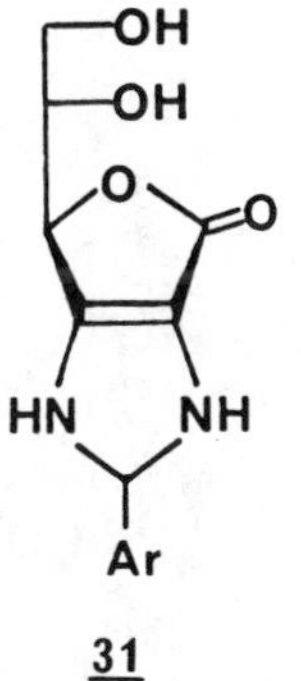   **31**

Side-Chain Oxidized Derivatives of Ascorbic Acid

Derivatives of ascorbic acid in which either or both of the C5 and C6 positions are in a higher oxidation state have achieved some importance as possible biochemical precursors or catabolites of ascorbic acid in vivo.

Saccharoascorbic acid, 35, has been proposed as a minor metabolite of ascorbic acid in animals (57–60). The isolation of ascorbic acid 2-O-sulfate, 18, in a variety of animal species and the remarkable oxidative stability of the 2-O-sulfate substituted enonolactone moiety have prompted suggestions (60) that saccharoascorbic acid 2-O-sulfate, 34, is a catabolite of 18 in vivo.

Stuber and Tolbert (61) utilized the oxidative stability of the 2-O-sulfate in a short synthesis of both saccharoascorbic acid and saccharoascorbic acid 2-O-sulfate. Oxidation of ascorbic acid 2-O-sulfate, 18, with platinum and oxygen afforded good yields of acid 34 under conditions in which ascorbic acid itself is oxidized to dehydroascorbic acid. Hydrolysis of the sulfate in acid afforded saccharoascorbic acid, 35, in good yield.

Side-chain oxidized derivatives of ascorbic acid are also implicated in the catabolism of ascorbic acid in plants. Loewus et al. (62) have established the intermediacy of ascorbic acid in the biosynthesis of tartaric acid in the grape. Labeling studies have established a metabolic pathway that must involve C5 and C6 oxidation of ascorbic acid.

33

Evidence from labeling studies (63, 64) has accumulated suggesting a dual pathway for ascorbic acid biosynthesis in plants involving not only the inversion of the glucose chain via glucuronic acid (65), but also via the inversion of stereochemistry at the C5 hydroxyl of glucose. Such an epimerization at the C5 position of glucose could occur through the stereoselective reduction of several possible biosynthetic intermediates including 5-ketogluconic, 2,5-diketogluconic, and 5-ketoascorbic acids (as well as by epimerization through 6-formyl and/or 4-keto derivatives).

Of the possible side-chain oxidized derivatives of ascorbic acid, all but 5-keto-ascorbic acid and 5-keto-6-formylascorbic acid have been reported. Bakke and Theander (66) formed 6-aldehydoascorbic acid, 37, as an unisolated intermediate in the reductive hydrolysis of 38 to ascorbic acid. Heyns and Linkies (67) synthesized 5-keto-saccharo-ascorbic acid, 40, via the oxidation and subsequent hydrolysis of man-narodilactone, 39. 5-Ketosaccharoascorbic acid appears to exist in solution as its enol tautomer.

As with previous 5,6-dehydro derivatives of ascorbic acid, configuration about the 5,6-olefin has not been established.

During the course of work directed toward the synthesis of ascorbic acid (68) via the stereo- and regioselective reduction of D-*threo*-2,5-hexo-dinlosonic acid, 41, we sought to synthesize 5-ketoascorbic acid directly by the lactonization of 41. Acid catalyzed lactonization of 41 and base catalyzed lactonization of the methyl ester of 41 both failed to produce the desired 5-ketoascorbic acid derivative. Lactonization of the 5,5-dimethyl ketal methyl ester, 42 (69), with sodium bicarbonate in refluxing methanol afforded the 5,5-dimethyl ketal of 5-keto-ascorbic acid, 43. Hydrolysis of the ketal protecting group with trifluoroacetic acid/water afforded 5-ketoascorbic acid, isolated as the hydrate 44. Compound 44 was shown by ^{13}C NMR spectroscopy to exist primarily (95%) as its hydrated keto tautomer in aqueous solution. The enol tautomer was not observed by ^{13}C NMR or UV spectroscopy; however, silylation of 44 with *t*-butyldimethylchlorosilane in DMF afforded the tetra-*t*-butyldi-methylsilyl derivative 45 as a single isomer, shown by ^{13}C NMR and UV analysis to be the 4,5-dehydro structure. The facile loss of the C4 proton of 44 in deuterium oxide and at pH 7; its rapid racemization in water at ambient temperature ($t_{1/2}$ = 2 h) argues strongly against the intermediacy of 5-ketoascorbic acid in the biosynthesis of ascorbic acid intermediates.

Deoxy Derivatives of Ascorbic Acid

The instability of ascorbic acid has limited its utility in a variety of applications and has been a major impetus for research into the chemistry of ascorbic acid. Goshima, Maezono, and Tokuyama (70) illustrated one possible decomposition pathway for ascorbic acid under acidic, anaerobic conditions that involved the initial Michael addition of the 6-hydroxyl function into the enonolactone. The epimeric lactones, 46 and 47, isolated in low yield from the reaction of ascorbic acid in methanol with boron trifluoride catalysis, have been proposed as intermediates in the further acid catalyzed degradation of ascorbic acid to furfural and polymeric materials. This hypothesis has prompted interest in ascorbic acid derivatives in which the C6 hydroxyl group is absent or blocked so as to prevent the initial Michael addition.

Recently the halogenation of ascorbic acid in acidic media has been reported by Kiss and Berg (71) and independently by Pedersen and coworkers (72, 73). The treatment of ascorbic acid with halogen acids in acetic or formic acids as solvent affords 5-halo-5-acyloxy derivatives

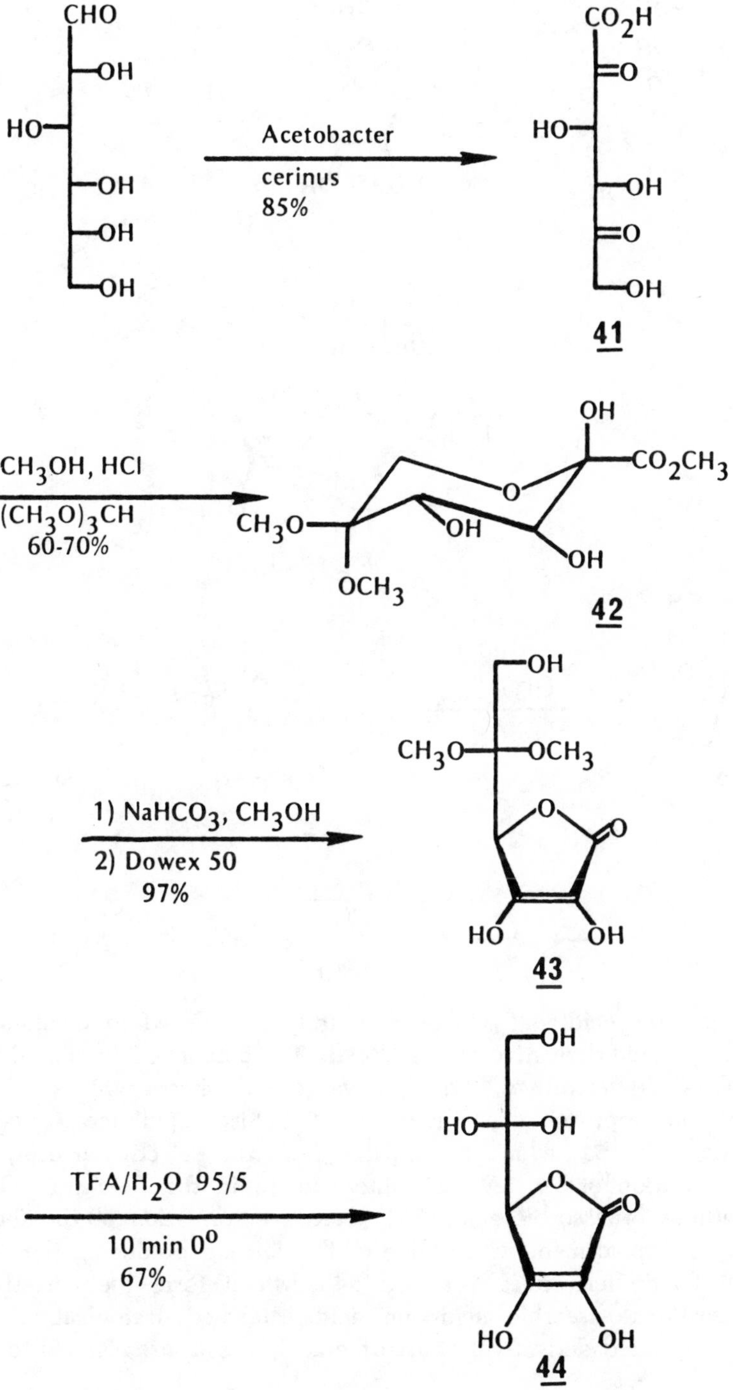

CHO
—OH
HO—
—OH
—OH
—OH

Acetobacter
cerinus
85%

CO_2H
=O
HO—
—OH
=O
—OH

41

CH₃OH, HCl
$(CH_3O)_3CH$
60-70%

OH
CO_2CH_3
CH₃O—
OH
OH
OCH₃

42

1) NaHCO₃, CH₃OH
2) Dowex 50
97%

—OH
CH₃O——OCH₃
O
O
HO   OH

43

TFA/H₂O 95/5
10 min 0°
67%

—OH
HO——OH
O
O
HO   OH

44

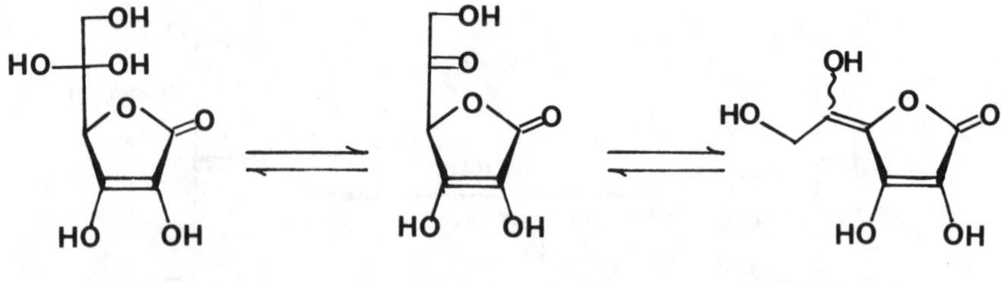

44

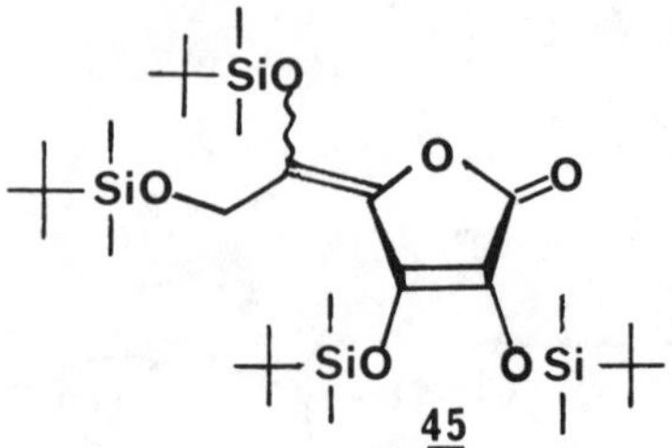

45

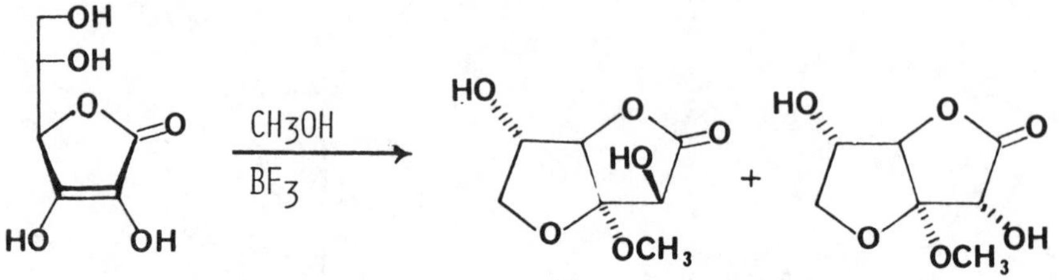

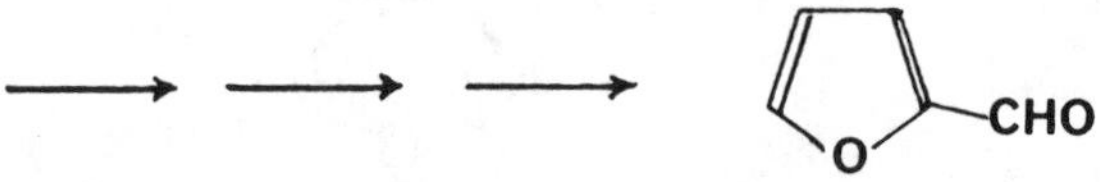

of ascorbic acid, **48**, which are readily hydrolyzed to 6-halo-6-deoxy-ascorbic acid derivatives **49c** and **49d**. The 6-fluoro-, 6-bromo-, 6-chloro-, and 6-iodo-derivatives, **49a–d**, have recently been synthesized by an alternate approach (74) via methyl 2,3-O-isopropylidine-D-*xylo*-furano-hexlosonate, **52**, which is available from the selective hydrolysis and esterification of **50**, an early intermediate in the Reichstein–Grussner synthesis of ascorbic acid (75). Selective formation of the 6-tosylate allows displacement with iodide or fluoride ion producing the 6-fluoro- and 6-iodo-derivatives **54a** and **54b**, which form the corresponding 6-deox-6-halo-ascorbic acids on acid catalyzed lactonization. These 6-halogenated derivatives of ascorbic acid, **49a–d**, are claimed to exhibit enhanced thermal stability (*71*). The 6-chloro-derivative has also shown high antiscurvy activity (*74*).

Pedersen further studied the reactivity of the intermediates **48** under dissolving metal conditions and synthesized the 5,6-dehydro-5,6-dideoxy derivative **55** which was catalytically reduced to the 5,6-dideoxy compound **56**.

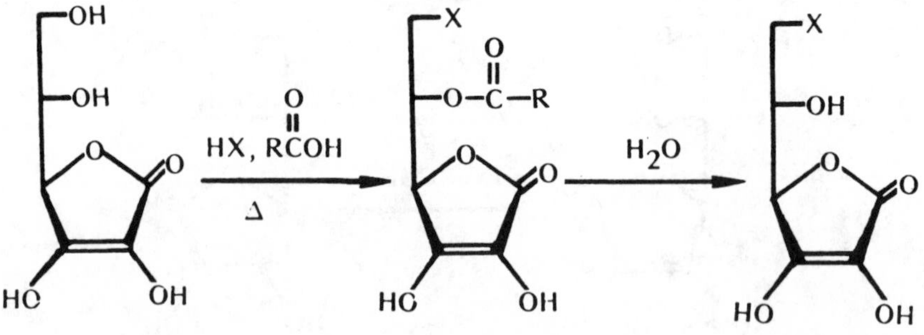

48 R = CH$_3$, H

49a X = F
49b X = Cl
49c X = I
49d X = Br

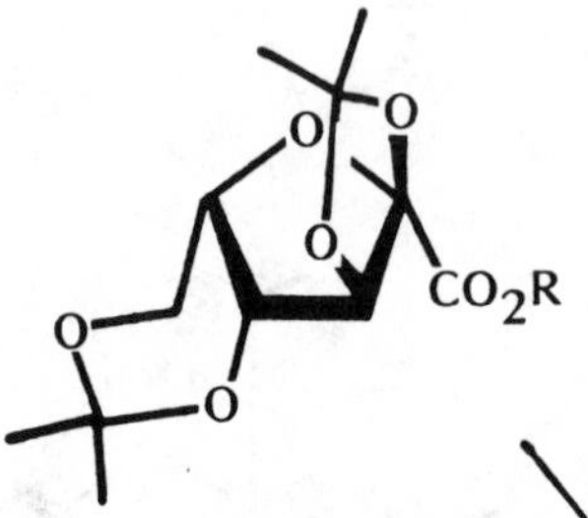

50 R = H
51 R = CH$_3$

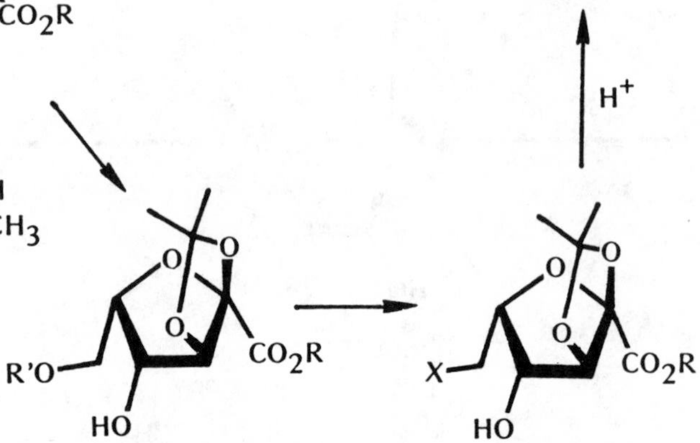

52 R = CH$_3$, R' = H
53 R = CH$_3$, R' = Tosyl

54a X = F
54b X = Cl
54c X = Br
54d X = I

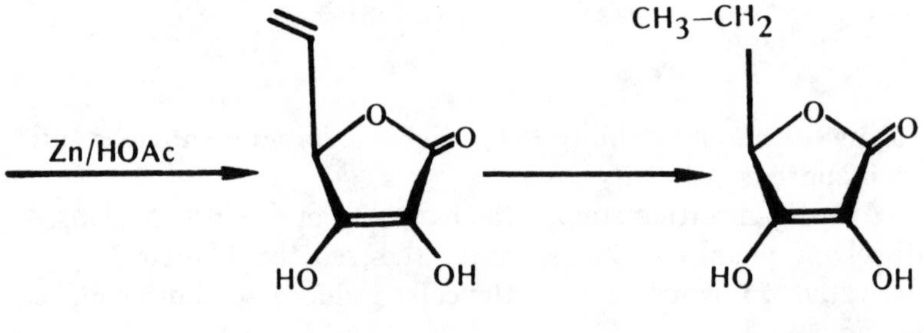

55

56

Literature Cited

1. Tolbert, B. M.; Downing, M.; Carlson, R. W.; Knight, M. K.; Baker, E. M. *Ann. N.Y. Acad. Sci.* **1975**, *258*, 48–69.
2. Jernow, J.; Blount, J.; Oliveto, E.; Perrotta, A.; Rosen, P.; Toome, V. *Tetrahedron* **1979**, *35*, 1483–1486.
3. Shrihatti, V. R.; Nair, P. M. *Indian J. Chem., Sect. B* **1977**, *15*(9), 861–863.
4. Jackson, K. G.; Jones, J. K. N. *Can. J. Chem.* **1965**, *43*, 450–457.
5. Veechi, M.; Kaiser, K. *J. Chromatogr.* **1967**, *26*, 22–29.
6. Radford, T.; Sweeny, J. G.; Iacobucci, G. A.; Goldsmith, D. J. *J. Org. Chem.* **1979**, *44*, 658–659.
7. Mutusch, R. *Z. Naturforsch., Teil B* **1977**, *32*(5), 562–568.
8. Berger, S. *Tetrahedron* **1977**, *33*, 1587–1589.
9. Seib, P.; Lee, C. H.; Liang, Y. T.; Hoseney, R. C.; Deyoe, C. W. *Carbohydr. Res.* **1978**, *67*, 127–138.
10. Seib, P. A.; Deyoe, C. W.; Hoseney, R. C. German Patent 2 719 303, 1977.
11. Gazave, J. M.; Truchard, M.; Parrot, J. L.; Achard, M.; Roger, C. *Ann. Pharm. Fr.* **1975**, *33*, 155–161.
12. Brenner, G. S.; Hinkley, D. F.; Perkins, L. M.; Weber, S. *J. Org. Chem.* **1964**, *29*, 2389–2392.
13. Bell, E. M.; Baker, E. M.; Tolbert, B. M. *J. Labelled Compd.* **1966**, *2*, 148–154.
14. Eitelman, S. J.; Hall, R. H.; Jordaan, A. *J. Chem. Soc., Chem. Commun.* **1976**, 923–924.
15. Liang, Y. T.; Lillard, D.; Seib, P. A.; Paukstelis, J. V.; Mueller, D. D., presented at the *178th Nat. Meet. Am. Chem. Soc., Washington, D. C., Sept., 1979.*
16. Szarek, W. A.; Kim, K. S. *Carbohydr. Res.* **1978**, *67*, C13–C16.
17. Suzuki, Y.; Miyake, T.; Uchida, K.; Mino, A. *Vitamins* **1973**, *47*(6), 259–267.
18. Brimacombe, J. S.; Murray, A. W.; Haque, Z. *Carbohydr. Res.* **1975**, *45*, 45–53.
19. Tsujimura, M.; Kitamura, S. *Vitamins* **1979**, *53*, 247–252.
20. Lillard, D. W.; Seib, P. A. *ACS Symp. Ser.* **1978**, *11*, 1–18.
21. Chu, T. T. M.; Slaunwhite, W. R. *Steroids* **1968**, *12*, 309–312.
22. Tsujimura, M.; Yoshikawa, H.; Hasegawa, T.; Suzuki, T. *Joshi Eiyo Daigaku Kiyo*, **1975**, *6*, 35–44.
23. Hayashi, E.; Fujimoto, Y.; Nezu, M. *Kokai Tokkyo Koho* **1977**, *83*, 946.
24. Nezu, Y.; Hayashi, E.; Sato, H.; Ishihara, E. *Kokai Tokkyo Koho* **1977**, *83*, 946.
25. McClelland, B. W. *Acta Crystallogr.* **1974**, *30*, 178–186.
26. Seib, P. A.; Liang, Y.-T.; Lee, C.-H.; Hoseney, R. C.; Deyoe, C. W. *J. Chem. Soc., Perkin Trans. 1* **1974**, 1220–1224.
27. Muccino, R. R.; Markezich, R.; Vernice, G. G.; Perry, C. W.; Liebman, A. A. *Carbohydr. Res.* **1976**, *47*, 172–175.
28. Nezu, Y.; Harakawa, M.; Shimizu, K.; Sato, H.; Takita, K. *Kokai Tokkyo Koho* **1976**, *6*, 956.
29. Ibid., *91*, 251.
30. Okuyama, T.; Sakurai, K.; Yamaguchi, T.; Kamohara, S. *Kokai Tokkyo Koho* **1975**, *64*, 267.
31. Fodor, G.; Butterick, J.; Springsteen, A.; Mathelier, H., presented at the *ACS–CSJ Chem. Congr., Honolulu, Apr., 1979.*
32. Fodor, G.; Butterick, J.; Mathelier, H.; Arnold, R., presented at the *2nd Chem. Congr. North American Continent, Las Vegas, Aug., 1980.*
33. Blaszczak, J. W. U.S. Patent 3 888 989, 1976.

34. Kamogawa, H.; Harmoto, Y.; Nanasawa, M. *Bull. Chem. Soc. Jpn.* **1979,** *52,* 846–848.
35. Seib, P. A.; Cousins, R. C.; Hoseney, R. C. German Patent 2 743 526, 1978.
36. Kobayashi, Y. *Kokai Tokkyo Koho* **1973,** *67,* 268.
37. Gruetzmacher, G.; Stephens, C. R. German Patent 2 584 353, 1979.
38. Cousins, R. C.; Seib, P. A.; Hoseney, R. C.; Deyoe, C. W.; Liang, Y. T.; Lillard, D. W. *J. Am. Oil Chem. Soc.* **1977,** *54,* 308–312.
39. Hoseney, R. C.; Seib, P. A.; Deyoe, C. W. *Cereal Chem.* **1977,** *54,* 1062–1069.
40. Koester, R.; Amen, K. R.; Dahlhoff, W. V. *Justus Liebigs Ann. Chem.* **1975,** 752–788.
41. Ruskin, S. L. U.S. Patent 2 635 102, 1953.
42. Ohmori, M.; Takagi, M. *Agric. Biol. Chem.* **1978,** *42,* 173–174.
43. Pfeilsticker, K.; Marx, F.; Bockisch, M. *Carbohydr. Res.* **1975,** *45,* 269–274.
44. Hvoslef, J.; Pedersen, B. *Acta Chem. Scand., Ser. B* **1980,** *34,* 285–288.
45. *Ibid.,* **1979,** *33,* 503–510.
46. Yagishita, K.; Takahashi, N.; Yamamoto, H.; Jennouchi, H.; Kiyoshi, S.; Miyakawa, T. *J. Nutr. Sci. Vitaminol.* **1976,** *22,* 419–427.
47. Roberts, G. A. F. *J. Chem. Soc., Perkins Trans. 1* **1979,** 603–605.
48. Soliman, R.; Elashry, E. S. H.; Elkholy, I. E.; Elkilany, Y. *Carbohydr. Res.* **1978,** *67,* 179–188.
49. Elashry, E. S. H.; Abdelrahman, M. M. A.; Nassr, M. A.; Amer, A. *Carbohydr. Res.* **1978,** *67,* 403–432.
50. Elashry, E. S. H. *Carbohydr. Res.* **1976,** *52,* 69–77.
51. Elashry, E. S. H.; Labib, G. H.; Elkilany, Y. *Carbohydr. Res.* **1976,** *52,* 251–254.
52. Mokhtar, H. M. *Pharmazie* **1978,** *38,* 709–711.
53. Sekily, M. A. E. *Pharmazie* **1979,** *34,* 531–534.
54. Pollet, P.; Gelin, S. *Tetrahedron* **1980,** *36,* 2955–2959.
55. Gross, B.; Sekily, M. A. E.; Mancy, S.; El Khadem, H. S. *Carbohydr. Res.* **1974,** *37,* 384–389.
56. Manousak, O. *Z. Chem.* **1971,** *11,* 18–19.
57. Hayashi, T.; Manou, F.; Namiki, M.; Tsuji, K. *Agroc. Biol. Chem.* **1981,** *45,* 711–716.
58. Tolbert, B. M.; Harkrader, R. J. *Biochem. Biophys. Res. Commun.* **1976,** *71,* 1004–1009.
59. Tolbert, B. M.; Harkrader, R. J.; Plunkett, L. M.; Stuber, H. A. *Fed. Proc., Fed. Am. Soc. Exp. Biol.* **1976,** *35,* 661.
60. Hornig, D. In "Vitamin C"; Birch, G.; Parker, K., Eds.; John Wiley & Sons: New York, 1974; pp. 91–103.
61. Stuber, H. A.; Tolbert, B. M. *Carbohydr. Res.* **1978,** *60,* 251–258.
62. Loewus, F. A.; Williams, M.; Saito, K. *Phytochemistry* **1979,** *18,* 953–956.
63. Loewus, F. A. *Ann. N.Y. Acad. Sci.* **1961,** *92,* 57–77.
64. Loewus, F. A. *Ann. Rev. Plant Physiol.* **1971,** *22,* 337–357.
65. Isherwood, F. A.; Mapson, L. W. *Ann. Rev. Plant Physiol.* **1961,** *92,* 6–20.
66. Bakke, J.; Theander, Ö. *J. Chem. Soc. D* **1971,** 175–176.
67. Heynes, K.; Linkies, A. *Chem. Ber.* **1975,** *108,* 3633–3644.
68. Andrews, G. C.; Bacon, B. E.; Crawford, T.; Breitenbach, R. *Chem. Commun.* **1979,** 740–749.
69. Andrews, G. C.; Bacon, B. E.; Bordner, J.; Hennessee, G. L. A. *Carbohydr. Res.* **1979,** *79,* 25–36.
70. Goshima, K.; Maezono, N.; Tokuyama, K. *Bull. Chem. Soc. Jpn.* **1973,** *46,* 902–904.
71. Kiss, J.; Berg, K. P. *U.S. Patent 3 043 937,* 1977.

72. Pedersen, C.; Bock, K.; Ludt, I. *Pure Appl. Chem.* **1978,** *50,* 1385–1400.
73. Bock, K. M.; Lundt, I.; Pedersen, C. *Carbohydr. Res.* **1979,** *68,* 313–319.
74. Kiss, J.; Berg, K. P.; Dirscherl, A.; Oberhansli, W. E.; Arnold, W. *Helv. Chim. Acta* **1980,** *63,* 1728–1739.
75. Rumpf, P.; Marlier, S. *Bull. Soc. Chem. Fr.* **1959,** 187–190.

RECEIVED for review February 9, 1981. ACCEPTED June 23, 1981.

Chemistry of Ascorbic Acid Radicals

BENON H. J. BIELSKI

Department of Chemistry, Brookhaven National Laboratory, Upton NY 11973

The chemistry of ascorbic acid free radicals is reviewed. Particular emphasis is placed on identification and characterization of ascorbate radicals by spectrophotometric and electron paramagnetic resonance techniques, the kinetics of formation and disappearance of ascorbate free radicals in enzymatic and nonenzymatic reactions, the effect of pH upon the spectral and kinetic properties of ascorbate anion radical, and chemical reactivity of ascorbate free radicals.

The most outstanding chemical characteristics of the ascorbate system (ascorbic acid/ascorbate, ascorbate free radical, dehydroascorbic acid) are its redox properties. Ascorbic acid/ascorbate can undergo a reversible Michaelis (1) two-step oxidation–reduction process with a free radical intermediate:

$$AH_2 \underset{+1e}{\overset{-1e}{\rightleftharpoons}} A^{\cdot} + 2H^+ \qquad (1, -1)$$

$$A^{\cdot} \underset{+1e}{\overset{-1e}{\rightleftharpoons}} A \qquad (2, -2)$$

Ascorbate is a reactive reductant, but its free radical is relatively nonreactive (2) (*see* Table I) and decays by disproportionation to ascorbic acid/ascorbate and dehydroascorbic acid:

$$2A^{\cdot} + H^+ \rightleftharpoons AH^- + A \qquad (3, -3)$$

$$2A^{\cdot} + 2H^+ \rightleftharpoons AH_2 + A \qquad (4, -4)$$

$$2AH\cdot \rightleftharpoons AH_2 + A \qquad (5, -5)$$

0065-2393/82/0200–0081$06.00/0

Table I.   Interaction of Ascorbate Radicals (A⁻)
with Various Biochemical Compounds

Reaction	pH	Rate Constant $(M^{-1}\,s^{-1})$
$A^{\overline{\cdot}} + A^{\cdot-}$	8.7	2.8×10^5
$A^{\overline{\cdot}} +$ dopamine	8.4	3.6×10^2
$A^{\overline{\cdot}} +$ cytochrome c	7.4	6.6×10^3
$A^{\overline{\cdot}} + O_2$	8.6	$< 5 \times 10^2$
$A^{\overline{\cdot}} +$ methanol	8.8	< 0.1
$A^{\overline{\cdot}} +$ lactate	8.6	< 10
$A^{\overline{\cdot}} +$ pyruvate	8.6	< 10
$A^{\overline{\cdot}} +$ fumarate	8.7	< 10
$A^{\overline{\cdot}} +$ L-α-ketoglutarate	9.7	< 10

Source: Reference 2.

The unusual biological protective properties of ascorbate against free radical damage are most likely due to the efficiency of ascorbate as a radical scavenger and the stability of its radical. The ascorbic acid radical reacts preferentially with itself (Reactions 3–5) thus terminating the propagation of free radical reactions. This concept is supported by early radiation studies (3–5) and more recent work (6), which demonstrated that the ascorbate free radical was the primary product when ascorbate reacted with several redox systems. These experiments not only show that ascorbate is a good reducing agent but also that its free radical was the most stable radical species in each of the systems studied. Because of its nonreactivity, the ascorbate radical is one of the very few species observed by electron spin resonance (ESR) in tissue (7–13). The stability and nonreactivity suggest that A⁻ is a relatively nontoxic species, a state consistent with the antioxidant role ascorbate plays in biological systems.

Research on ascorbate and dehydroascorbate can be performed by conventional biochemical methods, but study of the relatively short-lived ascorbate free radical requires methods such as flow techniques with rapid mixing or pulse radiolysis coupled with polarography, ESR, or spectrophotometry. Ascorbate free radicals have been generated preferentially by oxidation of ascorbic acid [enzymatic (14–17), chemical (18–20), radiation chemical (21–26), and photochemical (27)] because ascorbic acid is easily available in a high purity grade but dehydroascorbic acid is not.

The primary objective of this chapter is to present an up-to-date review of the basic chemistry of the ascorbate free radical in aqueous solutions. The discussion will include such topics as spectral and kinetic properties, ESR studies, the role of ascorbate free radicals in the auto-oxidation of ascorbate, and selected ascorbate free radical reactions.

Spectral and Kinetic Properties of the Ascorbate Radical Anion

The spectral and kinetic properties of the ascorbate free radical have been studied extensively by optical pulse radiolysis experiments (*21–24, 26*). When dilute aqueous solutions are exposed to ionizing radiation, essentially all of the energy is absorbed by the water yielding (*28*):

$$H_2O \leadsto \rightarrow OH\,(2.74),\, e_{aq}^-\,(2.76),\, H\,(0.55),\, H_2O_2\,(0.72),\, H_2\,(0.55)$$

$$(6)$$

The numerical values in parentheses are G values for high energy electrons and gamma rays; they represent the number of molecules formed per 100 eV of energy dissipated in the system.

Nitrous oxide added to neutral or alkaline aqueous solutions converts the hydrated electron to OH radicals that react with ascorbate at near diffusion-controlled rates (*see* Table II) to give a mixture of ascorbate radical anion and OH–radical adducts:

$$N_2O + e_{aq}^- + H_2O \rightarrow N_2 + \cdot OH + OH^- \qquad (7)$$

$$AH^- + \cdot OH \rightarrow A^\mathbf{\cdot} + H_2O \qquad (8)$$

$$AH^- + \cdot OH \rightarrow [AH^-(OH)\text{-adducts}] \rightarrow A^\mathbf{\cdot} + H_2O + \text{products} \qquad (9)$$

Early work (*21, 22*) on the absorption spectrum of the ascorbate radical failed to take into account the complex nature of the reaction between ascorbate and the OH radical, which was later shown by ESR studies (*18, 19*) and by optical pulse radiolysis using very short pulses (*23*).

The number of different hydroxyl radical adducts formed and the rate with which some of these species decompose to the ascorbate radical radical depends upon pH. The decomposition rates for the OH–radical adducts vary from 5 μs to 1.5 ms (*23*). Definite structure assignment to the various OH–radical adducts was obtained by ESR studies discussed in the next section.

The use of halide anion radical complexes (X_2^-) (*23*) as oxidizing agents to minimizes the difficulties encountered with the hydroxyl radical. Such complexes are generated in pulse radiolysis experiments by addition of relatively large concentrations of halide anions (X^- can be Cl$^-$, Br$^-$, I$^-$, or the pseudohalide CNS$^-$) to the solutions:

$$X^- + \cdot OH \rightarrow X \cdot + OH^- \tag{10}$$

$$X^- + X \cdot \rightarrow X_2^- \tag{11}$$

$$AH_2 + X_2^- \rightarrow adduct \tag{12}$$

$$adduct \rightarrow AH \cdot + HBr + Br^- \tag{13}$$

or

$$AH^- + X_2^- \rightarrow adduct \tag{14}$$

$$adduct \rightarrow A^{\cdot} + 2Br^- + H^+ \tag{15}$$

The halide anion radicals apparently also add to the ascorbate ring-carbon atoms to yield adduct(s), but these adducts are much shorter lived transients (few microseconds) and decompose to the ascorbate anion radical only (23, 26). The reaction rates of the halide anion radicsl with ascorbic acid/ascorbate are moderately fast (see Table III) and are sensitive to ionic strength.

The current best resolved absorption spectrum of the ascorbate anion radical (Figure 1) was determined (26) in a study of ascorbate oxidation by halide anion radicals (particularly Br_2^-) at pH 11. The spectrum shows a symmetrical Gaussian-type band with an absorption peak at 360 nm and a width at half-maximum of about 50 nm. The molar absorbance at 360 nm = 3300 $M^{-1}cm^{-1}$ is lower than earlier reported values (21, 23).

The ascorbate anion radical and the OH–radical adducts have similar absorption spectra with a maximum near 360 nm. The only significant spectral difference exists in the 300–340 nm wavelength region, where the absorbance of $A^{\cdot}$ is less than that of the OH-radical adducts, and at 560 nm, where one of the OH–radical adducts has an additional peak. This spectral similarity makes spectrophotometric resolution of the mixture into individual components difficult.

Table II. Rate Constants for Oxidation of Ascorbic Acid/Ascorbate ($pK_1 = 4.3$) by Hydroxyl Radicals

pH	k $(M^{-1}s^{-1})$	Reference
1.0	7.2×10^9	65
1.5	4.5×10^9	23
7.0	7.0×10^9	23
7.0	1.1×10^{10}	66
11.0	4.1×10^9	26

Table III. Rate Constants for Oxidation of Ascorbic Acid/Ascorbate (pK₁ = 4.3) by Halide Anion Radicals

Radical	pH	μ	k (M⁻¹s⁻¹)	Reference
Cl_2^-	2	0.10	6.8×10^8	23
	2	0.01	6.0×10^8	66
Br_2^-	2	0.10	1.1×10^8	23
	7	0.10	1.1×10^9	23
	11	0.01	8.7×10^8	66
	11	0.00	4.8×10^8	26
I_2^-	2	0.10	5.0×10^6	23
	7	0.10	1.4×10^8	23
	11	0.00	1.7×10^8	26
$(SCN)_2^-$	2	0.10	1.0×10^7	23
	7	0.10	6.0×10^8	23
	11	0.01	4.8×10^8	66
	11	0.00	3.1×10^8	26

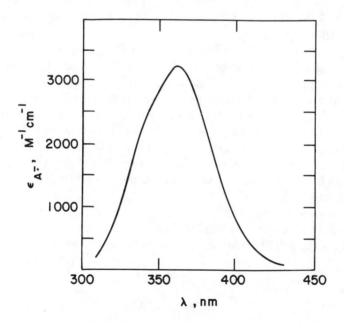

Figure 1. Absorption spectrum of the ascorbate radical anion at pH 11.0 (26).

The spectrum of $A^{\cdot}$ (measured 100 μs after termination of the electron pulse) is constant in the 1–10 pH range, suggesting a single species present over that pH range (23). This finding was later corroborated and explained in work (25) that demonstrated that the ascorbate radical is present in its anionic form in the 0–13 pH range, but protonates at pH < 0 (Reactions 16,–16), with pK = −0.45. Earlier reported pK values (22, 23) were incorrect and arose from misinterpretation of kinetic and spectral data.

$$(16, -16)$$

The ascorbate free radical decays by a strictly second-order disproportionation process to ascorbic acid and dehydroascorbic acid, independent of generation method. A product analysis (22) with L-ascorbate-1-^{14}C showed dehydroascorbate to be the only new product in an irradiated solution.

Figure 2 shows the combined results of decay data for runs in which the ascorbate radical was generated by the X_2^- method (23) and those from Reference 22, now reevaluated with an $\epsilon = 3300$ M^{-1} cm^{-1} (26) and assuming no change in molar absorbance between pH 1 and 10. The earler reported (22) extinction coefficient of the radical changed with pH, but this changing was an error resulting from the formation of different types of radicals from oxidation of ascorbate by OH. The two sets of data are in good agreement and show a strong pH dependence, with a 3000-fold change in rates between the respective plateau regions in the alkaline and acid range.

A new mechanism was proposed recently (29) for the second-order decay of $A^{\cdot}$ as a function of pH. This mechanism is consistent with a low pK_{AH}. and the observed pH profile in Figure 2:

$$2\,A^{\cdot} \rightarrow (A^{\cdot}A^{\cdot}) \tag{17}$$

$$(A^{\cdot}A^{\cdot}) \rightarrow 2\,A^{-} \tag{18}$$

$$(A^{\cdot}A^{\cdot}) + H^{+} \rightarrow AH^{-} + A \tag{19}$$

$$(A^{\cdot}A^{\cdot}) + H_2O \rightarrow AH^{-} + A + OH^{-} \tag{20}$$

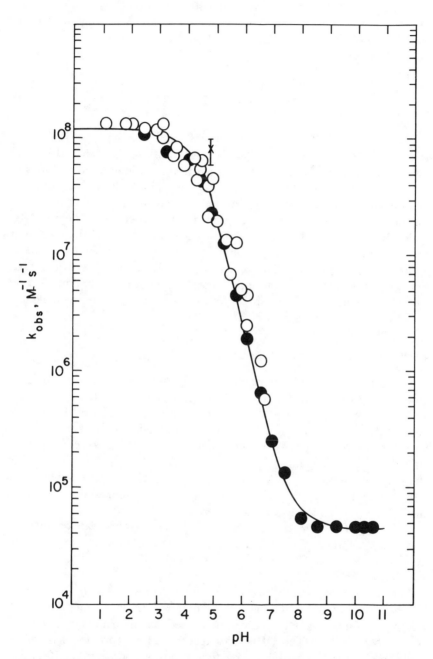

Figure 2.   Reaction rate, k_{obs}, as a function of pH for the decay of ascorbate radicals at ambient temperature. Key: ○, data from Ref. 23; ●,
data from Ref. 22; and ⚍, data from Ref. 14.

The complex $A \cdot A \cdot$ exists in a very low steady-state concentration during the reaction. The observed rate, $2k_{obs}(A \cdot)^2$, is given for this mechanism by the sum of the rates of Reactions 19 and 20; the steady-state approximation then yields:

$$k_{obs} = \left[\frac{k_{17}}{1 + k_{18}/[k_{20} + k_{19}(H^+)]} \right] \qquad (21)$$

The curve in Figure 2 is calculated from Equation 21 with $k_{17} = 1.2 \times 10^8 M^{-1}s^{-1}$, $k_{19}/k_{18} = 2.0 \times 10^4$, and $k_{20}/k_{18} = 3.92 \times 10^{-4}$, and gives an excellent fit to the data obtained in three different laboratories.

The effect of added salt on the decay rate (ionic strength effect) was determined at pH 3.3 and 9.0. Added salt should increase the rate of reaction between two ions of the same sign to a predictable degree (Reaction 19), and should have little or no effect on the rate of the first-order Reactions 18 and 20. At pH 9, where Reaction 19 does not occur appreciably and the salt effect is governed by Reaction 17, salt increased the decay rate (22) in quantitative agreement with expectation. At pH 3.3, where Reactions 17 and 19 affect the decay rate, no appreciable salt effect was found, again as predicted (29).

Electron Spin Resonance Studies

The first successful observation and characterization of the ascorbate free radical was carried out with ESR (14, 15). A 1.7-G ESR doublet was reported and it was correctly concluded that the observed spectrum represented the anionic form ($A \cdot$) of the radical. These measurements (14, 15) showed that the enzyme-generated radical (horseradish peroxidase–hydrogen peroxide–ascorbate) was present as a free radical and decayed by second-order kinetics (see Figure 2). Recent experiments (16, 17) have shown that ascorbate oxidase and dopamine-monooxygenase also generate unbound ascorbate radicals.

Studies (20) of the radical in oxygenated neutral or alkaline ascorbate solutions (pH 6.6–9.6) showed that the spectrum could be resolved into a doublet of triplets (1.7 and 0.17 G) with an intensity ratio close to 1:2:1.

The early ESR studies led to controversy (14, 15, 18–20, 30–33) over the exact structure of the radical, a situation that became even more confusing when the OH radical was used as an oxidizing agent for ascorbate (18–25). The OH radical can oxidize ascorbate to $A \cdot$ either by direct electron transfer or by first forming short-lived OH–radical adducts, some of which subsequently yield $A \cdot$. That ascorbate yields a mixture of radicals upon reaction with the OH radical was first observed in studies with Fenton reagents (*18, 19*). An ascorbate radical mixture was also observed in radicals generated by pulse radiolysis (*23*). To resolve the correct structure assignment, a very systematic ESR study of the ascorbate radical(s) and radicals formed from a number of ascorbate analogues was conducted (*25, 26, 34–37*). Good structure assignment for the ·OH adducts was obtained by time-resolved ESR (*37*).

Using in situ radiolysis–ESR, the ESR spectrum shown in Figure 3 was obtained (*25*); the spectral parameters were reported as g factor, 2.00518; a_{H_4}, 1.76 G; a_{H_5}, 0.07 G; and a_{H_6}, 0.19 G for the two protons on C6. These results showed that the radical is in its anionic form with the unpaired electron spread over a highly conjugated tricarbolyl system:

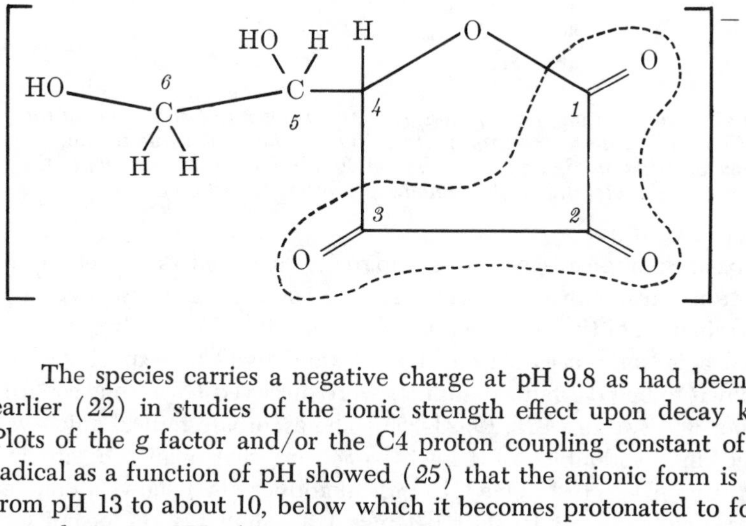

(22)

The species carries a negative charge at pH 9.8 as had been shown earlier (*22*) in studies of the ionic strength effect upon decay kinetics. Plots of the g factor and/or the C4 proton coupling constant of the A· radical as a function of pH showed (*25*) that the anionic form is present from pH 13 to about 10, below which it becomes protonated to form the neutral species AH· (*see* Reaction 16, −16).

Structure assignments to the various OH–radical adducts of ascorbate have been further elucidated and/or confirmed using time-resolved ESR coupled with pulse radiolysis (*37*). The complexity of the system becomes apparent when one considers that OH can form the ascorbate anion radical by direct electron transfer or it can add to either end of the double bond of either of the two tautomeric forms of ascorbate:

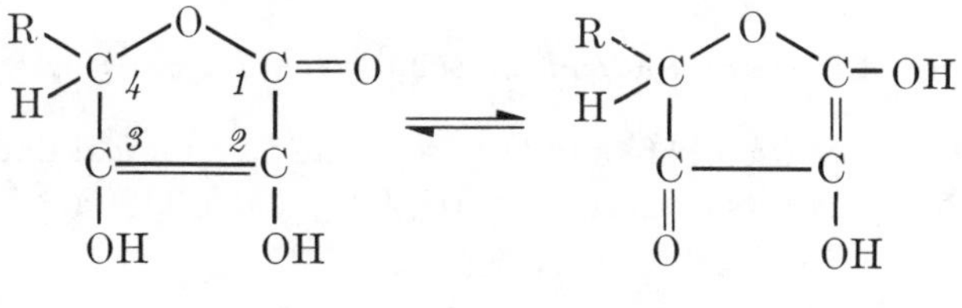

(23)

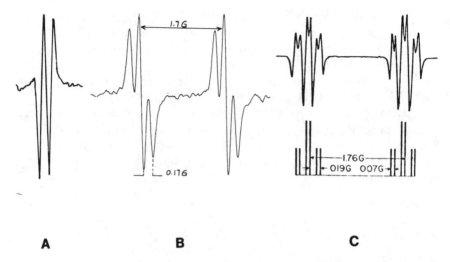

A   B   C

Figure 3.   Illustration of three stages of increasing resolution showing the 1.76-G doublet due to the proton at position 4, the triplet due to the two protons at position 6, and the completely resolved spectrum with the doublet due to the remaining proton at position 5.

In basic solutions ascorbate is apparently oxidized preferentially by the electron transfer process, which goes to completion in less than 2 μs after termination of the electron pulse (*see* Structure I). In nitrous-oxide-saturated acid solutions (pH 3.0–4.5), A⁻ and two other species which were shown to be OH–radical adducts were observed (*37*), thus confirming earlier observations (*18, 19, 23, 25*). The ascorbate radical anion was identified by its doublet of triplets spectrum that maintains its line position from pH 13 to 1. One OH–radical adduct (**IV**) shows a doublet, the lines of which start to shift below pH 3.0; it has a pK near 2.0, a decay period of about 100 μs, and probably does not lead to formation of A⁻. The other OH–radical adduct (**II**) is formed by addition of the OH radical to the C2 position; its ESR parameters are $a_H = 24.4 \pm 0.0002$ G and $g = 2.0031 \pm 0.0002$. Time growth studies suggest that this radical adduct converts to the ascorbate anion radical (**III**) with $\tau \sim$ 15 μs, and accounts for 50% of the A⁻ signal intensity 40 μs after termination of the electron pulse. The formation of the three radicals can be summarized as shown in Scheme 1.

The Role of Ascorbate Radical in the Autoxidation of Ascorbate

Reactions that ascorbate and the ascorbate free radical undergo with molecular oxygen or its derivatives (HO_2/O_2^-, ·OH, $^1O_2$) are biologically

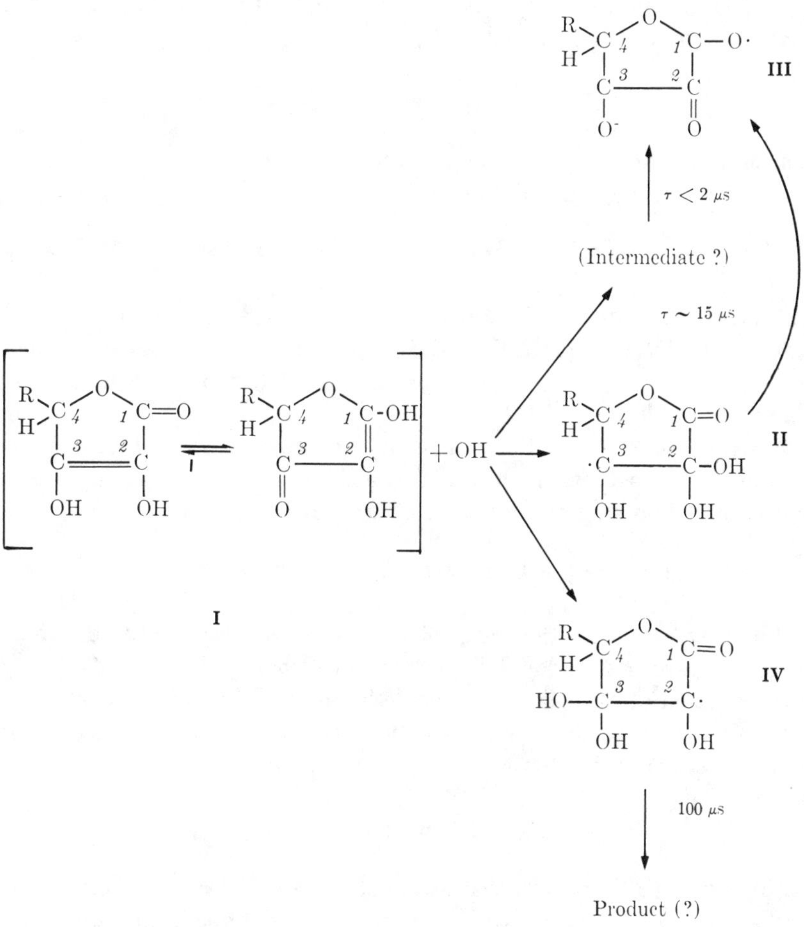

Scheme 1.

important because they may occur in living cells. Despite studies on autoxidation of ascorbate the mechanism(s) of electron transferral to oxygen or hydrogen peroxide remains obscure. ESR studies (14, 15, 20) have shown that a steady state concentration of ascorbate radicals is formed when ascorbate reacts with either hydrogen peroxide at pH 4.8 or molecular oxygen in the pH range 6.6–9.6; similar evidence for formation of HO_2/O_2^- in such mixtures is not well established.

Autoxidation of ascorbate at pH 7.8 is inhibited by addition of

superoxide dismutase (*38*), the enzyme that catalyzes the disproportionation of superoxide radicals (*39*):

$$O_2^- + O_2^- + 2H^+ \rightarrow H_2O_2 + O_2 \tag{24}$$

Such inhibition suggests that superoxide radical may be generated as an
intermediate during autoxidation:

$$AH^- + O_2 \rightarrow A^{\cdot} + O_2^- + H^+ \tag{25}$$

Studies (*40*) on indolylamine 2,3-dioxygenase suggested molecular
oxygen reduction to superoxide radical by ascorbate. Superoxide radicals
have also been implicated in ascorbate-simulated oxygen uptake by
isolated chloroplasts (*41, 42*).

Absence of superoxide radicals in oxygenated neutral or alkaline
solutions suggests that the oxidation mechanism involves a single two-
electron oxidation step as suggested earlier (*14*):

$$AH^- + O_2 + H^+ \rightarrow A + H_2O_2 \tag{26}$$

On the other hand, reaction rates of ascorbate/ascorbic acid with molecular oxygen are low and pH dependent [10^{-5}–5 $M^{-1}s^{-1}$ at pH 4–10 (*43,
44*)]; detection of O_2^- may be difficult because of its low concentration.
Ascorbate free radicals in such solutions could arise from a secondary
reaction between dehydroascorbic acid and ascorbate:

$$A + AH^- \rightleftharpoons 2 A^{\cdot} + H^+ \tag{27, -27}$$

An ESR study (*30*) showed that ascorbate free radicals are formed when
ascorbate and dehydroascorbic acid are mixed under anaerobic conditions.
The equilibrium constant $K = [AH\cdot]^2/[AH_2][A]$ is 4.85 $\pm$ 0.38 $\times$ 10^{-9}
at pH 6.4 and 25°C. Using the numerical values from Reference *30* and
Equation 28, which describe the same equilibrium in terms of concentrations of the ascorbate radical anion, ascorbic acid, and ascorbate ion at
any pH, the following value is obtained:

$$K_{27, -27} = \left[\frac{[A^{\cdot}]^2[H^+][1 + H^+/K_{AH_2}]}{[A][AH_2]_{total}} \right] = 2.0 \times 10^{-15}M^{-2} \tag{28}$$

where K_{AH_2} is the first dissociation constant for ascorbic acid, and
$(AH_2)_{total} = (AH_2) + (AH^-)$.

Radical-induced oxidation of ascorbate by molecular oxygen probably
involves a short chain (*45*). The overall mechanism or parts of it have
been studied primarily by high energy ionizing radiation (*45, 46*) or

photolysis of peroxide (27) containing ascorbate solutions. Because the mechanism has not been resolved, a number of selected reactions that have been proven or are most likely to occur in this system will be discussed next.

Radiolysis of oxygenated water or photolysis of hydrogen peroxide solutions yields two oxidative species, the ·OH radical and the perhydroxyl radical ($HO_2 \rightleftharpoons O_2^- + H^+$). As previously discussed, the final reaction product of hydroxyl radicals interaction with ascorbate above pH 6 is predominantly the ascorbate anion radical ($A^{\cdot}$). To account for the stoichiometry of ascorbic acid consumption in a ^{60}Co gamma ray study of oxygenated ascorbic acid solutions, the ascorbic acid free radical was thought (3) to react with molecular oxygen to yield a transient adduct:

$$A^{\cdot} + O_2 \rightarrow A^{\cdot}O_2 \tag{29}$$

A similar ^{60}Co gamma ray study (4) led to essentially the same conclusion.

Using the flow-radiolysis technique, the rate of Reaction 29 was determined by measuring the disappearance of $A^{\cdot}$ under pseudo first-order conditions at 360 nm (2). At pH 8.6, $k_{29} < 500\ M^{-1}s^{-1}$. This value is in relatively close agreement with $k_{29} \simeq 600\ M^{-1}s^{-1}$, which was determined at pH 6.0–6.5 in a ^{60}Co gamma ray study (45).

Formation of the Barr–King complex radical ($A^{\cdot}O_2$) is reportedly (46) slow and has to compete with other reactions, in particular Reaction 32. The ratios $k_{29}k_{30}/k_{32} = 0.23\ M^{-1}s^{-1}$ and $k_{29}k_{33}/k_{31} = 6.9 \times 10^{-2}\ M^{-1}s^{-1}$ were determined by varying the concentrations of ascorbic acid and oxygen as well as the dose rate. The particular rate constants represent the following equations:

$$AH_2 + HO_2 \rightarrow A^{\cdot} + H^+ + H_2O_2 \tag{30}$$

$$A^{\cdot} + A^-O_2 \xrightarrow{H^+} 2A + H_2O_2 \tag{31}$$

$$A^{\cdot} + HO_2 \xrightarrow{H^+} A + H_2O_2 \tag{32}$$

$$A^-O_2 + AH_2 \rightarrow A + A^{\cdot} + H_2O_2 \tag{33}$$

$$HO_2 + HO_2 \rightarrow H_2O_2 + O_2 \tag{34}$$

Using $k_{29} = 500\ M^{-1}s^{-1}$ (2) and $k_{30} = 1.25 \times 10^6\ M^{-1}s^{-1}$ (27), one can calculate $k_{32} = 2.7 \times 10^9\ M^{-1}s^{-1}$. Because this is a radical–radical reaction, the order of magnitude of k_{32} is not surprising and supports the suggestion that Reaction 32 effectively competes with Reaction 29. A similar substitution into $k_{29}k_{33}/k_{31}$ shows that A^-O_2 reacts approximately 10^4 times faster with A^- (because it is a radical–radical reaction) than with ascorbic acid. This difference in reaction rates is in agreement with the observation that Reaction 33 was not effective unless the ascorbic acid concentration was relatively high.

The oxidation of ascorbic acid/ascorbate by HO_2/O_2^- radicals was studied (27) in the pH range 2.75–7.78. The HO_2/O_2^- radicals were generated by flash photolysis of hydrogen peroxide in presence of ascorbic acid/ascorbate:

$$H_2O_2 + h\nu \rightarrow 2OH \tag{35}$$

$$OH + H_2O_2 \rightarrow HO_2 + H_2O \tag{36}$$

$$HO_2 \rightleftharpoons O_2^- + H^+ \tag{37,-37}$$

The pK_{HO_2} for Equation 37 is 4.7 (see Ref. 47). Based upon an observed stoichiometery of $2(HO_2):1(AH_2)$ for the overall oxidation of ascorbic acid by superoxide radicals and kinetic rate measurements carried out under pseudo first-order kinetics as a function of pH, the following mechanism was proposed:

$$HO_2 + AH_2 \rightarrow A^{\cdot} + H_2O_2 + H^+ \tag{30}$$

$$HO_2 + A^{\cdot} + H^+ \rightarrow A + H_2O_2 \tag{32}$$

Two limiting rate values, $k_{30} = 1.25 \pm 0.25 \times 10^6\ M^{-1}s^{-1}$ and $k_{38} = 5.75 \pm 0.35 \times 10^4\ M^{-1}s^{-1}$ were reported (27). The latter value is for the reaction of superoxide radicals with the ascorbate ion:

$$AH^- + O_2^- \rightarrow A^{\cdot} + HO_2^- \tag{38}$$

This value should be compared with earlier reported values: $k_{38} = 1.52 \pm 0.1 \times 10^5\ M^{-1}s^{-1}$ at pH 9.9 (2), $k_{38} = 2.7 \times 10^5\ M^{-1}s^{-1}$ (48), and $k_{38} = 8 \pm 2 \times 10^7\ M^{-1}s^{-1}$ (49).

Selected Ascorbate Free Radical Reactions

The involvement of the ascorbate free radical in biological reactions is so extensive that a thorough discussion of the subject is beyond the scope of this chapter. Because in many cases $A^{\cdot}$ is invoked with little or no experimental evidence, only a few selected systems will be discussed to illustrate the types of reactions ascorbate free radicals undergo.

The Catalysis of Ascorbate Autoxidation by Organic Compounds. While developing an in vitro reaction system for following oxygen consumption during autoxidation of 6-hydroxydopamine (6-OHDA),

6-aminodopamine (6-ADA), and dialuric acid (DA), researchers (50–54) discovered that these compounds were very efficient catalysts for autoxidation of ascorbate. These studies drew attention to the possibility that organic free radicals play a major role in the overall autoxidation mechanism.

The mechanism of the catalysis of ascorbate autoxidation by 6-OHDA, 6-ADA, DA, and other related compounds was studied in great detail (6) in double-mixer flow experiments coupled with ESR. These studies showed that the free radicals ($QH\cdot$) generated by oxidation of the catalyst, for example, 6-OHDA in mixer No. 1 could be converted quantitatively to the ascorbate radical in the tandem mixer No. 2 by addition of excess ascorbate. A simplified version of this mechanism [*see* Ref. 6 for details] in neutral or alkaline solutions is:

$$QH_2 + O_2 \rightarrow QH\cdot + O_2^- + H^+ \tag{39}$$

$$QH_2 + O_2^- \xrightarrow{H^+} QH\cdot + H_2O_2 \tag{40}$$

$$QH\cdot + AH^- \rightarrow QH_2 + A^{\frac{.}{}} \tag{41}$$

Reaction 41 was proved independently under anaerobic conditions by oxidizing QH_2 to $QH\cdot$ with ferricyanide in mixer No. 1 and scavenging $QH\cdot$ with ascorbate in mixer No. 2. Ascorbate is a powerful enough reducing agent to reduce $QH\cdot$ back to QH_2.

Interaction Between Vitamin E· Radicals and Ascorbate. Vitamin E and ascorbate probably act synergistically (55) that is, vitamin E acts as the primary antioxidant (particularly in biomembranes) and the resulting vitamin E· radical then reacts with ascorbate to regenerate vitamin E. That such a reaction can occur was subsequently demonstrated (56), and the reaction rate ($k_{42} = 1.55 \pm 0.2 \times 10^6$ $M^{-1}s^{-1}$) was measured in a pulse radiolysis study:

$$\text{vitamin E}\cdot + AH^- \rightarrow \text{vitamin E} + A^{\frac{.}{}} \tag{42}$$

The $A^{\frac{.}{}}$ radical can disproportionate to ascorbate and dehydroascorbic acid or be enzymatically reduced back to AH^- by an NADH-dependent system (57), therefore the following repair mechanism was proposed (56) for potentially damaging organic free radicals:

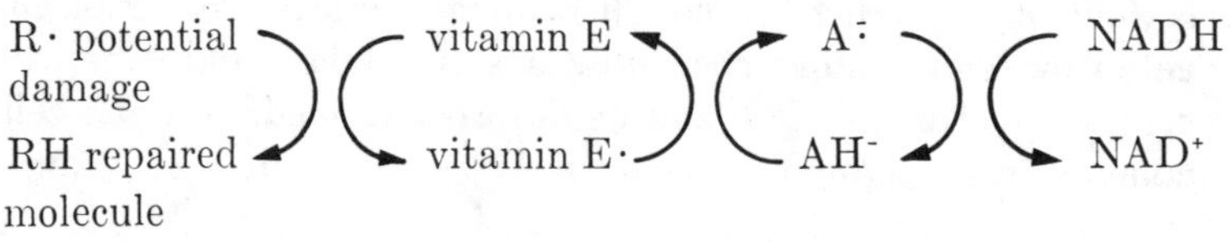

R· potential damage / RH repaired molecule   vitamin E / vitamin E· $A^{\frac{.}{}}$ / AH^- NADH / NAD$^+$ (43)

These observations (*56*) suggested that "the recycling of vitamin E at the expense of vitamin C may account in part for the fact that clinically overt vitamin E deficiency has not been demonstrated in man."

Ascorbate Potentiated Cytotoxicity of Nitroaromatic Compounds. Extensive research aimed at finding chemicals or chemical systems that will sensitize hypoxic cells, which are ordinarily very resistant to radiation or chemicals, is being conducted in the field of radiobiology. Of particular interest are the investigations (*58–61*) of the catalytic effect of certain carcinogens upon the oxidation of ascorbate. 4-Nitroquinoline N-oxide (4-NQO), which is one of many compounds (*52, 62, 63*) that mediate the ascorbate–oxygen reaction, is used as an example.

The overall reaction is initiated by an electron transfer from ascorbate to 4-NQO with the production of A⁻ and 4-NQO⁻ (Reaction 46, 1). The 4-NQO⁻ radical reacts rapidly [reported values for similar compounds range from 10^7 to 10^9 $M^{-1}s^{-1}$ (*62, 63*)] with molecular oxygen to yield superoxide radical (Reaction 46, 2), which dismutates to peroxide and oxygen (Reaction 46, 3) or reacts with ascorbate (Reaction 46, 4). Specific tests with superoxide dismutase and catalase suggest that OH radicals are formed in this system by a Haber–Weiss (*64*) and/or Fenton (*65*) type reaction:

$$HO_2 + H_2O_2 \rightarrow H_2O + O_2 + OH \tag{44}$$

$$M^{2+} + H_2O_2 \rightarrow M^{3+} + OH^- + OH \tag{45}$$

From this in vitro study, the 4-NQO mediated oxidation of ascorbate in presence of oxygen generates two radicals (·OH and 4-NQO⁻) that are potentially mutagenic to mammalian cells. The effect of this system in vivo is difficult to predict. Although hydroxyl radical production may be prevented by high cellular concentrations of catalase and superoxide dismutase, the effect of A-NQO⁻ and its nitroso intermediate upon cellular components and macromolecules nevertheless could be significant.

Miscellaneous Electron Transfer Processes. The electron transfer from ascorbate/ascorbic acid to a number of organic free radicals has been studied by the pulse radiolysis technique. The corresponding rate constants are summarized in Table IV.

The phenothiazine radical cations are particularly interesting because they have been implicated in charge transfer reactions with several neutral transmitter molecules (68):

$$(47)$$

Name	R	X
Promazine (PMZ)	$-(CH_2)_3N(CH_3)_2$	H
Chlorpromazine (ClPMZ)	$-(CH_2)_3N(CH_3)_2$	Cl
Promethazine (PMTZ)	$-CH_2CH(CH_3)N(CH_3)_2$	H

Table IV. Rate Constants for the Oxidation of Ascorbate by Organic Radicals

	pH	k $(M^{-1}s^{-1})$	Reference
Alcohol/Carboxylic Acid Radicals			
CH_2OH	11.0	10^6	26
$\cdot C(OH)(CH_3)_2$	5.7	1.2×10^6	67
$\cdot CH(CO_2^-)_2$	5.7	1.3×10^7	67
CO_3^-	11.0	1.1×10^9	67
Peroxy Radicals			
$Cl_3CO_2\cdot$	7.0	1.8×10^8	71
$Cl_2CHO_2\cdot$	7.0	2.2×10^8	71
$ClCH_2O_2\cdot$	7.0	9.2×10^7	71
$\cdot O_2CCl_2CO_2^-$	7.0	9.0×10^7	71
$\cdot O_2CHClCO_2^-$	7.0	5.1×10^7	71
$CH_3O_2\cdot$	7.0	2.2×10^6	71
$(CH_3)_2C(OH)CH_2O_2\cdot$	7.0	2.1×10^6	71
Phenoxyl Radicals			
Phenoxyl	11.0	6.9×10^8	26
p-Aminophenoxyl	11.0	5.1×10^7	26
p-Bromophenoxyl	11.0	8.3×10^8	26
m-Bromophenoxyl	11.0	8.9×10^8	26
o-Bromophenoxyl	11.0	7.7×10^8	26
p-Carboxyphenoxyl	11.0	4.6×10^8	26
o-Carboxyphenoxyl	11.0	8.3×10^7	26

Continued on next page.

Table IV. (Continued)

	pH	k $(M^{-1}s^{-1})$	Reference
p-Chlorophenoxyl	11.0	7.3×10^8	26
m-Chlorophenoxyl	11.0	1.25×10^9	26
o-Chlorophenoxyl	11.0	1.09×10^9	26
p-Cyanophenoxyl	11.0	2.0×10^9	26
o-Cyanophenoxyl	11.0	1.8×10^9	26
p-Fluorophenoxyl	11.0	4.6×10^8	26
m-Fluorophenoxyl	11.0	9.7×10^8	26
o-Fluorophenoxyl	11.0	9.5×10^8	26
m-Hydroxyphenoxyl	11.0	1.1×10^8	26
p-Iodophenoxyl	11.0	1.06×10^9	26
Phenothiazine Cation Radicals			
Promazine	5.9	4.9×10^8	70
Chlorpromazine	5.9	1.4×10^9	70
Promethazine	5.9	1.3×10^9	70
Semiquinones			
p-Semiquinone	11.0	$< 5.0 \times 10^6$	26
o-Semiquinone	11.0	$< 2.0 \times 10^7$	26

Some researchers (*68, 69*) favor the formation of a charge transfer complex between ascorbate anion (AH⁻) and the respective cation radical (e.g., ClPMZ·⁺); a pulse radiolysis study (*70*) concluded that if such a complex is formed, its lifetime is shorter than 70 ns. At pH 2.2–7.2 the radical cations are reduced by AH⁻ (*70*):

$$\text{ClPMZ}\cdot^+ + \text{AH}^- \rightleftharpoons \frac{k_{48} = 1.1 \times 10^5 \, M^{-1}s^{-1}}{k_{-48} = 5.0 \times 17^7 \, M^{-1}s^{1-}} \text{ClPMZ} + \text{A}^= + \text{H}^+$$

$$(48, -48)$$

In strongly acid solutions (1 M HCl) the reverse reaction occurs (Reaction −48), that is, the ascorbic acid radical (AH·) oxidizes N-alkyl-phenothiazine, for example, to the corresponding radical cation.

Acknowledgment

The author thanks A. O. Allen for constructive criticism of this manuscript and for many stimulating discussions and helpful suggestions.

The author thanks R. W. Fessenden and K. M. Morehouse for Figure 3B and R. H. Schuler for Figure 3C.

The research was carried out at Brookhaven National Laboratory under contract with the U.S. Department of Energy and was supported by its Office of Basic Energy Sciences.

Literature Cited

1. Michaelis, L. *J. Biol. Chem.* **1932**, *96*, 703.
2. Bielski, B. H. J.; Richter, H. W.; Chan, P. C. *Ann. N.Y. Acad. Sci.* **1975**, *258*, 231.
3. Barr, N. F.; King, C. G. *J. Am. Chem. Soc.* **1956**, *78*, 303.
4. Rao, B. S. N. *Radiat. Res.* **1962**, *5*, 683.
5. Ogura, H.; Murata, M.; Kondo, M. *Radioisotopes* **1970**, *19*, 89.
6. Borg, D. C.; Schaich, K. M.; Elmore, J. J., Jr.; Bell, J. A. *Photochem. Photobiol.* **1978**, *28*, 887.
7. Duke, P. S. *Exp. Mol. Pathol.* **1968**, *8*, 112.
8. Vaughan, W. M.; Henry, J. T.; Commoner, B. *Biochem. Biophys. Acta* **1970**, *329*, 159.
9. Floyd, R. A.; Brondson, A.; Commoner, B. *Ann. N.Y. Acad. Sci.* **1973**, *222*, 1077.
10. Dodd, N. J. F. *Br. J. Cancer* **1973**, *28*, 257.
11. Swartz, H. M.; Gutierez, P. L. *Science* **1977**, *198*, 936.
12. Gutierez, P. L.; Swartz, H. M. *Br. J. Cancer* **1979**, *39*, 24.
13. Gutierez, P. L.; Swartz, H. M.; Wilkinson, E. G. *Br. J. Cancer* **1979**, *39*, 330.
14. Yamazaki, I.; Mason, H. S.; Piette, L. *J. Biol. Chem.* **1960**, *235*, 2444.
15. Yamazaki, I.; Piette, L. H. *Biochim. Biophys. Acta* **1961**, *50*, 62.
16. Ljones, T.; Skotland, T. *FEBS Lett.* **1979**, *108*, 25.
17. Skotland, T.; Ljones, T. *Biochim. Biophys. Acta* **1980**, *630*, 30.
18. Kirino, Y.; Kwan, T. *Chem. Pharm. Bull.* **1971**, *19*, 718.
19. Ibid., **1972**, *20*, 2660.
20. Lagercrantz, C. *Acta Chem. Scand.* **1965**, *18*, 562.
21. Bielski, B. H. J.; Allen, O. A. *J. Am. Chem. Soc.* **1970**, *92*, 3793.
22. Bielski, B. H. J.; Comstock, D. A.; Bowen, R. A. *J. Am. Chem. Soc.* **1971**, *93*, 5624.
23. Schöneshöfer, M. *Z. Naturforsch., Teil B* **1972**, *27*, 649.
24. Bansal, K. M.; Schoneshofer, M.; Gratzel, M. *Z. Naturforsch., Teil B* **1973**, *28*, 528.
25. Laroff, G. P.; Fessenden, R. W.; Schuler, R. H. *J. Am. Chem. Soc.* **1972**, *94*, 9062.
26. Schuler, R. H. *Radiat. Res.* **1977**, *69*, 417.
27. Nadezhdin, A. D.; Dunford, H. B. *Can. J. Chem.* **1979**, *57*, 3017.
28. Bielski, B. H. J.; Allen, A. O. *Int. J. Radiat. Phys. Chem.* **1969**, *1*, 153.
29. Bielski, B. H. J.; Allen, A. O.; Schwarz, H. A. *J. Am. Chem. Soc.* **1981**, *103*, 3516.
30. Forster, G. V.; Weiss, W.; Staudinger, H. *Justus Liebigs Ann. Chem.* **1965**, *690*, 16.
31. Kluge, H.; Rasch, R.; Brux, B.; Frunder, H. *Biochim. Biophys. Acta* **1967**, *141*, 260.
32. Russell, G. A.; Strom, E. T.; Talaty, E. R.; Chang, K. Y.; Stephens, R. D.; Young, M. C. *Rec. Chem. Progr.* **1966**, *27*, 3.
33. Steenken, S. *Prog. Photobiol., Proc. Int. Congr.,* 6th Bochum, Germany, 1972, Abstr. No. 83.
34. Kirino, Y.; Schuler, R. H. *J. Am. Chem. Soc.* **1973**, *95*, 6926.
35. Kirino, Y.; Southwick, P. L.; Schuler, R. H. *J. Am. Chem. Soc.* **1974**, *96*, 673.
36. Schuler, M. A.; Bhatia, K.; Schuler, R. H. *J. Phys. Chem.* **1974**, *78*, 1063.
37. Fessenden, R. W.; Verma, N. C. "Proceedings of Meeting on Fast Biochemical Reactions in Solutions, Membranes, and Cells"; Rockefeller Univ. Press: New York, 1978; p. 93.
38. Puget, K.; Michaelson, A. M. *Biochimie* **1974**, *56*, 1255.
39. Fridovich, I. *Adv. Enzymol.* **1974**, *41*, 35.

40. Hirota, F.; Hayaishi, O. *J. Biol. Chem.* **1975**, *250*, 5960.
41. Elstner, E. F.; Kramer, R. *Biochim. Biophys. Acta.* **1973**, *314*, 340.
42. Allen, J. F.; Hall, D. O. *Biochem. Biophys. Res. Commun.* **1973**, *52*, 856.
43. Weissberger, A.; LuValle, J. E.; Thomas, D. S., Jr. *J. Am. Chem. Soc.* **1943**, *65*, 1934.
44. Blaug, S. M.; Hajratwala, B. *J. Pharm. Sci.* **1972**, *61*, 556.
45. Fedorova, O. S.; Berdnikov, V. M. *Khim. Vys. Energ.* **1978**, *12*, 463.
46. Sadat-Shafai, T.; Ferradini, C.; Julien, R.; Pucheault, J. *Radiat. Res.* **1979**, *77*, 432.
47. Bielski, B. H. J. *Photochem. Photobiol.* **1978**, *28*, 645.
48. Nikishimi, M. *Biochem. Biophys. Res. Commun.* **1975**, *63*, 463.
49. Greenstock, C. L.; Ruddock, G. W. *Int. J. Radiat. Phys. Chem.* **1976**, *8*, 367.
50. Heikkila, R. E.; Cohen, G. *Mol. Pharmac.* **1972**, *8*, 241.
51. Heikkila, R. E.; Cohen, G. *Science* **1973**, *181*, 456.
52. Heikkila, R. E.; Cohen, G. *Ann. N.Y. Acad. Sci.* **1975**, *258*, 221.
53. Heikkila, R. E.; Winston, B.; Cohen, G.; Barden, H. *Biochem. Pharmacol.* **1976**, *25*, 1085.
54. Cohen, G.; Heikkila, R. E. *J. Biol. Chem.* **1974**, *249*, 2447.
55. Tappel, A. L. *Geriatrics* **1968**, *23*, 97.
56. Packer, J. E.; Slater, T. F.; Willson, R. L. *Nature* **1979**, *278*, 737.
57. Schneider, W.; Staudinger, H. *Biochim. Biophys. Acta* **1965**, *96*, 157.
58. Biaglow, J. E.; Jacobson, B.; Koch, C. *Biochem. Biophys. Res. Commun.* **1976**, *70*, 1316.
59. Koch, C. J.; Biaglow, J. E. *J. Cell Physiol.* **1978**, *94*, 299.
60. Jacobson, B.; Biaglow, J. E.; Fielden, E. M.; Adams, G. E. *Cancer Clin. Trials* **1980**, *3*, 47.
61. Koch, C. J.; Howell, R. L.; Biaglow, J. E. *Br. J. Cancer* **1979**, *39*, 321.
62. Biaglow, J. E.; Nygaard, O. F.; Greenstock, C. L. *Biochem. Pharm.* **1976**, *25*, 393.
63. Mason, R. P.; Holzman, J. L. *Biochem. Biophys. Res. Commun.* **1975**, *67*, 1267.
64. Haber, F.; Weiss, J. *Proc. R. Soc. London, Ser. A* **1934**, *147*, 332.
65. Fenton, H. J. H.; Jackson, H. *J. Chem. Soc.* **1899**, *75*, 1.
66. Adams, G. E.; Boag, J. W.; Currant, J.; Michael, B. D. *"Pulse Radiolysis"*; Ebert, M. et al., Eds.; Academic: 1965; p. 131.
67. Redpath, J. L.; Willson, R. L. *Int. J. Radiat. Biol.* **1973**, *23*, 51.
68. Gutmann, F.; Smith, L. C.; Slifkin, M. A. *Adv. Biochem. Psychopharmacol.* **1974**, *9*, 15.
69. Klein, N. A.; Toppen, D. L. *J. Am. Chem. Soc.* **1978**, *100*, 4541.
70. Pelizzetti, E.; Meisel, D.; Mulac, W. A.; Neta, P. *J. Am. Chem. Soc.* **1979**, *101*, 6954.
71. Packer, J. E.; Willson, R. L.; Bahnemann, D.; Asmus, K. D. *J. Chem. Soc. Perkin Trans. 2* **1980**, *2*, 296.

RECEIVED for review January 22, 1981. ACCEPTED May 26, 1981.

Dehydroascorbic Acid

BERT M. TOLBERT and JONI B. WARD

Department of Chemistry, University of Colorado, Boulder, CO 80309

Dehydroascorbic acid (DHA) is the first stable oxidation product of L-ascorbic acid (AA). DHA can be easily and quantitatively prepared by air oxidation of AA over charcoal in ethanol. DHA is stable for days in aqueous solution of pH 2–4. ^1H NMR and ^{13}C NMR studies show that the principle species of DHA is the bicyclic hydrate, 3,6-anhydro-L-xylo-hexalono-1,4-lactone hydrate. This finding is confirmed by synthesis and spectral studies of related compounds. DHA contains equilibrium concentrations of various dehydrated and open side-chain forms, but these species are too small to detect using NMR spectroscopy. The DHA dimer is converted to the monomer when it is dissolved in water. The chemistry of DHA is reviewed, including the hydrolysis to diketogulonic acid and the reactions of the 2- and 3-oxo groups. DHA readily forms Schiff bases and undergoes a Strecker reaction with amino acids. The known enzymatic reactions of DHA are reviewed.

The first chemically stable product in the oxidation of L-ascorbic acid (AA) is L-dehydroascorbic acid (DHA). It is normally prepared from AA using a variety of oxidizing agents such as the halogens (*1–5*), oxygen (*6*), quinones (*7*), and potassium iodate (*8*). DHA is present in biological tissue and is a part of the AA/DHA oxidizing/reducing couple. In addition, DHA or AA/DHA ratios may be related to cell division and, therefore, may have a critical role in growth regulation.

The oxidized form of AA was first detected when Zilva (*9*) noticed that freshly oxidized solutions of AA retained their nutritional or physiological activity. At the same period Szent-Gyorgyi also recognized that the oxidized form of AA could be regenerated to AA (*10*). Further investigations of these discoveries led to conclusion that AA could be reversibly oxidized to DHA (*11*) without loss of nutritional activity (*12*). On the basis of the structure of AA, the structure of DHA was postulated as a 2,3-diketolactone with possibly one or more of the keto groups hydrated (*2*).

0065-2393/82/0200–0101$06.75/0

During the last 20 years a better understanding of the structure and chemical nature of DHA and the free radical intermediate that may be formed during the oxidation of AA has developed. These developments were based on modern instrumental techniques including ¹H NMR and ¹³C NMR spectroscopies and pulsed radiation electron spin resonance (ESR) spectroscopy. The chemistry and properties of monodehydroascorbic acid (AA⁻), a free radical intermediate that may be formed in the oxidation of AA, is covered elsewhere in this volume. This chapter concerns DHA, its reactions, structure, and physiological chemistry.

The fact that DHA possesses vitamin C activity was recognized early in studies of AA and was studied by several groups (13, 14). Enzymes that catalyze the reduction of DHA to AA have been demonstrated in many systems and are discussed later in this chapter. Dimeric DHA, or bisdehydroascorbic acid (BDHA), and DHA both are important in nutrition; this importance has been taken for granted in that the common assay of ascorbic acid, the dinitrophenylhydrazine (DNPH) method, does not distinguish between these forms.

The nomenclature of the oxidized forms of AA is badly in need of revision. Not only is dehydroascorbic acid a long and cumbersome name, but it is also confusing in inferring that the compound is an acid. As is discussed later in this chapter, the principle structure is a bicyclic compound containing both lactone and hemiketal groups. Names such as ascorbitone or dehydroascorbitone would be better trivial representations.

Preparation of DHA and BDHA

DHA has been prepared from AA using a great variety of oxidizing agents and conditions. The oxidizers include the halogens, Cl_2, Br_2, and I_2 (1–5); the quinones (7); iodate (8); and oxygen (6) as well as other reagents. Since AA is a good reducing agent that readily reacts with one-electron or two-electron oxidizing agents, the problem in the preparation of DHA is to find reagents that do not overoxidize AA and that give reaction products that are easily separated from DHA. DHA is only stable under certain conditions in water solution and is also easily oxidized. In general, equivalent amounts of AA and the halogens do not give quantitative yields of DHA because of partial overoxidization, and a complicated purification procedure is required to give pure DHA (1). Also, the purification procedures often lead to more decomposition than purification.

One of the more extensive reports on the preparation of DHA is by Pecherer (1) who worked out a large-scale preparation using iodine oxidation. Neither in this study, nor in any other has DHA been obtained in crystalline form, although there does not seem to be any good reason to believe it impossible. DHA is usually obtained as a thick syrup or as an amorphous or microcrystalline solid by solvent precipitation or lyophilization. Because DHA is very easy to prepare from AA, it is best prepared as needed using the following method.

A particularly useful preparation of DHA, described by Ohmori and Takagi, uses oxygen oxidation over a charcoal catalyst (6). The use of oxygen and charcoal to convert AA to DHA is a well-known reaction that has been used in AA assays for many years. The oxidation can be made in ethanol, methanol, water, or various mixtures of these solvents. We carry out this procedure as follows:

Ten grams of ascorbic acid is dissolved in 300 mL of solvent, and 15 g of activated charcoal is added. Oxygen or air is bubbled through the solution at a flow rate of 20 mL/min for 30–60 min while the solution is gently stirred with a magnetic stir bar. At the completion of the reaction the solution is filtered, first through a Whatman #2 filter paper and then by suction through a fine glass filter. The solvent is removed by a rotary evaporator with a bath temperature of 30°C. The resulting syrup is pure DHA with traces of the organic solvent used in the preparation. Addition of a small amount of water and repeated lyophilization will remove the traces of organic solvent.

Because the initial rotary evaporation is faster with the organic solvent, we have usually prepared DHA in 95% ethanol. In methanol the reaction gives up to 10–20% of a methanol complex of DHA that is only partly reconverted to free DHA on repeated evaporations from water. Extensive rotary evaporation with repeated additions of diethyl ether, followed by lyophilization, yields a more manageable, semisolid product. DHA in the syrup or semisolid form is stable for many weeks when stored at −10° to −20°C. Analysis of the products prepared as described above was done by ^{13}C NMR, one of the few analytical techniques that gives unambiguous results on the purity and identity of this compound.

Crystalline BDHA can be prepared from DHA by the method of Dietz (15): 10 g of DHA syrup, prepared by the method described above, is dissolved in 30 mL of nitromethane. After the syrup has dissolved, 100 mL more of ice-cold nitromethane is added. The solution is heated to boiling. A white precipitate of BDHA is formed and can be filtered off and dried. Hvoslef has prepared macrocrystalline BDHA from this material for x-ray crystallographic studies (16).

The dimer is stable in solid dry form. Several commercial firms sell "dehydroascorbic acid" that may or may not be identified as BDHA. We have analyzed several old commercial and privately prepared samples of BDHA using ^{13}C NMR, and have found large amounts of decomposition products in all of them. However the purity of the original product and storage conditions were not known.

Chemical Reactions of DHA

The ene–diol system of AA and its diketo oxidation product are well-known structures in organic chemistry. The lactone group in AA is quite stable in acid or alkaline solution; in contrast, the lactone group in DHA is rapidly hydrolyzed in alkaline or acid solution and is stable only in a limited pH range around 2–4.

As an effective ketone, DHA reacts readily with hydrazines to form a variety of 2- and 2,3-hydrazones. These reactions are characteristic of the 2,3-bisketobutyrolactone group. The standard assay of AA takes advantage of the reaction between DNPH and DHA to give a bishydrazone that exhibits a distinctive absorption band at 516 nm in dilute sulfuric acid solution (17). This reaction is not quantitative; a mixture of the hydrazone and decomposition products is formed. We have estimated that the derivative is formed in about 35% yield. The success of the DNPH reaction as a quantitative assay for AA is dependent on the use of adequate controls, representing a significant weakness of the method.

The bishydrazones of DHA and related compounds have been studied and used to synthesize a number of nitrogen derivatives of DHA (18–23). Thus the bisphenylhydrazone of DHA is reduced by hydrogen/platinum to 2,3-diamino-2,3-dideoxyascorbic acid, which in turn can be converted to a variety of acyl derivatives. The structure of DHA phenylosazone is a hexenonelactone (24).

Under proper conditions DHA reacts with amines to form Schiff bases. Dahn and Moll describe this reaction between o-phenylene-diamine and DHA as well as with other 2,3-diketobutyrolactones (25). With aliphatic amines and amino acids, the Schiff base is not favored in aqueous solution. The extent of the reversible formation of Schiff bases of DHA has not been extensively studied, and clearly needs more attention. DHA in biological fluids is probably in reversible equilibrium with amino groups of amino acids, proteins, and other amines. However, the extent of any such conjugation is unknown. If such bases are formed, they probably involve derivatization of the 2-position of DHA.

The browning reaction between carbohydrates and amino acids has attracted attention for many years. In the presence of amino acids, DHA undergoes a browning reaction that was described in 1956 (26) and later extensively studied (27–33). A distinctive early product of this reaction is the formation of a red chromophore, λ_{max} 515 nm, (1, 31), believed to be the product of a Strecker reaction between the amino acid and DHA. This reaction product seems to be quite specific for DHA.

The reaction itself is analogous to the reaction of ninhydrin with amino acids:

+ RCHN⁺H₃COO⁻ → + CO₂ + RCHO

Kurata et al. (*32*) have isolated this compound and obtained a ¹H NMR spectrum with shifts as follows: 3.74 ppm (doublet), 4.19 ppm (triplet), and 4.88 ppm (doublet). We have also examined a low purity sample of this red chromophore and obtained a similar ¹H NMR spectrum (*33*) as well as a ¹³C NMR spectrum. The results obtained show that the chromophore has an open side-chain and does not exist in a hemiketal form analogous to that observed in DHA and BDHA.

This color reaction has not been used to any extent in the assay of DHA. We have used it to identify DHA in thin-layer chromatography (TLC) with excellent results. The plate is sprayed with 1 *M* glycine and heated in an oven at 90–100°C for 4–5 min. A distinctive pink spot develops, and slowly turns brown in 1–2 d. Various qualitative studies were done to improve the sensitivity of this assay for DHA. Amines did not give the chromophore. There was little difference between different amino acids. Heating DHA and glycine in either water or methanol solution gives the chromophore. Although a better yield may be obtained in water, problems result in water due to the instability of the chromophore in this solvent. BDHA also gives this reaction in solution, presumably because it decomposes to DHA under the conditions of the reaction. The yield of the chromophore is low, and thus only moderate sensitivities for DHA assays were achieved. If the yield in this reaction could be substantially improved by appropriate choices of solvent and reaction conditions, the reaction has the potential for a good assay procedure. The reaction is specific and the product quite distinctive and easy to quantitate by spectroscopy.

Associated with the browning reaction are a number of fairly stable free radical compounds in which the unpaired electron is often associated with a nitrogen atom. A blue substance that displays an ESR triplet spectrum can be isolated by TLC; a red chromophore can also be isolated (34–39). Many of the radical compounds either may be related to the red chromophore or are intermediates in the synthesis of the chromophore (34–39).

Many decomposition products of DHA are probably the same as those observed in the decomposition of AA (40). Fifteen products from DHA decomposition in aqueous solution were reported (41). Of these fifteen, the five main volatile products were 3-hydroxy-2-pyrone, 2-furan-carboxylic acid, 2-furaldehyde, acetic acid, and 2-acetylfuran. DHA also undergoes a benzilic acid rearrangement in alkaline solution (42).

The reduction of DHA to AA is accomplished by a variety of reagents. Hydrogen sulfide, cysteine, and other thiols will reduce DHA. Hydrogen sulfide is frequently used since the excess reagent can be purged from the reaction solution and sulfur, the oxidized product, can be removed by filtration. Because the reaction with hydrogen sulfide is disagreeable to use because of the toxic and odorous hydrogen sulfide, this reduction has been used most often in differential assay procedures for DHA. Sodium dithionate rapidly and qualitatively reduces DHA to AA. Sodium borohydride and lithium aluminum hydride give complex mixtures of products with DHA.

Structural Studies of DHA and BDHA

The crystalline dimer of DHA was analyzed by x-ray crystallography (17), and the structure proposed by earlier chemical studies was confirmed (43).

The dimer is not readily soluble in water, although DHA is very soluble in water. Thus some questions have arisen as to the exact nature of BDHA in water. The dimer disassociates to a monomer in dimethyl formamide, dimethylacetamide, and pyridine (44) in agreement with earlier studies (45–47). A series of studies of AA and BDHA have now clarified many aspects of this problem. ^{13}C NMR studies of AA were published (48–51) that show the structure of AA in solution is essentially as proposed by classical carbohydrate chemistry and is the same as the structure found in crystalline ascorbic acid by x-ray crystallographic studies. Recent ^{13}C NMR studies of BDHA in dimethyl sulfoxide-d_6 (DMSO-d_6) show that in this solvent BDHA is a mixture of two forms, a symmetric and an asymmetric dimer (52). The asymmetric form is thermodynamically favored.

The best approach to the structure of monomeric DHA was through ^{1}H NMR and ^{13}C NMR studies. On the basis of ^{1}H NMR, DHA was proposed to exist in aqueous solution as a bicyclic hydrated species, that is, 3,6-anhydro-L-*xylo*-hexulono-1,4-lactone hydrate (53). We have made further studies on this structure using DHA prepared by oxygen oxidation in ethanol, or methanol or water using charcoal as a catalyst. The method is described earlier in this chapter.

^{13}C **NMR Studies.** DHA was dissolved in deuterium oxide and the ^{13}C NMR spectrum was obtained from a JOEL PFT-100 spectrometer using an external dioxane reference. The spectrum of BDHA was obtained in DMSO-d_6 instead of deuterium oxide.

Results on ^{13}C NMR shifts in parts per million from Me$_4$Si for DHA and BDHA are presented in Table I. For comparison, Hvoslef and Pederson's results (52) are given, including assignments of shifts to specific symmetric and antisymmetric structures for BDHA. Hvoslef's results are readily reproduced using the material prepared by the Ohmori oxidation and the Dietz dimerization procedure. The spectra from the two laboratories show a consistent difference in shifts, probably arising from differences in reference standards. The difference in shifts of C4 and C5 is caused by a difference in assignment of these shifts, and is discussed later.

The ^{13}C NMR shifts for DHA, presented in Table I, were studied and carbon assignments made by two methods: by proton–carbon decoupling experiments and by comparison of ^{13}C NMR spectra of various derivatives.

^{1}H **NMR Decoupling Experiments.** DHA was dissolved in deuterium oxide and the spectra were recorded from a Nicolet NT-360 spectrometer with an internal sodium 2,2-dimethyl-2-silapentane-5-sulfonate (DSS) standard. The shifts for the protons of DHA were determined from the ^{1}H NMR spectrum (Figure 1): C4, singlet at 4.76; C5,

Table I. ^{13}C NMR Data for DHA and BDHA

Sample Identification	C1	C2	C3	C4	C5	C6
DHA (*52*)	174.2	92.0	106.3	73.5	88.6	76.2
DHA prepared in absolute methanol[a]	173.6	91.4	105.7	87.6	73.0	76.2
DHA prepared in 95% ethanol[a]	173.3	91.1	105.7	87.3	72.6	76.2
DHA prepared in H$_2$O[b]	173.5	91.3	105.6	87.4	72.8	76.1
BDHA symmetric (*52*)[b]	169.1	91.6	105.6	73.0	90.3	76.3
BDHA antisymmetric (*52*)[b]	168.1	99.1	103.4	73.2	88.3	74.5
	168.7	104.2	113.9	73.4	89.1	76.7
BDHA symmetric[c]	169.3	91.9	105.9	89.6	73.3	75.6
BDHA antisymmetric[c]	168.4	99.8	103.7	88.4	73.3	74.7
	168.8	104.0	114.1	89.4	73.8	76.6

[a] Solvent, D$_2$O; reference, external dioxane.
[b] Solvent, DMSO-d_6; reference, internal Me$_4$Si.
[c] Solvent, DMSO-d_6; reference, external dioxane.

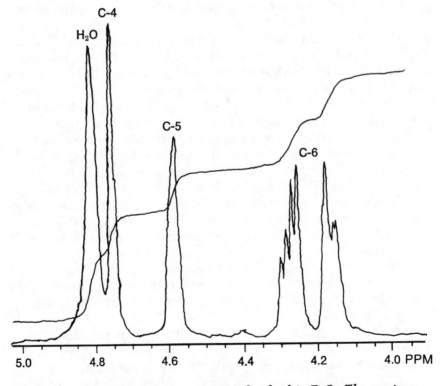

Figure 1. ^{1}H NMR spectrum of DHA dissolved in D$_2$O. The spectrum was recorded on a Nicolet NT-360 spectrometer with an internal DSS reference.

singlet at 4.6; C6, multiplet at 4.2. The interpretation of the ¹H NMR spectrum as an ABCD pattern suggests that the protons on C6 are different from one another; these protons split one another. The fact that these protons appear as different peaks in the ¹H NMR suggests that there is not free rotation of C6. In the proton–proton decoupling experiments (Figure 2), the splitting of the proton on C4 by the proton on C5 is very small. This observation suggests that the orbitals for these protons are separated by an angle of approximately 90°, and therefore cannot interact with each other to cause splitting.

Proton–Carbon Decoupling Experiments. Having obtained correct values for the proton shifts, a series of proton–carbon decoupling experiments were performed (Figures 3–5). The experiments performed involved combining two types of decoupling: off-resonance and single-frequency. In off-resonance decoupling experiments ¹H irradiation is kept at high power levels. The center of frequency is moved 500–1000 Hz away from the protons to be irradiated, and the excitation bandwidth generator is switched off. Carbons having zero, one, two, or three

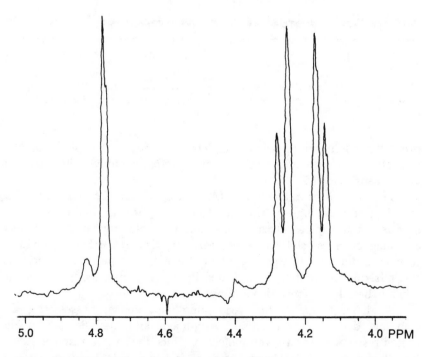

Figure 2.   ¹H NMR spectrum of DHA. The proton on C5 has been decoupled.

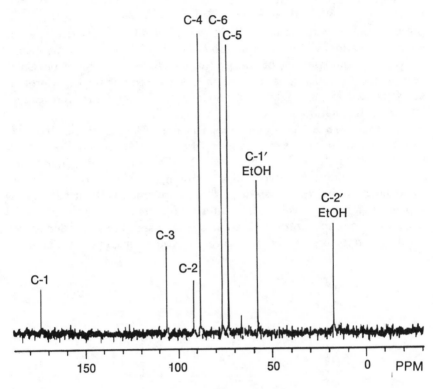

Figure 3. ^{13}C *NMR spectrum of DHA dissolved in* D_2O. *The spectrum was recorded on a Nicolet NT-360 spectrometer with an internal DSS reference.*

protons bonded now appear as singlets, doublets, triplets, and quartets, respectively. Coupling information is therefore retained without much loss of sensitivity (*54*).

The carbons of interest in DHA are C4, C5, and C6. Carbons-1, -2, and -3 appear as singlets. Carbons-4 and -5 appear as doublets, and C6 appears as a triplet. Because C4 and C5 both appear as doublets, assigning chemical shifts to these carbons without further information would be difficult. It was important, therefore, to perform a series of single-frequency proton–carbon decoupling experiments, while maintaining the off-resonance decoupling.

Single-frequency proton decoupling, also known as selective decoupling, depends upon proper assignment and identification of the proton resonances for a given molecule. Once the proton resonances are identified in an ^1H NMR spectrum, it is possible to irradiate specific protons at low radiofrequency power. The result as seen in the ^{13}C NMR spectrum is the collapse to a singlet of the multiplet associated with the carbon attached to that proton. The other protonated carbons retain some C–H coupling (*54*).

In these experiments, each proton resonance was irradiated, and the resulting ^{13}C NMR spectrum was observed to see which multiplet collapsed to a singlet. Proper assignment of the chemical shifts can be made for C4, C5, and C6 (Figures 4 and 5).

The assignment of proton chemical shifts is also supported by carbon-13 chemical shifts obtained for the 5,6-isopropylidene derivatives of DHA, D-*erythro*-DHA and 6-bromo-6-deoxy-L-DHA. All the dehydro compounds were prepared by oxidation using oxygen over charcoal in 95% ethanol. The preparation of the isopropylidene derivatives follows.

L-5,6-O-Isopropylidene AA. In a 5-L reaction flask equipped with an efficient paddle stirrer and a water-cooled condenser with a drying tube, and heated by a steam bath, was placed 250 g of L-AA (1.4 mol),

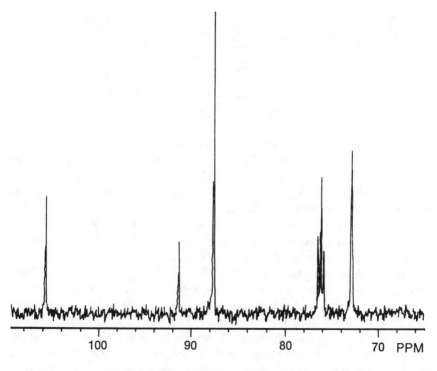

Figure 4. ^{13}C NMR spectrum of DHA obtained when the proton on C4 was selectively decoupled.

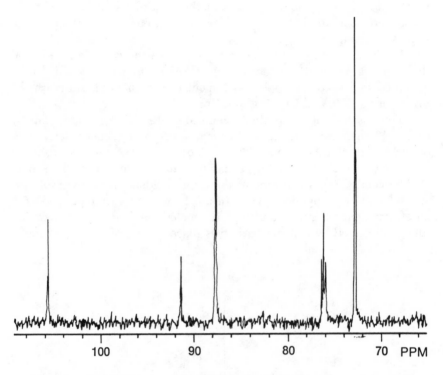

Figure 5. ¹³C NMR *spectrum of DHA obtained when the proton on C5 was selectively decoupled.*

437 g of 2,2-dimethoxypropane (4.2 mol), 880 mL of *p*-dioxane, and 6 mL of trifluoroacetic acid (TFA). The reaction is stirred and heated to reflux. After 15 min, the white voluminous product begins to precipitate. Heating and stirring are continued for another 45 min, at which time the reaction has solidified into a copious white mass. The reaction mixture is cooled, slurried in several liters of petroleum ether, and filtered. The product is dried in a vacuum desiccator. The product is obtained as a white solid in 95–100% yield.

D-5,6-O-Isopropylidene IsoAA. The proportion of reactants and the reaction conditions are the same for preparing this isomer as for preparing AA. However, the reaction takes 2–3 h to complete. The D-isopropylidene isoAA does not precipitate from the reaction mixture, even on cooling to room temperature. The solvents are removed by rotary evaporation (water aspiration, bath temperature of 35°C)· and the resulting red-brown oil is poured into four times its volume of efficiently stirred petroleum ether to precipitate the product as a tan powder. The powder must be filtered and quickly dried under vacuum to prevent reconversion into an oil. The D-isopropylidene isoAA can be obtained as white flakes by precipitating with petroleum ether from a chloroform–acetone solution.

Discussion of Structural Studies. Collected data from the ^{13}C NMR spectra are shown in Table II. L-DHA and D-isoDHA have similar chemical shifts, suggesting a similar structure. They both show an assigned shift for C6 that is further downfield than for the C6 of the respective starting materials. One would expect the C6 to be shifted downfield if the compound is in the hemiketal form. This fact, with the information from the preceding proton experiments, supports a proposed hemiketal structure.

The assigned shift for C2 of L-DHA and D-isoDHA is further upfield than would be expected if C2 were a keto group, indicating hydration at this carbon.

For L-isopropylidene-DHA, D-isopropylidene isoDHA, and 6-bromo-6-deoxy-L-DHA, the assigned shifts for C2 and C3 are upfield from values expected for keto groups. This observation indicates that these carbons are hydrated. In these compounds the C6 hydroxy group has either been derivatized or replaced, preventing the formation of the hemiketal. These compounds readily form an open-chain form of DHA, suggesting a reasonable stability for the hydrated diketo structure.

D-IsoDHA, which readily forms the hemiketal, has an *endo*-5-hydroxyl group, but L-DHA is an *exo*-5-hydroxyl compound. The *endo*-hydroxyl does not cause sufficient steric hindrance to prevent the formation of the hemiketal ring.

The most important inference to be drawn from the data is that DHA can exist as a mixture of various structures. An equilibrium of major and minor forms of DHA in aqueous solution undoubtedly exists, with the hydrated hemiketal being the favored form (Scheme 1, A). Most of these forms have been postulated for many years (2). The only form detected by ^{13}C NMR spectroscopy in aqueous solution is the hydrated hemiketal form (Scheme 1, A). Assuming that 99% of the DHA is the hydrated hemiketal form, this form is calculated to be favored by 2.5 kcal/mol. When the side-chain is derivatized as in L-isopropylidene-DHA, D-isopropylidene isoDHA, or 6-bromo-6-deoxy-L-DHA, the open-chain dihydrate is seen. This finding suggests a reasonable stability for the hydrated hemiketal form and is evidence for an open side-chain compound in the equilibrium mixture of DHA (Scheme 1, C). This compound has been suggested as a major product in aged solutions of DHA (52). Although small concentrations ($< 1\%$) may exist in solution, the principle compound formed in aged solutions of DHA has ^{13}C NMR shifts that correspond to diketogulonate (DKG).

Table II. ¹³C NMR Data on DHA and Related Compounds

Compound Identification	C1	C2	C3	C4	C5	C6	Carbonyl Isopropylidene	-CH₃	-CH₃
Reduced Forms									
L-AA	173.8	118.3	156.1	76.7	69.4	62.6	—	—	—
D-IsoAA		118.2	155.6	74.4	71.0	61.4	—	—	24.4
Isopropylidene-L-AA		118.2	152.9	74.9	73.3	64.8	109.8	25.0	25.7
Isopropylidene-D-isoAA	170.6	118.7	152.6	74.7	73.9	65.3	109.4	26.2	
6-Bromo-6-deoxy-L-AA	173.1	118.1	155.2	76.8	69.0	32.8	—	—	—
Oxidized Forms									
L-DehydroAA	173.6	91.4	105.7	87.6	73.0	76.2	—	—	—
L-IsoDHA	173.5	91.5	104.8	83.1	71.9	69.5	—	—	25.0
Isopropylidene-L-DHA	173.9	91.3	96.0	84.6	74.2	64.4	110.5	26.1	24.6
Isopropylidene-D-isoDHA	173.9	91.3	95.7	84.4	73.9	65.2	110.4	25.8	
6-Bromo-6-deoxy-L-DHA	173.6	91.3	96.0	83.5	68.2	34.2	—	—	—

Note: Shifts in ppm from Me₄Si.

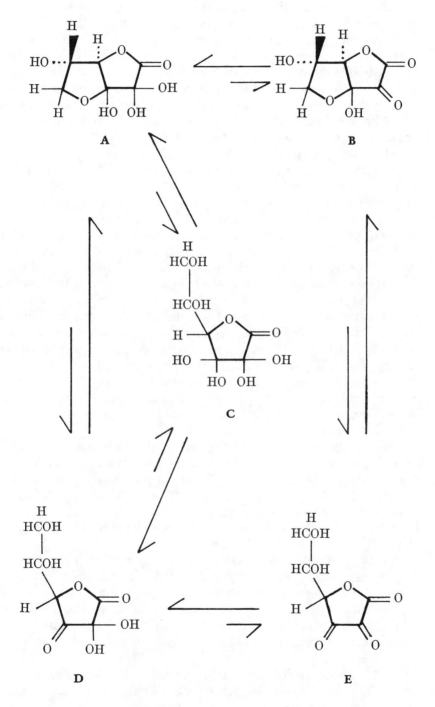

Scheme 1.   Equilibrium mixture of the various forms of DHA.

The evidence for the other forms of DHA shown in Scheme 1 is based on theory of reaction mechanisms. The fact that DHA reacts with DNPH to form a hydrazone is supportive evidence for the existence of a 2- or 3-monoketo compound. A 3-monoketo compound is required by any reasonable mechanism for the formation of the hydrated hemiketal form. The 2,3-diketo compound would be very unstable due to the high positive charge associated with the carbonyl carbons. These carbons would be very susceptible to nucleophilic attack. However, a small concentration of the 2,3-diketo form should exist in equilibrium mixtures. Direct oxidation of AA should give the 2,3-diketo form.

A proposed mechanism for the acid-catalyzed formation of the hydrated hemiketal is shown in Scheme 2. On the basis of analogy with hemiketal ring formation and mutarotation in sugars, opening and closing of the hemiketal ring is expected to be fast compared with other reactions of DHA, such as hydrolytic cleavage to DKG. Hydration of the carbonyl groups should also be rapid. It thus appears that there is a rapid equilibrium of all the postulated forms of DHA in aqueous solution. Which of these forms are active in biological reactions is unknown.

The facile formation of the hydrated and hemiketal forms of DHA, as well as the alcohol complexes, opens the critical question of whether DHA in biological fluids is to any great extent conjugated with other compounds such as amino acids and proteins. At pH 7, DHA is rapidly converted to DKG, but there is no evidence that DHA in biological fluids is rapidly hydrolyzed. It is therefore appropriate to question whether DHA, as such, exists in any significant concentration in biological fluids. Further studies of DHA in tissue are needed to clarify the nature of this compound in biological systems.

The UV spectra of the DHA used in the experiments described shows a weak broad transition at 225 nm leading into a strong absorbance below 200 nm. The transition at 225 nm can be used in liquid chromatography of DHA if the sample is fairly pure. Unfortunately, many compounds absorb in this region, so direct spectrophotometric assay of DHA by UV with high pressure liquid chromatography (HPLC) probably is not possible in most experiments.

Stability of DHA and BDHA. BDHA is not stable in aqueous solution (33, 44). In the solid form dry BDHA is quite stable, although it appears to decompose slowly to a complex mixture of products. Because BDHA dissociates to the monomer in water, and DHA has 80–100% of the vitamin C activity of AA, BDHA is an interesting form of this vitamin with properties of low solubility in water and good resistance to air oxidation.

DHA is hydrolyzed in aqueous solutions to yield DKG. The reaction velocity is pH dependent, subject to both acid and base catalysis. The

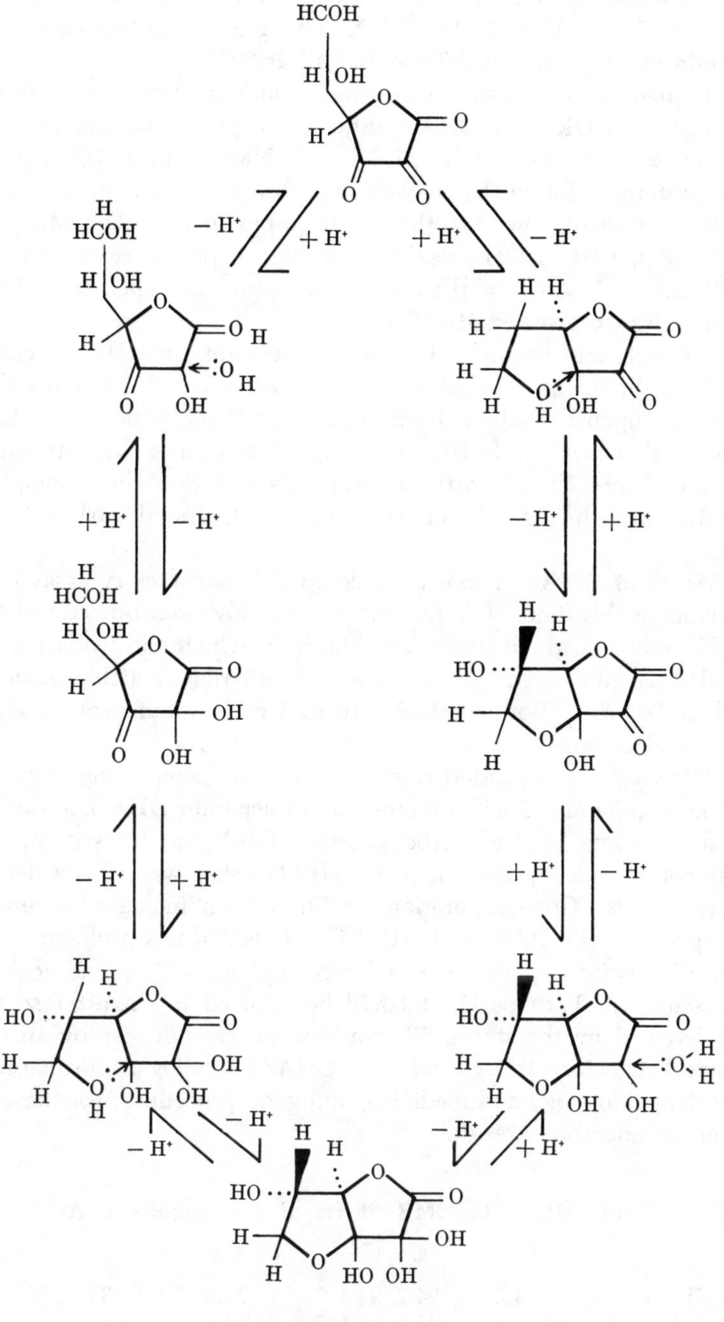

Scheme 2. *Acid-catalyzed formation of the hydrated hemiketal form of DHA.*

kinetics were reported to be first order with respect to H⁺ (55, 56) with a K_{vel} of 7.6 × 10^{-4} at pH = 7.2. The specific rate constant for this reaction was reported as 2.08 × 10^{-5} s⁻¹ at 30°C.

In neutral and alkaline aqueous solutions, DHA is very rapidly hydrolyzed to DKG. If DHA is adjusted to pH 7.0 in buffered solution and immediately assayed by TLC or ¹³C NMR, only DKG is observed. In unbuffered solution the conversion is slow because hydrolysis of DHA produces an acid, lowering the pH to approximately 2.5. Many of the ¹³C NMR spectra of DHA described in this chapter were run on samples at 30°C over 12–24 h, and these spectra could be repeated 3 d later if the samples were stored at 4°C.

Hvoslef suggests that the hemiketal form of DHA is converted slowly to the open side-chain form in water. Ward (33) shows that the presumed open side-chain form is actually DKG, which has ¹³C NMR shifts as shown in Table III. In the NMR spectra of DKG the shifts of C2 and C3 are characteristic of *gem*-diols and thus the principal form of DKG in aqueous solution is with fully hydrated carbonyls on C2 and C3.

Assay of DHA. There is no completely satisfactory assay of DHA available at this time. The two most commonly used procedures are the DNPH reaction, done under conditions in which the oxidation of AA to DHA is minimized (58, 59) and the differential dichloroindophenol method (60, 61). Both methods are subject to interference and rather large random errors.

DHA can be separated from AA and most ionic compounds by ion exchange columns. Such columns do not separate DHA from other AA metabolites and neutral carbohydrates. DHA can be separated from these compounds by reverse phase HPLC using water or water–acetonitrile eluants. Good separations of DHA from biological samples can be expected to be achieved by HPLC. Detection is a problem since UV absorption is inadequate. The red chromophore with amino acids is not very sensitive. Perhaps DHA could be reduced to AA after separation and detected by the strong 263-nm absorption of AA or by an electrochemical detector. DHA levels and DHA/AA ratios are probably quite important in biology and medicine, and good procedures for these assays are of considerable interest.

Table III.   ¹³C NMR Shifts of Diketogulonic Acid

	C1	C2, C3 [a]	C4	C5	C6
pH 7.0	174.5	94.7, 94.4	74.6	68.6	62.5
pH 2.0	171.2	94.5, 96.1	74.3	68.0	62.4

[a] Shifts for C2 and C3 are too similar to assign to specific carbons.

Biochemistry of DHA

A number of enzymes have been characterized that catalyze reactions involving DHA. In addition, other aspects of DHA biochemistry can be deduced from metabolic studies of ascorbic acid. Experiments demonstrating the biological oxidation of AA and reduction of DHA were first made in 1928 (*10*) and during the next decade several groups studied these reactions. By 1941 Crook (*62*) was able to separate the ascorbic acid oxidase and DHA reductase activities and to show that glutathione was used in the reductase reaction.

The best characterized of the enzymes involving DHA is ascorbic acid oxidase (L-ascorbate: O_2 oxidoreductase, EC 1.10.3.3). This plant enzyme catalyzes the reaction of AA and oxygen to give DHA and 1 mol of water (*63*).

Ascorbate oxidase is a dimer containing two identical subunits, and appears to be accompanied by smaller amounts of oligomeric forms (*64–66*). This compound contains 8–10 atoms of copper and is blue colored. The copper may be removed to give an inactive apoenzyme. Ascorbate oxidase contains Cu^{2+} in three different environments (*63, 67, 68*). The enzyme also catalyzed the oxidation of *o*-catechols, although the K_m is less favorable than that for AA: K_m, (+)-catechin, 3.08 mM; K_m, L-AA, 0.24 mM (*69*). The role of ascorbate oxidase in plants is not known.

Two other copper enzymes possess ascorbate oxidase activity, human ceruloplasm and *Polyporus* laccase (*70, 71*). Ceruloplasm may function as an AA oxidase in vivo. Both ceruloplasm and laccase are 10^4 times less active toward AA oxidation than is ascorbate oxidase. However, the reaction is definitely enzymic, and water is produced.

In recent years DHA reductase has been purified from several sources and characterized. DHA reductase (EC 1.8.5.1) purified from carp hepatopancreas was specific for glutathione as a reducing agent (*72*). K_m values were 5.7×10^{-4} M for DHA and 1.5×10^{-3} M for glutathione. The enzyme was not affected by metal ion chelating agents. DHA reductase from spinach leaves has a MW of about 25,000 daltons and a pH optimum of 7.5. K_m values were 4.4 mM for glutathione and 0.34 mM for DHA (73). DHA reductase appears to be widely distributed in plant and animal tissue, and to consistently use glutathione as the reducing agent (74, 75).

A DHA lactonase has been described (76, 77) in the ox, rabbit, rat, and guinea pig. In the ox the lactonase is present in several tissues but is most abundant in the liver. The enzyme appears to be absent in human and monkey tissue. This result is consistent with the observation that primates and fishes do not catabolize labeled ascorbic acid to carbon dioxide. AA and DHA appear to be metabolized into a series of water soluble products that are excreted in the urine, but 2,3-DKG is decarboxylated and otherwise degraded to intermediates that enter the C_5 and C_4 carbohydrate pools (78).

DHA and AA can react to form the free radical intermediate, monodehydroascorbate ion (AA$^-$), also called semidehydroascorbate. Enzymes that reduce AA$^-$ were demonstrated in animals (79, 80), plants (81), and microorganisms (82).

Other than the three enzymes (AA oxidase, DHA reductase, and DHA lactonase) no other enzymes have been demonstrated that directly involve DHA. DHA may be produced by a number of oxygenases that use AA as a cofactor, and it seems reasonable that much of the DHA formed in vivo is produced by these reactions.

Intravenous injection of DHA in rats at 40–60 mg/kg produces excitation, salivation, lacrimation, and elevated blood pressure (83–85). Most of the responses originated with the central nervous system. At higher doses, respiratory arrest occurs (86). The LD_{50} appears to be about 300 mg/kg. When repeated injections of DHA are given to rats at about 20 mg/kg, marked hyperglycemia is observed in many of the rats after 3 weeks (87). This diabetogenic effect was confirmed (88) and seems to be associated with abnormalities of the beta cells of the islets of Langerhans of the pancreas. Unlike alloxan diabetes, necrosis of the beta cells is not seen. Alloxan and DHA are structural analogues in that both have a potential 1,2,3-triketo structure. The doses of DHA required to produce these physiological effects are so large that the toxicity of DHA does not have any noticeable significance in the nutritional use of AA. DHA is a minor by-product of storage and is a normal component of both foods and tissue. Normal blood levels of DHA are probably around 0.2 mg/100 mL, and tissue levels may be comparable.

DHA is rapidly transported across cell membranes. Autoradiographic studies using labeled DHA show that DHA is more rapidly absorbed by guinea pigs than is AA (89). Injected DHA is not rapidly absorbed from the blood (90–92) and the observations suggest that DHA is not favored as a physiological transport form. Only in the brain and bone marrow are DHA taken up more rapidly than AA. Both leucocytes and erythrocytes are readily permeable to DHA as well as AA (93, 94). After uptake of DHA by leucocytes, only AA is found, showing an active DHA reductase system. The reduction of DHA in red blood cells is less rapid and incomplete, suggesting that a DHA reductase system is either absent or of low activity.

A general belief, supported by a limited amount of experimental evidence, is that DHA levels or alternatively, DHA/AA ratios, are sensitive indications of cell physiology, including pathogenic states and mitotic index (95–98). Because glutathione (GSH) is the reducing agent for DHA reductase, the DHA/AA ratio may reflect the GSSG/GSH ratio, and this ratio was related to the NADPH/NADP ratio. Assuming the DHA/AA ratio reflects the oxidation state of the metabolism of the cell, including the NADPH/NADP ratio, the correlation appears to have merit. Certainly more experimental studies are important in this area.

Acknowledgments

We thank Paul Seib for the samples of D-*erythro*-dehydroascorbic acid and 6-bromo-6-deoxy-L-dehydroascorbic acid.

Literature Cited

1. Pecherer, B. *J. Am. Chem. Soc.* **1951**, *73*, 3827–3830.
2. Kenyon, J.; Munro, H. *J. Chem. Soc.* **1948**, 158–161.
3. Muller–Mulot, W. *Hoppe–Seylers Z. Physiol. Chem.* **1970**, *351*, 52–55.
4. Patterson, J. W. *J. Biol. Chem.* **1950**, *183*, 81–88.
5. Weis, W.; Staudinger, H. *Liebigs Ann. Chem.* **1971**, *754*, 152–153.
6. Ohmori, M.; Takagi, M. *Agric. Biol. Chem.* **1978**, *42*, 173–174.
7. Sjostrand, S. E. *Acta. Physiol. Scand.* **1970**, *Suppl. 356*, 1–79.
8. Penney, J. R.; Zilva, S. S. *Biochem. J.* **1945**, *29*, 1–4.
9. Zilva, S. S. *Biochem. J.* **1927**, *21*, 689.
10. Szent–Gyorgi, A. *Biochem. J.* **1928**, *22*, 1387.
11. Schultze, M.; Stotz, E.; King, C. G. *J. Biol. Chem.* **1937**, *122*, 395–405.
12. Tillmans, J.; Hirsh, P.; Dick, H. *Z. Unters. Lebensm.* **1932**, *63*, 267.
13. Fox, F. W.; Levy, L. F. *Biochem. J.* **1936**, *30*, 211.
14. Todhunter, E.; McMillan, T.; Ehmke, D. *J. Nutr.* **1950**, *42*, 297–308.
15. Dietz, H. *Justus Liebigs Ann. Chem.* **1970**, *738*, 206–208.
16. Hvoslef, J. *Acta Cryst. Scand.* **1970**, *24*, 2238–2239.
17. Roe, J. H. In "Methods of Biochemical Analysis"; Vol. 1 Glick, D., Ed., Interscience: New York, 1954, 126.
18. Michael, M.; Brode, G.; Siebert, R. *Chem. Ber.* **1937**, *70*, 1862–1866.
19. El Khadem, H.; El Ashry, S. H. *J. Chem. Soc.* **1968**, 2247–2251.
20. El Khadem, H.; El Ashry, S. H. *Carbohydr. Res.* **1970**, *13*, 57.
21. El Khadem, H.; Meshreki, M.; Ashry, S.; El Sekeili, M. *Carbohydr. Res.* **1972**, *21*, 430–439.
22. El Sekeily, M. et al. *Carbohydr. Res.* **1977**, *59*, 141–149.
23. El Sekeily, M.; Mancy, S. *Carbohydr. Res.* **1979**, *68*, 87–93.
24. Roberts, G. *J. Chem. Soc. Perkin Trans. 1* **1979**, 603–605.
25. Dahn, H.; Moll, H. *Helv. Chim. Acta*, **1964**, *47*, 1860–1869.

26. Dulkin, S. I.; Friedeman, T. E. *Food Res.* **1956**, *21*, 519–527.
27. Ranganna, S.; Setty, L. *J. Agric. Food Chem.* **1974**, *22*, 1139–1142.
28. Nomura, D.; Okamura, T. *Nippon Nogei Kagaku Kaishi* **1972**, *46*, 67–72.
29. Yu, M. H.; Wu, M.; Wang, D.; Salunkhe, D. *J. Inst. Can. Sci. Technol. Aliment.* **1974**, *7*, 279–283.
30. Kurata, T.; Fujimaki, M. *Agric. Biol. Chem.* **1976**, *40*, 1429–1430.
31. Ranganna, S.; Setty, L. *J. Agric. Food Chem.* **1974**, *22*, 719–722.
32. Kurata, T.; Fujimaki, M.; Sakurai, Y. *Agric. Biol. Chem.* **1973**, *37*, 1471–1477.
33. Ward, J. B., M. S. Thesis, Univ. of Colorado, Boulder, CO, 1980.
34. Yano, M.; Hayashi, T.; Namiki, M. *Agric. Food Chem.* **1976**, *24*, 815–819.
35. Yano, M.; Hayashi, T.; Namiki, M. *Agric. Biol. Chem.* **1976**, *40*, 1209–1215.
36. Ibid., **1978**, *42*, 809–817.
37. Ibid., 2239–2243.
38. Kurata, T.; Fujimaki, M. *Agric. Biol. Chem.* **1974**, *38*, 1981–1988.
39. Namiki, M.; Yano, M.; Hayashi, T. *Chem. Letters* **1974**, 125–128.
40. Mikova, K.; Davidek, *Chem. Listy* **1974**, *68*, 715.
41. Velicek, J.; Davidek, J.; Kubelka, V.; Zelinkova, Z.; Porkorny, J. Z. *Lebensm.-Unters. Forsch.* **1976**, *162*, 285–290.
42. Lowendahl, L.; Peterson, G. *Anal. Biochem.* **1976**, *72*, 623–628.
43. Hvoslef, J. *Acta Crstallogr.* **1972**, *28*, 916–923.
44. Dietz, H. *Justus Liebigs Ann. Chem.* **1970**, *738*, 206–208.
45. Albers, H.; Muller, E.; Dietz, H. *Hoppe–Seyler's Z. Physiol. Chem.* **1963**, *334*, 243–258.
46. Muller–Mulot, W. *Hoppe–Seyler's Z. Physiol. Chem.* **1970**, *351*, 56–60.
47. Ibid., 52–60.
48. Matusch, R. *Z. Naturforsch.* **1977**, *Teil 32b*, 562–568.
49. Berger, S. *Tetrahedron* **1977**, *33*, 1587–1589.
50. Radford, T.; Sweeny, J.; Iacobucci, G.; Goldsmith, D. *J. Org. Chem.* **1979**, *44*, 658–659.
51. Ogawa, T.; Uzawa, J.; Matsui, M. *Carbohydr. Res.* **1979**, *59*, C32–35.
52. Hvoslef, J.; Pedersen, B. *Acta Chem. Scand.* **1979**, *B33*, 503–511.
53. Pfeilstricker, K.; Marx, F.; Bochisch, M. *Carbohydr. Res.* **1975**, *45*, 269–274.
54. Levy, G. C.; Nelson, G. L. "C–13 NMR"; Wiley Intersciences: New York, 1972; Chap. 1.
55. Kazuko, T.; Ōhmura, T. *Nippon Nogei Kagaku Kaishi*, **1966**, *40*, 196–200.
56. Velicek, J.; Davidek, J.; Janicek, G. *Collect. Czech. Chem. Commun.* **1972**, *37*, 1465–1470.
57. Dutta, S. K. *Indian J. Pharm. Sci.* **1978**, *40*, 85–87.
58. Roe, H. H.; Kuether, C. A. *J. Biol. Chem.* **1943**, *147*, 399.
59. Schaffert, R. R.; Kingsley, G. R. *J. Biol. Chem.* **1955**, *212*, 59.
60. Bessey, D. A. *J. Biol. Chem.* **1938**, *126*, 771–784.
61. Sauberlich, H. E. *Ann. N.Y. Acad. Sci.* **1975**, *258*, 438–449.
62. Crook, E. M. *Biochem. J.* **1941**, *35*, 226–236.
63. Dawson, C. R.; Strothkamp, K.; Krul, K. *Ann. N.Y. Acad. Sci.* **1975**, *258*, 209–220.
64. Strothkamp, K. G.; Dawson, C. R. *Biochemistry* **1974**, *13*, 434–440.
65. Lee, M. H.; Dawson, C. R. *J. Biol. Chem.* **1973**, *248*, 6596–6602.
66. Amon, A.; Markakis, P. *Phytochemistry* **1973**, *12*, 2127–2132.
67. Deinum, J.; Reinhammer, B.; Marchesini, A. *FEBS Lett.* **1974**, *42*, 241–245.
68. Avigliano, L.; Gerosa, P.; Rotilio, G.; Finazzi Agro, A.; Calabrese, L.; Mondovi, B. *Ital. J. Biochem.* **1972**, *21*, 248–255.
69. Marchesini, A.; Capelletti, P.; Canonica, L.; Danieli, B.; Tollari, S. *Biochem. Biophys. Acta* **1977**, *489*, 290–300.

70. Osaki, S.; McDermott, J.; Frieden, E. *J. Biol. Chem.* **1964**, *239*, 3570–3575.
71. Osaki, S.; Johnson, A.; Frieden, E. *J. Biol. Chem.* **1971**, *246*, 3018.
72. Yamamoto, Y.; Sato, M.; Ikeda, S. *Bull. Jpn. Soc. Sci. Fish.* **1977**, *43*, 59–67.
73. Foyer, C. H.; Halliwell, B. *Phytochemistry* **1977**, *16*, 1347–1350.
74. Hughes, R. E. *Nature* **1964**, *203*, 1068–1069.
75. Christine, L.; Thompson, G.; Iggs, B.; Brownie, A.; Stewart, C. *Clin. Chim. Acta* **1956**, *1*, 557–569.
76. Kagawa, Y.; Takiguchi, H. *Biochem.* **1962**, *51*, 197–203.
77. Kagawa, Y.; Takiguchi, H.; Shimazono, N. *Biochim. Biophys. Acta* **1961**, *51*, 413–415.
78. Kagawa, Y.; Mano, Y.; Shimazono, N. *Biochim. Biophys. Acta* **1960**, *43*, 348–349.
79. Kersten, H.; Kersten, W.; Staudinger, H. J. *Biochim. Biophys. Acta* **1958**, *27*, 598–608.
80. Gliss, D.; Schulze, H–U. *FEBS Lett.* **1975**, *60*, 374–379.
81. Yamauchi, N.; Ogata, K. *Jpn. Soc. Horticult. Res.* **1978**, *47*, 121–127.
82. Schulze, H–U.; Schott, H–H; Standinger, H. J. *Hoppe–Seylers J. Physiol. Chem.* **1972**, *353*, 1931–1942.
83. Wegman, A. *Acta Physiol. Scand.* **1954**, *42*, 363–370.
84. Patterson, J.; Mastin, D. *Am. J. Physiol.* **1951**, *167*, 119–126.
85. Sjostrand, S. E. *Acta Physiol. Scand.* **1970**, *Suppl. 356*, 1–79.
86. Patterson, J. W. *J. Biol. Chem.* **1950**, *183*, 81–85.
87. Merlini, D.; Caramia, F. *J. Cell. Biol.* **1965**, *26*, 245–261.
88. Pillsbury, S.; Watkins, D.; Cooperstein, S. *J. Pharm. Exper. Therap.* **1973**, *185*, 713–718.
89. Hornig, D.; Weber, F.; Wiss, O. *Int. J. Vitam. Nutr. Res.* **1974**, *44*, 217–229.
90. Ibid., *42*, 223–241.
91. Ibid., *42*, 511–523.
92. Hammarstrom, L. *Acta Physiol. Scand.* **1966**, *70 Suppl 289*, 1–84.
93. Hornig, D.; Weiser, H.; Weber, F.; Wiss, O. *Clin. Chim. Acta* **1971**, *32*, 33–39.
94. Ibid. *31*, 25–35.
95. Edgar, J. A. *Nature* **1970**, *227*, 24–26.
96. Edgar, J. A. *Experientia* **1979**, *25*, 1214–1215.
97. Warden, J.; Ferreira, T.; Contreiras, J. *Genet. Iber.* **1972**, *24*, 283–303.
98. Banerjee, S. *Indian J. Physiol. Pharmacol.* **1977**, *21*, 85–93.

RECEIVED for review February 3, 1981. ACCEPTED September 2, 1981.

6

NMR Spectroscopy of Ascorbic Acid and Its Derivatives

J. V. PAUKSTELIS—Department of Chemistry, Kansas State University, Manhattan, KS 66506

D. D. MUELLER—Department of Biochemistry, Kansas State University, Manhattan, KS 66506

P. A. SEIB and D. W. LILLARD, JR.[1]—Department of Grain Science, Kansas State University, Manhattan, KS 66506

^{13}C resonances of L-ascorbic acid (I) at 25.2 MHz were identified from proton-coupled spectra, spin-lattice relaxation times, changes in chemical shifts with ionization, and 4-D isotopic substitution. ^{13}C NMR spectroscopy was used to differentiate 2-O- from 3-O-, and 5-O- from 6-O-substituted derivatives of I. The ^1H NMR spectra of I, 4-D-L-ascorbic acid, 5-D-L-ascorbic acid, D-isoascorbic acid, and 5-D-D-isoascorbic acid were recorded at 600.2 MHz. The proton–proton vicinal coupling constants showed the conformation of the side-chain of I in water to be the same as that in its crystalline state. Unlike the solid state, however, the conformation did not change when I ionized at OH3. In the proton-coupled ^{13}C NMR spectrum of I at 25.2 MHz, virtual coupling occurred between H6, H6', and C4. To resolve $^3J_{C4,H6'}$, spectra must be measured at a field strength exceeding 2.3 T.

The detailed structure of L-ascorbic acid is important in understanding its biological and chemical properties. The formula of L-ascorbic acid (I) was first deduced in 1933 by Herbert et al. (1), and was later confirmed using x-ray crystallography (2). Hvoslef (3), who also examined the structure of sodium L-ascorbate (II), concluded, as others had previously proposed (4,5,6), that the monoanion of I is formed by ionization of OH3, and that the predominant resonance form of the monoanion is the 2,3-enolate form. Data from ^{13}C NMR studies (7) on II also were in accord with those conclusions.

[1] Current address: Spring and Durum Wheat Quality Research Laboratory, SEA, U.S. Department of Agriculture, North Dakota State University, Fargo, ND 58105.

0065-2393/82/0200–0125$07.75/0
© 1982 American Chemical Society

CH₂OH structures:

$$
\begin{array}{c}
\text{CH}_2\text{OH} \\
| \\
\text{H—C—OH}
\end{array}
$$

I   II

From the crystal structure data the ring in the free acid (I) was found to be nearly planar and contain a slight distortion of the lactone atoms out of the ene–diol plane. In the singly charged anion (II), the situation was reversed, and the ene–diol atoms were puckered, whereas the lactone group was virtually planar. Some delocalization of electron density over the ring was evidenced in II by changes in bond lengths and angles when I ionized. In addition, the primary alcohol group (OH6) in II rotated more than 100° from its position in I. Thus, the conformation about the C5–C6 bond changed from that in I where O5 and O6 are nearly antiparallel to a *gauche* orientation in the anion (II). Conformational change may reflect preferential interactions in the crystal that are not necessarily available to the molecule in solution. No intramolecular hydrogen bonds were found in the crystals of I or II (2, 3).

The objectives of this work were to verify the assignments of carbon-13 resonances in L-ascorbic acid (I), to use the carbon-13 chemical shifts to assign positions of substitution in derivatives of I, and to determine the conformational preference of I and its sodium salt (II) in aqueous solution.

¹³C NMR Studies of L-Ascorbic Acid (I)

Commensurate with the biological and chemical importance of I, investigators have studied the NMR properties of this molecule and several of its derivatives (7–10). The investigators generally have agreed to the assignments originally put forth (7,8). However, no complete proof of assignments has been reported.

The {¹H} ¹³C NMR spectrum of L-ascorbic acid is shown in Figure 1A. The most upfield resonance arose from the primary alcohol group at C6 because of its triplet pattern in proton-coupled spectra, and because the chemical shift of 63.1 ppm is typical of primary alcohols in carbohydrates (11). Of the remaining two protonated carbons, which are doubles when proton coupled, C4 would be expected to occur at lower field than C5 because of the ene–diol group in a β-position. This hypothe-

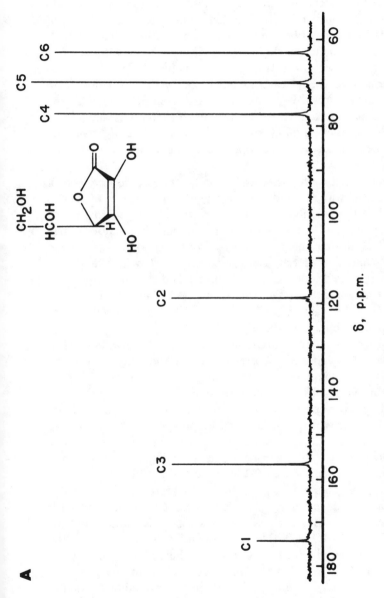

Figure 1A. Proton-decoupled ^{13}C NMR spectrum of L-ascorbic acid in H_2O, pH 2.0, 33°C. Short-range multiplicities arising from proton coupling are C1 (S), C2 (S), C3 (S), C4 (D), C5 (D), and C6 (T), where S, D, and T refer to singlet, doublet, and triplet, respectively. The direct and long-range ^1H–^{13}C coupling constants are summarized in Table VII.

sis was confirmed by preparation of the 4-deutero compound (Figure 1B), which showed only a weak triplet centered at 76.7 ppm. These assignments agree with those given by earlier workers (7, 8).

The assignments for the three nonprotonated carbons in the downfield portion were not as easily deduced. The long-range coupling patterns of those resonances were complex and probably ambiguous (vida infra). Nevertheless, the resonance at 156.4 ppm (Figure 1) had the largest proton coupling constant (∼ 6 Hz) and reasonably could be assigned to C3. Furthermore, carbonyl carbons are typically the most downfield resonances in compounds like L-ascorbic acid, and lactone carbonyl carbons in particular are known to fall in the 170–180-ppm range (11). Therefore, the resonance at 174.0 ppm was assumed initially to correspond to C1. The peak at 118.8 ppm could be assigned to C2 by difference.

To help confirm the proposed assignments, the pH dependence of the chemical shifts was studied. A pH dependence study of I was reported (9), but the solutions apparently were not purged to remove atmospheric oxygen, and under alkaline conditions the solutions may have changed pH during the recordings of the spectra. We repeated the experiment under an inert atmosphere to avoid oxidative degradation of L-ascorbic acid. Our data (Figure 2) and that of Berger (9) are in excellent agreement between pH 2 and 7, but in less than satisfactory agreement between pH 7 and 11. The earlier data show considerably smaller shifts over the higher pH range.

The signal at 156.4 ppm undergoes a 19.3-ppm downfield shift between pH 2 and 6 (Figure 2A), corresponding to the range over which OH3 ionizes (12). Although such a shift is much larger than the 4–5-ppm downfield shift normally observed for ionization of carboxylic acids (11), it almost certainly arose from C3. Over the same pH range, C1 was deshielded by 3.9 ppm, which was enough to prevent C3 from moving downfield of C1 (Figure 2A). Similarly, C4 was shifted downfield by 2.1 ppm (Figure 2B). On the other hand, C2 moved upfield by 4.6 ppm, and the side-chain carbons C5 and C6 were deshielded by 0.55 and 0.46 ppm, respectively. Consequently, ionization of L-ascorbic acid at C3 also shifts the signals of the other ring carbons more than is observed for adjacent carbons in simple carboxylic acids. This is caused by the lengthening of the C2–C3, C3–C4, C1–O1, and C2–O2 bonds in the monoanion (II) compared with I, as well as the shortening of the C1–C2 and C3–O3 bonds (2, 3). Furthermore, delocalization of electron density throughout the ene–diol and carbonyl groups probably is mainly responsible for the abnormally large downfield shift of C3 upon ionization.

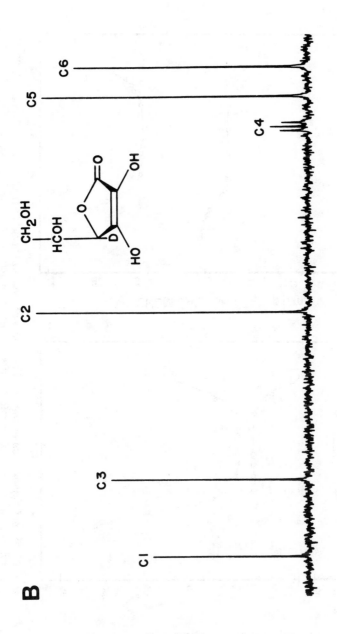

Figure 1B. Proton-decoupled ^{13}C *NMR spectrum of 4-D-ʟ-ascorbic acid in* H_2O, *pH 2.3, 33°C. Deuteration at C4 produced a 0.41-ppm upfield shift in the C4 peak. Shifts are relative to internal* Me_4Si.

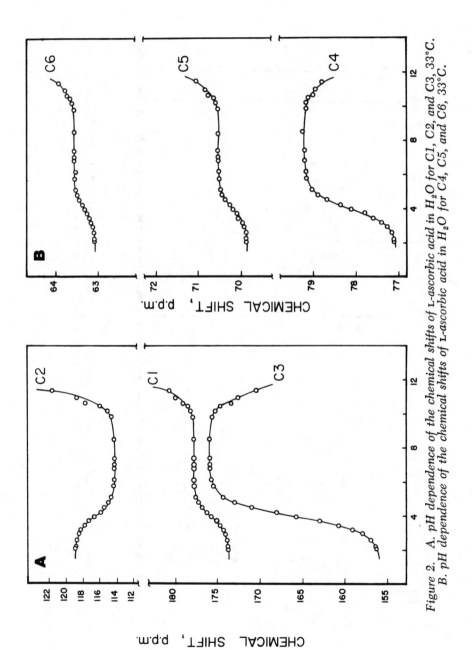

Figure 2. A. pH dependence of the chemical shifts of L-ascorbic acid in H_2O for C1, C2, and C3, 33°C. B. pH dependence of the chemical shifts of L-ascorbic acid in H_2O for C4, C5, and C6, 33°C.

Between pH 6 and 9 no substantial shifts in the carbon resonances of II were noted. Above pH 10, OH2 began to ionize and the C2 resonance moved downfield rapidly with increasing pH, while the C3 and C4 peaks shifted upfield, which reversed the trend seen between pH 2 and 7. Carbons C1, C5, and C6 continued to show increased deshielding at pH values above 10. Perhaps the tendency toward increased delocalization seen with the first ionization was reversed somewhat when C2 ionized. The continued downfield shift of C1, however, would not fit that explanation.

Further confirmation of the assignments of the nonprotonated carbons was obtained from measurement of spin-lattice relaxation times (T_1). Relaxation times for the carbons of I determined in deuterium oxide solution at 33°C and pH 1.6 are summarized in Table I. The relaxation times of C4, C5, and C6 are typical of protonated carbon atoms in an isotropically tumbling molecule of this size, but the relaxation times of nonprotonated carbons are unusually long. However, the trend among the relaxation times of the nonprotonated carbons was of increasing time with increasing distance from H4. This trend would be expected if the assignments were correct and H4 made the major contribution to the dipolar relaxation of the ring carbons. The unusually inefficient relaxations of the nonprotonated carbon atoms in I will be discussed elsewhere (13). Again the assignments for nonprotonated carbons agree with those reported earlier (7, 8).

NMR Studies of Derivatives of L-Ascorbic Acid.

Researchers have used ^{13}C NMR spectroscopy to assign structure to several ester and ether derivatives of I. That method is particularly useful to differentiate 2-O- and 3-O-substituted derivatives of I because ionization of the OH3 induces the large downfield shift of C3, as previously discussed. Thus, 2-O-methyl-L-ascorbic acid, but not 3-O-methyl-L-ascorbic acid, showed a 16-ppm change in the chemical shift of C3 when the pH values of their solutions were changed from 2 to 7 (Table II). At pH 7, the chemical shifts of the C3 carbons in L-ascorbate (II) and in its 2-sulfate and 2-phosphate esters were similar in magnitude (Table II).

Table I.   Spin-Lattice Relaxation Times for the Carbon Atoms of L-Ascorbic Acid

Carbon Atom	1	2	3	4	5	6
NT_1 (sec)[a]	132	98	38	1.60	1.44	2.02

Note: In D_2O under N_2, pH 1.6 (meter reading in D_2O using a glass electrode), 33°C.

[a] N, number of directly bonded protons, if not zero.

Table II. Chemical Shifts[a] for Carbons in L-Ascorbic Acid and Several Derivatives

Derivative of L-Ascorbic Acid	Carbon Atom					
	1	2	3	4	5	6
	pH 2.0–2.1[b]					
Unsubsituted (this work)	174.0	118.8	156.4	77.1	69.9	63.1
2-O-Methyl[c] (14)	173.7 (−0.3)[d]	122.5 (3.7)	162.1 (5.7)	77.0 (−0.1)	69.7 (−0.2)	62.8 (−0.3)
3-O-Methyl[c] (14, 10)	174.1 (0.1)	119.2 (0.4)	155.9 (−0.5)	76.9 (−0.2)	69.8 (−0.1)	62.8 (−0.3)
	pH 6.5–7.0[b]					
Unsubsituted (this work)	178.0	114.1	176.2	79.2	70.6	63.6
2-O-Methyl[c] (14)	179.4 (1.4)[d]	119.3 (5.2)	178.1 (2.1)	79.3 (0.1)	70.4 (−0.2)	63.3 (−0.3)
3-O-Methyl[c] (14, 10)	174.8 (−3.2)	120.4 (6.3)	155.0 (−21.2)	76.8 (−2.4)	70.0 (−0.6)	63.0 (−0.6)
2-Sulfate (10, 15)	181.1 (3.1)	111.6 (−2.5)	176.7 (0.5)	79.9 (0.7)	70.7 (0.1)	63.5 (0.1)
2-Phosphate (10, 15)	177.4 (−0.6)	113.2[f] (−0.9)	177.0 (0.8)	78.7 (−0.5)	70.1 (−0.5)	62.9 (−0.7)

[a] Chemical shifts (δ from Me_4Si).
[b] pH meter reading in D_2O using a glass electrode.
[c] Signal of OMe at 61.2 and 61.6 ppm, pH 2 and 7, respectively.
[d] Difference between chemical shift of parent compound (I or II) and derivative.
[e] Signal of OMe at 60.2 and 60.1 ppm at pH 2 and 7, respectively.
[f] Doublet with splitting 7.3 Hz (^{13}C–^{31}P coupling).

The monoanion (II) involves OH3 (3); therefore, 2-substitution of the phosphate and sulfate groups is indicated.

The ^{13}C NMR spectrum of 3-O-methyl-L-ascorbic acid and that of its parent compound (I) were almost identical at pH 2 (Table II). The 3-methyl derivative is a vinyl ether, and it could have been hydrolyzed at pH 2 during recording of the spectrum. However, hydrolysis did not occur since the methyl signal was observed at 60.2 ppm and no methanol signal was found at 48 ppm.

Because the signal of H4 moves upfield by approximately 0.5 ppm when OH3 ionizes, ^1H NMR spectroscopy also can be used to differentiate between 2-O- and 3-O-substituted derivatives of I. The upfield shifts for H4 in several 2-O-substituted derivatives of I are given in Table

Table III.   Proton Magnetic Resonances of
L-Ascorbic Acid and Several Derivatives

Derivative of L-Ascorbic Acid	pH	Chemical Shift[a] (δ)			
		H4	$\Delta H4$[b]	H5	H6, H6'
Free acid (16)	2	4.97	—	4.09	3.76
	7	4.50	0.47	4.02	3.74
3-O-Methyl[c] (14)	2	4.91	—	4.02	3.71
	7	4.90	0.01	4.01	3.71
2-O-Methyl[d] (14)	2	4.90	—	4.01	3.76
	7	4.49	0.41	4.00	3.71
2-Sulfate (16)	1	5.02	—	4.20	3.76
	7	4.57	0.45	4.05	3.73
2-Phosphate (16)	1	5.00	—	4.16	3.74
	7	4.60	0.40	4.05	3.70
2,2'-Phosphoric diester (16)	1	5.00	—	4.15	3.78
	12	4.50	0.50	4.02	3.68

[a] Determined in D_2O at 60 or 100 MHz. Chemical shifts in ppm from internal DSS. Chemical shifts of H5 and H6 are reported as the center of the recorded peaks.
[b] $\Delta H4$ is the upfield shift of H4 on changing the pH of the medium.
[c] Signal of OMe was 4.18 ppm at pH 2 and 7. At pH 10, the spectrum showed degradation of the 3-methyl ether.
[d] Signal of OMe was 3.69 ppm at pH 2 and 3.62 ppm at pH 7.

III. The H4 signal of the 3-methyl ether failed to shift to higher field at pH 7.

Data from UV spectroscopy are helpful in distinguishing 2- and 3-derivatives of L-ascorbic acid. The ionization of OH3 is accompanied by a bathochromic shift of approximately 20 nm (Table IV).

Workers have used ^{13}C NMR spectroscopy to assign structures to the 5- and 6-sulfate esters of L-ascorbic acid and to the 4Z and 4E isomers of 2-sulfo-2,3,4,6-tetrahydroxyhexa-2,4-dienoate-δ-lactone (Table V). Sulfonation at C6 (C5) of L-ascorbic acid shifted the signal of C6 (C5) downfield by 7–8 ppm; the signal(s) of the adjacent carbon(s) moved slightly upfield (18). Those shifts were noted previously by others (19) in sugar sulfates. When I was dissolved in concentrated sulfuric acid-d_2, ^{13}C NMR shows approximately 90% monosulfonation at C6 (18).

The 2-sulfate ester of 4Z-2,3,4,6-tetrahydroxyhexa-2,4-dienoate-δ-lactone (4,5-dehydroascorbate 2-sulfate) was characterized largely by ^{13}C NMR and ^1H NMR. The data in Table V show that the signals of C4 and C5 were shifted downfield 70 and 38 ppm, respectively, compared to their positions in the spectrum of L-ascorbate at pH 7. In addition, the resonances of C1 and C3 moved upfield approximately 5 ppm upon introduction of the 4,5-double bond.

Table IV. UV Spectral Properties of L-Ascorbic
Acid and Several Derivatives

Derivative of L-Ascorbic Acid	Acid (pH 2.0)		Neutral (pH 7.0)		Base (pH 10.0)	
	λ_{max}	ϵ_{mM}	λ_{max}	ϵ_{mM}	ϵ_{mM}	λ_{max}
Free acid (17)	243	10	265	16.5	—	—
2-O-Methyl (14)	239	8.5	260	12.3	—	—
3-O-Methyl (17)	244	9	244	9	—	—
2-O-(Phenylphosphono)[a]	233	9.6	257	14.5	258	15
3-O-(Phenylphosphono)[a]	237	8	238	8	263	8
2-Sulfate (16)	232	11	255	16.3	255	16.3
2-Phosphate (16)	238	9	258	11.5	264	16.0
2,2'-Phosphoric diester (16)	236	17.3	258	21.6	259	30.2

[a] 5,6-Isopropylidene acetal; data from Bond et al. (17).

Tentatively, the Z-configuration was assigned to the 4,5-ene bond in the derivative prepared from L-ascorbic acid. This assignment was based on the stereochemical argument that in the transition state of the elimination reaction, H4 and O5 assume an antiparallel orientation. Using the same argument the E-configuration was assigned to the isomer prepared from D-isoascorbic acid (III). The ^{13}C data in Table V show that both isomers have been isolated. The scheme used to prepare the

III

4,5-dehydro derivatives is shown in Scheme 1. Other 4,5-dehydro derivatives of I are known (20).

The structure of the 4,5-dehydro compounds was verified using ^1H NMR spectroscopy; the spectrum of the Z-isomer at pH 6.2 is shown in Figure 3. The signal of H5 was a triplet centered at 5.59 ppm with $J_{H5,H6}$ = 7.3 Hz, and H6 was a doublet at 4.34 ppm. For the E-isomer at pH

Table V. ¹³C NMR and UV Data for Several Monosulfate Esters

Derivative of L-Ascorbic Acid	¹³C Chemical Shifts (δ-Values in H₂O at pH 6.5–7.0)			¹³C Chemical Shifts (δ-Values in H₂O at pH 6.5–7.0)			UV (λmax in H₂O)	
	C1	C2	C3	C4	C5	C6	pH 2	pH 7
Sodium salt (this work)	178.0	114.1	176.2	79.2	70.6	63.6	244	265
5-Sulfate (18)	177.6 (−0.4)	113.9 (−0.2)	175.7 (−0.5)	77.6 (−1.6)	77.4 (6.8)	61.4 (−2.2)	245	267
6-Sulfate (18)	179.4 (1.4)	116.1 (2.0)	176.1 (−0.1)	80.5 (1.3)	69.8 (−0.8)	71.5 (7.9)	244	266
(Z)-4,5-Dehydro-2-sulfate (this work)[a]	172.7 (−5.3)	114.2 (0.1)	171.2 (−5.0)	149.4 (70.2)	108.2 (37.6)	57.7 (−5.4)	260	244
(E)-4,5-Dehydro-2-sulfate (this work)[b]	172.6 (−5.4)	116.0 (1.9)	170.2 (−6.0)	148.4 (69.2)	108.6 (38.0)	58.4 (−5.2)	260	247

[a] Prepared starting from L-ascorbic acid.
[b] Prepared starting from D-isoascorbic acid.

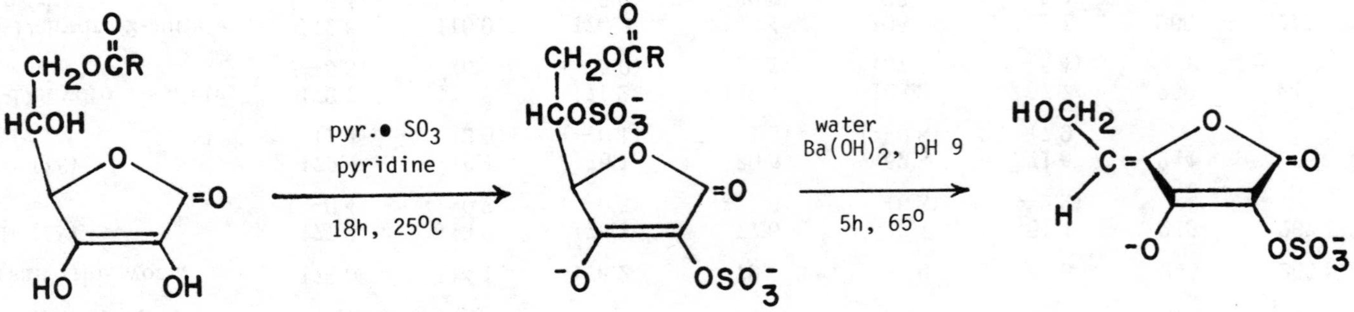

Scheme 1. Synthesis of 4,5-dehydroascorbate 2-sulfate.

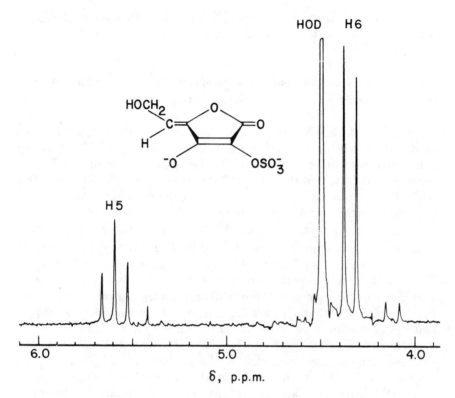

Figure 3.   100-MHz ¹H NMR spectrum of 4Z-2-sulfo-2,3,4,6-tetrahydroxyhexa-2,4-dieonate-δ-lactone (4,5-dehydroascorbate 2-sulfate) in D_2O, pH (meter reading) 6.2, 33°C. Shifts are from internal Me_4Si.

5.9, H5 was a triplet at 5.80 ppm with $J_{H5,H6} = 6.6$ Hz, and H6 was a doublet at 4.59 ppm.

As mentioned previously, ionization of OH3 in L-ascorbic acid is accompanied by a shift in λ_{max} to longer wavelengths. However, the opposite is true in the case of the 4,5-dehydro-2-sulfate derivatives (Table V). At pH 0.5–1.0 those derivatives gave λ_{max} of 260–262 nm, but at pH 7 λ_{max} was 244–247 nm. Apparently most of the charge in the anion is on O1 (Scheme 2), whereas most of the charge on the ascorbate monoanion (**II**) is on O3 (3).

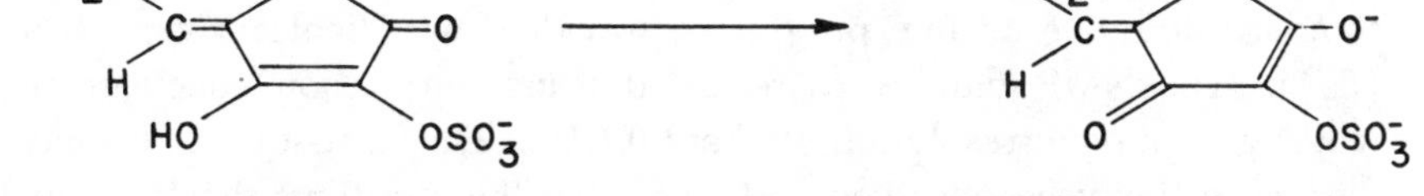

Scheme 2.   Ionization of 4,5-dehydroascorbate-2-sulfate.

Tolbert and Ward have reviewed the ^{13}C NMR data on dehydro-L-ascorbic acid in chapter 5 in this book.

^{1}H NMR Spectroscopy and the Conformations of L-Ascorbic Acid and D-Isoascorbic Acid in Aqueous Solution

In 1977 ^{13}C NMR spectroscopy was used to assign a conformation to the side-chain of L-ascorbic acid (I) in water (21). That report stimulated us to measure the 600-MHz ^{1}H NMR spectra of I and D-iso-ascorbic acid (III) and their 4- and 5-deutero derivatives. The 600-MHz ^{1}H NMR spectra were analyzed, and the vicinal coupling constants were used to predict preferred conformations.

The ^{1}H NMR spectrum of L-ascorbic acid at low fields has been observed by many groups and was published (22). The results at 100 MHz gave $^3J_{H4, H5}$ of 1.8 Hz, but the coupling constants between H5, H6, and H6′ could not be obtained by inspection because they were strongly coupled. However, the 100-MHz spectrum of I can be simulated by machine computation with a high degree of correlation when $^3J_{H5, H6}$ and $^3J_{H5, H6'}$ are assumed to be 6.6 Hz, which is a typical value in ethane derivatives (23). But if H6 and H6′ have different chemical shifts and different coupling constants, that is, $^3J_{H5, H6}$ does not equal $^3J_{H5, H6'}$, the computer simulation with the assumed equivalent coupling constants would still arrive at an apparently correct solution because at 100 MHz it is very difficult to experimentally measure all the spectral lines. To detect the difference between the two coupling constants in question, the spectrometer would have to record spectral lines that are 0.1% of the most intense lines. That sensitivity would require a signal-to-noise ratio in excess of 2000:1, which is not readily obtainable at 100 MHz. No high-field spectra of L-ascorbic acid have been published, although some preliminary spectra at 360 MHz were made available to us (24).

We have examined L-ascorbic acid and its 4-D and 5-D derivatives at 600.2 MHz at the Carnegie–Mellon NMR Facility for Biomedical Studies. We also obtained data on D-isoascorbic acid and its 5-D derivative. The simulated and observed spectra for H5, H6, and H6′ of I are shown at pH 2 and 7 in Figures 4 and 5. Table VI presents the coupling constants obtained from computer simulation of the spin system using a standard iterative fitting program [provided by Nicolet Corporation (25)]. The NMR data were recorded using correlation spectroscopy, which gave a point resolution of about 0.1 Hz. The least-squares fits gave differences between observed and computed line positions that averaged 0.04 Hz. Consequently, the J values are accurate to at least ± 0.1 Hz.

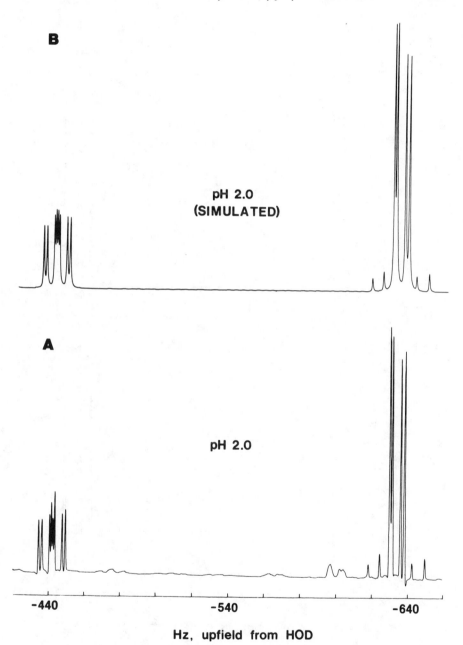

Figure 4.   A. Observed 600.2-MHz [superscript]1*H NMR spectrum for H5, H6, and H6′ of* L*-ascorbic acid in* D_2O*, pH (meter reading) 2.1.   B. Computer simulated spectrum giving the calculated* [superscript]1*H–*[superscript]1*H coupling constants listed in Table VI.*

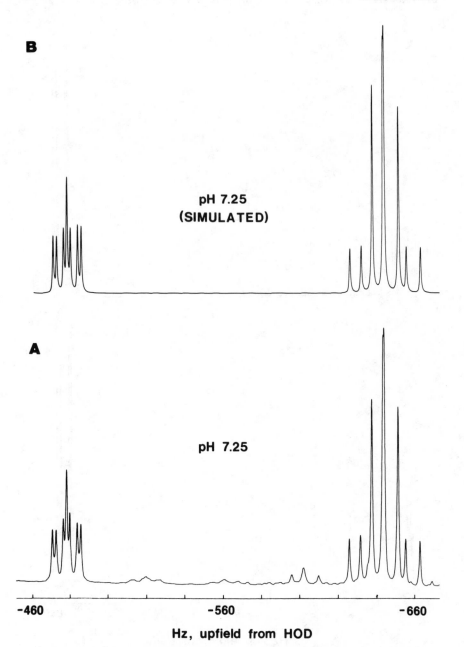

Figure 5.   A.   Observed 600.2-MHz ^{1}H NMR spectrum for H5 and
H6,H6' of L-ascorbic acid in D_2O, pH (meter reading) 7.25.   B. Computer
simulated spectrum giving the calculated ^{1}H–^{1}H coupling constants listed
in Table VI.

Table VI.   Proton–Proton Coupling Constants and $\Delta\delta_{6,6'}$ for L-Ascorbic and D-Isoascorbic Acids

Compound	pH	$^3J_{4,5}$	$^3J_{5,6}$	$^3J_{5,6'}$	$^2J_{6,6'}$	$\Delta\delta_{6,6'}$
L-Ascorbic	2.06[a]	1.83	5.81	7.34	−11.55[b]	6.48
	7.25	1.93	5.65	7.63	−11.60	14.77
4-D-L-Ascorbic	2.04	—	5.76	7.36	−11.55	6.29
	7.09	—	5.74	7.65	−11.73	14.42
5-D-L-Ascorbic	2.35	—	—	—	−11.61	6.37
	7.20	—	—	—	−11.58	14.63
D-Isoascorbic	NR[c]	NR	NR	NR	NR	NR
	7.09	2.96	3.24	7.93	−11.99	6.19
5-D-D-Isoascorbic	2.45	—	—	—	−11.85	12.62
	7.76	—	—	—	−11.95	6.25

Note: Data computed from spectra obtained at 600.2 MHz in D_2O. Probable error in $J \sim 0.10$ Hz.
[a] pH meter readings in D_2O using a glass electrode.
[b] Assumed to be negative in the simulation, and all vicinal coupling constants assumed to be positive.
[c] Not recorded.

The information in Table VI may be summarized as follows: $^3J_{H5,H6}$ did not equal $^3J_{H5,H6'}$ for either isomer; no changes in geminal or vicinal coupling constants occurred between pH 2 and 7 for L-ascorbic acid, except for a slight change in $^3J_{H5,H6'}$, which was barely outside the error limits; at pH 2 the difference in chemical shifts between H6 and H6' for L-ascorbic acid was 6.4 Hz but at pH 7 it was 14.6 Hz; and the difference in chemical shifts between H6 and H6' was reversed for D-isoascorbic, that is, the difference was 12.6 Hz at pH 2 and 6.2 Hz at pH 7.

The fact that $^3J_{5H,H6}$ did not equal $^3J_{H5,H6'}$ indicated that it might be possible to determine the conformation of the side-chain in L-ascorbic acid. Furthermore, the NMR data gave no evidence of conformation change between pH 2 and 7, in contrast with x-ray data (3). The conformation previously assigned (21) to the C5–C6 bond of **I** in water is not consistent with the 600-MHz ^1H NMR data.

The values of $^3J_{H5,H6}$ and $^3J_{H5,H6'}$ observed for **I**, which were 5.7 and 7.5 Hz, respectively, did not appear at first glance to be consistent with the theoretical values of approximately 3 Hz and 10 Hz normally observed for gauche and antiparallel conformations of vicinal protons. However, electronegative substituents modify the magnitude of vicinal coupling constants (26). In cyclic compounds, such as steroids (27) or 4-t-butylcyclohexanols (28), coupling values of 5.5 ± 1 Hz vs. 2.5–3.2 Hz are possible for protons separated by identical dihedral angles of 60°.

The difference in magnitude is attributed to the orientation of a coupled proton with respect to an adjacent OH group. The orientation effect was shown by Booth (29) to be maximal (smallest J) when an electronegative substituent is antiparallel to each of the coupled protons.

If the electronegativity effect is taken into account, the observed coupling constant of 1.83 Hz for $^3J_{H4, H5}$ in I may be assigned to rotamer A (Figure 6) where H4 is antiparallel to O5 and H5 is antiparallel to O4. Rapid rotation (averaging) around the C4–C5 bond in I would be expected to make $^3J_{H5, H4}$ larger, not smaller, than the observed value. Thus, the value of 1.83 Hz is quite reasonable for the conformation shown in Figure 6A, which is identical with the original assignment of the side-chain in L-ascorbic acid (21).

The increased magnitude of $^3J_{H4, H5}$ (2.94 Hz) for D-isoascorbic acid (III) compared to 1.8 Hz in I provides support for rotamer 9A in L-ascorbic acid. The value of 2.94 Hz for $^3J_{H4, H5}$ also suggests a *gauche* orientation of H4 and H5 in III (rotamers B and C, Figure 7). Those rotamers contain only one proton antiparallel to an oxygen, and $^3J_{H4, H5}$ would be expected to be greater in magnitude in III than it is in I.

The three staggered rotamers around the C5–C6 bond of L-ascorbic acid are shown in Figure 8. Compound I at pH 2 (Table VI) gave the coupling constants $^3J_{H5, H6}$, $^3J_{H5, H6'}$, and $^2J_{H6, H6'}$ equal to 5.81, 7.34, and -11.55 Hz, respectively. Rotamer 9C can be ruled out since the coupling constants are unequal for H5–H6 and H5–H6'. Rotamer 9B appears to fit the NMR data better than rotamer 9A. Both rotamers have a pair of antiparallel protons that can be assigned to the coupling constant 7.34 Hz, but the other coupling constant of 5.81 Hz is better assigned to the *gauche* coupling in rotamer 9B, where neither of the protons is antiparallel to an adjacent oxygen. The observed value of 5.81 Hz is just slightly greater than the range (4.5–5.5 Hz) proposed (29) for this type of coupling.

Application of the same arguments to the C6–C5 bond III (Figure 9) shows rotamer 10A to be the most probable. The calculated coupling constants for III at pH 7.09 were 3.24, 7.93, and -11.99 Hz for $^3J_{H5, H6}$, $^3J_{H5, 'H6'}$, and $^3J_{H6, H6'}$, respectively. The coupling constants for H5–H6' and H6–H6' were almost identical to those observed for I. The only value that differed substantially was $^3J_{H5, H6}$, which was 3.24 Hz. Based on these values, rotamer 10B can be eliminated immediately. Of the remaining two rotamers, 10A is preferred over 10C because 10A should have a smaller value of $^3J_{H5, H6}$ than rotamer 10C. Furthermore, rotamer 10C contains no oxygens antiparallel to either H5 or H6.

Different coupling constants between H5–H6 and H5–H6' can occur only if there is a preferred conformation for L-ascorbic acid around the C5–C6 bond. The C4–C5 bond of I also exists in a preferred conforma-

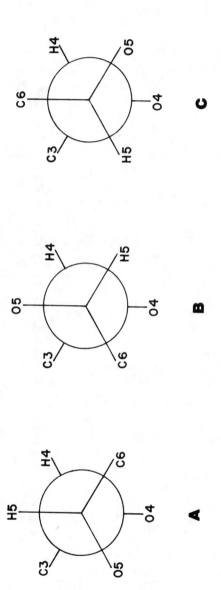

Figure 6. Newman projection viewed down the C5–C4 bond of L-ascorbic acid.

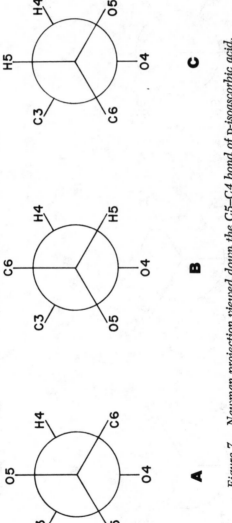

Figure 7. Newman projection viewed down the C5–C4 bond of D-isoascorbic acid.

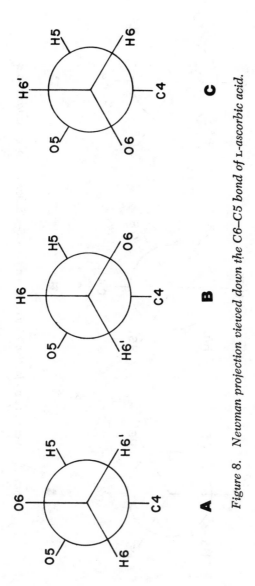

Figure 8. Newman projection viewed down the C6–C5 bond of L-ascorbic acid.

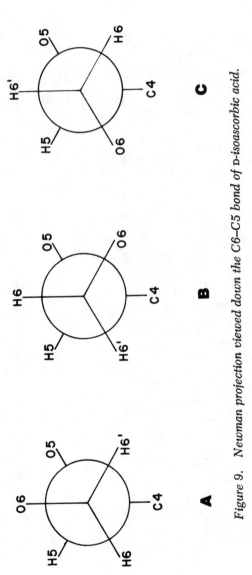

Figure 9.   Newman projection viewed down the C6–C5 bond of D-isoascorbic acid.

tion in solution, as evidenced by the small value for $^3J_{H4,H5}$ of 1.83 Hz. This value is too low to result from time-averaging, and therefore requires a preferred conformation. The preferred rotamer 7A around C4–C5 and rotamer 9B around the C5–C6 bond are essentially the same conformations found by Hvoslef (2) in crystalline L-ascorbic acid. Since no intramolecular hydrogen bonds occur in the crystal (2), none would be expected when I is dissolved in a hydrogen-bonding solvent such as water. Thus, our result is not surprising. What is surprising is that no change in the conformation of the side-chain is apparent when a solution of I is changed from pH 2 to 7. One might expect a conformational change corresponding to that observed in the crystalline state (3). Vicinal coupling constants however, in ^1H NMR data do not indicate any appreciable change in side-chain conformation upon ionization at OH3.

^{13}C NMR Spectroscopy and the Conformation of L-Ascorbic Acid

The paper of Ogawa et al. (21) prompted us to examine the use of ^{13}C NMR spectroscopy to verify the conformation of I determined by ^1H NMR. Those workers (21) reported that $^3J_{C4,H6}$ and $^3J_{C4,H6'}$ equal 2.4 Hz, which would fix the conformation around the C5–C6 bond of I as shown in rotamer 9A. They also concluded that rotamer 7A was required to explain the observed coupling constants. Spoormaker and de Bie (30) suggested that no conformation was preferred around the C5–C6 bond, but instead that equal rotamer populations explained the observed data.

We recently recorded the proton-coupled ^{13}C NMR spectrum of I. Our $^1H–^{13}C$ coupling constants and the literature values are presented in Table VII. The ^1H NMR data at 600 MHz affirmed that rotamer 9B is the preferred conformation at the C5–C6 bond. The $^1H–^{13}C$ coupling data have led to a different conformational assignment than the $^1H–^1H$ coupling data because virtual coupling is involved in the ABX spin system formed by H6, H6', and C4. The virtual coupling yields a deceptively simple spectrum at 25.2 MHz; this spectrum shows too few lines and yields (31) an average value of $^3J_{C4,H6}$ and $^3J_{C4,H6'}$. The conditions for virtual coupling involving H6 and H6' are present in L-ascorbic acid. The H6 and H6' nuclei are nearly isochronous yet are not magnetically equivalent, as shown in the 600 MHz spectra. The chemical shift difference between H6 and H6' at 2.3 T field is about 1.1 Hz with a coupling constant of about 11 Hz. Thus $\Delta\delta/J$ equals approximately 0.1 and the coupling constants cannot be determined by inspection (32). To determine if virtual coupling is the cause of the discrepancy, coupled ^{13}C NMR spectra need to be obtained at the highest possible field. At 9.4 T, $\Delta\delta/J = 0.4$ and if an experiment were run at elevated pH, such as 7, the

Table VII. Carbon–Proton Coupling Constants for L-Ascorbic Acid

^{13}C

Proton	C1	C2	C3	C4	C5	C6
H4	1.87[a]	1.96	5.70	153.1	0.2	1.4
	(2.0)[b]	(2.0)	(5.9)	(152.8)	—	(1.0)
H5	< 0.5[c]	< 0.5[c]	1.20[c]	1.85	145.6	5.40
	—	—	(1.5)	(2.0)	—	(5.4)
H6	—	—	—	2.55	—	144.3
	—	—	—	(2.0–2.4)	—	(145.0)
H6′	—	—	—	2.55	—	144.3
	—	—	—	(2.0–2.4)	—	(145.0)

Note: Data given as Hz; pH 2.31 (pH meter reading in D_2O with a glass electrode).
[a] Probable error of $J = 0.1$ Hz.
[b] Data taken from Ref. 21; reported precision $\pm$ 0.24 Hz.
[c] From 4-D-L-ascorbic acid.

value of $\Delta\delta/J$ would be greater than 1. Under those circumstances $^3J_{C4, H6}$ and $^3J_{C4, H6'}$ without ambiguity might be determined. Such an experiment is in progress.

Experimental

NMR.   Most ^{13}C NMR and ^1H NMR spectra of L-ascorbic acid and its derivatives were recorded from aqueous solutions using a Varian Model XL-100-15 spectrometer interfaced to a Nicolet 1180 digital computer and to a Nicolet 1093B pulse Fourier transform system with quadrature phase detection. Some ^1H NMR spectra were also obtained at 600.2 MHz in deuterium oxide on the Carnegie–Mellon instrument. All ^{13}C NMR samples were in 12-mm, and all ^1H NMR in 5-mm, sample tubes. In most cases dioxane was used as an internal reference for ^{13}C NMR spectroscopy and the shifts were calculated as follows: $\delta_{Me_4Si} = \delta_{dioxane} + 67.40$ ppm. For ^1H NMR spectroscopy, and in a few instances for ^{13}C NMR, sodium 2,2-dimethyl-2-silapentan-5-sulfonate (DSS) was used as the internal reference and its shift was assumed to equal that of tetramethylsilane. All shifts are reported relative to tetramethylsilane. Full-range ^{13}C NMR spectra normally were acquired using 16K time domain data points with 40–50 degree pulse widths and 3–5 s delays between pulses. Some partial-range proton-coupled spectra were collected under higher point resolution (2–4 points/Hz) to give more accurate coupling constants. The ^1H NMR spectra were acquired routinely at 4 spectral points/Hz resolution on the XL-100.

The pH dependence of the ^{13}C NMR chemical shifts was determined on 0.5-M samples of L-ascorbic acid in water using a 5-mm concentric capillary tube containing deuterium oxide and DSS to provide the lock and reference signals, respectively. The pH of an initially acidic solution was adjusted upward with 1 M sodium hydroxide directly in the NMR tube while purging with nitrogen. The pH was measured with a Beckman Centry-SS meter equipped with a 3-mm diameter Ingold combination electrode (Wilmad Glass Co., Inc.). All pH values were obtained following data acquisition. The values did not vary by more than 0.15 units, however, from the initial readings. The shifts reported were corrected for the 1.75-ppm difference between external DSS in deuterium oxide and internal DSS in water with the external signal occurring more upfield.

Spin-lattice relaxation times for the carbon atoms of L-ascorbic acid treated with Chelex-100 (Bio-Rad Laboratories) were determined on 0.25 M solutions in deuterium oxide purged with nitrogen. The inversion–recovery method (*33–35*) with alternating phases and 8–10 τ values was used for the protonated carbons, and the homo-spoil technique with 6–8 τ values was used for the nonprotonated atoms. The spin-lattice relaxation times (T_1) were calculated from the data using the appropriate Nicolet (*25*) digital computer programs. The T_1-values for the nonprotonated carbon atoms were repeated using the inversion recovery method and were virtually identical to those reported in Table 1.

Barium 4Z- and 4E-2-Sulfo-2,3,4,6-tetrahydroxyhexa-2,4-dienoate-δ-lactone. The procedure of Cousins et al. (*36*) was used to prepare L-ascorbyl 6-valerate (mp 89–92°C). The valerate ester (15 g, 57.6 mmol) was dissolved in pyridine (250 mL) at 25°C and pyridine–sulfur trioxide complex (25 g, 2.5 equivalents) was added. After stirring 18 h at room temperature, water (500 mL) was added, and the mixture was placed in a water bath at 70°C. The pH of the mixture was maintained at 9–9.5 by periodic addition of saturated barium hydroxide solution. The elimination reaction at 65°C was complete in 4–6 h, as evidenced by the constancy of the reaction pH. The reaction mixture was adjusted to pH 10 by addition of saturated barium hydroxide, and at that point the total volume of the mixture was 1.5 L. Pyridine was removed by evaporation under vacuum to 300 mL, and the evaporation step repeated twice after addition of water (250 mL). The mixture was adjusted to pH 2 by addition of sulfuric acid (1 M), and barium sulfate was removed by filtration. The filtrate was extracted with ethyl ether (3 × 500 mL) to remove valeric acid, and the aqueous layer (∼ 300 mL) was adjusted to pH 7 by addition of barium hydroxide. After evaporation to 50 mL, barium sulfate was removed, and an equal volume of acetonitrile was added to the filtrate. The desired compound crystallized in the cold to give 12.0 g (55%) of crude material with mp 215–225°C. The crystals were dissolved in water (30 mL) and were decolorized with charcoal; after addition of acetonitrile, analytically pure crystals were obtained [yield, 5 g with mp 220–225°C (decomposed)].

Analysis. Calculated for $C_6H_4O_8SBa \cdot \frac{1}{2}H_2O$: C, 18.85; H, 1.31. Found: C, 18.95; H, 1.29. UV data: pH 0.5–1.0, λ_{max} 260 nm; pH 6.5 λ_{max} 244; ε_{mM}, 14.6. The ionization of OH3 had a pK_a of 2.0, determined from the change in λ_{max} between pH 0.5 and 7.0.

The *E*-isomer was prepared in the same manner starting from D-isoascorbic acid (III, 26 g). The 6-valerate ester of III was a syrup, and the yields of crude and pure crystals of the *E*-isomer were 8.1 g and 2.3 g, respectively. The mp of the pure material was 235–240°C (decomposed).

Analysis. Calculated for $C_6H_4O_8SBa$: C, 19.30; H, 1.08; S, 8.58; and Ba, 36.77. Found: C, 19.40; H, 1.25; S, 8.58; and Ba, 37.01. UV data: pH 7, λ_{max} 248; ε_{mM}, 11.6.

Acknowledgments

We thank J. Dadok at the Carnegie–Mellon NMR Facility for Biomedical Studies for help in obtaining the 600-MHz NMR data, and National Institutes of Health for support of the Facility. We also thank Thomas C. Crawford and Glenn C. Andrews of Pfizer, Incorporated, for samples of 5-D-L-ascorbic acid and 5-D-D-isoascorbic acid; and the Kansas State Agricultural Experiment Station for support of the campus NMR facility.

Literature Cited

 1. Herbert, R. W.; Hirst, E. L.; Percival, E. G. V.; Reynolds, R. J. W.; Smith, F. *J. Chem. Soc.* **1933**, 1275.
 2. Hvoself, J. *Acta Crystallogr. Sect. B* **1968**, *24*, 23.
 3. Hvoself, J. *Acta Crystallogr. Sect. B* **1969**, *25*, 2214.
 4. Von Euler, H.; Eistert, B. "Chemie und Biochemie der Reduktone und Reducktonate"; F. Enke: Stuttgart, 1957.
 5. Eigen, M.; Ilgenfritz, G.; Kruse, W. *Chem. Ber.* **1965**, *98*, 1623.
 6. Hurd, C. D. *J. Chem. Educ.* **1970**, *47*, 481.
 7. Billman, J. H.; Sojka, S. A.; Taylor, P. R. *J. Chem. Soc. Perkin Trans. 2* **1972**, 2034.
 8. Matwiyoff, N. A.; Tolbert, B. M., private communication.
 9. Berger, S. *Tetrahedron* **1977**, *33*, 1587.
10. Radford, T.; Sweeney, J. G.; Iacobucci, G. A.; Goldsmith, D. J. *J. Org. Chem.* **1979**, *44*, 658.
11. Stothers, J. B. "Carbon-13 NMR Spectroscopy"; Academic: New York, 1972.
12. Bell, R. P.; Robinson, R. R. *Trans. Faraday Soc.* **1961**, *57*, 965.
13. Mueller, D. D.; Seib, P. A.; Paukstelis, J. V., unpublished data.
14. Lillard, D. W., Jr., Ph.D. Dissertation, Kansas State Univ., Manhattan, 1980.
15. Lee, C. H. Ph.D. Dissertation, Kansas State Univ., Manhattan, 1976.
16. Lee, C. H.; Seib, P. A.; Liang, Y. T.; Hoseney, R. C.; Deyoe, C. W. *Carbohydr. Res.* **1978**, *67*, 127.
17. Bond, A. D.; McClelland, B. W.; Einstein, J. R.; Finamore, F. J. *Arch. Biochem. Biophys.* **1972**, *153*, 207.
18. Lillard, D. W., Jr.; Seib, P. A. In "Carbohydrate Sulfates," Schweiger, R. G., Ed.; *ACS Symp. Ser.* **1978**, 77.
19. Honda, S.; Yuki, H.; Takiura, K. *Carbohydr. Res.* **1973**, *28*, 150.
20. Eitelman, S. J.; Hall, R. H.; Jordon, A. *J. Chem. Soc., Chem. Commun.* **1976**, 923.
21. Ogawa, T.; Uzawa, J.; Matsui, M. *Carbohydr. Res.* **1977**, *59*, C32.
22. "Sadler Standard Spectra, ¹H NMR No. 3126," Sadler Research Laboratories, Inc., Philadelphia, 1972.
23. Jackman, L. M.; Sternhell, S. "Applications of Nuclear Magnetic Resonance Spectroscopy in Organic Chemistry"; 2nd ed.; Pergamon: New York, 1969.
24. Tolbert, B. M., private communication.
25. Nicolet Technology Corporation, 300 Pioneer Way, Mountain View, CA 94041.
26. Hall, L. D. In "The Carbohydrates: Chemistry and Biochemistry", 2nd ed.; Pigman, W.; Horton, D., Eds.; Academic: New York, 1980; pp. 1306–1308.

27. Williams, D. H.; Bhacca, N. S. *J. Am. Chem. Soc.* **1964,** *86,* 2742.
28. Anet, F. A. L. *J. Am. Chem. Soc.* **1962,** *84,* 1053.
29. Booth, H. *Tetrahedron Lett.* **1965,** 411.
30. Spoormaker, T.; de Bie, M. J. A. *Recl. Trav. Chim. Pays-Bas.* **1979,** *98,* 59.
31. Abraham, R. J.; Berstein, H. J. *Can. J. Chem.* **1961,** *39,* 216.
32. Diehl, P. *Helv. Chim. Acta* **1964,** *47,* 1.
33. Vold, R. L.; Waugh, J. S.; Klein, M. P.; Phelps, D. E., Jr. *J. Chem. Phys.* **1968,** *48,* 3831.
34. Freeman, R.; Hill, H. D. W. *J. Chem. Phys.* **1969,** *51,* 3140.
35. Ibid., **1970,** *53,* 4103.
36. Cousins, R. C.; Seib, P. A.; Hoseney, R. C.; Deyoe, C. W.; Liang, Y. T.; Lillard, D. W., Jr. *J. Am. Oil Chem. Soc.* **1977,** *54,* 308.

RECEIVED for review April 17, 1981. ACCEPTED July 14, 1981.

Chelates of Ascorbic Acid

Formation and Catalytic Properties

ARTHUR E. MARTELL

Department of Chemistry, Texas A&M University, College Station, TX 77843

Ascorbic acid, H_2L, is a relatively weak bidentate ligand, which coordinates metal ions, M^{n+}, to form chelates, MHL^{+n-1} at low and intermediate pH values, and unprotonated chelates, ML^{+n-2} at high pH. Metal ions capable of undergoing redox reactions catalyze the autoxidation of ascorbic acid through the formation of intermediate metal–ascorbate–dioxygen complexes. Catalysis of autoxidation by metal chelates seems to occur through the formation of ternary ascorbate complexes of the metal chelates. Ascorbic acid is assigned a significant catalytic role in Udenfriend's system through the formation of an initial ascorbate–Fe(III)–dioxygen complex in which electron transfer to dioxygen results in oxygen activation and oxygen atom insertion.

Ascorbic acid, **1**, is a dibasic acid with a bifunctional ene–diol group built into a heterocyclic lactone ring (*1*). Although the dissociation constants of the ene–diol hydroxyls are increased somewhat over normal values by the electron-withdrawing oxygen atoms on the adjacent 1- and 4-positions, the acidity of ascorbic acid is due mainly to resonance stabilization of the monoanion (*2*), which distributes the negative charge between the oxygens at the 1- and 3-positions, as indicated by **2a** and **2a'**. Such stabilization is not possible when the 3-hydroxyl is not ionized. Formula **2b** therefore represents a higher energy form that does not contribute appreciably to the structure of the monoanion. The undissociated hydroxyl group of the monoanion may be hydrogen bonded to either of the adjacent negatively charged oxygens at the 1- and 3-positions, as indicated by **2a** and **2a'**. The high acidity of the 3-hydroxyl group can be readily understood by analogy with carbonic acid mono esters, with which it has a vinylogous relationship. The nature of the monoanion has been well-characterized by x-ray crystallographic studies

0065-2393/82/0200–0153$06.00/0

of its salts (2, 4) and its metal complexes (3, 5) as well as by IR (6) and NMR (7) studies of the ligand and its metal complexes.

The second pK corresponding to the conversion of 2a to 3 is relatively high ($\sim$ 11.3) because of the negative charge on 2a, and hydrogen bonding to the negative oxygens at the 1- and 3-positions. Both effects tend to increase the stability of the monoanion relative to the completely dissociated form.

The binegative ene–diol anion of ascorbic acid, L^{2-}, is a bidentate ligand and is capable of reacting with metal ions M^{n+} of coordination number 4 or 6 to form a series of complexes ML^{+n-2}, ML_2^{+n-4}; or ML^{+n-2}, ML_2^{+n-4}, and ML_3^{+n-6}; respectively. Comparison with analogous ligands having similar pK's indicates that the stabilities of the 1:1 ascorbate chelates of divalent transition metals should be in the range of 10^5–10^{10}. The stability constant data available for ascorbic acid, listed in Table I, indicate that only relatively very weak chelates have been reported. For the "normal," fully deprotonated chelates, the stabilities of only the 1:1 chelates of Ca(II), Fe(II), Cd(II), and Ag(I) are indicated. The formation constants listed are in the range of $10^{1.4}$ to $10^{3.6}$, orders of magnitude below what would be expected for complexes of the type indicated by formula 5.

Table I.   Stabilities of Metal Chelates of L-Ascorbic Acid (H₂L)

Metal Ion	*Equilibrium Quotient*	*Log Formation Constant* ($\mu = 0.10$ M; t = 25°C)	
H^+	$[HL^-]/[H^+][L^{2-}]$	11.34	
H^+	$[H_2L]/[H^+][HL^-]$	4.03	
Ca^{2+}	$[CaHL^+]/[Ca^{2+}][HL^-]$	0.2 [a]	
	$[CaL]/[Ca^{2+}][L^{2-}]$		1.4 [b]
Sr^{2+}	$[SrHL^+]/[Sr^{2+}][HL^-]$	0.3 [a]	
Mn^{2+}	$[MnHL^+]/[Mn^{2+}][HL^-]$	1.1 [c]	
Fe^{2+}	$[FeHL^+]/[Fe^{2+}][HL^-]$	0.21 [b]	
	$[FeL]/[Fe^{2+}][L^{2-}]$		2.0 [b]
Ni^{2+}	$[NiHL^+]/[Ni^{2+}][HL^-]$	1.1 [c]	
Cu^{2+}	$[CuHL^+]/[Cu^{2+}][HL^-]$	1.6	
Zn^{2+}	$[ZnHL^+]/[Zn^{2+}][HL^-]$	1.0 [c]	
Cd^{2+}	$[CdHL^+]/[Cd^{2+}][HL^-]$	0.42 [b]	
Pb^{2+}	$[PbHL^+]/[Pb^{2+}][HL^-]$	1.8	
Al^{3+}	$[AlHL^{2+}]/[Al^{3+}][HL^-]$	1.9	
	$[Al(HL)_2^+][Al^{3+}][HL^-]^2$	3.6	
Ag^+	$[AgL^-]/[Ag^+][L^{2-}]$	3.66	
UO_2^{2+}	$[UO_2HL^+]/[UO_2^{2+}][HL^-]$	2.35	
	$[UO_2(HL)_2]/[UO_2^{2+}][HL^-]^2$	3.32	

[a] 25°C, $\mu = 0.16$ M.
[b] 25°C, $\mu = 3.0$ M.
[c] 25°C, $\mu \sim 0$.
Source: Reference 1.

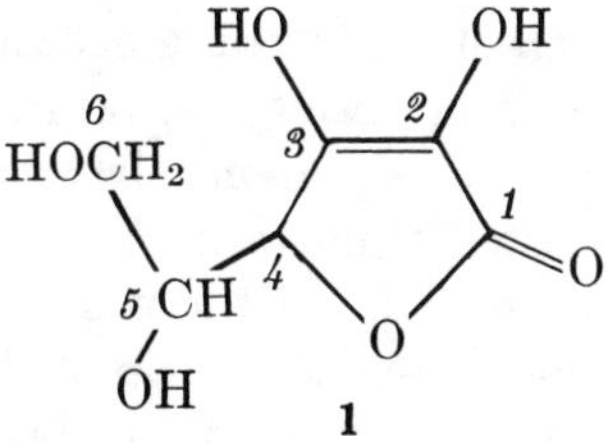

1

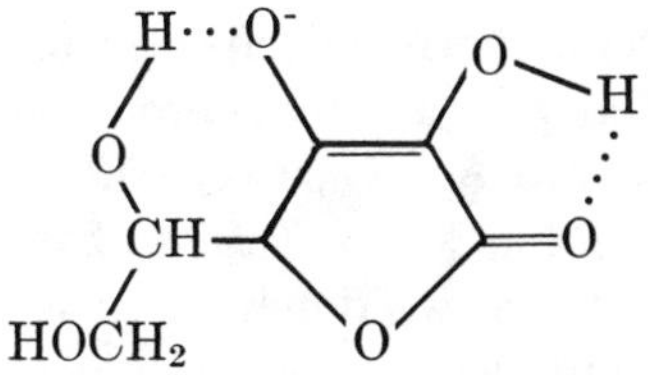

2a

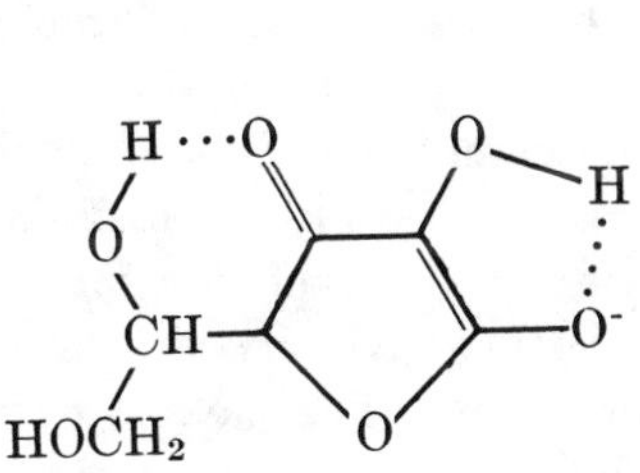

2a′

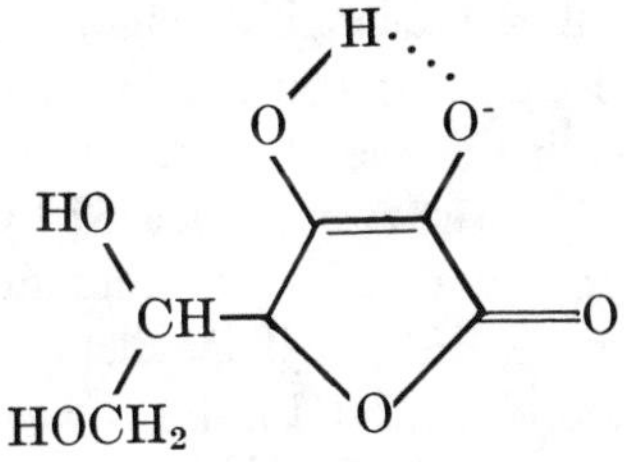

2b

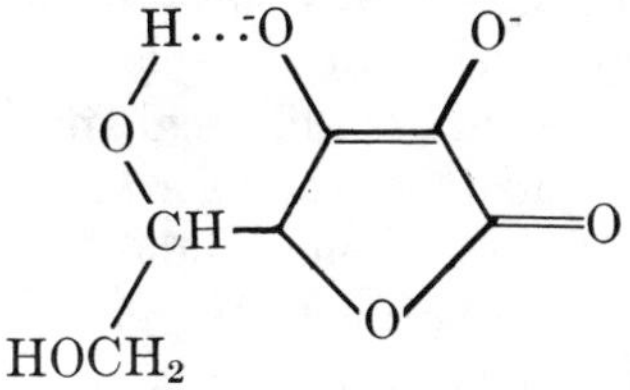

3

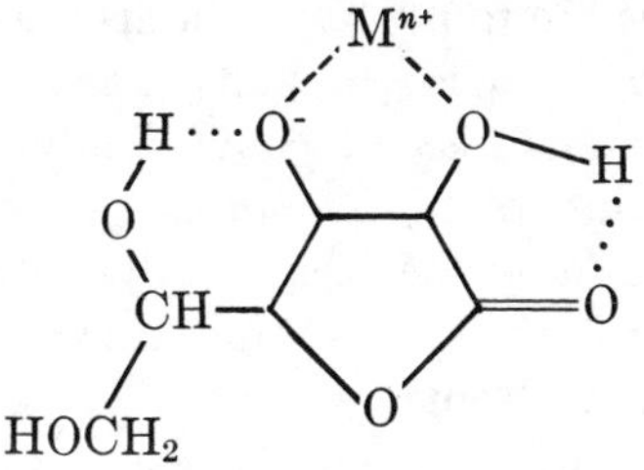

4a

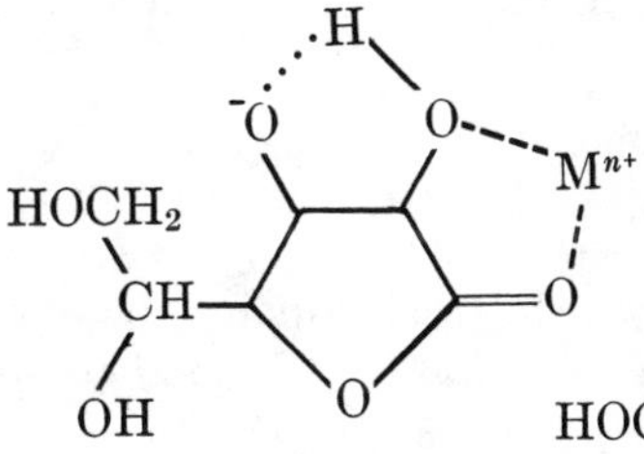

4b

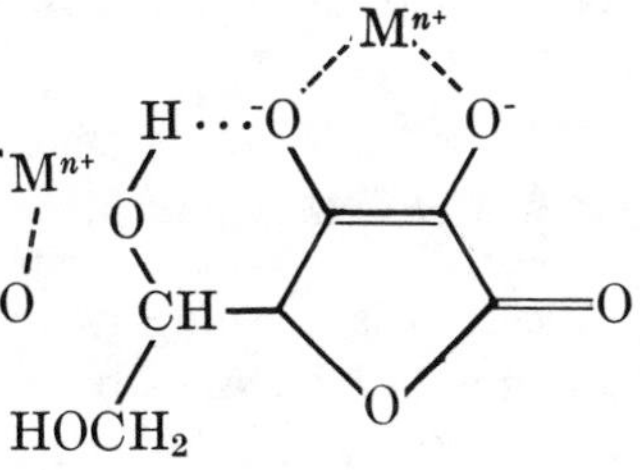

5a

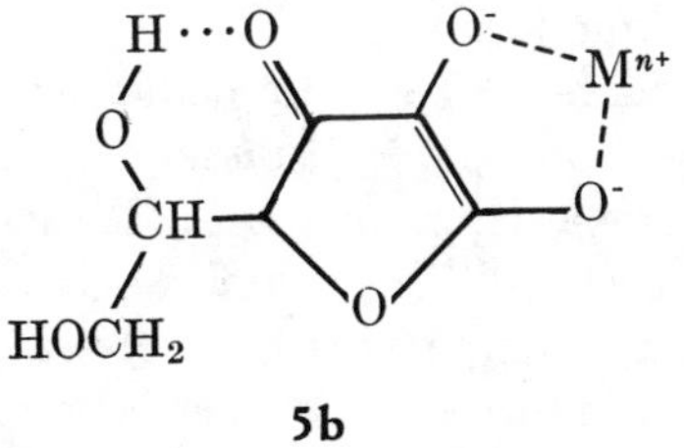

5b

Most of the metal chelates for which stability constants have been reported are the 1:1 monoprotonated chelates corresponding to formula **4**. These are quite weak, with log K values ranging from 0.2–2.35, because of the low negative charge on the ligand anion and the fact that one of the two donor oxygens is protonated. Of the possible ligand donor group arrangements indicated by formulas **4a** and **4b**, **4a** is generally accepted and agrees with the x-ray data thus far obtained for this type of chelate compound. The bonding arrangement in **4b**, however, is still a reasonable possibility because of the delocalization of negative charge between the oxygens at the 1- and 3-positions.

Although the metal chelates of the completely deprotonated ligand are generally written as indicated by **5a**, there is also a possibility of the formation of coordinate bonding modes of the type illustrated by **5b**, again because of the delocalization of negative charge between the oxygens bound to the 1- and 3-carbon atoms. The lack of data in the literature on the "normal" metal chelates in which the ligand is fully deprotonated is probably due to the fact that for most metal ions such chelates are formed only in alkaline solution. Interesting redox reactions of ascorbic acid, its salts, and its metal chelates take place in acid solution and may be conveniently studied at moderately low to low pH. In alkaline solution the rate of autoxidation of ascorbic acid and the effect of trace impurities that catalyze such oxidation reactions increase many fold, and the precautions necessary to carry out studies in alkaline solution are somewhat inconvenient. There seems to be no fundamental reason, however, why chelate formation by ascorbic acid with non-oxidizing metal ions could not be studied at moderately to high pH under such conditions that the metal ions do not hydrolyze extensively or precipitate.

Oxidation by Metal Ions and Metal Chelates

Ascorbic acid is a strong two-electron reducing agent that is readily oxidized in one-electron steps by metal ions and metal complexes in their higher valence states. An inner sphere mechanism for the stoichiometric oxidation of ascorbic acid by ferric ion in acid solution is illustrated by Scheme 1 (8). The first step in the reaction is the formation of a mono-protonated Fe(III) complex similar to the monoprotonated ascorbate complexes listed in Table I. The intermediate monoprotonated Fe(III) complex is short-lived and rapidly undergoes an intramolecular one-electron transfer to give a deprotonated Fe(II) complex of the ascorbate radical anion, indicated by **7**. This complex dissociates to the free radical anion, which may then combine with a second ferric ion to form the complex **9**. Complex **9** in turn undergoes a second intramolecular electron

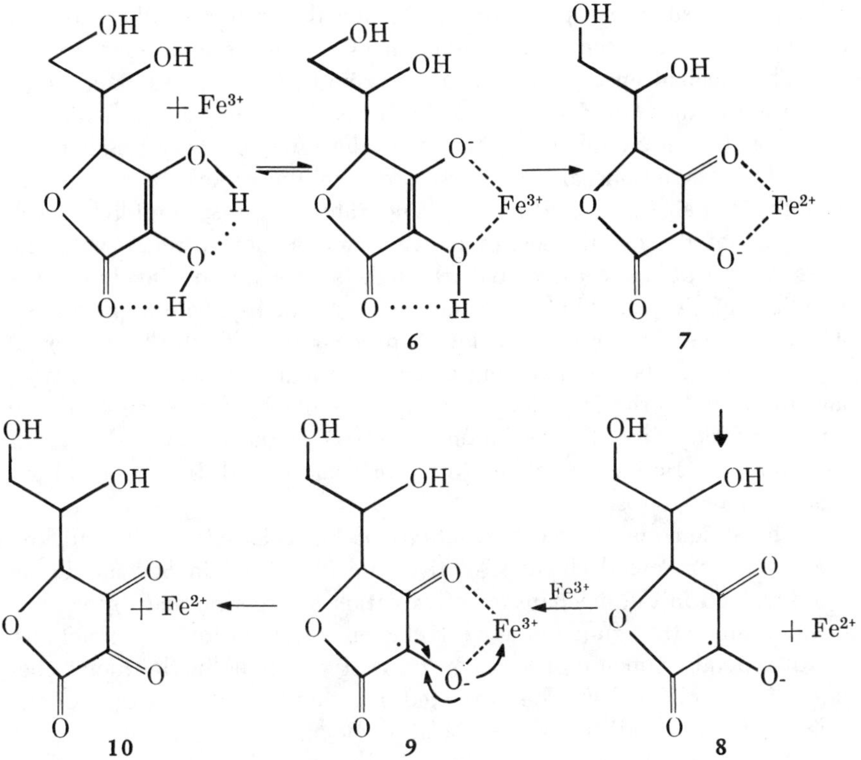

Scheme 1.   *Direct oxidation of ascorbic acid by ferric ion.*

transfer to give the final product, dehydroascorbic acid, formula 10. The monoprotonated complex 6 has been identified as the starting material for both Cu(II)- and Fe(III)-catalyzed oxidation of ascorbic acid on the basis of the pH dependence of the reaction rate for oxidation with both metal ions, and by rapid equilibrium measurements of chelate formation with Cu(II) ion. The postulation in Scheme 1 that ascorbate radical anion 8, and its Fe(II) chelate 7, as well as its Fe(III) chelate 9, are completely deprotonated, is based on Chapter 4 in this volume.

The oxidation of ascorbic acid by Cu(II) ion is somewhat less rapid than the rate of oxidation by Fe(III), but is considered to proceed by the same type of mechanism. As may be seen from that data in Table I, the monoprotonated metal chelates of ascorbic acid are generally quite weak and tend to be extensively dissociated in solution. Moreover, as electrons are withdrawn from the ligand to give first the radical anion and finally the neutral dehydroascorbic acid, the affinities of these oxidized forms for metal ions are further decreased with each oxidation step. Therefore, with the possible exception of 6, the metal complexes illustrated in Scheme 1 may represent rather minor species in the reaction mixture.

The mechanism of oxidation of ascorbic acid by various metal chelates such as those of Fe(III) and Cu(II) is similar to the mechanism of oxidation by the metal ion, except that the rates are very much lower (9). These reactions are also first order in the ascorbate monoanion and first order in metal chelate. The rates decrease rapidly as the stabilities of the metal chelates increase but do not correlate with the rates that would be predicted through a mechanism involving the equilibrium dissociation of the metal chelate to the free (aquo) metal ion. Therefore, the reactions are believed to occur through the formation of a mixed ligand chelate involving ascorbate anion as a secondary ligand, and the rate-determining electron transfer would be dependent not only on the stability (i.e., the oxidation potential) of the metal chelate itself but also on steric factors related to the orientation and dimensions of the ligand donor groups.

The stoichiometric redox reactions of ascorbic acid with oxidizing metal ions and metal chelates, of the type illustrated in Scheme 1, are also involved in the mechanisms of oxidation of ascorbic acid by various oxidants since they function as very efficient catalysts for such reactions. Further details concerning electron transfer processes in the metal chelates of ascorbic acid will be presented in the following discussion of the role of simple metal ascorbate chelates and of mixed ligand ascorbate chelates in the oxidation of ascorbic acid by molecular oxygen.

Catalysis of the Autoxidation of Ascorbic Acid by Metal Ions and Metal Chelates

The systems described above by which metal ions and metal chelates accomplish two-electron oxidation of ascorbic acid, may be employed in catalytic systems in which the metal ion or chelate is only a minor constituent. Any oxidizing agent capable of reoxidizing the metal ion or chelate from its lower valent state to its higher valent state may be employed. While in the following treatment the oxidant is molecular oxygen, it should be possible to set up analogous reaction systems with other oxidants such as hydrogen peroxide, halogens, nitrite ion, and many others.

Metal-Ion-Catalyzed Autoxidation. Figure 1 illustrates the variation of the first-order rate constants for the autoxidation of ascorbic acid by molecular oxygen with the concentration of the Cu(II) ion, which is present in catalytic (i.e. low) concentrations (8). The linear relationship indicates second-order behavior [first order in ascorbic acid and first order in Cu(II)]. The catalytic effect of Cu(II) is also seen to decrease

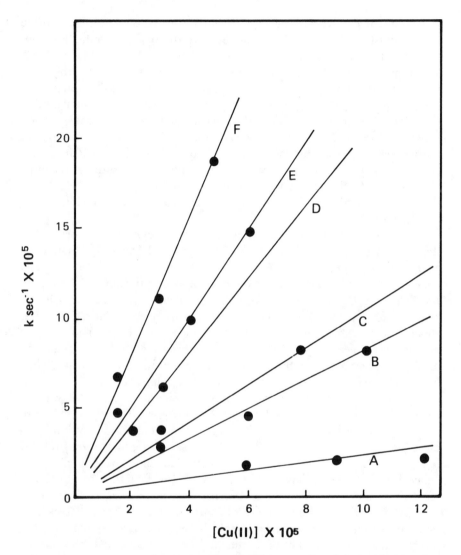

Figure 1. Rate constants for the Cu(II)-ion-catalyzed autoxidation of ascorbic acid as a function of Cu(II) concentration at $-\log [H^+]$ values of: A, 1.50; B, 2.00; C, 2.25; D, 2.50; E, 2.85; and F, 3.45; t = 25°C; $\mu = 0.10M$ (KNO$_3$).

rapidly as hydrogen ion concentration is increased. This variation of the second-order rate constant with pH may be eliminated if the concentration of the substrate is replaced by that of the monoanion, indicating that the latter, or the corresponding monoprotonated Cu(II) chelate, is the reactive species in the oxidation reaction.

A similar catalytic effect (8) of Fe(III) on the oxidation of ascorbic acid is illustrated in Figure 2. In this case the observed rates are considerably higher than those illustrated in Figure 1 for Cu(II) catalysis. The pseudo first-order rate constants for the oxidation of ascorbic acid illustrated in Figure 2 are seen to vary in a linear fashion with the concentration of Fe(III), which is present in catalytic amounts. The rates indicated in Figure 2 are also seen to increase with hydrogen ion concentration, and here again the pH variation in the rate indicates that the monoanion, or its monoprotonated iron chelate, is formed in a pre-equilibrium step prior to the rate-determining electron transfer reaction. From the data illustrated in Figure 2, second-order rate constants for the Fe(III)-catalyzed oxidation of the ascorbic acid monoanion may be calculated.

The second-order rate constants for the autoxidation of ascorbic acid determined from data of the type illustrated in Figures 1 and 2 were found to be proportional to the dioxygen concentration. At low oxygen concentrations this dependence on oxygen concentration was found to level off indicating a change in reaction mechanism. Also the rates in the presence of oxygen were found to be much more rapid than the direct stoichiometric rates of oxidation by the Cu(II) and Fe(III) ions in the absence of molecular oxygen. Figure 3 illustrates the dependence on oxygen concentration of the specific rate constants (i.e., rate constants based on concentration of the monoprotonated anion) for the autoxidation of ascorbic acid in the presence of catalytic amounts of Fe(III). Similar relationships were obtained for Cu(II) catalysis. The data therefore indicate third-order behavior for Cu(II) and Fe(III) catalysis of the autoxidation of ascorbic acid—first order in substrate, first order in metal ion, and over a limited range of concentration, first order in dioxygen concentration. This behavior, together with the fact that the observed reaction is much more rapid in the presence of dioxygen than in its absence, provides evidence for the formation of an intermediate ascorbate–copper–dioxygen complex in which the rate-determining electron transfer takes place. The experimental observation that the metal-catalyzed oxidation by molecular oxygen is much more rapid than the stoichiometric oxidation of ascorbic acid by the metal ion or chelate in the absence of molecular oxygen, was noted some time ago by Dekker and Dickinson (10) but this observation was interpreted in terms of the reactivity of the ascorbate radical anion, and its involvement in a free radical chain reaction.

A reaction mechanism for the metal-ion-catalyzed autoxidation of ascorbic acid, involving the formation of an intermediate ternary ascorbate–metal ion–dioxygen complex, is illustrated in Scheme 2. Although the bonding between the metal ion and the dioxygen in the intermediate

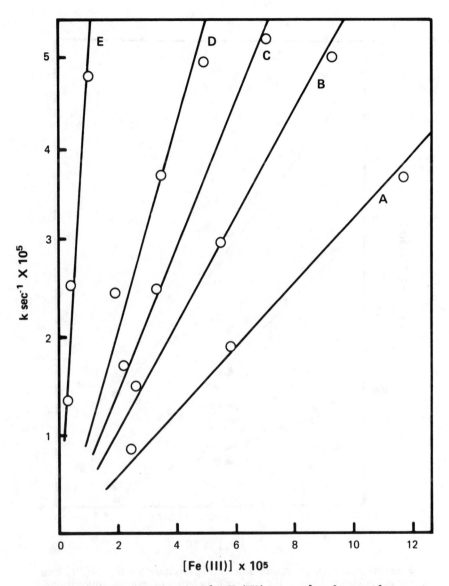

Figure 2. Rate constants for the Fe(III)-ion-catalyzed autoxidation of ascorbic acid as a function of Fe(III) concentration at $-\log [H^+]$ values of: A, 1.50; B, 2.00; C, 2.42; D, 2.94; E, 3.44; t = 25°C; $\mu = 0.10M$ (KNO_3).

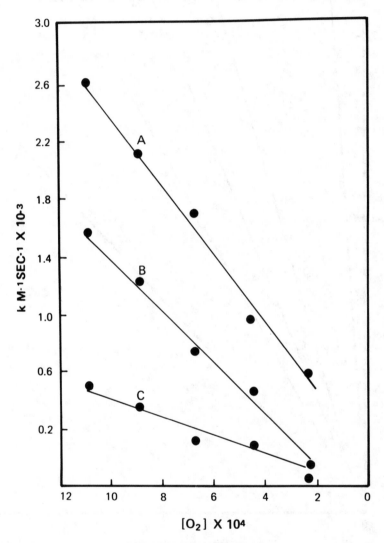

Figure 3.   Variation of second-order rate constants for the Fe(III) catalyzed autoxidation of ascorbic acid as a function of oxygen concentration
at $-\log [H^+]$ values of: A, 3.85; B, 3.45; C, 3.00; t = 25°C; μ = 0.10M
(KNO₃).

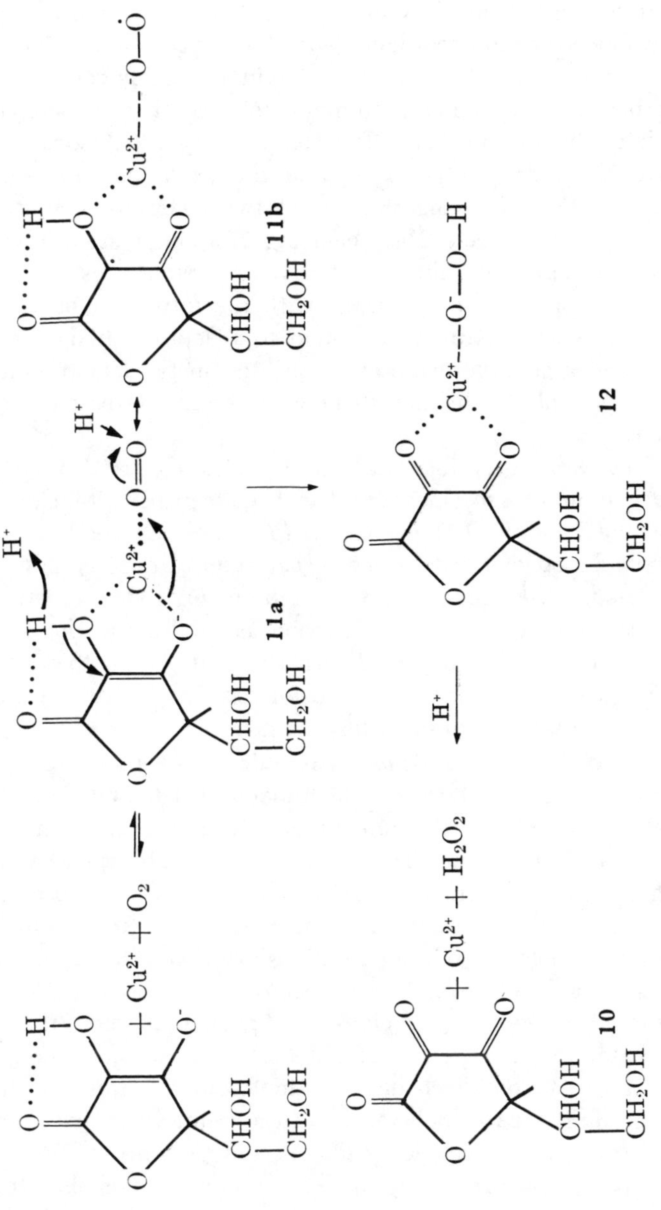

Scheme 2. Cu(II)-ion-catalyzed oxidation of ascorbic acid.

dioxygen complex would seem to be extremely weak, it may be stabilized by resonance of the type indicated by **11a** and **11b** (Scheme 2) as suggested by Hamilton (*11*). The rate-determining electron transfer step illustrated in Scheme 2 is indicated as occurring through an ionic shift of two electrons in accordance with the suggestion of Hamilton (*11*) to give directly a Cu(II) complex containing weakly coordinated dehydroascorbic acid and a more strongly coordinated hydroperoxide donor, as indicated by formula **12**. This complex rapidly dissociates to the free metal ion, hydrogen peroxide, and the oxidation product. While the redox reaction involving transfer of two electrons is illustrated in the mechanism in Scheme 2 as occurring in a single step, it would also be quite reasonable to illustrate the redox reaction as occurring in two successive one-electron transfers with the formation of an intermediate complex in which Cu(II) is bound to a deprotonated ascorbate radical anion and a superperoxide anion. With kinetic data presently available it is impossible to distinguish between these alternative reaction mechanisms.

The work described here on the Cu(II)- and Fe(III)-catalyzed autoxidation of ascorbic acid has been extended to catalytic systems involving vanadyl (*12*) and uranyl (*13*) ions. On the basis of the results described above it would seem that there are potentially many other metal ions that are capable of undergoing redox reactions with the ascorbate ion, and that may function as catalysts in the autoxidation of ascorbic acid. Analogous mechanisms may also apply to systems involving metal-ion catalysis of ascorbate oxidation in which the primary oxidant is a reagent other than molecular oxygen.

Metal-Chelate-Catalyzed Autoxidation of Ascorbic Acid. Kinetic data for reaction systems in which metal chelates rather than metal ions serve as catalysts for the autoxidation of ascorbic acid are illustrated in Figures 4, 5, and 6 (*9*). The rate constants are independent of molecular oxygen concentration and are much lower than those observed for autoxidation of ascorbic acid in the presence of free (aquo) metal ions. The metal-chelate-catalyzed reactions are therefore expected to proceed through single electron transfer steps, with the first electron transfer followed by metal ion dissociation and recombination of the deprotonated ascorbate radical anion with the higher valence form of the metal chelate. Thus the reaction mechanism is similar to the stoichiometric reaction scheme illustrated in Scheme 1 with a metal chelate replacing the free metal ion. In a catalytic system in the presence of excess molecular oxygen and only a relatively small amount of metal chelate the generation of the lower valence form of the metal chelate by oxidation of ascorbic acid is counter-balanced by rapid reoxidation of the metal chelate to the higher valence form by molecular oxygen, resulting a cyclic catalytic

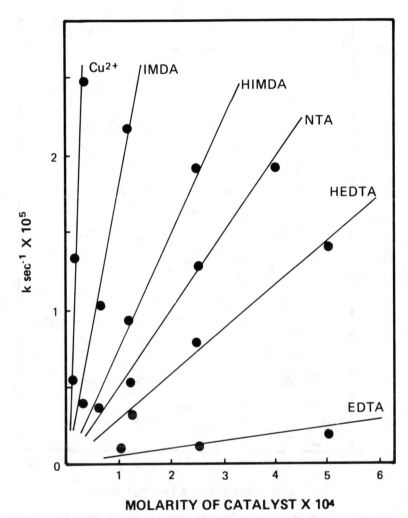

Figure 4. Variation of rate constants for the autoxidation of ascorbic acid as a function of concentration of Cu(II) chelates at 25°C and −log [H⁺] of 3.45: EDTA = ethylenediaminetetraacetic acid; HEDTA = hydroxyethylethylenediaminetetraacetic acid; NTA = nitrilotriacetic acid; HIMDA = hydroxyethyliminodiacetic acid; IMDA = iminodiacetic acid.

process of the type illustrated in Scheme 3. The pseudo first-order rate constants plotted in Figures 4 and 5 show linear dependence of the rate constants on copper chelate and on iron chelate concentrations, respectively, thus indicating the formation of a mixed ligand complex with ascorbate as the reactive intermediate in which the slow rate-determining electron transfer occurs. The reaction rates are also seen to decrease rapidly with an increase in the stabilities of the copper and iron chelates

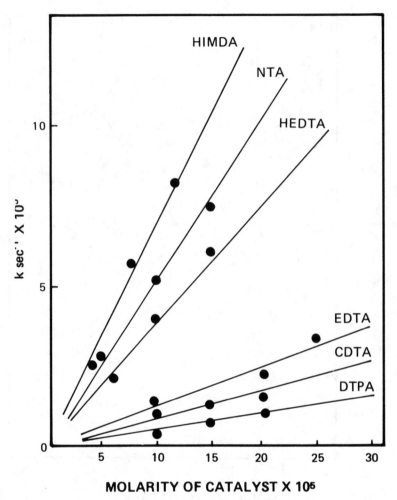

Figure 5. Variation of rate constants for the autoxidation of ascorbic acid as a function of concentration of Fe(III) chelates at 25°C and −log [H⁺] of 2.45; DTPA = diethylenetriaminepentaacetic acid; CDTA = trans-1,2-diaminocyclohexanetetraacetic acid; other terms as in caption of Figure 4.

involved. This effect may be interpreted in one of two ways: (i) that the reaction occurs through a dissociative mechanism releasing a small amount of the free metal ion, which then acts as a catalyst for ascorbic acid oxidation, in the manner illustrated in Scheme 2; or (ii) that the redox potential of the copper ion in the mixed ligand–ascorbate–carrier ligand complex stabilizes the higher valent form of the metal ion to a greater extent when a more highly stable metal chelate is involved as the catalyst.

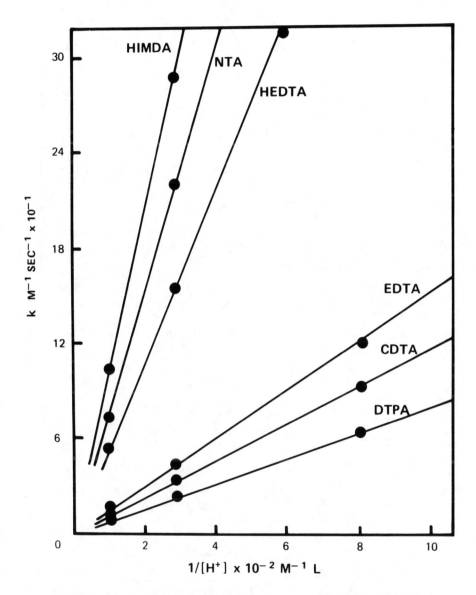

Figure 6.   Dependence of second-order rate constants for Fe(III)-chelate-catalyzed autoxidation of ascorbic acid on hydrogen ion concentration at 25°C. Abbreviations are those given in Figures 4 and 5.

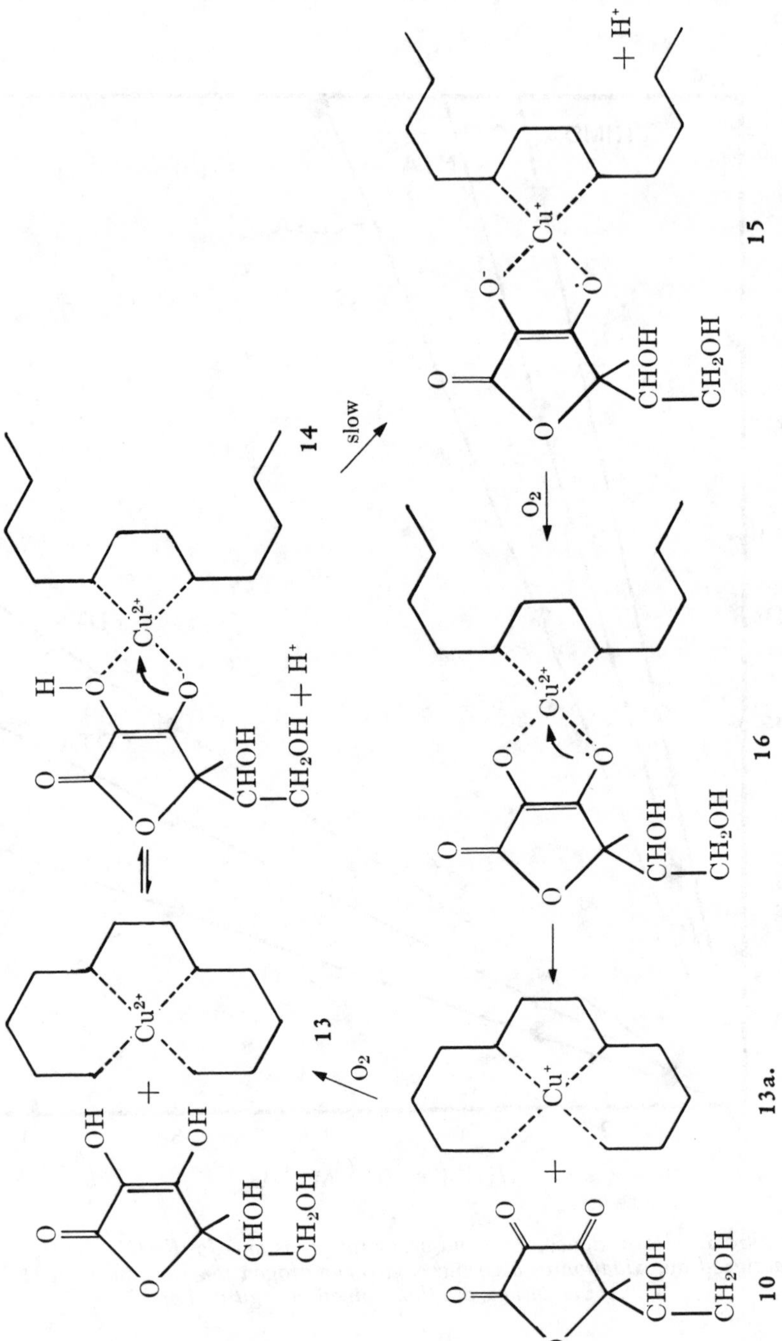

Scheme 3. Proposed mechanism for: metal-chelate-catalyzed autoxidation of ascorbic acid.

The possibility that the decreased catalytic activity with increase in metal chelate stability represents a dissociative mechanism in which the free metal ion is actually the catalyst was explored by comparing the observed rates with the concentrations of free metal ion in equilibrium with the various chelates investigated. Since the rate constants for free-metal-ion catalysis are known it was possible to calculate and predict the observed catalytic rate constants, since the equilibrium constants for dissociation of the metal chelates are also known. The values calculated in this manner did not correlate with the observed rates, indicating that the observed catalysis probably proceeds by electron transfer from the reductant to the metal ion in the mixed ligand chelates of the type illustrated in Scheme 3. In such a mechanism the metal chelates are visualized as remaining intact in both the oxidized and reduced forms through the entire catalytic cycle. Thus the deprotonated ascorbate radical anion and the carrier-ligand are visualized in formula 15 as remaining simultaneously bound to the reduced metal ion and remain combined with the metal ion when it is reoxidized to the higher valence state [i.e., from Cu(I) to Cu(II)]. After the second electron transfer, however, as indicated in 16, the dehydroascorbic acid finally formed is such a weak ligand that it readily dissociates and the simple metal chelate in which the metal ion is again in its lower valence state and is reoxidized by molecular oxygen to regenerate the catalyst 13.

In the first mixed ligand complex formed in the reaction mixture, 14, the coordinated ascorbate ion is indicated in its monoprotonated form. Experimental evidence for the degree of protonation of this species was obtained from the variation of the calculated second-order rate constants with hydrogen ion concentration in the low pH range in which these reactions were carried out. The substrate was primarily in its neutral diprotonated form and the equilibrium involving mixed ligand complex formation results in displacement of one of the two protons present on the ene–diol groups. Thus the concentration of intermediate 14 will increase as the hydrogen ion concentration decreases. This effect is clearly observed in the plots of the second-order rate constants as a function of pH in Figure 6. Similar effects were obtained for both iron- and copper-chelate-catalyzed oxidation reactions. Since the tendency of a metal ion in a metal chelate compound to exist in its higher valence state increases with the stability of the metal chelate compound, and in fact its redox potential can be calculated from the stability constant of the metal chelate itself, it would be expected that increasing the stability of the metal chelate would decrease its catalytic activity for the autoxidation of ascorbic acid, as is seen in Figures 4 and 5. While it is clear that this trend exists, there is no linear correlation between chelate stability and catalytic activity because, if such a correlation existed, it would not have been possible to eliminate the dissociative mechanism involving an alternate catalytic route involving the free aquo metal ion in its higher valence state. It is obvious that the more stable metal chelates will have a larger number of donor groups coordinated to the metal ion and will have coordinate bonds that are more difficult to break, a process that would be necessary for the complexes with multidentate ligands in which the metal ion is nearly or fully coordinated. This type of displacement is indicated schematically by formulas 13 and 13a in Scheme 3 in which the metal ions [Cu(II)] are represented as being tetra-coordinated. The formation of a mixed ligand complex required for an inner-sphere electron transfer of the type indicated in formulas 14, 15, and 16 would involve displacement of one or more of the coordinated donor groups of the carrier ligand. It is expected that considerable steric effects would be associated with such displacement processes and that these effects would vary in a very complex way with the nature of the ligand in the catalytic metal chelate.

Finally it should be pointed out that there is an alternate mechanism for the two successive electron transfer processes indicated by the sequence 14 → 15 → 16 → 13a. It is quite possible that the ascorbate radical anion dissociates from the mixed ligand complex 15, prior to reoxidation of the Cu(I) ion, and recombines with another Cu(II) chelate prior to the final electron transfer step indicated by 16 → 17 + 10. This represents a slight modification of the mechanisms in Scheme 3, and involves an alternate branch for reaction sequence 15 → 16 → 17.

The main difference between the Fe(III) and Cu(II) ion-catalyzed autoxidation of ascorbic acid on one hand, and the Fe(III) and Cu(II) chelate-catalyzed oxidation reactions is the lack of dependence of the latter systems on the concentration of molecular oxygen, and the absence of a ternary metal substrate–carrier ligand–dioxygen complex as an intermediate in the proposed reaction mechanism. The absence of such an intermediate may be considered to be due at least in part to the occupation of all or nearly all the coordination positions of the metal ion by the carrier ligand, thus crowding out the dioxygen, which is at best a relatively weak monodentate ligand. It should also be noted that the proposed mechanism in Scheme 3 involves two successive electron transfers rather than a single ionic type two-electron shift of the type indicated in Scheme 2. It is not intended at this stage to favor one mechanism over the other; both should be considered alternatives. A factor in ascorbate autoxidation that may not apply to many other substrates is the resonance stabilization of the one-electron oxidation intermediate, the ascorbate radical anion. In cases where one-electron reduction of oxidation products are stabilized by resonance or other constitutional factors, the one-electron transfer process may be favored over two-electron redox reactions.

Ascorbic Acid Oxidase

Ascorbic acid oxidase is activated by Cu(II) ion and is believed to function in a manner similar to the mechanism indicated in Scheme 3 involving a series of two successive one-electron transfer steps in which the ascorbic acid is oxidized to an intermediate free radical anion coordinated at the active site in a manner similar to that indicated by formula 15. In the enzymic system it seems likely that the intermediate ascorbate free radical would remain coordinated to the metal ion in both Cu(I) and Cu(II) forms, rather than undergo successive dissociation and reassociation steps that would tend to greatly slow down the enzymic reaction process. In this respect the enzymic mechanism may differ from that suggested in Scheme 3 for metal chelate catalysis of the autoxidation of ascorbic acid, since there is no evidence in the latter case that the weak Cu(I) intermediate complex would hold together long enough for the reoxidation step to occur (*see* discussion later). Since the metal ion would remain bound to the active site of the enzyme, its reoxidation by molecular oxygen may very well occur through the formation of a dioxygen complex, thus providing an additional reaction intermediate. As mentioned before, the free radical ascorbate anion is resonance-stabilized and its formation in these systems in appreciable quantities therefore seems reasonable. Another probable difference between the enzymic mechanism and the mechanism suggested in Scheme 3 for metal chelate catalysis is the displacement of some of the ligand donor groups from the coordination sphere of the metal ion that would be required for the formation of the mixed ligand complexes in which the electron transfer process takes place. Such displacement reactions would greatly slow down and inhibit the reaction rate and it is believed that the enzyme certainly would eliminate such reaction barriers by the design of a coordination sphere that would make available at least two labile coordination sites of Cu(II) for combination with the substrate.

Rate Laws for Metal-Ion- and Metal-Chelate-Catalyzed Autoxidation of Ascorbic Acid

On the basis of kinetic data of the type illustrated in Figures 1, 2, and 3 the rate law of autoxidation of ascorbic acid is represented by Equation 1, involving a third-order rate constant and a reaction rate that is first order in substrate monoanion, metal ion, and molecular oxygen. Since the rate-determining step involves electron transfer in a ternary complex, third-order behavior involves two pre-equilibria, Equations 2 and 3, for the formation of the ternary complex, and a final slow step, Equation 4, in which the coordinated oxygen undergoes a two-electron reduction to hydrogen peroxide. As pointed out by Taqui Khan and Martell (9), the hydrogen peroxide rapidly disappears and is not detected in the final reaction mixture. The hydrogen peroxide formed may be reconverted to oxygen and water through the catalase-like action of the cupric ion or of some of its complexes.

$$-\frac{d[HL^-]}{dt} = k[HL^-][Cu^{2+}][O_2] \tag{1}$$

$$Cu^{2+} + HA^- \rightleftharpoons CuHA^+ \tag{2}$$

$$CuHA^+ + O_2 \rightleftharpoons CuHAO_2^+ \tag{3}$$

$$CuHAO_2^+ + H^+ \xrightarrow{\text{slow}} Cu^{2+} + A + H_2O_2 \tag{4}$$

The metal-chelate-catalyzed autoxidation of ascorbic acid is not dependent on the concentration of molecular oxygen. On the basis of the data illustrated in Figures 4, 5, and 6 the rate expression suggested for this type of reaction is given by Equation 5, which indicates that the disappearance of the monoanion of the substrate is first order in both metal chelate and the ascorbate monoanion. Thus the reaction sequences indicated by Equations 6, 7, and 8 consist of a pre-equilibrium involving the formation of a mixed ligand metal–carrier ligand–substrate mono-anion complex. Following the rate-determining electron transfer reaction within the mixed ligand complex (Equation 7), the lower valence form of the metal complex is rapidly reoxidized in solution by molecular oxygen, thus regenerating the catalyst. H_nA represents a multidentate ligand, and H_2L is ascorbic acid.

$$-\frac{d[HL^-]}{dt} = k[HL^-][CuA^{(2-n)+}] \tag{5}$$

$$Cu^{II}A^{(2-n)+} + HL^- \rightleftharpoons Cu^{II}(A)(HL)^{(1-n)+} \tag{6}$$

$$Cu^{II}(A)(HL)^{(1-n)+} \xrightarrow{\text{slow}} Cu^IA^{(1-n)+} + L^- + H^+ \tag{7}$$

$$\text{Free radicals} \xrightarrow[CuA^{(2-n)+},\ O_2]{\text{fast}} A + H_2O_2 \tag{8}$$

Recently Jameson and Blackburn (14, 15, 16) have suggested an alternate mechanism for the copper-catalyzed autoxidation of ascorbic acid, involving the formation of a binuclear Cu(II) complex (17) of the ascorbate anion, and the subsequent formation of an intermediate peroxo type Cu(II)–dioxygen–ascorbate complex (18). Their kinetic data suggested a variety of rate behavior depending on the nature of the supporting electrolyte. Formula 17, which was postulated for nitrate

Initial binuclear complex, $(CuHL)_2^{2+}$, **17**

Intermediate dioxygen complex, $CuHLO_2CuHL$, **18**

media, seems to suggest the rate indicated by Equation 9. Thus the reaction sequence suggested consists of two pre-equilibria, Equations 10 and 11, which result in the formation of the dinuclear peroxo type dioxygen complex, **18**. This is followed by a rate-determining electron transfer (Equation 12), which results in the formation of two free radicals that are converted to final products in subsequent steps that seem to be partially rate determining. In chloride media [and probably in the

$$\frac{-d[O_2]}{dt} = k'[Cu^{2+}][HL^-][O_2]^{1/2} \tag{9}$$

$$2CuHL^+ \rightleftharpoons (CuHL)_2^{2+} \tag{10}$$

$$(CuHL)_2^{2+} + O_2 \rightleftharpoons CuHLO_2CuHL^{2+} \tag{11}$$

$$CuHLO_2CuHL^{2+} \overset{slow}{\longrightarrow} LCuO_2H\cdot + Cu^{2+} + L\cdot \tag{12}$$

$$\text{free radicals} \rightarrow \text{products} \tag{13}$$

presence of other anions that coordinate Cu(II)] the chloride ion seems to participate in binuclear complex formation, and further complicates the kinetics.

The half-order dependence of the rate of autoxidation of ascorbic acid on molecular oxygen that was found by Blackburn and Jameson and that was the basis for their suggestion of binuclear intermediates 17 and 18, is quite interesting, especially in view of the fact that peroxo bridged dioxygen complexes analogous to 18 have also been observed for cobalt dioxygen complex systems (17). As noted above, the first-order dioxygen dependence observed by Taqui Khan and Martell (9) undergoes a transition at low oxygen concentrations to lower order dependence and finally zero-order dependence as indicated in Figure 3. Thus it may very well be that at low oxygen concentrations binuclear complexes of the kind observed by Blackburn and Jameson become the reaction intermediates for autoxidation of ascorbic acid, resulting in the observed half-order dependence of the reaction rates on oxygen concentration. On the other hand, binuclear complexes of the type illustrated, 17 and 18, tend to form only in solutions in which the metal ion concentration is at least moderately high. Therefore in solutions in which the catalytic species, either the Cu(II) or Fe(III) ions, or their metal chelates, are present at very low concentrations the formation of binuclear complex intermediates is not very likely. Under such conditions, catalysis by mononuclear complexes of the types indicated in Schemes 2 and 3 would seem to be favored.

It is interesting to note that the +3 oxidation state of copper has been invoked by Jameson and Blackburn (15, 16) in the formation of dioxygen complexes. Although this is an attractive idea in view of recent investigations reported by Margerum et al. (18), the formation of stable Cu(III) complexes in aqueous solution would require coordination with ligands having very special properties. Here again it seems somewhat unlikely that appreciable concentrations of Cu(III) complexes are formed in these reaction systems. On the other hand, Cu(III) may be invoked for explaining the stabilities of Cu(II)–dioxygen complexes of the type illustrated in Scheme 2, and 18. Thus the dioxygen complex intermediates formed in trace amounts in these reaction systems may be considered to involve oxidation of copper to an intermediate oxidation state between Cu(II) and Cu(III).

Role of Ascorbic Acid in a Mono-oxygenase Model (Udenfriend's System)

Recently ascorbic acid has been assigned a significant function in the reactions involving oxygen insertion by model oxygenase and peroxidase systems in which ferric ion or a ferric chelate is considered to be the catalyst. Although reaction mechanisms suggested by earlier workers involved ascorbic acid merely as a reductant to convert Fe(III) to Fe(II), which would then in turn interact with the oxidant, Hamilton

(*11*) suggested that ascorbate or similar reductants such as catechol are involved in the formation of a ternary complex in which the metal ion is coordinated simultaneously to the reductant and the oxidant.

The reaction sequences originally suggested for oxygen insertion in a substrate such as salicyclic acid in Udenfriend's System (*19–22*) in which molecular oxygen is the oxidant and an iron chelate such as Fe(II)-EDTA is the catalyst and ascorbic acid is the reductant, is indicated by Equations 14–18. In this reaction sequence oxygen insertion is considered to occur by direct reaction of the aromatic compound with $HO_2 \cdot$ and $OH \cdot$ free radicals, and the ascorbate reductant merely serves the purpose of regenerating the Fe(II) chelate as indicated by Equations 16 and 17.

$$Fe^{II}\text{-EDTA} + O_2 + H_2O \rightarrow Fe^{III}\text{-EDTA} + OH^- + HO_2 \cdot \quad (14)$$

$$(15)$$

$$Fe^{III}\text{-EDTA} + H_2A + OH^- \rightarrow Fe^{II}\text{-EDTA} + HA \cdot + H_2O \quad (16)$$

$$Fe^{III}\text{-EDTA} + HA \cdot + OH^- \rightarrow Fe^{II}\text{-EDTA} + A + H_2O \quad (17)$$

$$Fe^{II}\text{-EDTA} + H_2O_2 \rightarrow Fe^{III}\text{-EDTA} + OH \cdot + OH^- \quad (18)$$

On the basis of the facts that oxygen insertion occurs preferentially at the *ortho* and *para* positions relative to the activating hydroxyl group on the aromatic ring, and that the reaction did not seem to involve free radicals, Hamilton (*11*) suggested an ionic mechanism involving a ternary ascorbate metal dioxygen complex of the type illustrated by **19** in Scheme 4. In the proposed mechanism a concerted shift of electron pairs results in the insertion of an oxygen atom into the substrate and a concomitant two-electron reduction of ascorbate to dehydroascorbic acid. An alternate electron transfer sequence is, of course, possible involving two single electron transfer steps and the formation of an intermediate complex in which the ascorbate anion radical is coordinated to the metal ion. The mechanism proposed in Scheme 4 is somewhat more satisfying than the previously recommended free radical mechanism (Equation 14–18) be-

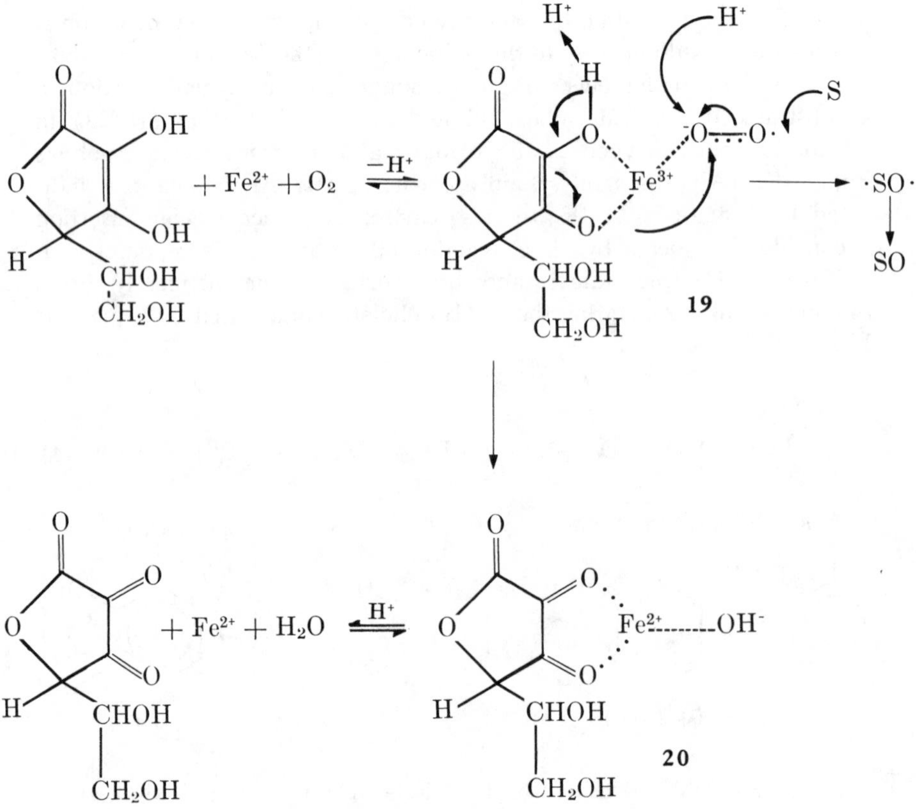

Scheme 4. *Proposed mechanism for Fe(II)-catalyzed oxygen insertion (Udenfriend's system).*

cause it assigns a more important role to the metal ion that is an essential catalyst in these enzyme model systems.

A similar mechanism illustrated in Scheme 5 has been suggested by Hamilton (*11*) for peroxidase model systems (*22*) in which the oxidant is hydrogen peroxide, the reductant is ascorbic acid or an analogous reagent such as catechol, and the catalytic metal ion is Fe(III). In this system the intermediate ternary complex undergoes an intramolecular electron transfer involving fission of the oxygen–oxygen bond of the peroxide ligand to give water and an intermediate complex that essentially involves coordination of atomic oxygen with Fe(III). This intermediate is somewhat stabilized by several resonance forms (**21a-c**) in which some negative charge is seen to reside on the oxygen atom, thus accounting for its ability to remain briefly coordinated with the metal ion. Insertion of atomic oxygen into an appropriate substrate results in regeneration of

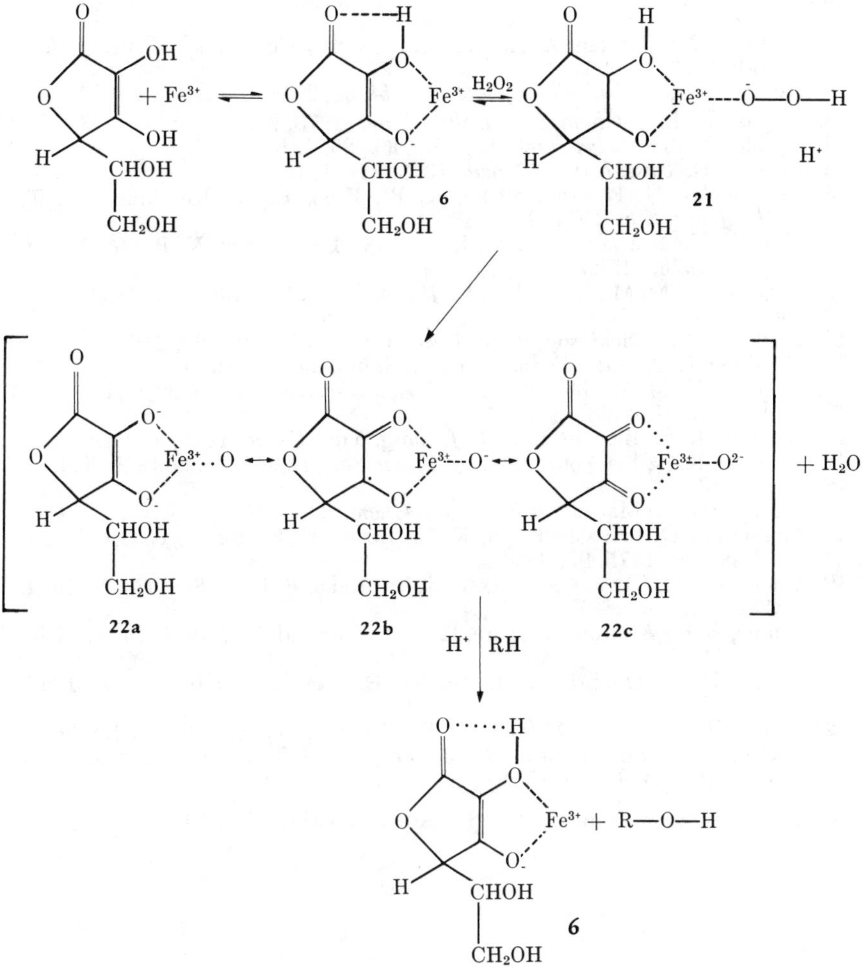

Scheme 5. Proposed mechanism for a model peroxidase system.

the Fe(III) complex **6** of the reducing ligand. Reduction of Fe(III) by the ascorbate ligand is prevented by the oxidant, hydrogen peroxide, to regenerate the original reactive ternary complex, **21**. Hamilton's mechanism for these peroxidase model reactions is of interest because of its similarity to the reactions occurring in catalase and peroxidase enzymic systems in which resonance forms of the iron porphyrin ring system stabilize a two-electron oxidant intermediate believed to involve a coordinated oxygen atom.

Literature Cited

1. Smith, R. M.; Martell, A. A. "Critical Stability Constants"; Plenum: New York, 1977.
2. Hvoslef, J. *Acta Crystallogr., Sect. B* **1974**, *30*, 2711.
3. Hughes, D. L. *J. Chem. Soc., Dalton Trans.* **1973**, 2209.
4. Hvoslef, J. *Acta Crystallogr., Sect. B* **1969**, *25*, 2214.
5. Kriss, E. E. *Russ. J. Inorg. Chem.* **1978**, *23* (7), 1004.
6. Evtushenko, N. P.; Yatsimirskii, K. B.; Kriss, E. E.; Kurbatova, G. T. *Zh. Neorg. Kim.* **1977**, *22*, 1543.
7. Kriss, E. E.; Kurbatova, G. T.; Kuts, V. S.; Prokopenko, V. P. *Zh. Neorg. Khim.* **1976**, *21*, 2978.
8. Taqui Khan, M. M.; Martell, A. E. *J. Am. Chem. Soc.* **1967**, *89*, 4176.
9. Ibid., 7104.
10. Dekker, A. O.; Dickinson, R. G. *J. Am. Chem. Soc.* **1940**, *62*, 2165.
11. Hamilton, G. A. *Adv. Enzymol. Delat. Subj. Biochem.* **1969**, *32*, 55.
12. Taqui Khan, M. M.; Martell, A. E. *J. Am. Chem. Soc.* **1968**, *90*, 6011.
13. Ibid., **1969**, *91*, 4468.
14. Jameson, R. F.; Blackburn, N. J. *J. Inorg. Nucl. Chem.* **1975**, *37*, 809.
15. Jameson, R. F.; Blackburn, N. J. *J. Chem. Soc., Dalton Trans.* **1976**, 534.
16. Ibid., 1596.
17. McLendon, G.; Martell, A. E. *Coord. Chem. Rev.* **1976**, *19*, 1.
18. Margerum, D. W.; Chellappa, K. L.; Bossu, F. P.; Burce, G. S. *J. Am. Chem. Soc.* **1975**, *97*, 6894.
19. Udenfried, S.; Clark, C. T.; Axelrod, J.; Brodie, B. B. *J. Biol. Chem.* **1954**, *208*, 731.
20. Brodie, B. B.; Axelrod, J.; Shore, P. A.; Udenfriend, S. *J. Biol. Chem.* **1954**, *208*, 741.
21. Mason, H. S.; Onoprienko, I.; Buhler, E. *Biochim. Biophys. Acta* **1957**, *24*, 225.
22. Taqui Khan, M. M.; Martell, A. E. "Homogeneous Catalysis by Metal Complexes: Activation of Small Inorganic Molecules"; Academic: New York, 1974; Vol. 1, p. 151.

RECEIVED for review January 22, 1981. ACCEPTED May 11, 1981.

Nitrogen Derivatives of L-Ascorbic Acid

EL SAYED H. EL ASHRY

Chemistry Department, Faculty of Science, Alexandria University, Alexandria, Egypt

The nitrogen derivatives of L-ascorbic acid or its dehydro derivative, and the rationale for interest in these derivatives, are reviewed. In particular, the reactions of dehydro-L-ascorbic acid (DHA) with o-phenylenediamine or its substituted derivatives are surveyed as well as the reactions of DHA with hydrazines, which yield monohydrazones or bishydrazones. Further conversion of these initial derivatives into a variety of nitrogen heterocyclic compounds is evaluated. The reactions of L-ascorbic acid with amino acids are also examined.

The role of L-ascorbic acid as a vitamin probably involves its participation in oxidation–reduction reactions. In those reactions dehydro-L-ascorbic acid (DHA) is the first stable oxidation product; DHA is often the first product in the degradation of L-ascorbic acid. Because of its three adjacent carbonyl groups, DHA would be expected to undergo nucleophilic reactions with a number of functional groups, including amines. Nitrogen compounds arise in biological systems either from naturally occurring amino acids and proteins or from added chemotherapeutic agents such as sulfa drugs, isoniazide, and hydralazine; therefore, the study of the products of amine reactions with DHA is important. Moreover, L-ascorbic acid in foods is converted to DHA when it acts as an antioxidant. Thus, the survival of vitamin C during food processing depends in part on its involvement, and the involvement of DHA, in reactions with amines in foods, giving products mostly incapable of regenerating the vitamin.

Nitrogen derivatives of L-ascorbic acid are important because they have been used extensively for the vitamin's determination (1) in the form of the bis(2,4-dinitrophenylhydrazone) of dehydro-L-ascorbic acid (1). In addition, because of the commercial availability of L-ascorbic acid with a relatively low price as well as the widespread use of hetero-

0065-2393/82/0200–0179$06.00/0

cycles, L-ascorbic acid could be used as a precursor in the synthesis of a variety of heterocyclic compounds with or without carbohydrate substituents.

Reaction of DHA with o-Phenylenediamine

In its oxidized form, L-ascorbic acid is more reactive than are aldo-2-uloses (osones); this greater reacitvity is caused by the carboxylic group adjacent to the dicarbonyl groups. Because of these three adjacent functional groups, DHA reacts with amines or o-phenylenediamine to yield a variety of products; the product is determined by the molecular proportions of the reactant (2–7). The product resulting from the condensation of one molar equivalent of o-phenylenediamine with the C1 and C2 carbons reacted (5) with phenylhydrazine to give 2,2'-anhydro-[2-hydroxy-3-(1-phenylhydrazono-L-*threo*-2,3,4-trihydroxybutyl)quinoxaline] (2) in its hydrated form. The structure of 2 was based on the formation of its diacetate (3) upon acetylation. More recently, the structure of 2 was revised (8–10) to the acyclic form 3-[(1-phenyl-

1

2 R' = H
3 R' = Ac

hydrazono)-L-*threo*-2,3,4-trihydroxybutyl]-2-quinoxalinone (4, where R = Ph). Those reactions have been extended using a variety of arylhydrazines and aroylhydrazines (9, 11) as well as semicarbazide and thiosemicarbazide (12) instead of phenylhydrazine. The structure of 4 was based on spectroscopic studies (mass and IR spectra) as well as periodate oxidation studies (10, 13). Periodate oxidation afforded the corresponding aldehydes whose structures were confirmed to be 3-(1-substituted hydrazono)glyoxal-1-yl]-2-quinoxalinones (6) rather than 5, as was expected from the cyclic structures. These aldehydes provide a simple route to glyoxalylquinoxalinone derivatives (6), which are potential precursors to other heterocyclic compounds such as 7–12. Compounds 7–12 are monosubstituted glyoxal monohydrazones, which would be difficult to obtain if we started with the possible, but unknown, pre-

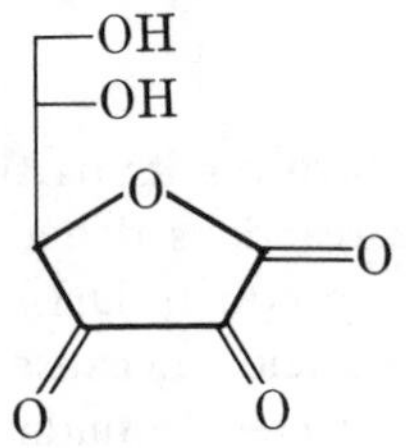

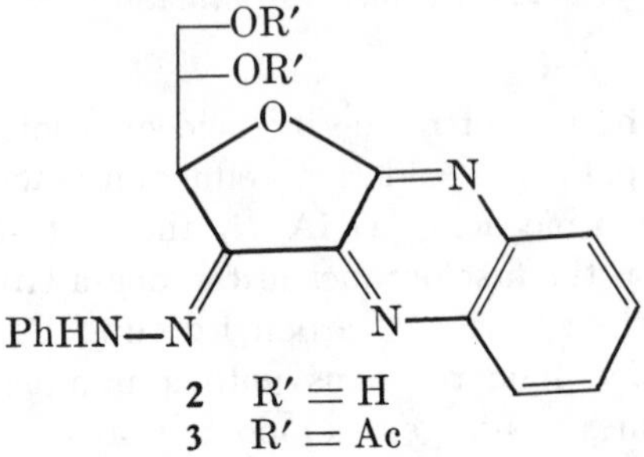

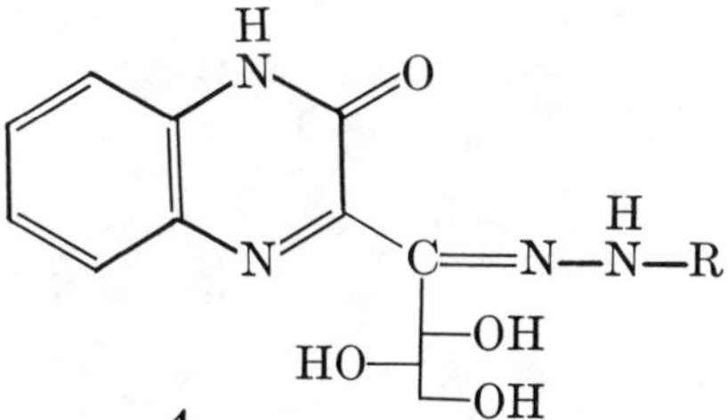

4

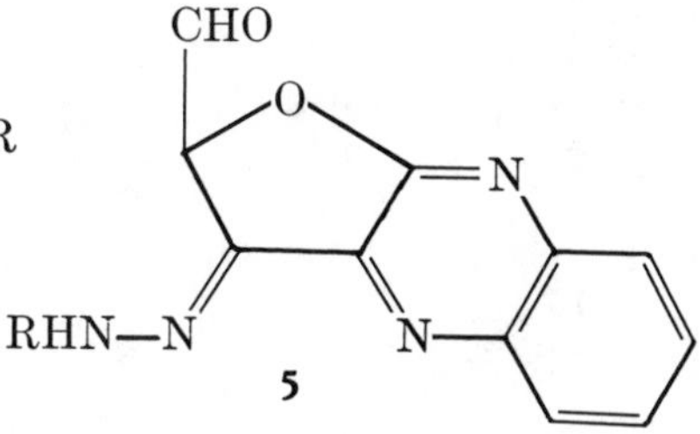

5

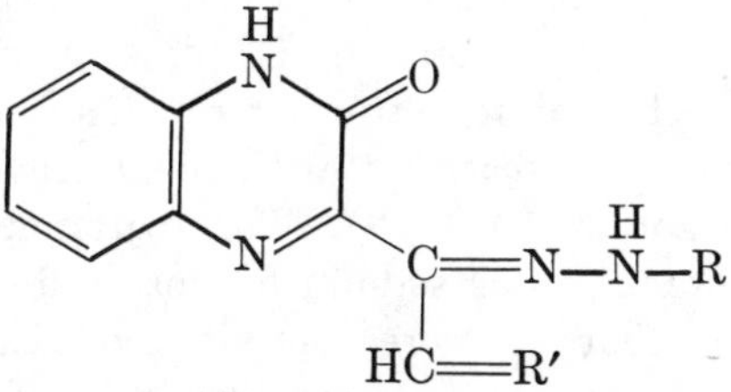

6 R' = O
7 R' = NOH
8 R' = NNHR″

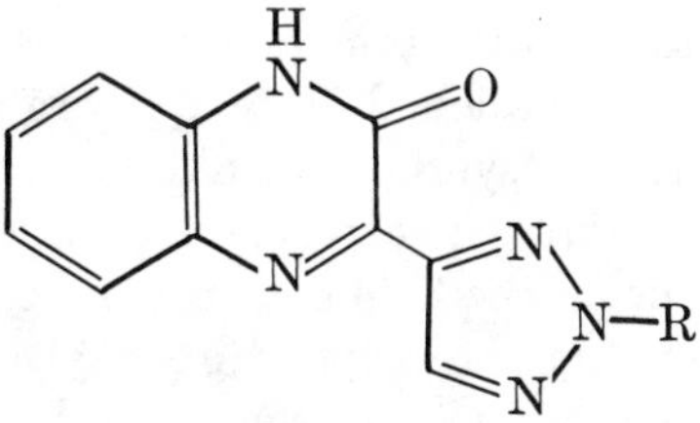

9

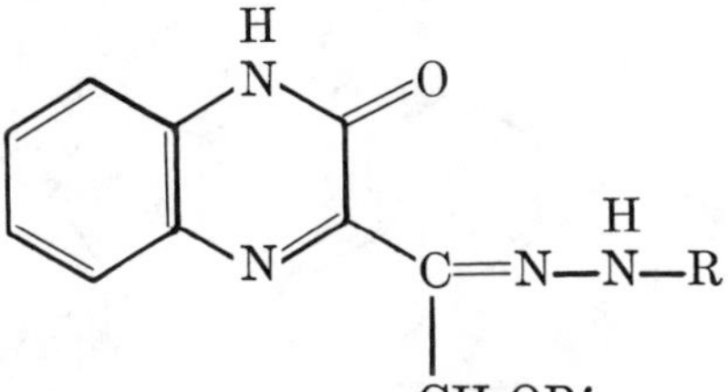

10 R' = H
11 R' = Ac

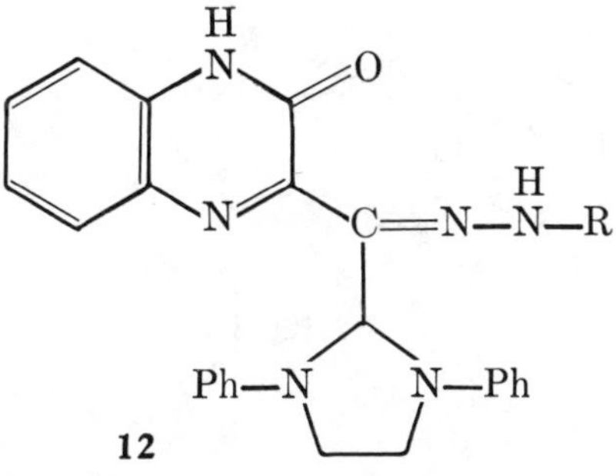

12

cursor, 3-(glyoxal-1-yl)-2-quinoxalinone, and allowed it to react with hydrazines. The only possible monohydrazone upon such direct condensation is the hydrazone on the C2 carbonyl. Reaction of **6** with carboethoxymethylidene triphenylphosphorane gave **13**, which was successfully cyclized to **14**. This reaction (**6** to **14**) was applied to other monohydrazones of 1,2-dicarbonyl compounds, indicating its use as a general method for pyridazinones synthesis.

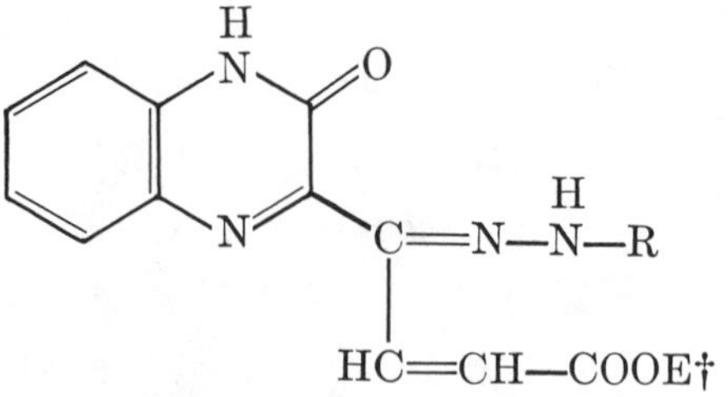

13

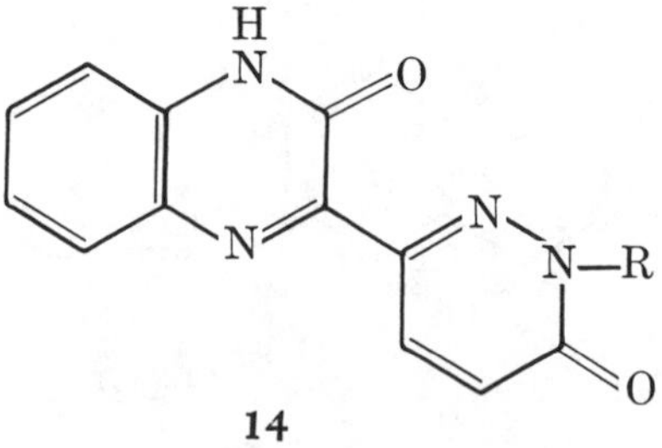

14

The formation of 1-phenylflavazole from reducing sugars not substituted on O2 and O3 is a general reaction (*14–18*), which proceeds
through the formation of an arylhydrazono group on C3 of a sugar
moiety attached to a quinoxaline. This prerequisite intermediate in
flavazole synthesis could be **4**, which on treatment with alkali gave
3-(L-*threo*-glycerol-1-yl)-1-arylflavazole (**15**) (5,9). The rearrangement proceeds in 1 h in boiling, dilute, aqueous sodium hydroxide, but
fission of the polyhydroxyalkyl chain occurs in more concentrated alkaline solution. On the other hand, dissolution of **4** in alkali, followed
immediately by acidification, regenerates the starting material. Formation of flavazoles from L-ascorbic acid is an inexpensive and simple route
to flavazoles otherwise obtained from L-galactose or L-talose. Reactions
of these flavazoles were studied (9); derivatives such as **16–18** can be
prepared.

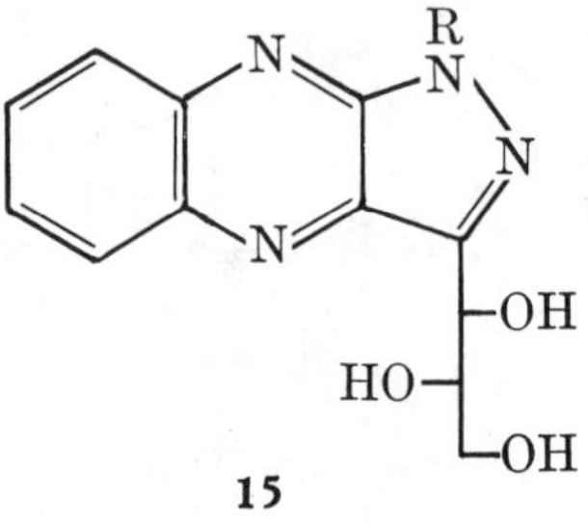

15

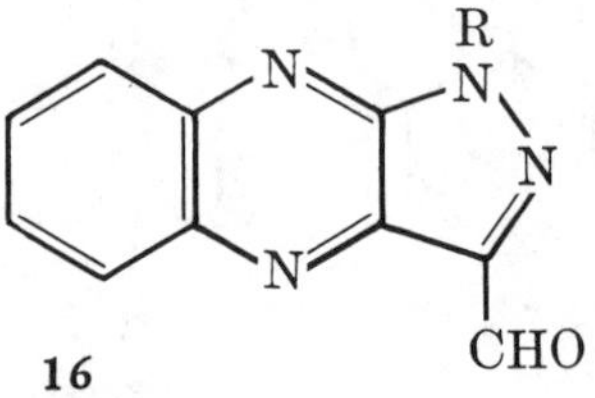

16

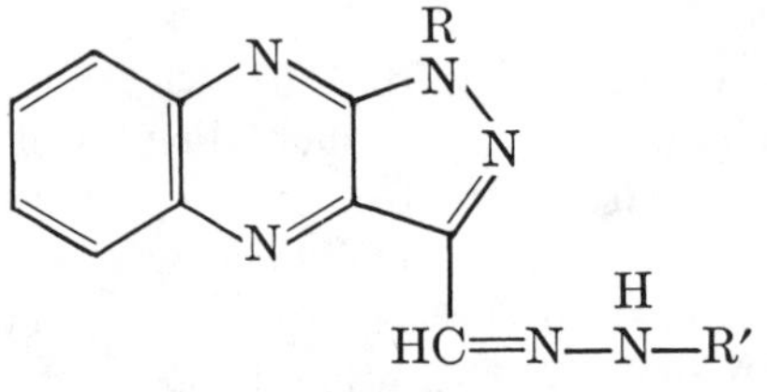

17

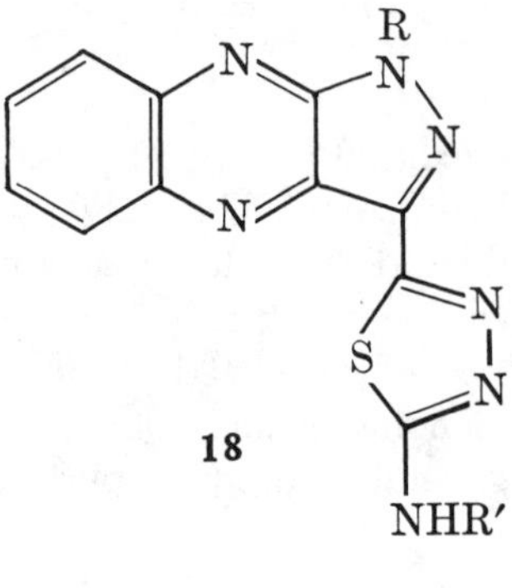

18

After the acyclic structure of 4 had been assigned, the behavior of similar compounds, which are presumably incapable of existing in a cyclic form [such as 19, which was prepared by the methylation (*19*) of 4], was studied. Periodate oxidation of 19 gave the corresponding aldehyde that could be converted into various other derivatives.

During acetylation with boiling acetic anhydride (*8,9*), the alditol portions in the molecules 4 and 19 dehydrate with simultaneous ring closure to give pyrazoles 23 and 21, respectively. Deacetylation of 23 afforded 20, which could also be obtained from 4 using hydroxylamine hydrochloride. The structures of the products were confirmed by IR, NMR, and mass spectra, and a mechanism for the formation of such pyrazoles was also suggested (*9*). An extension of this work using substituted o-phenylenediamines such as those with chloro, methyl, or dimethyl groups has also been completed (*8, 20*).

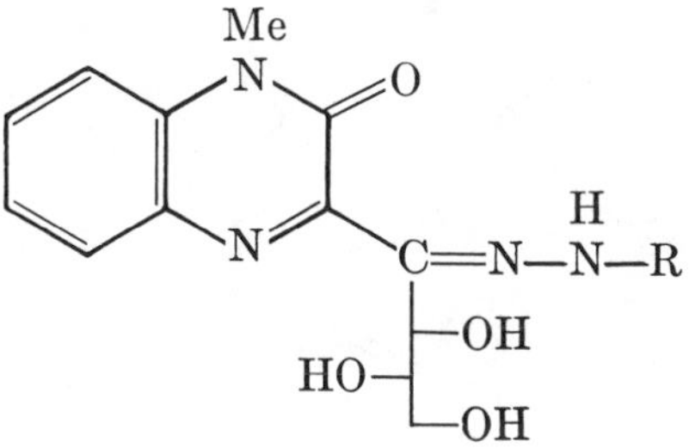

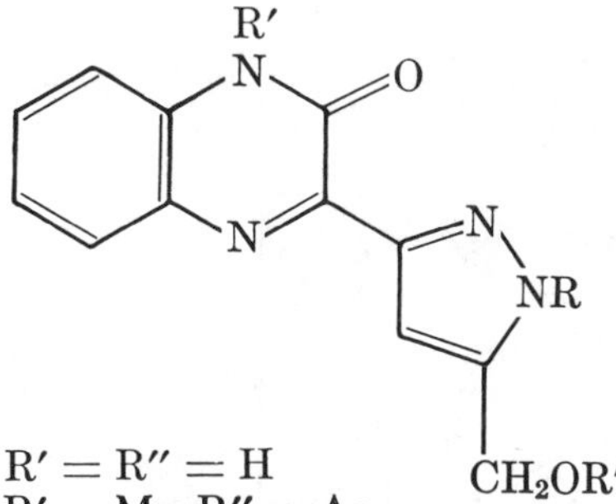

20   R' = R'' = H
21   R' = Me, R'' = Ac
22   R' = R'' = Me
23   R' = H, R'' = Ac

The reaction of 2 mol of o-phenylenediamine with DHA was reported (*2*) to give 26, which produced colorless crystals from water and yellow crystals from ethanol. Treatment of 26 with cold mineral acid gave the monoquinoxaline derivative 24, which upon acetylation gave the diacetate 25 and upon reaction with o-phenylenediamine gave 26 again. Treatment of 24 with alkali gave the sodium salt 27, which on acidification gave the γ- and δ-lactones (24 and 29), respectively, indicating that the two nitrogen atoms are present on C2 and C3. On the other hand, Hasselquist (*21*) assigned the structures 28 and 30 to the colorless and yellow crystals, respectively, one of which was converted into the di-*N*-acetyl derivative (*31*). Later, the structure of the reaction product was reported to be 32 (*22*). Compound 32 gave the mono-*N*-acetyl derivative (*33*) and, upon treatment with hydrochloric acid, gave 24. Further studies to clarify these structures are now underway in our laboratory.

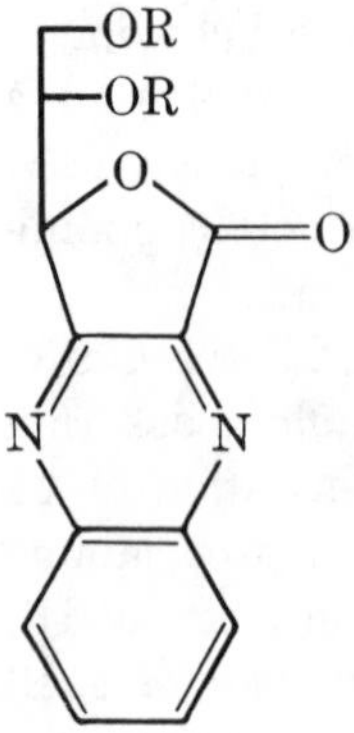

24 R = H
25 R = Ac

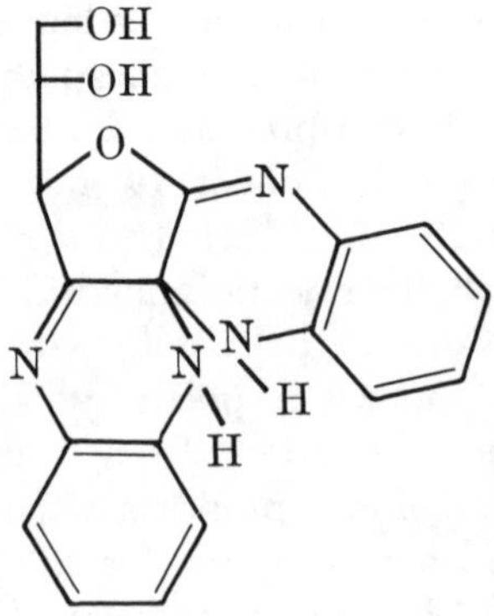

26

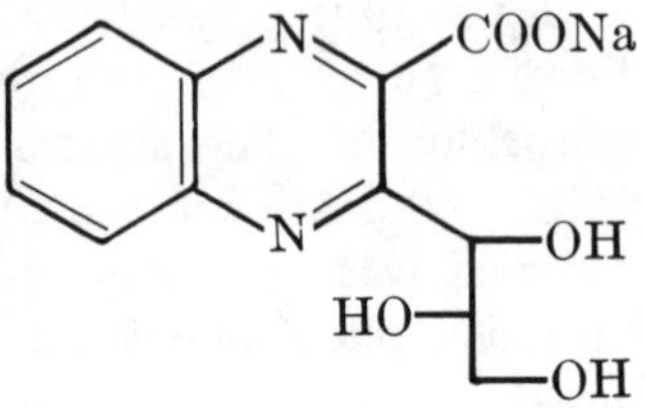

27

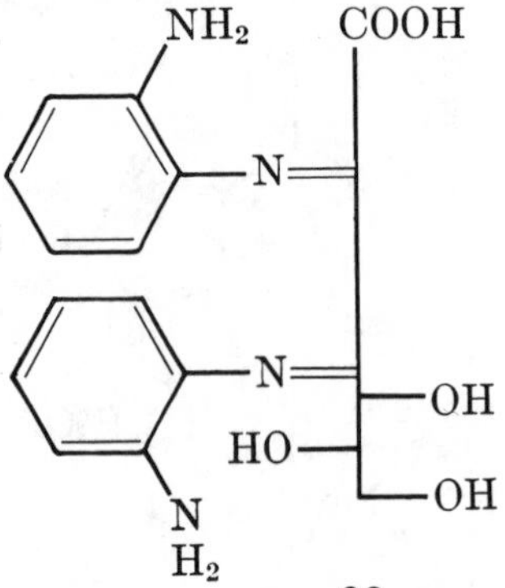

28

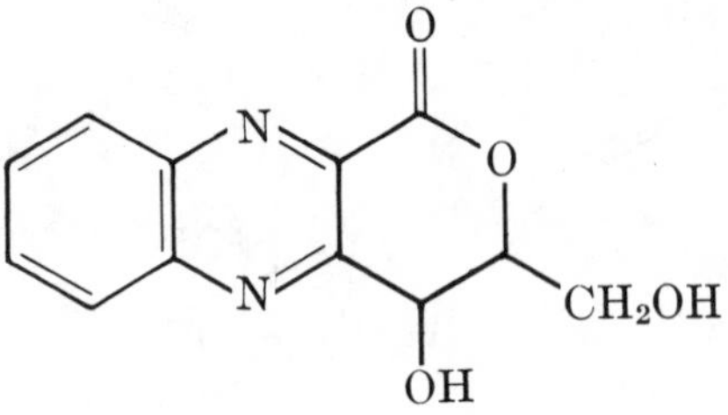

29

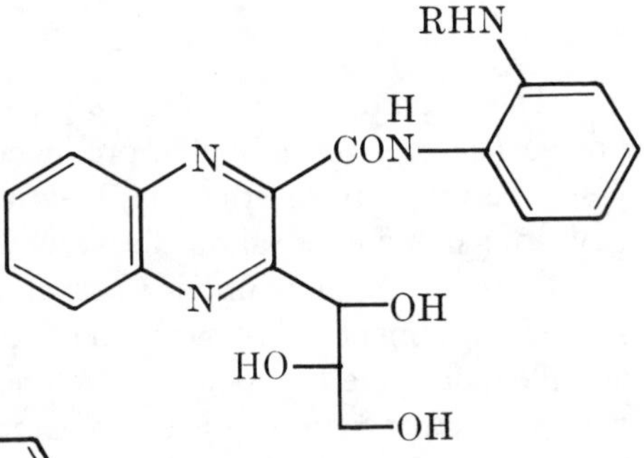

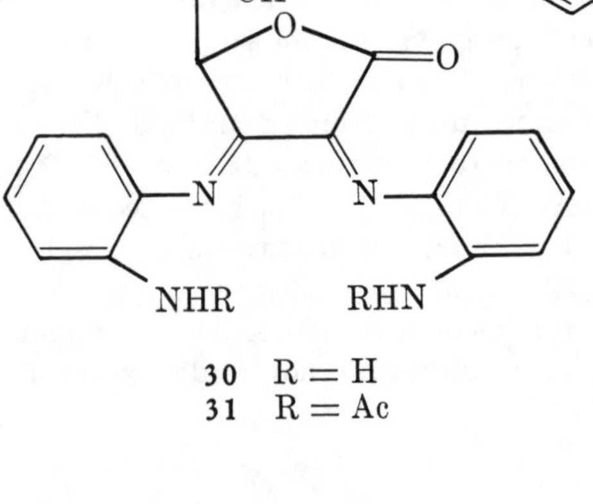

30 R = H
31 R = Ac

32 R = H
33 R = Ac

DHA Monohydrazones

L-*threo*-2,3-Hexodiulosono-1,4-lactone 2-(phenylhydrazone) (38, R = Ph), was first prepared (23) by reacting 34 with the sodium derivative of diethyl malonate to give 35. Hydrolysis of the adduct 35 gave 36, which upon treatment with alcoholic alkali afforded 37. Reaction of 37 with benzene diazonium chloride gave 38 (R = Ph), which was conveniently prepared (24) by reaction of DHA with N-acetyl-N-phenyl-hydrazine in the presence of iodine. Controlled reaction (25, 26) of substituted phenylhydrazine with DHA gave the corresponding mono-hydrazones (38), although the phenyl derivative was not isolated by this method. X-ray crystallography confirmed the structure (37) of the corresponding *p*-bromo derivative.

Acetylation and benzoylation of 38 caused a simultaneous dehydration with the formation of an optically inactive olefinic compound (40), probably through the formation of the diacylated derivative (39); the structures were confirmed (24) by spectroscopic methods. Compound 40 can also be prepared from the corresponding D-analogue (28, 29).

The reaction of 38 with various hydrazines gave the corresponding mixed bishydrazones (42), which could be rearranged into other heterocycles (25, 26). The bishydrazones could not be isolated with

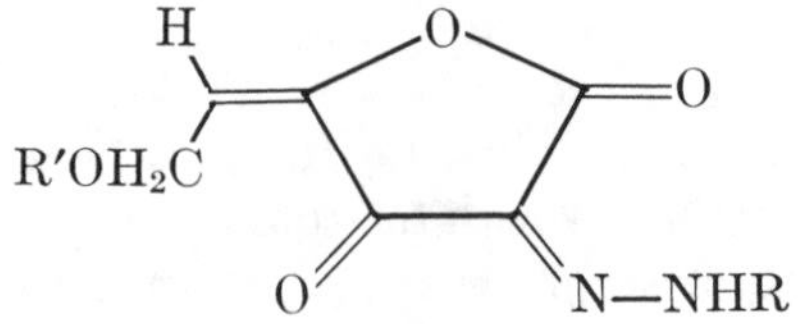

40

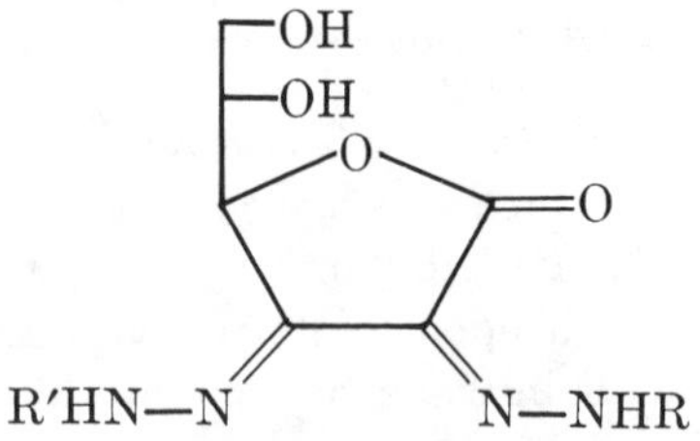

41 R = R'
42 R ≠ R'

methylhydrazine, and a pyrazole derivative (43) was directly obtained (30, 31). The reaction of 40 with methylhydrazine was more complicated, affording a product whose elemental analysis and spectral data indicate that 2 mol of methylhydrazine was consumed in the reaction to give 45 (Scheme 1). The structure 45 and not 44 was assigned on the basis of x-ray crystallography (32). Spectroscopic methods agreed with both structures.

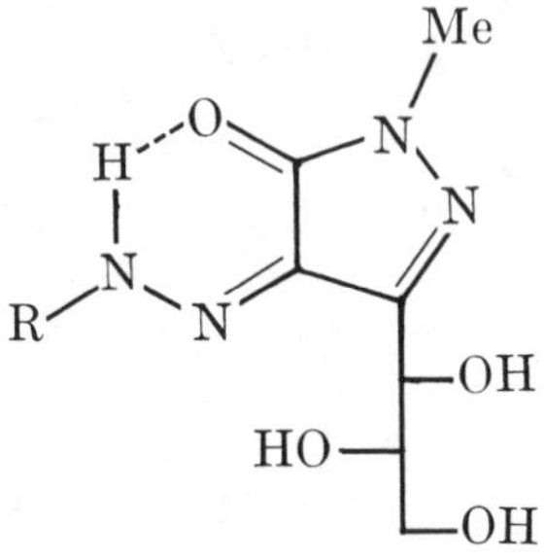

43

DHA Bishydrazones

Treatment of DHA or 38 with the corresponding arylhydrazine afforded the bis(arylhydrazone) (41) (33–40). Similarly, aroylhydrazines and semicarbazide condensed readily with DHA to give the corresponding bishydrazone (41, 42) and bis(semicarbazone) (43, 44). A series of derivatives related to sulfa drugs (45) was prepared by the reaction of DHA with hydrazines having such moieties.

The bishydrazones are now known to be in the 1,4-lactone form, showing that no opening of the lactone ring in DHA occurred during the reaction. However, at one time (38) the 1,5-lactone was the preferred form, since the IR spectra of the bishydrazones showed a carbonyl lactone band at a frequency lower than that expected for a

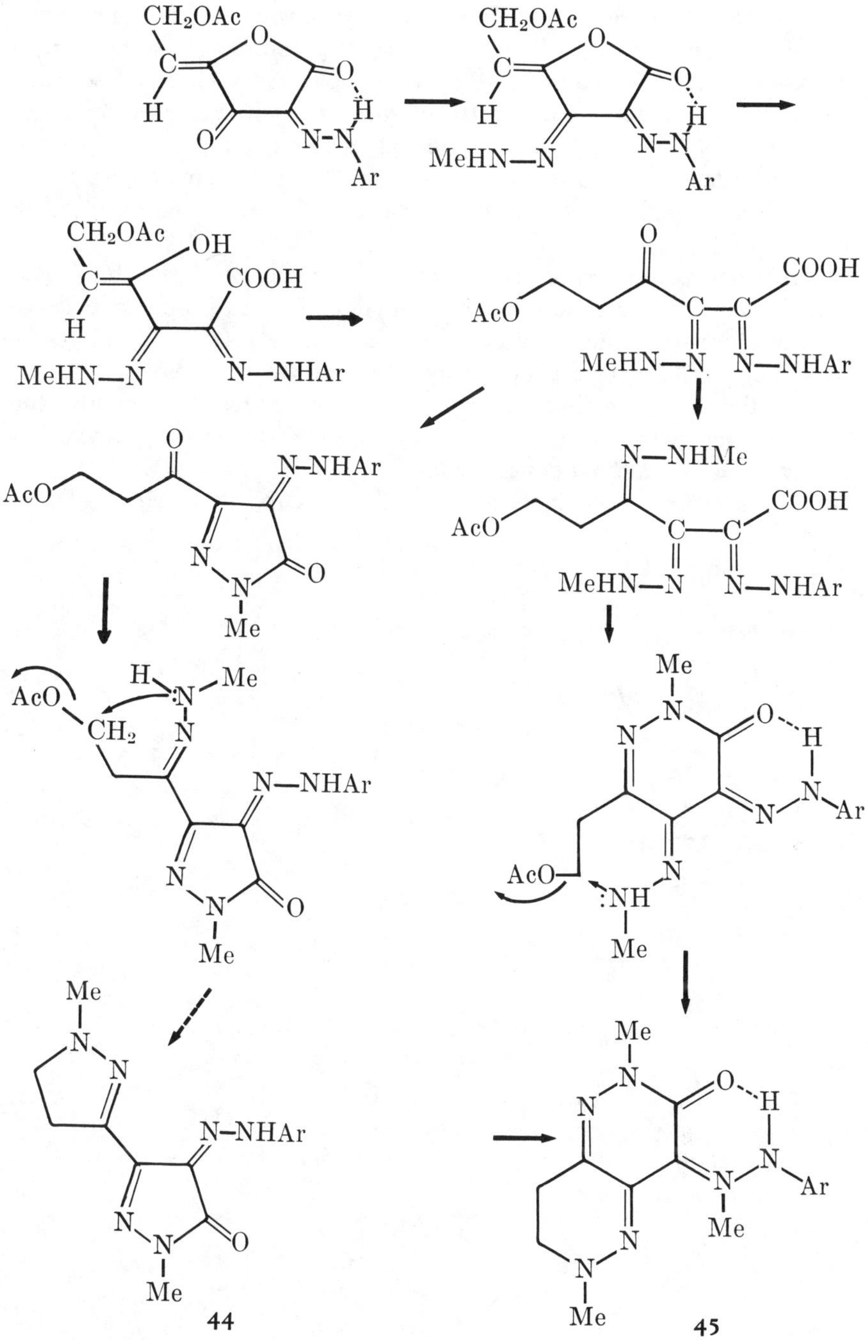

Scheme 1.

1,4-lactone. The observed low frequency is probably caused by hydrogen bonding of the lactone carbonyl with the imino proton of the hydrazone residue on C2, as shown by NMR spectroscopy. The same low frequency band also appeared in the spectra of the bis(arylhydrazones) of other analogues (42, 46) such as the phenyl analogue of DHA [4-phenyl-butano-1,4-lactone 2,3-bis(phenylhydrazone)], which cannot form a 1,5-lactone. Finally, the lactone ring size was also deduced from its chemical reactions (24).

Another controversial aspect of the bishydrazone structure concerns the hydrazone residues. The bishydrazone was proposed to have the structure 46, which mutarotates in solution to 47 (47). More recently, on the basis of a comparative study of the spectroscopic properties of the bis(phenylhydrazone) with some related compounds, the bishydrazone was assigned the structure 2,3-dideoxy-3-phenylazo-2-phenylhydrazino-L-*threo*-hex-2-enone-1,4-lactone (48) (48). However, this latter structure was inconsistent with its ^{13}C NMR spectra (49).

46   47

48

Reactions of the Bishydrazones

Rearrangement into Pyrazolediones. L-*threo*-2,3-Hexodiulosono-1,4-lactone 2,3-bis(phenylhydrazone) rearranged to 1-phenyl-4-phenylazo-3-(L-*threo*-glycerol-1-yl)-pyrazoline-5-one (**49**) when its solution in alkali was acidified with acetic acid (*50*). The reaction was further extended to other bis(arylhydrazones) (*51*). The structure of the phenyl analogue (**49**) was established by oxidation to the known 3-carboxy-1-phenyl-4-phenylazopyrazolin-5-one (*50*). Later, on the basis of NMR data (*39*), the structure of this group of compounds was formulated as the hydrazones (*51*). Acylation of **51** afforded the tri-O-acylated derivatives (*51*), while periodate oxidation of **51** gave 3-formyl-1-aryl-4,5-pyrazoledione-4-(arylhydrazone) (**54**), which could be transformed into a variety of derivatives (*29, 51*) upon reaction with amines, hydrazines, semicarbazide, or thiosemicarbazide. The thiosemicarbazones were cyclized to the thiadiazoles, which are of chemitherapeutic interest (*52*).

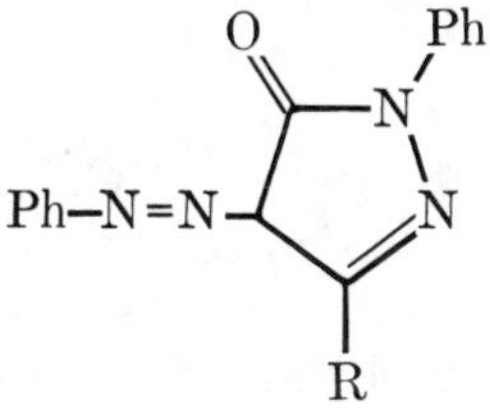

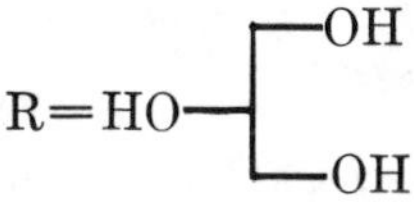

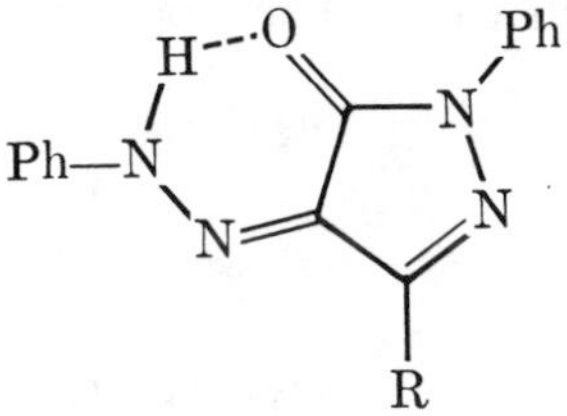

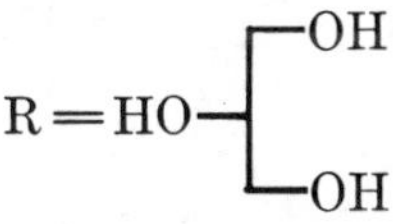

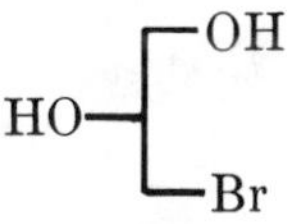

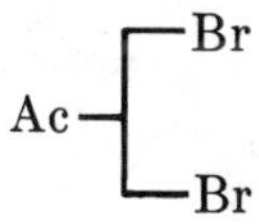

54   R=CHO

55   R=CH=N—NHR′

Reduction of the phenyl analogue 51 with zinc in acetic acid in etha-
nolic solution afforded substituted rubiazonic acid (56), whose structure
was confirmed by IR and NMR spectroscopy (53). Upon reaction of 51
with hydrogen bromide in acetic acid, the major product was isolated
and its structure was confirmed (54) to be that of 53. The monobromo-
deoxy derivative (52) was prepared from the bromodeoxy-L-ascorbic
acid.

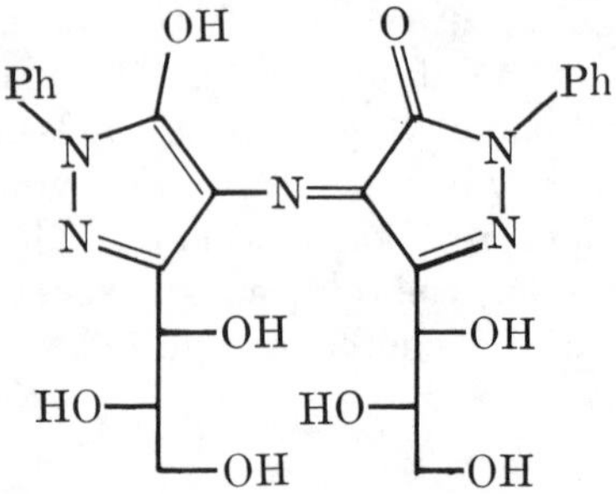

56

Treatment of L-*threo*-2,3-hexodiulosono-1,4-lactone 2,3-bis(semicarbazone) with dilute sodium hydroxide solution afforded the sodium salt
of L-*threo*-2,3-hexodiulosonic acid 2,3-bis(semicarbazone) (43, 44), which
upon heating yielded 57. The bis(semicarbazone) afforded the pyrazole
(59) on dissolution in liquid ammonia and acidification with dilute
sulfuric acid to pH 4, whereas acidification to pH 2 afforded 58.

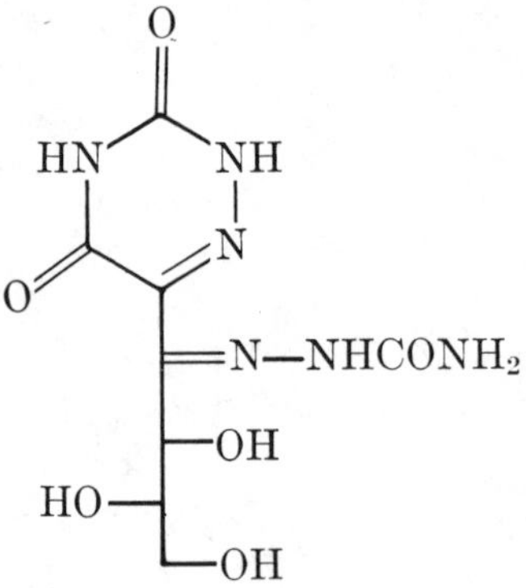

57

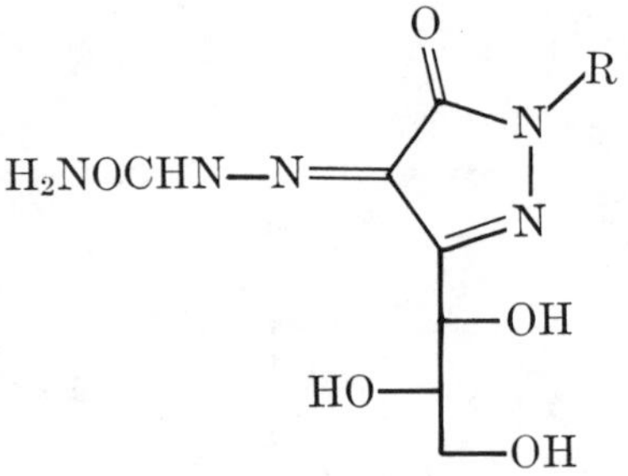

58   R = H
59   R = CONH$_2$

Conversion into Pyrazine Derivatives. Pyrazine derivatives are examples of 1,2-diazines in the carbohydrate series (*24*). The derivative was prepared by partial tosylation of **41** to give the mono-*p*-toluenesulfonyl derivative (**60**), which upon treatment with sodium iodide in acetone gave the bicyclic diazine derivative (**62**). However, the di-*p*-toluenesulfonyl derivative (**61**) afforded, under conditions similar to those specified, the 6-deoxy-6-iodo **63**. The 6-bromodeoxy **64** was prepared (*54*) by reacting phenylhydrazine with 6-bromo-6-deoxy-L-ascorbic acid.

60   R = Ts, R′ = H
61   R = R′ = Ts

62

63   R = I, R′ = Ts
64   R = Br, R′ = H

Oxidation of Bishydrazones. Mild oxidation of the bishydrazones (**41**) with cupric chloride yielded yellow bicyclic compounds (**66**) and not the anticipated triazoles (**72**). The structures were confirmed by both degradative and spectroscopic (*55–60*) methods. Thus, upon treatment with alkali and acidification of the phenyl analogue of **66**, the monophenylhydrazide of mesoxalic acid (**68**) was obtained. This compound gave **69** upon acetylation (*57*). Acetylation of **66** afforded a mono-*O*-acetyl derivative whose NMR spectrum showed only one imino proton instead of two in its precursor. The structure has been confirmed by detailed mass spectroscopy, and ^{13}C NMR and ^{15}N NMR spectroscopy. The structure was questioned when electron impact mass spectroscopy detected a molecular ion peak two mass units higher than expected. Careful experiments at low temperature revealed that the molecular ion disproportionates when heated, giving an ion of 65 (58, 59).

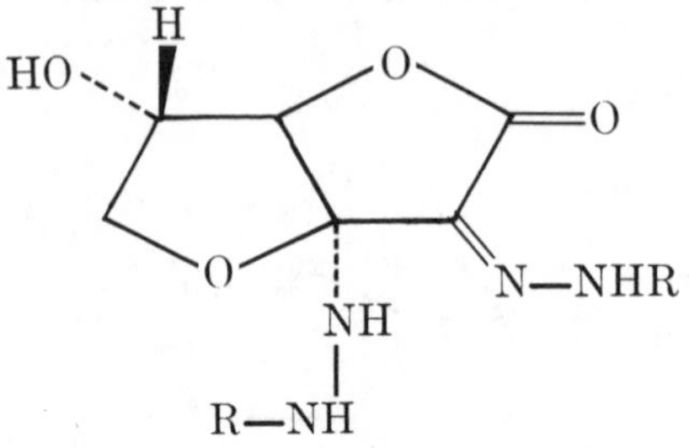

65

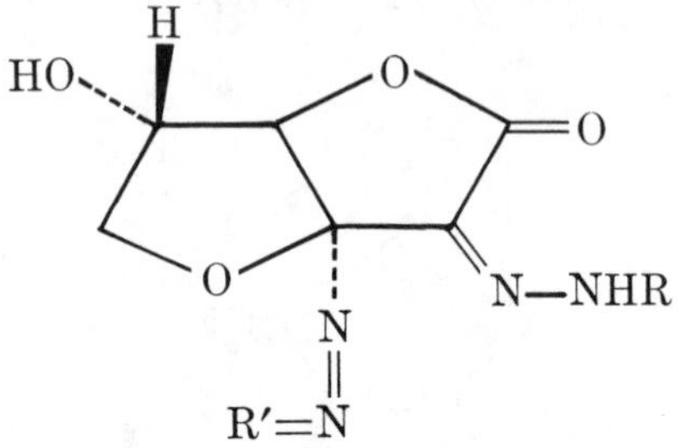

66   R = R′
67   R ≠ R′

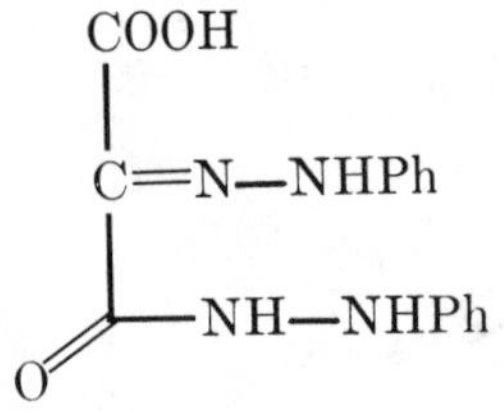

68

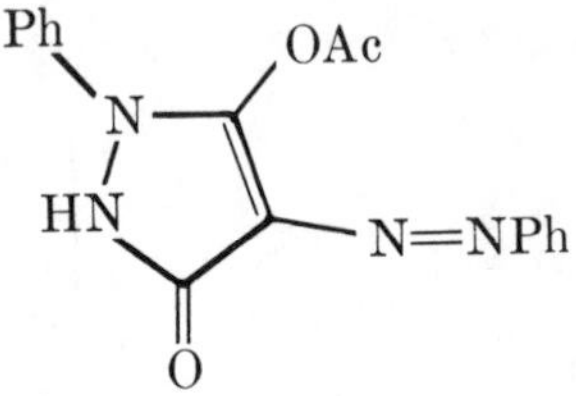

69

Mixed bishydrazones (25, 26, 61) of type 42 were similarly transformed into 67 upon treatment with cupric chloride (30). The bis(o-chlorophenyl) analogue of 41 gave the corresponding o-chloro derivative of 66 without loss of chlorine atoms (40), as was anticipated from previous studies in the carbohydrate series. Bromination of the bis(phenylhydrazone) (41) afforded the p-bromophenyl analogue (66) (62).

To synthesize the triazole (71), another approach (63) was used, where dehydration of the mixed hydrazone oxime (70) (61) with acetic anhydride afforded the triazole (71).

Reduction of Bishydrazones. Catalytic hydrogenation (64) of the bis(phenylhydrazone) (41) gave the diamino derivative (73). Derivatives of the latter were prepared by reacting it with different aldehydes to give imidazoline derivatives (74) (65). Reduction of 41 with lithium aluminum hydride afforded a product tentatively formulated as 75 (53).

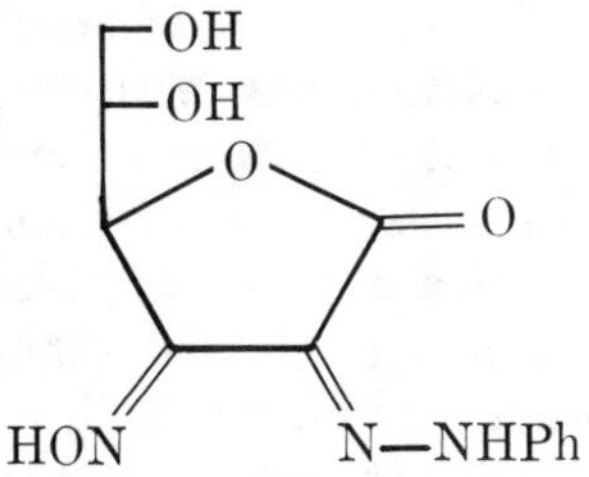

70

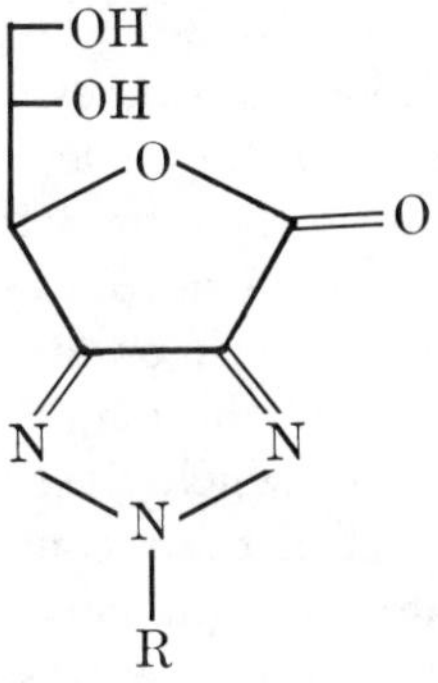

71 R = Ph
72 R = Ar

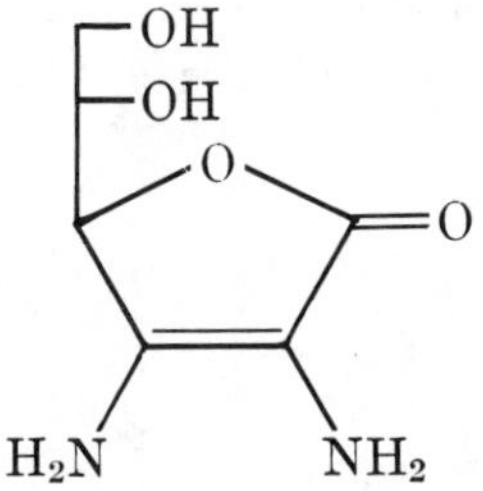

73

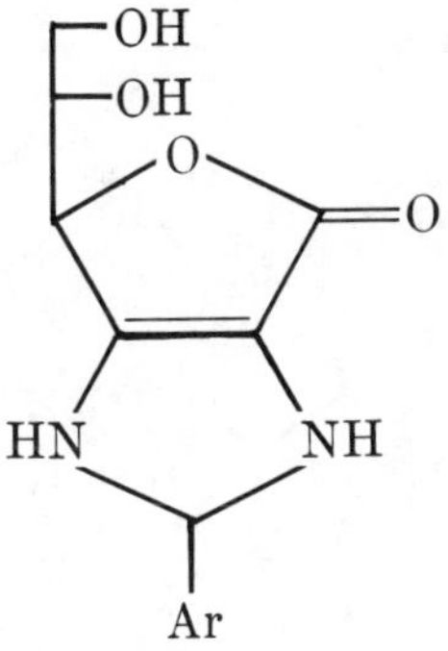

74

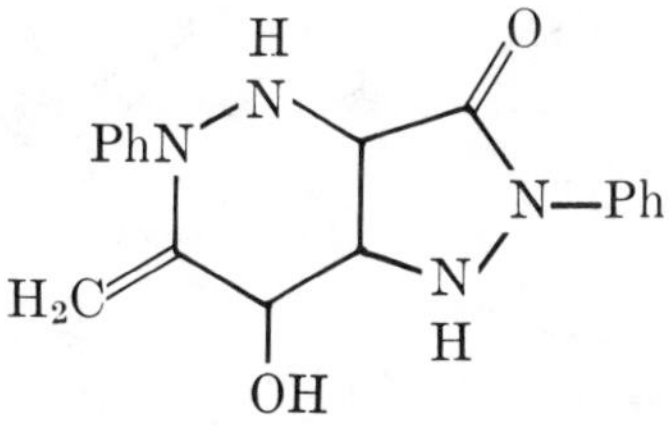

75

Reaction of DHA with Amino Acids

Amino acids are quickly deaminated by L-ascorbic acid, leading to browning reactions (*66*). In the presence of oxygen, iron, and ascorbic acid or DHA, the amino acids gave ammonia, carbon dioxide, and an aldehyde with one carbon less than the original acid (*67, 68*). The aldehydes are isolated as dimedone derivatives and are useful for identification of the amino acids. In the presence of copper and UV light, the deamination is increased. The red color (*69–73*) formed upon reaction of DHA with amino acids was used for their detection. Recent studies (*74–78*) of the reaction of DHA with amino acids led to the isolation of a product that changes readily to a novel, stable, free radical species identified as tri(2-deoxy-2-L-ascorbyl)amine (*76*). Chemical studies using acetone derivatives and analogous compounds (*79*) confirmed the structure of *76*; the structure of the free radical, obtained upon its oxidation, retained the symmetrical structure. Electrochemical studies (*80*) show that *76* is oxidized in aqueous solution in two reversible, one-electron transfer steps on mercury or platinum electrodes. The first step occurs through the dianion and its product is an unusually stable blue anion radical, which gives a characteristic electron spin resonance signal. The product of the second step of oxidation is labile and is slowly converted into a red pigment, whose structure is formulated as the oxidized form of bis(2-deoxy-2-L-ascorbyl)amine (*81*), presumably by hydrolysis with splitting of L-ascorbic acid.

DHA reacted with *p*-aminobenzoic acid in the presence of hydrochloric acid affording 6-carboxy-2-hydroxy-4-hydroxymethylquinoline (*77*) (*82*).

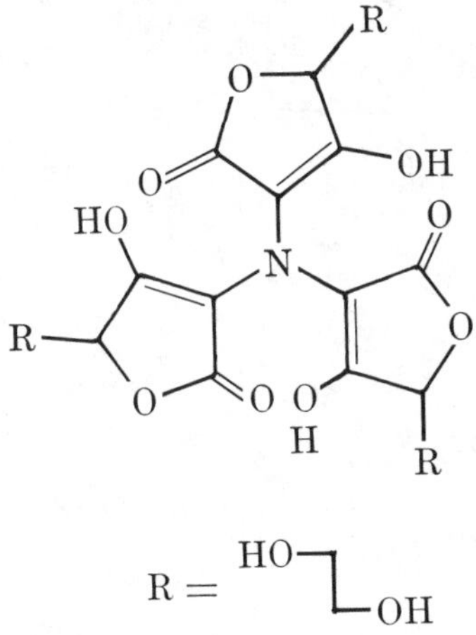

76

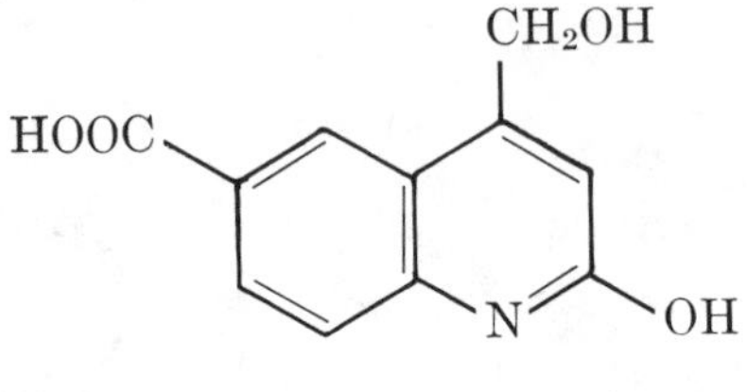

77

Bound Form of L-Ascorbic Acid

After the characterization of vitamin C as ascorbic acid, it was observed that the content of ascorbic acid in some vegetables (*83, 84*) increases when boiled or cooked. The increase is believed to be caused by liberation of bound ascorbic acid (*85, 86, 87*). The name ascorbigen (*87*) was given to that substance that was later separated (*88*) and synthesized (*89, 90, 91*). Ascorbigen was synthesized either from 3-hydroxy indole and ascorbic acid or from indole, formaldehyde, and ascorbic acid.

Acknowledgments

I am indebted to C. Schuerch and H. El Khadem for their encouragement. I express my sincere thanks to all participants in this study: Y. El Kilany, N. Rashed, A. Amer, A. Moussad, M. Shoukry, and F. Singab.

Literature Cited

1. Roe, J. H. *Ann. N.Y. Acad. Sci.* **1961**, *92*, 277.
2. Erlbach, H.; Ohle, H. *Ber. Dtsch. Chem. Ges.* **1934**, *67*, 555.
3. Ogawa, S. *Yakugaku Zasshi* **1953**, *73*, 309.
4. Henseke, G.; Dose, W.; Dittrich, K. *Angew. Chem.* **1957**, *69*, 479.
5. Henseke, G.; Dittrich, K. *Chem. Ber.* **1959**, *92*, 1550.
6. Henseke, G.; Lehmann, D.; Dittrich, K. *Chem. Ber.* **1961**, *94*, 1743.
7. Henseke, G. *Z. Chem.* **1966**, *6*, 329.
8. El Ashry, E. S. H.; El Kholy, I. E.; El Kilany, Y. *Int. Symp. Carbohydr. Chem., London, 1978,* A19.
9. El Ashry, E. S. H.; El Kholy, I. E.; El Kilany, Y. *Carbohydr. Res.* **1978**, *60*, 303.
10. Ibid., *67*, 495.
11. El Ashry, E. S. H.; Nassr, M. M.; Shoukry, M. *Carbohydr. Res.* **1980**, *83*, 79.
12. El Ashry, E. S. H.; El Kilany, Y.; Amer, A.; Zimmer, H., unpublished data.
13. El Ashry, E. S. H.; El Kholy, I. E.; El Kilany, Y. *Carbohydr. Res.* **1978**, *60*, 396.
14. Ohle, H.; Melkonian, G. *Ber. Dtsch. Chem. Ges.* **1941**, *74*, 279.
15. Ibid., 398.
16. Ohle, H.; Liebig, R. *Ber. Dtsch. Chem. Ges.* **1942**, *75*, 1536.
17. Ohle, H., Kruyff, J. *Ber. Dtsch. Chem. Ges.* **1944**, *77*, 507.
18. French, D.; Wild, G. W.; James, W. J. *J. Am. Chem. Soc.* **1953**, *75*, 3664.
19. El Ashry, E. S. H.; El Kholy, I. E.; El Kilany, Y. *Carbohydr. Res.* **1978**, *64*, 81.
20. El Ashry, E. S. H.; Abdel Rahman, M. M. A.; Nassr, M.; Amer, A. *Carbohydr. Res.* **1978**, *67*, 403.
21. Hasselquist, H. *Ark. Kemi* **1952**, *4*, 369.
22. Dahn, H.; Moll, H. *Helv. Chem. Acta* **1964**, *47*, 1860.
23. Micheel, F.; Mittag, R. *Naturwissenschaften* **1937**, *25*, 158.
24. El Khadem, H.; El Ashry, E. S. H. *Carbohydr. Res.* **1970**, *13*, 57.
25. El Ashry, E. S. H.; El Kholy, I. E.; El Kilany, Y. *Carbohydr. Res.* **1977**, *59*, 417.
26. El Ashry, E. S. H.; El Kilany, Y.; Singab, F. *Carbohydr. Res.* **1978**, *67*, 415.
27. Hvoslef, J.; Pedersen, B. *Acta Chem. Scand.* **1979**, *33*, 503.
28. Ozawa, T.; Nakamura, Y. *Yakugaku Zasshi* **1973**, *93*, 304.
29. El Ashry, E. S. H.; El Kilany, Y.; Singab, F. *Carbohydr. Res.* **1977**, *56*, 93.
30. El Ashry, E. S. H.; El Ashry, Y. *Chem. Ind. (London)* **1976**, 372.
31. El Ashry, E. S. H.; *Carbohydr. Res.* **1976**, *52*, 69.
32. Stam, C.; El Ashry, E. S. H.; El Kilany, Y.; Van der Plas, H. C. *J. Heterocycl. Chem.* **1980**, *17*, 617.
33. Herbert, R. W.; Hirst, E. L.; Percival, E. G. V.; Reynolds, R. J. W.; Smith, J. *J. Chem. Soc.* **1933**, 1270.
34. Antener, I. *Helv. Chem. Acta* **1947**, *20*, 742.
35. Drevon, B.; Nofr, C.; Cier, A. *Compt. Rend.* **1956**, *243*, 607.
36. Szotyori, K. S. *Nahrung* **1967**, *11*, 129.

37. El Khadem, H.; El Ashry, E. S. H. *Carbohydr. Res.* **1968**, 7, 501.
38. El Khadem, H.; El Ashry, E. S. H. *J. Chem. Soc.* **1968**, 2248.
39. El Khadem, H.; Meshreki, M. H.; El Ashry, E. S. H.; El Sekeili, M. *Carbohydr. Res.* **1972**, 21, 430.
40. El Ashry, E. S. H.; Labib, G. H.; El Kilany, Y. *Carbohydr. Res.* **1976**, 52, 200.
41. Fischer, R. *Pharm. Ztg.* **1934**, 79, 1207.
42. El Ashry, E. S. H.; Nassr, M.; Singab, F. *Carbohydr. Res.* **1977**, 56, 200.
43. Provost, C.; Fleury, M. *Compt. Rend.* **1964**, 258, 587.
44. Fleury, M. *Bull. Soc. Chim. Fr.* **1966**, 522.
45. Soliman, R.; El Ashry, E. S. H.; El Kholy, I. E.; El Kilany, Y. *Carbohydr. Res.* **1978**, 67, 179.
46. El Khadem, H.; El Sahfei, Z. M.; El Ashry, E. S. H.; El Sadek, M. *Carbohydr. Res.* **1976**, 49, 185.
47. Rao, J. M.; Nair, P. M. *Tetrahedron* **1970**, 26, 3833.
48. Roberts, G. A. F. *J. Chem. Soc.* **1979**, 603.
49. Pollet, P.; Gelin, S. *Tetrahedron* **1980**, 36, 2955.
50. Ohle, H. *Ber. Dtsch. Chem. Ges.* **1934**, 67, 1750.
51. El Khadem, H.; El Ashry, E. S. H. *J. Chem. Soc.* **1968**, 2248.
52. El Ashry, E. S. H.; Abdel Rahman, M. M.; Hazah, A.; Singab, F. *Sci. Pharm.* **1980**, 48, 13.
53. El Khadem, H.; El Shafei, Z. M.; El Sekeili, M. *J. Org. Chem.* **1972**, 22, 3523.
54. El Ashry, E. S. H.; El Kilany, Y. *Carbohydr. Res.* **1980**, 80, C8.
55. El Khadem, H.; El Ashry, E. S. H. *Carbohydr. Res.* **1968**, 7, 507.
56. El Khadem, H.; El Ashry, E. S. H. *J. Chem. Soc.* **1968**, 2251.
57. El Khadem, H.; El Ashry, E. S. H. *J. Heterocycl. Chem.* **1973**, 10, 1051.
58. El Khadem, H.; El Ashry, E. S. H.; Kreishman, G. P., presented at the 2nd Chem. Congr. North Am. Continent, San Francisco, 1980, Carb-11.
59. El Khadem, H.; El Ashry, E. S. H.; Jaeger, D. L.; Kreishman, G. P.; Foltz, R. L. *J. Heterocycl. Chem.* **1980**, 17, 1181.
60. El Khadem, H.; Coxon, B. *Carbohydr. Res.*, in press.
61. El Ashry, E. S. H.; Abdel Rahman, M. M. A.; Mancy, S.; El Shafei, Z. M. *Acta Chim. Acad. Sci. Hung.* **1977**, 95, 409.
62. El Ashry, E. S. H.; El Kilany, Y.; Singab, F. *Carbohydr. Res.* **1980**, 82, 25.
63. El Sekeili, M.; Mancy, S.; El Kholy, I. E.; El Ashry, E. S. H.; El Khadem, H. S.; Swartz, D. L. *Carbohydr. Res.* **1977**, 59, 141.
64. Micheel, F.; Bode, G.; Siebert, R. *Ber. Dtsch. Chem. Ges.* **1937**, 70, 1862.
65. Gross, B.; El Sekeili, M. A.; Mancy, S.; El Khadem, H. *Carbohydr. Res.* **1974**, 37, 384.
66. Abderhalden, E. *Wien. Klin. Wochenschr.* **1937**, 50, 815.
67. Abderhalden, E. *Fermentforschung* **1937**, 15, 285.
68. Ibid., **1938**, 15, 522.
69. Wurtz, B.; North, J. C. *Compt. Rend.* **1963**, 256, 1388.
70. Mori, Y.; Kumano, S.; Nango, I.; Kano, M.; *Eiyo To Shokuryo*, **1967**, 20, 211.
71. Ibid., 216.
72. Shamanna, R.; Lakshiminarayana, S. *J. Agric. Food Chem.* **1968**, 16, 528.
73. Pohloudek-Fabini, R.; Fuerting, W. *J. Chromatogr.* **1964**, 13, 139.
74. Namiki, M.; Yano, M.; Hayashi, T. *Chem. Lett.* **1974**, 125.
75. Yano, M.; Hayashi, T.; Namiki, M. *Chem. Lett.* **1974**, 1973.
76. Yano, M.; Hayashi, T.; Namiki, M. *J. Agric. Food Chem.* **1976**, 24, 815.
77. Yano, M.; Hayashi, T.; Namiki, M. *Agric. Biol. Chem.* **1978**, 42, 2239.
78. Hayashi, T.; Namiki, M. *Tetrahedron Lett.* **1979**, 4476.
79. Hayashi, T.; Manou, F.; Namiki, M.; Tsuji, K., unpublished data.
80. Tsuji, T.; Hayashi, T.; Namiki, M. *Electrochim. Acta* **1980**, 25, 605.

81. Kurata, T.; Fujimaki, M.; Sakurai, Y. *J. Agric. Food Chem.* **1973**, *21*, 676.
82. Hasselquist, H. *Ark. Kemi* **1964**, *7*, 121.
83. Ahmad, B. *Biochem. J.* **1935**, 275.
84. McHenry, E. W.; Graham, M. L. *Nature* **1935**, *135*, 871.
85. Guha, B. C.; Pal, J. C. *Nature* **1936**, *137*, 946.
86. Ibid., **1937**, *139*, 844.
87. Sen-Gupta, P. N.; Guha, B. C. *Nature* **1938**, *141*, 974.
88. Prochazka, Z.; Sanda, V.; Sorm, F. *Collect. Czech. Chem. Commun.* **1957**, *22*, 333, 654.
89. Gimelin, R.; Virtanen, A. I. *Ann. Acad. Sci. Fenn., Ser. A2* **1961**, *107*.
90. Piironen, E.; Virtanen, A. I. *Acta Chem. Scand.* **1962**, *16*, 1286.
91. Virtanen, A. I.; Piironen, E. *Suom. Kemistil.* **1962**, *35*, 104.

RECEIVED for review January 22, 1981. ACCEPTED June 2, 1981.

Determination of Ascorbic Acid and Dehydroascorbic Acid

HOWERDE E. SAUBERLICH, MARTIN D. GREEN,
and STANLEY T. OMAYE[1]

U.S. Department of Agriculture–SEA Western Human Nutrition Research
Center and Letterman Army Institute of Research, Presidio of
San Francisco, CA 94129

*Advantages and limitations of commonly used and recently
developed methods for the analysis of ascorbic acid and
dehydroascorbic acid in foods and biological samples have
been reviewed. Various procedures based on titrimetric,
spectrophotometric, or fluorometric principles have been
used for this purpose. Depending upon the procedure
selected, dehydroascorbic acid, hydroascorbic acid, or total
ascorbic acid levels may be measured. Although often quite
accurate, these techniques can be laborious and time-consuming. Recently, the usefulness of high performance
liquid chromatography (HPLC) in the measurement of
ascorbic acid in multivitamin products has been extended
to foods and biological materials, including plasma, and
liver, brain, and adrenal glands. Advantages of the technique include fast analysis times, high sensitivity, and
minimum sample preparation.*

There are many methods for determining the α-ketolactone, L-ascorbic
acid (1-*threo*-2,4,5,6-pentohexane-2-carboxylic acid lactone), activity
in animal tissue extracts and fluids (*1, 2*) and food extracts (*3, 4*). With
the exception of outdated bioassays, most of the analytical procedures
used for the measurement of ascorbic acid fall into two categories: (i)
the determination of the reduced form of ascorbic acid, usually based
upon the oxidation–reduction properties of the vitamin; or (ii) the
determination of total ascorbic acid based upon the oxidation of ascorbic

[1] Current address: U.S. Department of Agriculture–SEA Western Regional Research Center, Berkeley, CA 94710.

acid followed by the formation of a hydrazone or fluorophor (5). The situation regarding chemical analyses for the vitamin remains dynamic, very much like the search for the biochemical mechanism of action of ascorbic acid. The complex biological relationship between the compound(s) possessing vitamin C activity, as well as the chemical similarity of these compounds to others that are inactive, has made the existence of a single, simple, and specific method close to impossible. This has led to a proliferation of method papers that has continued to the present.

Recently, due to the advancements in high performance liquid chromatography (HPLC), quantitative measurements of unmodified L-ascorbic acid and its metabolites have become possible. Soon the measurement of L-ascorbic acid and L-dehydroascorbic acid and other ascorbate metabolites simultaneously should be forthcoming. These methods will be of particular interest in research, since recent findings suggest a biological significance for dehydroascorbic acid and other ascorbate metabolites (6, 7, 8, 9). In the following paragraphs various techniques often used to measure ascorbic acid content will be briefly reviewed and some of the more recent developments in high performance liquid chromatographic techniques used in ascorbic acid analysis will be explored.

Bioassays

Bioassays have the distinct advantage of measuring the summation of chemical entities that possess only vitamin C activity and exclude material devoid of vitamin C activity. At the present time, bioassays are used only on occasion in comparative studies to establish the biological specificity of chemicals and in the determination of the antiscorbutic activity of individual products. However, bioassays are time-consuming, expensive, and lack precision; therefore, their applicability is limited. Rats cannot be used as test animals because of their ability to synthesize the vitamin; however, guinea pigs with their high requirement for vitamin C have been proved satisfactory. Unfortunately, there are no microbiological organisms that have an absolute requirement for ascorbic acid that can be used as the basis for a bioassay.

One of the first bioassay methods used defined the amount of test material just sufficient to prevent scurvy in the guinea pig as equivalent to one Sherman unit or 0.5–0.6 mg ascorbic acid (10). Test animals are fed a basal diet containing all known nutrients except ascorbic acid and supplemented with graded amounts of the test sample. At the end of 6–10 weeks, the degree of protection against scurvy is determined by autopsy findings and survival rates (11). Several bioassays have used dental histology as an end point (4, 12, 13). After 2 weeks on a given basal diet, supplemented with graded levels of the test substance or ascorbic acid, the guinea pigs are killed, the lower jaws removed and sections made of the decalcified incisors. The degree of protection is assessed by microscopic examination for histologic changes such as disorganization of the odontoblasts, the width of irregularity, and the structure of the dentine and the degree of calcification of the predentine. There is also a simple curative method based on weight changes in guinea pigs during scurvy (*14*). A quantitative bioassay based upon serum levels of alkaline phosphatase has been worked out for ascorbate activity (*15*). In this method, the level of serum alkaline phosphatase in the test animal is first reduced 1–5 units by ascorbate depletion, and then the test sample is administered at varying ascorbic acid levels. The details and the numerous precautions that one should take in bioassays have been reviewed elsewhere (*4*). In 1931, the unit of vitamin C adopted was the activity in 0.1 mL of freshly squeezed lemon juice. Subsequently, one International Unit (I.U.) or one U.S.P. XIV unit of vitamin C was adopted as the antiscorbutic activity of 0.05 mg of ascorbic acid, the approximate amount in 1 mL of lemon juice. Therefore, 1 g of ascorbic acid is equivalent to 20,000 I.U.

Chemical and Physical Methods of Analysis

Optical Absorbance and Spectrophotometric Methods.   Direct spectrophotometric methods involving light absorption have some limited value for very high potency material. The absorbance spectrum of ascorbic acid in neutral aqueous solutions has a peak value at 265 nm with E between 7500 and 16,650 as reported in the literature. The differences are due to nonanaerobic conditions (*16, 17*). The maximum is shifted towards 245 nm in acidic solutions. Dehydroascorbic acid is transparent in the region of 230 nm to 280 nm, but has a weak absorption, $E_{max} = 720$ at 300 nm (*18*). A basic drawback to the successful application of spectrophotometric methods to the estimation of ascorbic acid is that the well-defined absorption band in the UV region of the spectrum is subject to interference from many substances, which would present a problem when applied to food and tissue extracts.

Colorimetric Methods.   The most frequently used colorimetric methods have been recently reviewed by Omaye et al. (*5*). Several methods of analyses are based upon the fact that ascorbic acid and dehydroascorbic acid possess certain chemical properties characteristic of sugars such as formation of osazones and conversion to furfural. Colorimetric determination of furfural, an aniline derivative, has been used to a limited extent for the estimation of ascorbic acid in certain materials. These methods have generally been found to be unsatisfactory for the measurement of ascorbic acid in food. For some time, methods for the determination of ascorbic acid based on the reduction of 2,6-dichlorophenolindophenol or the formation of a colored dinitrophenyl-hydrazine derivative by the vitamin, were the most satisfactory. Although introduced in 1927 (19, 20), dichlorophenolindophenol has remained useful because ascorbate is essentially the only substance in acid extracts that reduces the indophenol at pH 1 to 4 to the colorless leuco form. For high sensitivity and specificity the dinitrophenylhydrazine method, where the 2- and 3-carbon keto group of diketogulonic acid forms a bis-2,4-dinitrophenylhydrazone, was often used. The osazone rearranges in acid to form a stable red product. Thiosulfate; certain metal ions, for example, copper and iron; and reductones may interfere. Depending upon the analytical conditions used, fructose, glucose, and glucuronic acid may also interfere in the dinitrophenylhydrazine method to yield high values (21). The dichlorophenolindophenol method measures only reduced ascorbate, while the dinitrophenylhydrazine method will measure dehydroascorbic acid and total ascorbic acid, with the difference reflecting the reduced ascorbic acid (22, 23). Dehydroascorbic acid can be reduced to ascorbic acid by agents such as 2,3-dimercaptopropanol (BAL) permitting the measurement of total ascorbic acid with dichlorophenolindophenol (24). Because of technical reasons, the procedure appears to have limited use. Several automated procedures for the measurement of ascorbic acid in serum have been described (25, 26, 27, 28).

The colorimetric methods often provide measures to stabilize the lactone ring of ascorbic acid from hydrolysis by decreasing the pH. Although the dry pure crystals of ascorbic acid are stable on the exposure to air and light at room temperature for long periods of time, aqueous solutions of the vitamin are oxidized on exposure to air, alkali, and certain traces of metals (1). Below pH 4.0, ascorbic acid and its biologically occurring oxidative product, dehydroascorbic acid, are stable. Once dehydroascorbic acid has been oxidized to diketogulonic acid and other compounds, its value as an antiscorbutic agent has been lost. In vivo, dehydroascorbic acid is reduced to ascorbic acid; however, further oxidation is irreversible.

The use of metaphosphoric acid solutions for the extraction of ascorbic acid from plant and animal tissues was first proposed in 1935 (29). Metaphosphoric acid, along with trichloroacetic acid, remain as the reagents of choice. Besides the decreased tendency for hydrolysis of the lactone ring, metaphosphoric acid inhibits the catalytic oxidation of ascorbic acid by metal catalysts, such as copper and iron ions, and it inactivates the enzymes that oxidize ascorbic acid. Oxidation of ascorbic acid, which apparently is the result of the action of oxyhemoglobin, may occur when animal tissues are ground with metaphosphoric acid. This oxidation is proportional to the blood content of the tissue, but is not a serious objection except in the case of whole blood or isolated red blood cells. To a certain extent, the problem of oxidation by oxyhemoglobin can be reduced by prior treatment of blood samples with carbon monoxide (30).

Other colorimetric methods include the official method of the United States Pharmacopeia, which is an iodometric determination (31). Various titrimetric procedures have been described (32). Recently, a sensitive rate assay method for the determination of ascorbic acid was described that used a stopped-flow apparatus (33). Several methods based upon coupling ascorbic acid to diazonium compounds have been proposed (34, 35). The deep blue derivative is determined colorimetrically. A quantitative reaction between selenious acid (1 mol) and ascorbic acid (2 mol) to form selenium has been reported (36). Stable selenious colloids can be formed when food extracts containing ascorbic acid are treated with selenious acid, and the resulting turbidity is proportional to the ascorbic acid content. There is also a chemical test for the determination of ascorbic acid that depends upon the reduction of ferric ion to ferrous ion by ascorbic acid followed by the determination of the ferrous ion as the red orange α-α'-dipyridyl complex. In the presence of orthophosphoric acid at pH 1–2, other reducing or interfering materials are inhibited. This simple method is fast and has gained considerable usage (5, 37, 38).

Attempts have been made to adapt the centrifugal analyzer to provide an automated method for determining ascorbic acid in serum and urine (39). The method is based on the reduction of ferric iron by ascorbic acid, producing dehydroascorbic acid, and the formation of a color between the resulting ferrous ion and the chromogenic reagent, ferrozine [3-(2-pyridyl)-5,6-bis-(4-phenylsulfonic acid)-1,2,4-triazine disodium salt] (40). Although the method was reported to be highly precise and specific, additional validation appears necessary.

Enzyme methods using ascorbic acid oxidase have not been widely used but several versions of reagents based on diazotized nitroanilines have been reported (41). The reaction is complicated and the ascorbic acid molecule is partly destroyed in forming the colored product. A chromatographic separation stage must precede the color development reaction (42). The procedure is time-consuming and there is no provision for reducing any dehydroascorbic acid in the sample extract to ascorbic acid.

Fluorometric Methods. One of the most specific methods for the determination of ascorbic acid and its biologically active oxidation product, dehydroascorbic acid, is the fluorometric method introduced by Deutsch and Weeks (43), which is an official AOAC method (44). It is based on the oxidation of ascorbic acid to dehydroascorbic acid and the condensation of dehydroascorbic acid with *ortho*-phenylenediamine to form the fluorophor, quinoxaline. Deutsch and Weeks (*43*) rigorously examined the sensitivity and specificity of the method and concluded that the procedure was suitable for samples containing large amounts of reducing substances or highly colored materials. For the initial oxidation of ascorbic acid to dehydroascorbic acid, various chemical oxidants, such as iodine, ferricyanide, chloramine-T, 2,6-dichloroindophenol, methylene blue, *N*-bromosuccinimide, and charcoal (Norit) have been reported in the literature. Several problems have been encountered when charcoal was used to oxidize ascorbic acid present in the extracts from meats, dairy products, and other complex mixtures of foods (*45*). The analytical results were affected by the grades of the charcoal used and by the method of activation. This is understandable, since the catalytic performance of the charcoal in many redox reactions depends upon the presence of unsaturated sites on the carbon surfaces, which can vary from source to source. *N*-Bromosuccinimide has been reported to serve as a replacement for Norit in the smooth oxidation of ascorbic acid to dehydroascorbic acid in an automated fluorometric assay of total vitamin C in food products (*45*). It appears to serve as an oxidizing agent that is selective (*46, 47*). The reagent is immune to reductones and reductic acids, which are generally present in fruits and vegetables.

Several adaptations of the basic fluorometric method are now available for specific application to plasma (*48*), and to food extracts (*49, 50*). A spectrophotofluorometric assay procedure also has been devised using DEA-Sephadex column to separate erythorbic (isoascorbic acid) and ascorbic acid (*51*). This is of particular importance since erythorbic acid, a very common food additive, has been suggested to be an antagonist of ascorbic acid (*52, 53, 54*). In general, the spectrofluorometric assay procedures involve measurements of fluorescence on solvent extracts of the acidified samples at 365–348 nm and 435–450 nm, as the wavelengths of maximum excitation and emission, respectively (*48, 50, 51*).

Chromatographic Methods. The methods mentioned for ascorbic acid analysis suffer from lack of specificity to varying degrees. Several attempts have been made to correct this by the addition of masking agents or the use of column and/or thin layer chromatography. Although combining chromatographic separations with the analytical methods described above complicates the analyses considerably, this is compensated for by the increased specificity. In many cases, particularly natural products, where interference is high, the use of a chromatographic separation is unavoidable. The selection of the specific method or combination of methods to be used depends upon a variety of factors including the information desired and the nature of the sample.

Many publications have dealt with modifications of the work of Mapson and Partridge (55) as applied to the qualitative and quantitative determination of ascorbic acid and various breakdown products (8) by paper chromatography. The location of ascorbic acid on the chromatograms can be revealed by several development agents including 2,6-dichlorophenolindophenol, ammoniacal silver nitrate tetrazolium salts, iodine vapor, ammonium molybdate, and molybdophosphoric acid. Other chromatographic methods, such as column and thin layer chromatography have been tried out in ascorbic acid studies (56, 57, 58). Such chromatographic procedures have been very valuable in special investigations such as the occurrence of breakdown products or metabolites of the vitamin (9, 59). Chromatographic procedures are also useful to provide confirmatory evidence when testing food for which the specificity of the method is not known. As mentioned before, the isomer of ascorbic acid, erythorbic acid (isoascorbic acid), is particularly difficult to identify when present in foods. Interference by isoascorbic acid in ascorbic acid analyses has been corrected by chromatographic means (60).

Several investigators have reported that ascorbic acid can be analyzed by gas–liquid chromatography following conversion of the parent compound to its trimethylsilyl ether (61–66). The procedures have been found to be reliable and to produce results comparable with those obtained by colorimetric procedures. In most cases, however, measurement of only the reduced form of the vitamin is possible (67). One method is suitable for microanalytical work and has the advantage that several other carbohydrates and carbohydrate derivatives can be measured simultaneously in the same extract (67).

The recent development of commercial HPLC systems has provided a powerful instrumentation for the separation, characterization, identification, and quantitation of minute amounts of essential dietary components (68, 69). Developments in hardware and packings for HPLC have overcome the problems of nonreproducible behavior and low efficiency separations previously associated with column chromatography (70). HPLC has already been applied to the quantitative analysis of analgesics, pesticides, and fat-soluble vitamins with precision and accuracy and a minimum of sample clean-up. Such instrumentation provides a rapid, accurate, and sensitive technique for the separation and analysis of subnanomole quantities of a wide range of complex high-molecular-weight, nonvolatile, thermally labile, compounds that are vital for metabolic and nutritional studies.

Several reports have described the use of HPLC in the analyses of ascorbic acid in foods and vitamin products (71, 72, 73, 74) and in tissue samples (75). Procedures vary in the type of column, mobile-phase, detection systems and means of stabilization of extracts. Reversed-phased,

Bondapak C columns (Water Associates, Milford, Massachusetts) with fixed wavelength detector (254 nm) and the sample or standards stabilized in 0.8% metaphosphoric acid have been used with urine samples (76). In that study 0.8% metaphosphoric acid served as the mobile phase. Other mobile phases, such as methanol–water (50:50) or ammonium salts in methanol–water, were tried but resulted in ascorbic acid values that were too high when compared with titrimetric measurements (76). A similar procedure, substituting an ion exchange column, has been used for multivitamin product analyses (77). With the addition of electrochemical detection, liquid chromatography analysis of ascorbic acid becomes quite specific and sensitive (77, 78, 79). These coupled detector systems (liquid chromatography electrochemical detector, LCEC) have been applied with excellent success to the analyses of ascorbic acid content in food and animal tissues (78, 79). Figure 1 represents a chromatogram for human urine obtained with the use of HPLC and an amperometric electrochemical detector (72). The ascorbic acid peak represents 19 ng. Figure 2 represents the analysis of ascorbic acid in a mouse brain tissue extract also employing HPLC and an electrochemical detector (75). The ascorbic acid peak corresponds to approximately 15 ng. Although the above procedures for the analysis of ascorbic acid content by HPLC have been very useful for determining the reduced

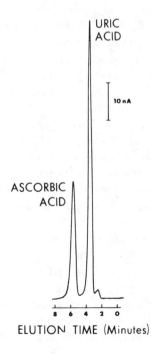

Figure 1. Analysis of ascorbic acid in urine employing HPLC and an amperometric electrochemical detector (72): column, Zipax SAX, 2.1 mm × 50 cm glass; mobile phase, 0.05M acetate buffer, pH 4.75; flow rate, 0.33 mL/min.

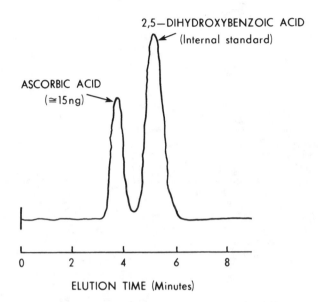

Figure 2. Analysis of ascorbic acid in a mouse brain tissue extract employing HPLC and an electrochemical detector. (Reproduced, with permission, from Ref. 75. Copyright 1975, Pergamon Press, Inc.)

form of the vitamin, they were not useful for determining other forms of ascorbate. Recently, conditions were described for the high performance liquid chromatographic separation of ascorbic acid from dehydroascorbic acid when in pure solutions (*80*). Dehydroascorbic acid was monitored at 228 nm and ascorbic acid at 268 nm (Figure 3). Unfortunately, the minimum detection limits were 500 ng per injection for dehydroascorbic acid compared with 10 ng per injection for ascorbic acid. Finley and Duang (*81*) have also described recently a high performance liquid chromatographic method that will separate and estimate ascorbic acid, dehydroascorbic acid, and 2,3-diketogulonic acid in fruit and vegetable extracts. Subsequent methods for measuring the three forms of ascorbate in animal tissue extracts should be soon forthcoming.

Other Chemical and Physical Methods. Polarography has been tried in special investigations, such as studies of the bound form of ascorbic acid. But because of limited specificity, the procedure has not seen wide application (*82, 83*). Ascorbic acid is oxidized at the dropping mercury electrode, the basis of the polarographic determination. Dehydroascorbic acid is not measured, however, since it is not reducible at the dropping mercury electrode. Mason et al. (*84*) have developed a method for the determination of ascorbic acid based on electrochemical oxidation at the tubular carbon electrode that has been modified to measure water-

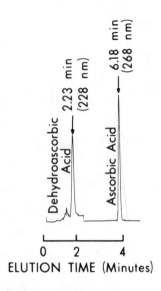

Figure 3. Simultaneous analysis for ascorbic acid and dehydroascorbic acid with the use of a gradient analysis HPLC method. The minimum detectable quantities were 10 ng/injection for ascorbic acid and 500 ng/injection for dehydroascorbic acid (80): column, LiChrosorb NH2, 10 μm; mobile phase, 0.005M KH2PO4, pH 3.5 and CH3CN; detection, ascorbic acid, 268 nm and dehydroascorbic acid, 228 nm. (Reproduced, with permission, from Hewlett-Packard.)

soluble vitamins (thiamin, riboflavin, pyridoxine, nicotinamide, and ascorbic acid) in pharmaceutical preparations.

Other methods for the determination of ascorbic acid include a qualitative spot test (85) and high voltage electrophoresis (86).

Applications

Blood and Animal Tissues. The most commonly used and practical procedure for evaluating vitamin C nutritional status is the measurement of serum (plasma) levels of ascorbic acid (87). Low plasma levels of ascorbic acid do not necessarily indicate scurvy, although scorbutic patients invariably have low or no plasma ascorbic acid, but continued low levels of plasma ascorbate of less than 0.10 mg/100 mL would eventually lead to signs and symptoms of scurvy. In general, serum ascorbic acid concentrations are usually more reflective of recent intakes rather than of total body stores (88).

Whole blood ascorbic acid values may be a less sensitive indicator of vitamin C nutriture than serum or plasma levels of the vitamin because the vitamin C content in erythrocytes never falls to the low levels found in serum or plasma (89, 90). Also there are no well-established classifications available relating blood vitamin C values to the nutritional status of this vitamin in a population (88).

Leukocyte ascorbic acid concentrations are generally considered to provide a better reflection of tissue stores than other blood components. Supporting evidence for this belief includes observations such as: (i) leukocyte ascorbate levels drop slowly during ascorbic acid deficiency, reaching zero just before the onset of clinical symptoms of scurvy (91); (ii) leukocyte ascorbate levels correlate well with ascorbic acid retention on diets with a fixed, inadequate level of ascorbic acid (92); (iii) studies correlating plasma ascorbate levels with leukocyte ascorbate levels suggest that the leukocyte levels reflect the amount of ascorbic acid for storage while plasma levels reflect its metabolic turnover rate (93, 94); and (iv) direct evidence indicates that leukocyte ascorbate levels reflect total body ascorbate pool better than any other blood component (95).

Prompt stabilization of ascorbic acid is especially important in the case of plasma or serum samples. Metaphosphoric acid is often used for this purpose because it also serves as a protein precipitant. Such properties are desirable in the inactivation of oxidase and the catalytic effect of copper. Oxalic acid is an attractive stabilizer for ascorbic acid analysis because of its lower cost and greater stability; however, it is not a protein precipitant, therefore, it has a limited use for the extraction of animal tissues. The use of ethylenediaminetetraacetic acid (EDTA) in addition to the metaphosphoric acid has been recommended (96). EDTA would chelate divalent cations, and a study has shown it will stabilize ascorbic acid in the presence of copper for several days (96). Perchloric acid has been used also but because of its inherent dangerous properties its use is generally avoided. Trichloroacetic acid and EDTA also seem appropriate extractants for ascorbate in plant materials (97).

As noted earlier, plasma from blood samples must be promptly stabilized and, if necessary, the acidified samples may be stored frozen at $-65°C$. Because of the existence of oxyhemoglobin in whole blood or red cell suspensions, some consideration must be given to inactivate oxyhemoglobin or use an assay for total ascorbic acid content. With respect to tissue analysis, some discretion must be considered as to the degree of blood contamination.

Foods. The distribution of ascorbic acid within one individual fruit or vegetable or between various foods is often extremely variable. Significant difference can be found in the skin as compared with the pulp of fruit. Seed-containing tissues show striking changes in concentration of ascorbic acid during maturation, but in storage organs such as potatoes and leaves, the average level remains relatively constant throughout the growth period. Post-harvest storage will affect the vitamin content of the raw fruit or vegetable commensurate with the time and temperature of storage, extent of cellular tissue damaged, and the presence of ascorbic acid oxidase. Temperature changes, slicing, cutting, or bruising of fruits and vegetables, such as is likely to occur in processing, can all contribute to ascorbate loss. Significant losses also occur with cooking because of the temporarily accelerated action of enzymes. In these instances, extraction takes place and the concentration of vitamin in the liquor approximates that of the tissues. However, when fruit is boiled with sugar, as in the making of jam, the vitamin C content is remarkably stable. Freezing is a good method of preserving fruits and vegetables only after proper precautions have been taken to blanch and remove enzymes that might oxidize ascorbic acid. Also thawing of the food before cooking may result in progressive loss of the vitamin, especially if enzymes are present.

For ascorbic acid analysis, metaphosphoric acid is very useful in the inactivation of the catalytic effect of ascorbic acid oxidase as well as other catalytic oxidizing agents discussed previously. Foods such as fruits and vegetables also have a tendency to have a larger proportion of dehydroascorbic acid than animal tissues; consequently, methods that assay for only the reduced form of ascorbate may provide misleading low values.

Pharmaceuticals. In commerce, ascorbic acid is produced exclusively by synthesis (98). Because of its rather pure nature and high concentrations in vitamin–multivitamin tablets, analysis by conventional or sophisticated procedures can be performed easily. The USP provides a reference standard of L-ascorbic acid for assay purposes. The methods used can be chosen from the many discussed above. The method officially approved by the Association of Official Analytical Chemists is the microfluorometric procedure developed by Deutsch and Weeks (44).

A Method for the Determination of Ascorbic Acid in Biological Tissues by HPLC

Introduction. As noted earlier, several investigators have reported methods for the determination of ascorbic acid in various substances using HPLC (71–75). Different groups of investigators have employed a variety of columns and elution conditions to achieve the separation of ascorbic from interfering substances. Both reversed-phase and ion exchange columns have been used to achieve an HPLC assay. The samples used in these ascorbic acid assays have represented mainly nonmammalian materials. In some instances, the samples have required various pre-column treatments. Among the desirable characteristics of an HPLC analytical assay are minimal sample handling and modification particularly with regard to complex biological tissues. A simple assay used to determine the ascorbic acid content of serum, liver, brain, and adrenal gland of the guinea pig is described in the following section.

Methods. All tissues were collected and stabilized by the addition of 3% metaphosphoric acid in the ratio of 1 part tissue to 3 parts metaphosphoric acid (w/v). Samples were then centrifuged at 3×10^3 g to remove precipitated proteins. Samples were then transferred to clean tubes, frozen, and stored at $- 65°C$ until assayed. Samples were analyzed on commercially available HPLC columns and equipment (Waters Associates). Samples were injected directly into the column in 1 μL aliquots using an auto-injector (Waters Associates). No deterioration in column performance was observed over a 6-month interval. Flow rate was maintained at 1 mL/min under all conditions throughout the assays. Ascorbic acid was measured in UV absorbance units at 254 nm and quantitated by measuring peak heights. Standard curves were prepared by the addition of known amounts of ascorbic acid to solutions of 3% metaphosphoric acid. In the development of this assay, the use of perchloric acid was avoided while trichloroacetic acid was found to be unsuitable as a stabilizer because of its UV characteristics. Standard curves were prepared for each assay. The final assay as adapted used 0.125% citrate made from the trisodium salt at pH 7.3 as the eluant.

Results. In the development of this assay, several reverse-phase columns as well as the μPorasil column were examined for their separatory ability. From among the following columns the Porasil column was judged as giving the best elution pattern with plasma: μBondapak CN, μBondapak phenyl, μBondapak C_{18}. Although retention times for both metaphosphoric acid and ascorbic acid remained approximately the same (Table I), the quality of the chromatogram was judged superior for the μPorasil column. This decision was based on overall peak shape and symmetry as well as baseline stability.

Table I. Effect of Column Types on the HPLC Retention Time of Ascorbic Acid Dissolved in 3% Metaphosphoric Acid

	Retention Time (min) [a]	
Column Type	*Ascorbic Acid*	*Metaphosphoric Acid*
μBondapak CN	2.67	2.09
μBondapak phenyl	2.68	2.15
μBondapak C_{18}	2.36	1.84
μPorasil	2.31	1.84

[a] Elution buffer was 0.125% citrate, trisodium salt, pH 7.3. All other conditions used are stated in text. Values are the average of three trials.

Subsequent to the selection of an appropriate column various characteristics of the buffer were examined. Both pH and buffer strength were varied and retention time was measured. The results are presented in Table II. Generally it was found that a decrease in buffer strength or an

Table II. Effect of Various Concentrations of Citrate Buffer and
pH on HPLC Retention Time and Chromatographic Pattern
for Ascorbic Acid and Metaphosphoric Acid

Buffer Concentration (% Citrate)	pH	Retention Time (min)[a]	
		Ascorbic Acid	Metaphosphoric Acid
1.000	7.3	2.73	2.47, 2.52 (2)
0.500	7.3	2.68	2.20, 2.36 (2)
0.125	7.3	2.20	1.78 (1)
0.062	7.3	1.94	1.68 (1)
1.000	5.5	3.10	2.68 (1)
0.500	5.5	2.83	2.57, 2.73 (2)
0.125	5.5	2.47	1.99, 2.15 (2)
0.062	5.5	2.26	1.78, 1.89 (2)
1.000	3.0	3.10	2.78 (1)
0.500	3.0	3.10	2.73 (1)
0.125	3.0	2.83	2.26, 2.41 (2)
0.062	3.0	3.10	2.20 (2)

[a] All values are the average of three trials. Values in parentheses indicate the number of peaks observed for metaphosphoric acid. Analytical conditions employed: μPorasil column; flow rate, 1.0 mL/min; sample size, 1 μL.

increase in pH decreased the retention time. Further, the number of peaks observed for metaphosphoric acid varied from 2 to 1 with changes in buffer strength or pH. At pH 3.0, any changes in buffer strength caused a shift in baseline.

To determine the stability of ascorbic acid under the various concentrations of citrate buffer and pH, the following experiment was performed with the use of a double wavelength, double beam, spectrophotometer (Perkin–Elmer 557).

Various concentrations of ascorbic acid (0.2, 2.0, and 20 μM) were incubated in a cuvette with the various buffers listed in Table II and monitored at 254 nm. The concentration of ascorbic acid was selected to approximate the sample ascorbic acid coming into contact with a buffer volume determined by its time in transit through the column. No detectable losses were observed over the 5-min incubation time for any concentration of ascorbic acid under any concentration of citrate buffer or pH.

To quantitate the ascorbic content of various tissues, a standard curve (3.0–50 μg/mL ascorbic acid) was prepared in 3% metaphosphoric for each analytical run. A typical standard curve is shown in Figure 4. Correlation coefficients of 0.998 or better were consistently obtained for the standard curve. Pooled serum samples were used to measure day-to-day and within-run precision. The coefficient of variation for within-run

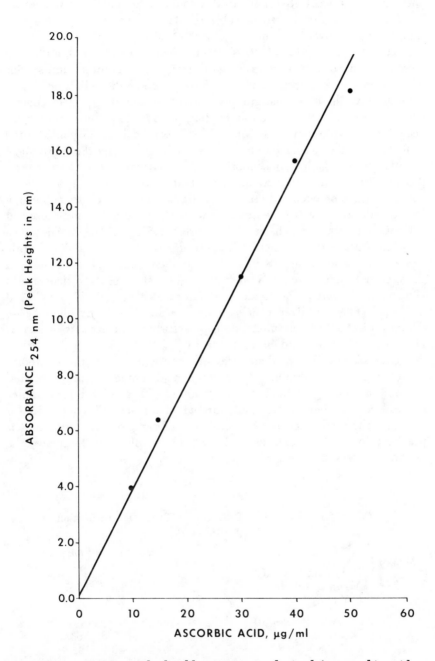

Figure 4. HPLC standard calibration curve obtained for ascorbic acid dissolved in 3% metaphosphoric acid; see text for conditions used; for ascorbic acid: $y = 0.3547x + 0.620$, $r = 0.9983$.

determinations was 0.78% and for day-to-day determinations was 4.6%. Precision data are presented in Table III. Ascorbic acid added to serum samples was recovered in the range of 90–93%.

The ascorbic acid contents of serum, liver, adrenal gland, and brain were determined in two groups of guinea pigs. One group of guinea pigs was fed an ascorbic acid adequate guinea pig chow diet (Ralston Purina No. 5022), while the second group was fed the Reid–Briggs (99) vitamin C deficient diet. After an 18-day feeding period, the animals were sacrificed by decapitation and trunk blood was collected, chilled, and centrifuged. The serum fraction was then stabilized by the addition of 3 parts (v/v) 3% metaphosphoric acid, centrifuged at 4°C to remove the precipitate, transferred, and stored at $-$ 65°C until assayed. All tissues were homogenized in 3% metaphosphoric acid to achieve a fourfold dilution (w/v), centrifuged at 4°C, transferred, and stored at $-$ 65°C until assayed. The results are presented in Table IV. All guinea pigs fed the ascorbate deficient Reid–Briggs diet contained significantly less ascorbic acid in each tissue examined when compared to animals fed the ascorbate adequate chow diet. The greatest percentage decrease in ascorbic acid content was found in the adrenal gland (92.4%) followed by brain (66.9%), liver (56.9%), and serum (43.5%). Figures 5–8 depict typical HPLC chromatograms of ascorbic acid extracts of serum, liver, adrenal gland, and brain, respectively.

Discussion. The method presented provides a fast and reproducible means of determining the ascorbic acid content of various tissues. In addition to a high rate of sample handling (12 samples/h for complex tissues such as liver, brain, and adrenal gland and 15 samples/h for plasma), the method requires a minimum of sample preparation and is practical for routine analysis of biological samples. Furthermore, the method utilizes equipment available to each laboratory with a rudimentary HPLC system.

Table III.   Precision Data for HPLC Determination of Ascorbic Acid

Parameter	Ascorbic Acid (mg/dL)[a]
Within Run ($n = 10$)	
Mean ± s.d.	8.5 ± 0.067
C.V., %	0.78
Day-to-Day ($n = 10$)	
Mean ± s.d.	13.8 ± 0.63
C.V., %	4.6

[a] Pooled guinea pig serum samples were employed. Analytical conditions employed: column, μPorasil; eluant, 0.125% citrate trisodium salt, pH 7.3; flow rate, 1.0 mL/min; sample size, 1 μL.

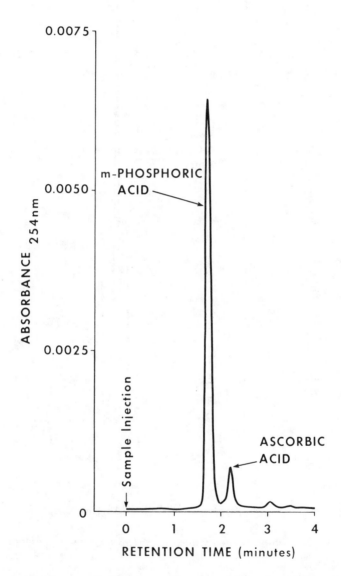

Figure 5. Chromatograms of serum extract stabilized in 3% metaphosphoric acid (v/v): column, μPorasil; eluent, 0.125% citrate trisodium salt; pH 7.3; flow rate, 1.0 mL/min; sample volume, 1 μL. Ascorbic acid and metaphosphoric acid identified at arrows.

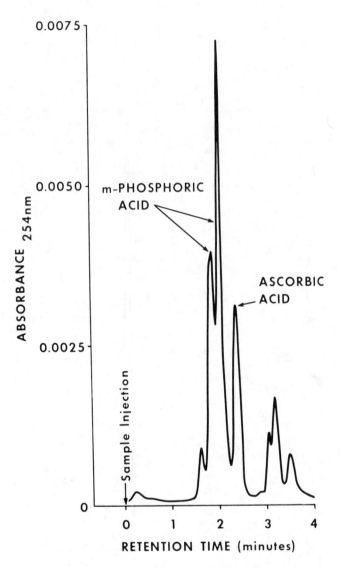

Figure 6.   Chromatogram of liver extract; conditions as in Figure 5.

Summary

The determination of ascorbic acid in biological materials, including foods and feeds, is beset with numerous technical problems. Hence, the methods used should be selected and conducted with extreme care with respect to reliability, specificity, sensitivity, and reproducibility. Depending upon the procedure selected, dehydroascorbic acid, hydroascorbic acid, or total ascorbic acid levels may be measured. At present, colori-

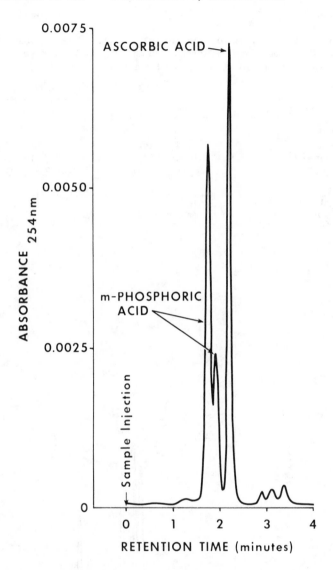

Figure 7. Chromatogram of adrenal gland extract; conditions as in Figure 5.

metric methods, using 2,6-dichloroindophenol or dinitrophenylhydrazine as the reactant, and fluorometric procedures have been the methods of choice. With further development, HPLC should provide a suitable, specific alternative. A need exists for a simple, sensitive, direct method for the measurement of erythorbic acid (isoascorbic acid) in foods and other biological materials.

Table IV.   Ascorbic Acid Content of Various Tissues from Guinea
Pigs Fed Two Different Diets (mg/100 g or per
100 mL of Tissue) as Determined by HPLC

	Type of Diet Fed[a]	
Tissue	*Chow-Fed*[b]	*Reid–Briggs*[c]
Serum	1.71 ± 00.25	0.967 ± 0.05
Liver	20.50 ± 05.0	8.840 ± 2.48
Adrenal gland	101.80 ± 20.2	7.720 ± 2.08
Brain	16.00 ± 04.81	5.300 ± 2.42

[a] Mean and standard deviation for results on 10 animals per group. *See* Table
III for analytical conditions employed.
[b] Ralston Purina complete guinea pig chow diet No. 5025.
[c] Reid–Briggs ascorbic acid deficient diet (*99*).

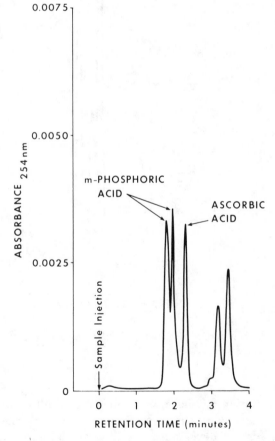

Figure 8.   Chromatogram of brain extract; conditions as in Figure 5.

Acknowledgments

Appreciation is expressed to Anne Regh and Richard Wheeler for their assistance in the preparation of this chapter.

Disclaimer

The opinions or assertions contained herein are the private views of the authors and are not to be construed as official or as reflecting the views of the Department of the Army, the Department of Defense, or the Department of Agriculture.

Literature Cited

1. Roe, J. *Methods Biochem. Anal.* **1954**, *1*, 115.
2. Hajratwala, B. R. *Aust. J. Pharm. Sci.* **1974**, *3*, 32.
3. Cooke, J. R. In "Vitamin C"; Birch, G.; Parker, K., Eds.; John Wiley & Sons: New York, 1974; p. 31.
4. Olliver, M. "The Vitamins"; Academic: New York, 1967; Vol. I, p. 338.
5. Omaye, S. T.; Turnbull, J. D.; Sauberlich, H. E. *Methods Enzymol.* **1979**, *62*, 3.
6. Mann, G. V.; Newton, P. *Ann. N.Y. Acad. Sci.* **1975**, *258*, 243.
7. Okamura, M. *J. Nutr. Sci. Vitaminol.* **1979**, *25*, 269.
8. Hornig, D. In "Vitamin C"; Birch, G.; Parker, K., Eds.; John Wiley & Sons: New York, 1974; p. 91.
9. Tolbert, B. M.; Campbell, W. T.; Ward, J. B. *Fed. Proc., Fed. Am. Soc. Exp. Biol.* **1980**, *39*, 796.
10. Sherman, H. C.; LaMer, V. K.; Campbell, H. L. *J. Am. Chem. Soc.* **1922**, *44*, 165.
11. Hojer, A. *Br. J. Exp. Pathol.* **1926**, *7*, 356.
12. Crampton, E. W. *J. Nutr.* **1947**, *33*, 491.
13. Key, K. M.; Elphick, G. K. *Biochem. J.* **1931**, *25*, 888.
14. Harris, L. J.; Olliver, M. *Biochem. J.* **1942**, *36*, 155.
15. Gould, B. S.; Shwachman, H. *J. Biol. Chem.* **1943**, *151*, 439.
16. Lawendel, J. J. *Nature* **1956**, *178*, 873.
17. Hewitt, E. J.; Dicks, G. J. *Biochem. J.* **1961**, *78*, 384.
18. Mattock, G. L. *J. Chem. Soc.* **1965**, *Part IV*, 4728.
19. Tillmans, J.; Hirsch, P.; Hirsch, W. *Z. Unters. Lebensm.* **1932**, *63*, 1.
20. Bessey, O. A.; King, C. G. *J. Biol. Chem.* **1933**, *103*, 687.
21. Roe, J. H. *J. Biol. Chem.* **1961**, *236*, 1611.
22. Zobel, M. *Ernaehrungsforschung* **1971**, *16*, 257.
23. Pelletier, O. *J. Lab. Clin. Med.* **1968**, *72*, 674.
24. Gero, E.; Candido, A. *J. Int. Vitaminol.* **1969**, *39*, 252.
25. Koch, P.; Sidloi, M.; Tonks, D. B. *Clin. Biochem.* **1980**, *13*, 73.
26. Garry, P. J.; Owen, G. M. *Autom. Anal. Chem., Technicon Symp.* **1968**, *1*, 507 (Mediad, Inc., Tarrytown, N.Y.).
27. Pelletier, O.; Brassard, R. *Adv. Autom. Anal., Technicon Int. Congr.* **1973**, *9*, 73.
28. Sauberlich, H. E.; Goad, W. C.; Skala, J. H.; Waring, P. P. *Sel. Methods Clin. Chem.* **1976**, *8*, 191.
29. Bradley, D. W.; Emery, G.; Maynard, J. E. *Clin. Chim. Acta.* **1973**, *44*, 47.
30. Owen, J. A.; Iggo, B. *Biochem. J.* **1956**, *62*, 675.

31. Finholt, P.; Paulssen, R. B.; Higuchi, T. *J. Pharm. Sci.* **1963**, *52*, 948.
32. Krishna Murty, N.; Rama Rao, K. *Methods Enzymol.* **1979**, *62*, 12.
33. Hiromi, K.; Kuwamoto, C.; Ohnishi, M. *Anal. Biochem.* **1980**, *101*, 421.
34. Scudi, J. V.; Ratish, H. D. *Ind. Eng. Chem., Anal. Ed.* **1938**, *10*, 420.
35. Ibid. **1939**, *11*, 98.
36. Ralls, J. W. *J. Agric. Food Chem.* **1975**, *23*, 609.
37. Zannoni, V.; Lynch, M.; Goldstein, S.; Sato, P. *Biochem. Med.* **1974**, *11*, 41.
38. Sicki, B. I.; Mimnough, E. G.; Gram, T. E. *Biochem. Pharmacol.* **1977**, *26*, 2037.
39. Butts, W. C.; Mulvihill, H. J. *Clin. Chem.* **1975**, *21*, 1493.
40. Stookey, L. L. *Anal. Chem.* **1970**, *42*, 779.
41. Schmall, M.; Pifer, C. W.; Wollish, E. G. *Anal. Chem.* **1953**, *25*, 1486.
42. Crossland, I. *Acta. Chem. Scand.* **1960**, *14*, 805.
43. Deutsch, M. J.; Weeks, C. E. *J. Assoc. Off. Anal. Chem.* **1965**, *48*, 1248.
44. "Official Methods of Analysis," 12th ed.; Association of Official Analytical Chemists: Washington, D.C., 1975; Sects. 43.056–43.062.
45. Roy, R. B.; Conetta, A.; Salpeter, J. *J. Assoc. Off. Anal. Chem.* **1976**, *59*, 1244.
46. Barakat, M. Z.; Abdel-Wahale, M. F. A.; El-Sadr, M. M. *Anal. Chem.* **1955**, *57*, 536.
47. Evered, D. F. *Analyst (London)* **1960**, *85*, 515.
48. Brubacher, G.; Vuilleumer, J. P. In "Clinical Biochemistry"; Curtins, H. C.; Roth, M., Eds.; de Gruyter: Berlin, 1974; Vol. 2, p. 989.
49. Egberg, D. C.; Potter, R. H.; Heroff, J. C. *J. Assoc. Off. Anal. Chem.* **1977**, *60*, 126.
50. Dunmire, D. L.; Reese, J. D.; Bryan, R.; Seegers, M. *J. Assoc. Off. Anal. Chem.* **1979**, *62*, 648.
51. Vuilleumier, J. P.; Pongraoz, G. *Alimenta.* **1976**, *77*, 27.
52. Hornig, D.; Weiser, H. *Int. J. Vitam. Nutr. Res.* **1976**, *46*, 40.
53. Omaye, S. T.; Green, M. D.; Turnbull, J. D.; Amos, W. H.; Sauberlich, H. E. *J. Clin. Pharmacol.* **1980**, *20*, 172.
54. Turnbull, J. D.; Sauberlich, H. E.; Omaye, S. T. *Int. J. Vitam. Nutr. Res.* **1978**, *49*, 92.
55. Mapson, L. W.; Partridge, S. M. *Nature* **1949**, *164*, 479.
56. Kadin, H.; Osadca, M. *J. Agric. Food Chem.* **1959**, *7*, 358.
57. Dittrich, S. *J. Chromatogr.* **1963**, *12*, 47.
58. Hasselquist, H.; Jaarma, M. *Acta Chem. Scand.* **1963**, *17*, 529.
59. Saari, J. C.; Baker, E. M.; Sauberlich, H. E. *Anal. Biochem.* **1967**, *18*, 173.
60. Mitchell, L. C.; Patterson, W. I. *J. Assoc. Off. Anal. Chem.* **1953**, *36*, 1127.
61. Schlack, J. E. *J. Assoc. Off. Anal. Chem.* **1974**, *57*, 1346.
62. Sweeley, C. C.; Bentley, R.; Makita, M.; Wells, W. W. *J. Am. Chem. Soc.* **1963**, *85*, 2497.
63. Roberts, R. N.; Johnston, J. A.; Fuhr, B. W. *Anal. Biochem.* **1965**, *10*, 282.
64. Dalgleish, C. E.; Horning, E. C.; Horning, M. G.; Knox, K. L.; Yarger, K. *Biochem. J.* **1968**, *101*, 792.
65. Horning, M. G.; Boucher, E. A.; Moss, A. M. *J. Gas Chromatogr.* **1967**, *5*, 297.
66. Vecchi, M.; Kaiser, K. *J. Chromatogr.* **1967**, *26*, 22.
67. Allison, J. H.; Stewart, M. A. *Anal. Biochem.* **1971**, *43*, 401.
68. Clifford, A. J. *Adv. Chromatogr.* **1976**, *14*, 1.
69. Williams, R. C.; Schmit, J. A.; Henry, R. A. *J. Chromatogr. Sci.* **1972**, *10*, 494.
70. Kissinger, P. T.; Felice, L. J.; King, W. P.; Pachla, L. A.; Riggin, R. M.; Shoup, R. E. *J. Chem. Educ.* **1977**, *54*, 50.
71. Sood, S. P.; Sartori, L. E.; Wittmer, D. P.; Haney, W. G. *Anal. Chem.* **1976**, *48*, 796.

72. Pachla, L. A.; Kissinger, P. T. *Anal. Chem.* **1976**, *48*, 364.
73. Williams, R. C.; Baker, D. R.; Schmit, J. A. *J. Chromatogr. Sci.* **1973**, *11*, 618.
74. Wills, R. B. H.; Shaw, C. G.; Day, W. R. *J. Chromatogr. Sci.* **1977**, *15*, 262.
75. Trivikvaman, K. V.; Refshauge, C.; Adams, R. N. *Life Sci.* **1975**, *15*, 1335.
76. Wagner, E. S.; Lindley, B.; Coffin, R. D. *J. Chromatogr.* **1979**, *163*, 225.
77. Brunt, K.; Bruins, C. H. P. *J. Chromatogr.* **1979**, *172*, 37.
78. Pachla, L. A.; Kissinger, P. T. *Methods Enzymol.* **1979**, *62*, 15.
79. Kissinger, P. T.; Felice, L. J.; Riggin, R. M.; Pachla, L. A.; Wenke, D. C. *Clin. Chem.* **1974**, *20*, 992.
80. Tweeten, T. "Hewlett–Packard Application Brief," Library File Code: 1-3-4-100, August, 1979.
81. Finley, J. W.; Duang, E., personal communications, 1980.
82. Olliver, M. "The Vitamins"; Academic: New York, 1967, Vol. I, p. 359.
83. Lindquist, J.; Farroha, S. M. *Analyst (London)* **1975**, *100*, 377.
84. Mason, W. D.; Gardner, T. D.; Stewart, J. T. *J. Pharm. Sci.* **1972**, *61*, 1301.
85. Kutter, D. *Aertzl. Lab.* **1966**, *12*, 180.
86. Letzig, E. *Nahrung* **1965**, *9*, 357.
87. Sauberlich, H. E. *Ann. N.Y. Acad. Sci.* **1975**, *258*, 438.
88. Sauberlich, H. E.; Dowdy, R. P.; Skala, J. H. "Laboratory Tests for the Assessment of Nutritional Status"; CRC: Cleveland, 1974; p. 13.
89. Baker, E. M.; Hodges, R. E.; Hood, J.; Sauberlich, H. E.; March, S. C.; Canham, J. E. *Am. J. Clin. Nutr.* **1971**, *24*, 444.
90. Hodges, R. E.; Hood, J.; Canham, J. E.; Sauberlich, H. E.; Baker, E. M. *Am. J. Clin. Nutr.* **1971**, *24*, 432.
91. Crandon, J. E.; Lund, C. C.; Dill, D. B. *N. Engl. J. Med.* **1960**, *223*, 353.
92. Lowry, O. H.; Bessey, O. A.; Brock, M. J.; Lopez, J. A. *J. Biol. Chem.* **1946**, *166*, 111.
93. Loh, H. S.; Wilson, C. W. M. *Br. Med. J.* **1971**, *3*, 733.
94. Loh, H. S. *Int. J. Vitam. Nutr. Res.* **1972**, *42*, 86.
95. Omaye, S. T.; Turnbull, J. D.; Sudduth, J. H.; Sauberlich, H. E. *Fed. Proc., Fed. Am. Soc. Exp. Biol.* **1980**, *39*, 796.
96. Jager, H. *Pharmazie* **1948**, *3*, 536.
97. Freebairn, H. T. *Anal. Chem.* **1959**, *31*, 1850.
98. Osol, A. "Remington's Pharmaceutical Sciences"; Mack Publ. Co.: Easton, PA, 1970; p. 1036.
99. Reid, N. E.; Briggs, G. M. *J. Nutr.* **1953**, *51*, 341.

RECEIVED for review January 22, 1981. ACCEPTED June 2, 1981.

Ascorbate Oxidase: Molecular Properties and Catalytic Activity

PETER M. H. KRONECK, FRASER A. ARMSTRONG[1],
HELLMUT MERKLE, and AUGUSTO MARCHESINI[2]

Universität Konstanz, Fakultät für Biologie, D-7750 Konstanz,
Federal Republic of Germany

Ascorbate oxidase (E.C. 1.10.3.3) of the squash C. pepo medullosa was investigated by electron paramagnetic resonance (EPR); redox titrations of the different copper sites were carried out anaerobically by following the absorbance at 610 and 330 nm, or the fluorescence at 335 nm. The kinetics of ascorbate oxidase reduction by L-ascorbate were studied by stopped-flow and rapid-freeze techniques. The enzyme contains eight copper atoms/M_r, four detectable by EPR (three type 1, one type 2), and four that are EPR silent (type 3). Potentiometric titrations showed equivalence among the three type 1 copper atoms (average midpoint potential 350 mV, 25°C); the midpoint potential of type 3 copper was slightly higher than that of type 1. At 10°C, increased differences between the two copper types were observed. On reduction, a free L-ascorbate radical, which was not bound to a paramagnetic copper, was formed. Type 1 and type 3 copper were reduced at similar rates, whereas the type 2 copper reacted more slowly.

The copper enzyme ascorbate oxidase (L-ascorbate:O_2 oxidoreductase, E.C. 1.10.3.3) was originally discovered (1) in cabbage leaves and named "hexoxidase," and has been the subject of numerous chemical and biological investigations. The literature published prior to 1963 has been

---

[1] Current address: Inorganic Chemistry Laboratory, University of Oxford, South Parks Road, Oxford OX 13QR, England.
[2] Current address: Istituto Sperimentale Per La Nutrizione Delle Piante, Sezione Periferica Operativa Di Torino, Via Ormea 47, 10125 Torino, Italy.

0065-2393/82/0200–0223$07.50/0

reviewed (2). More recent results concerning structural and catalytic properties of the metalloenzyme have been summarized (3,4), and reviewed in connection with copper proteins (5–8). In addition, Lee and Dawson (9) have recently published an article summarizing the copper content and activity data of 137 purified samples of ascorbate oxidase prepared in Dawson's laboratory during 1951–1977.

Ascorbate oxidase belongs to the class of blue oxidases that also includes the laccases and ceruloplasmin (5). All three proteins contain at least four copper atoms and are capable of catalyzing the four-electron reduction of dioxygen, yielding two molecules of water. As its name implies, L-ascorbate:O_2 oxidoreductase displays its greatest specificity towards L-ascorbic acid (vitamin C). The substrate is oxidized to L-dehydroascorbate with the production of 1 mol of water/mol of L-ascorbate oxidized. As will be discussed later in this chapter, many other reductants may serve as electron donors to ascorbate oxidase, making this enzyme not only a valuable diagnostic agent for the determination of vitamin C in medicine and food chemistry (10), but also a powerful chemical reagent, performing redox reactions with structurally complicated organic molecules (11,12).

Ascorbate oxidase, which has been found only in plant tissues, is generally isolated from green or yellow squash. Considerable caution must be used when evaluating the ascorbate activity of plant extracts (2). Many metal-containing proteins, or free Cu^{2+} ions in solution, can undergo oxidoreduction in the presence of ascorbate, generally producing hydrogen peroxide instead of water. There are also reports mentioning a fungal enzyme from *Myrothecium verrucaria* (13) that is termed an "atypical ascorbate oxidase" because it is unaffected by inhibitors of heavy metal catalysis, in contrast to the copper enzymes from higher plants. We have repeated the purification procedure of White and Krupka (13) and subjected the yellow-brown material, collected after diethylaminoethyl cellulose chromatography, to spectrophotometry and electron paramagnetic resonance (EPR) spectroscopy. Neither a typical absorbance in the 350–1000-nm region nor a characteristic EPR signal could be detected under oxidizing and reducing conditions; only a very weak EPR signal at a g of approximately 4, indicative of nonspecifically bound iron from a denatured protein, was detected.

Ascorbate oxidase is mostly found in the peripheral part of the plant, as shown in Figure 1 for cauliflower and apple that had been cut through the middle and pressed on a piece of paper coated with a solution of L-ascorbate and the redox dye dichloroindophenol (14). The close association with the cell-wall material gives some support to the theory that the enzyme might be important for plant growth and ripening of

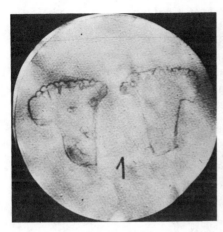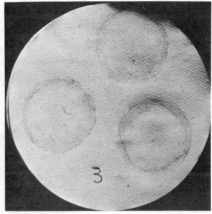

Figure 1. Peripheral location of ascorbate oxidase in cauliflower (left) and apple (right). The fruit was cut through the middle and pressed onto a piece of filter paper soaked with a mixture of L-ascorbate and dichloroindophenol, phosphate buffer (pH 6.0).

the fruit (2). Because of the high reactivity of reduced ascorbate oxidase towards dioxygen, the enzyme has also been linked to plant respiration by analogy with cytochrome oxidase in mammalian tissues.

In contrast to tree and fungal laccase, whose molecular parameters and mechanisms of action have been thoroughly investigated (8), few such studies have been reported for ascorbate oxidase. This is mainly because of the relatively difficult isolation and purification procedure of ascorbate oxidase in comparison with laccase. Furthermore, this enzyme appears to be more sensitive to environmental factors such as ionic strength of the buffer medium, its pH, or the presence of extraneous metal ions. Consequently, many samples isolated over a long period were found to be homogeneous from the standpoint of the protein biochemist but appeared inhomogeneous with respect to the catalytically active copper sites (9).

This chapter summarizes some recent developments in the purification of ascorbate oxidase, the number of copper atoms per active molecule, and the stoichiometry of the different copper sites with reference to the classification introduced by Malkin and Malmström (5). Furthermore, physical properties of the metal centers are discussed in relation to other simple copper proteins that have been characterized in recent years. Finally, kinetic investigations of ascorbate oxidase reduction are presented as studied by anaerobic stopped-flow and rapid-freeze techniques.

Purification of the Enzyme and Copper Content

A homogeneous sample of ascorbate oxidase was first prepared in 1951. Since then, the specific activity and the copper content of homogeneous preparations greatly increased (9) from 740 units/μg of copper and six copper atoms/M_r to 1000 units and ten to twelve copper atoms. The chronological correlation of the specific activity of the enzyme as a function of copper content documents impressively the difficulties associated with the preparation of "pure" ascorbate oxidase. Although drastic changes of these activity values per copper atom have been observed by Dawson and coworkers (2, 3, 9), other criteria, such as molecular weight (M_r) or homogeneity analyzed by ultracentrifugation, or amino acid composition, have remained relatively constant. This experimental fact is hypothesized to result from varying degrees of prosthetic copper loss occurring during the purification steps (9).

A procedure was developed (15) that yielded a 14% recovery of the total enzymatic activity present in the crude juice extract from green squash. The optimum specific activity was in the range of 4025 ± 50 units/mg protein in a preparation containing 0.46–0.52% copper (10–12 Cu atoms/140,000 M_r).

Three other purification methods have been described in the literature—for cucumber (16) and for the enzyme from green squash (17, 18). Table I summarizes the salient molecular properties of ascorbate oxidase purified according to the different procedures mentioned above. A detailed purification table is presented in References 15 and 18, and includes the enzyme yield calculated on the basis of total protein present in the crude juice. The yield is 14% for the method of Lee and Dawson

Table I. Physical and Chemical Properties

Source	Reference	M_r	Specific Activity (Units/mg of Protein)	Cu/M_r	Cu EPR/M_r (%)	A_{330}/A_{610}
Yellow squash	48	140,000	3600	8	—	>1
Cucumber	16	132,000	3500	8	—	0.79
Green squash	17	140,000	—	8	45	1.9
Green squash	15	140,000	3800–4250	8–10	—	1.8
Green squash	28	140,000	3609	8	47 ± 3	0.68
Green squash	17	—	—	5.4–6.5	59	0.87
				7.5–8.0	48	
Green squash	18	140,000	3930	8	48 ± 2	0.65

^{a} g values (g_z, g_y, g_x) obtained from computer simulations.

(9) vs. 34% for the method of Marchesini and Kroneck (18). Nakamura et al. (16) recover 0.093 g of pure enzyme from 15 kg of fresh cucumber vs. 0.015 g from fresh squash by Avigliano et al. (17). The preparations of Lee and Dawson (9) and of Avigliano et al. (17) exhibit relatively high variations in copper/M_r (Table I), ranging from 5.4 to 10 Cu atoms/140,000 M_r. A constant value of 7.95 ± 0.1 Cu atoms/140,000 M_r can be achieved by the method of Marchesini and Kroneck (18).

Among the blue oxidases only laccase appears to exhibit reproducible values for the copper/M_r ratio. Thus, it is generally agreed that laccase contains four copper atoms per enzyme molecule (5), whereas in ceruloplasmin (19) and ascorbate oxidase the metal is much more labile and sensitive towards various agents and environmental factors. This sensitivity towards extraneous agents is also evident from the data reported by Avigliano et al. (20), who removed varying amounts of type 2 and type 3 copper (5) by treatment with ethylenediaminetetraacetic acid (EDTA) or a combination of EDTA and dimethylglyoxime (DMG). According to these authors, ascorbate oxidase contains only five to six prosthetic copper atoms/M_r, whereas two to three of the eight copper atoms originally present are extremely labile. Unfortunately, no precise activity values are specified for the several enzyme preparations containing eight, six to seven (after EDTA), and five (after EDTA plus DMG) copper atoms per enzyme molecule.

In investigations on the so-called "reaction inactivation" of ascorbate oxidase by hydrogen peroxide (21, 22), essentially no prosthetic copper became bound to the resin during 64-copper exchange experiments on an Amberlite IR-100 column, at pH 5.6.

of Ascorbate Oxidase from Different Sources

			Type 1 Copper				Type 2 Copper		
$Cu/$ M_r	λ (nm)	ϵ (M^{-1} cm^{-1})	$g_\parallel$	$g_\perp$	$A_\parallel$ (mT)	$Cu/$ M_r	$g_\parallel$	$g_\perp$	$A_\parallel$ (mT)
—	608	10,400	—	—	—	—	—	—	—
—	607	9,680	2.22	2.06	5.0	—	—	—	—
2	610	10,700	2.22	2.05	5.4	2	2.22	2.05	19.5
—	610	9,600	2.24	2.07	6.0	—	—	—	—
3	610	9,680	2.227[a]	2.036 2.058	5.6	1	2.242[a]	2.053	19.0
3	610	11,000	2.229	—	5.8	1	2.248	—	18.8
3	610	9,700	2.227[a]	2.036 2.058	5.6	1	2.242[a]	2.053	19.0

The copper content and enzyme activity is also markedly dependent on the pH of the solution. Extensive studies (23, 24) show a rapid loss of the metal below pH 4.6; this loss is temperature dependent and accompanied by an irreversible unfolding of the protein moiety. At pH 11, dissociation of a subunit ($M_r \sim$ 65,000) is observed by ultrafiltration. This process is not accompanied by loss of copper, and residual activity ($\sim$ 25%) is detectable.

Apart from prosthetic copper loss due to environmental factors, coordination site structural changes that are detectable by spectroscopic techniques can occur. These changes are discussed later in the section on spectroscopic properties.

Molecular Properties of the Protein

The most extensive studies on the molecular properties of ascorbate oxidase have been carried out in Dawson's laboratory. Sedimentation equilibrium experiments have confirmed a molecular weight of 140,000; a value of 137,000 was determined for the apoprotein. The enzyme isolated and purified according to the different methods (Table I) is homogeneous by electrophoretic methods and ultracentrifugation ($s_{20,w}$ = 7.52) in the pH range 5.2–10. Above pH 11 dissociation occurs as reported earlier (23, 24). When exposed to sodium dodecyl sulfate (SDS) or guanidinium chloride, the enzyme dissociates into two equivalent subunits of 65,000 M_r accompanied by the loss of prosthetic copper. In the presence of a strong reducing agent, such as 2-mercaptoethylamine (or its corresponding ethanol derivative), and SDS, two other subunits are found. These subunits are termed chain α (M_r 38,000) and chain β (M_r 28,000). On the basis of these results ascorbate oxidase is proposed to be a tetramer composed of two α and two β chains, where each $\alpha\beta$ pair is covalently connected by disulfide bonds (25). A quaternary structure similar to that of the native enzyme is believed to exist for the copper-free apoprotein, which is obtained by exhaustive dialysis against cyanide (26). Reincorporation of the metal into the apoprotein causes the protein molecule to dimerize, because with gel filtration techniques a M_r of 285,000 ($s_{20,w}°$ = 9.79) was obtained. Unfortunately neither optical nor EPR spectra of the different protein species (which might have given some structural information about the reconstituted copper sites, particularly with respect to the ratio of type 1 to type 2 copper) were presented.

A quaternary structure consisting of two identical, laccase-like, active sites per molecule, each containing four copper atoms, was suggested for the native enzyme (27). In the enzyme the subunits α and β are arranged in a symmetrical way, $\alpha\beta/\beta\alpha$, whereas in the apoenzyme an asymmetrical geometry, $\alpha\alpha/\beta\beta$, is assumed. This interpretation of the quaternary structure of native ascorbate oxidase and its apoprotein is somewhat contradictory to reported results (*18, 28*). Evidence was provided for an "asymmetric" stoichiometry of the three different copper classes (*5*), that is, only one type 2 copper out of eight copper atoms, and not two as predicted for two laccase-like subunits.

Like laccase and ceruloplasmin, ascorbate oxidase is an acidic protein, with aspartic acid and glutamic acid in excess over histidine, lysine, and arginine. For the amino acid composition see the detailed data in References 3 and *18*. Unlike laccase, ascorbate oxidase has a relatively low carbohydrate content, 2.4% vs. approximately 45% (*29*).

A special interest has been directed towards the number and accessibility of cysteine (RSH) sulfur and cystine (RSSR) sulfur groups, which have been proposed as binding sites for the blue type 1 copper, and as potential electron accepting sites (*30–34*). For ascorbate oxidase from yellow squash, ten to twelve cysteine residues plus six to eight cystine residues were found; none of the SH groups was accessible to mercurials (*35*). These results are in good agreement with the data reported (*18*) for the enzyme from green squash. Only three to four half-cystine residues were determined for the laccases (*36*).

Spectroscopic Properties and Stoichiometry of the Copper Types

Optical Spectra. The absorption spectrum of the pure enzyme in phosphate buffer (pH 7.0) exhibits the typical blue maximum at 610 nm, assigned to the blue or type-1 copper, and the shoulder at 330 nm, assigned to the EPR-nondetectable type 3 copper (*5*) (Figure 2, Table I). Table I also includes molecular parameters from previous preparations by Lee and Dawson (*15*), and other authors. A notable feature is the absence of a distinct absorption maximum around 800 nm, reported by Lee and Dawson for their purest preparation. According to our standards (*18*) pure ascorbate oxidase is characterized by the optical indices $A_{280}/A_{610} = 25 \pm 0.5$, $A_{330}/A_{610} = 0.65 \pm 0.05$, and $A_{610}/A_{500} = 7.00 \pm 0.25$. Deviations from these values indicate the loss of the type 1 copper, as is also supported by the corresponding EPR spectra. An increase of the absorbance at 500 nm is associated with a denaturation of the protein, as observed at the end of titrations with hydrogen peroxide (*18*). Upon addition of a reductant, for example, L-ascorbate or reductate, the blue chromophore and the absorbance at 330 nm are both bleached. Nearly identical electronic spectra have been reported for the two other multicopper oxidases, ceruloplasmin and laccase (*5–8*). In the latter case the optical properties have been elucidated in much greater detail using low-temperature spectroscopy (*37,*

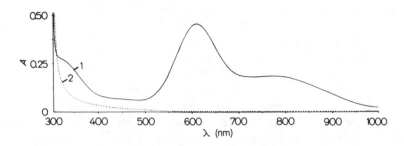

Figure 2. Absorption spectra of pure ascorbate oxidase. Enzyme 48 μM in 0.1 M phosphate buffer (pH 7.0), 20°C, 1.0-cm cell. Key: 1, oxidized enzyme; 2, reduced enzyme, slight excess of L-ascorbate. (Reproduced, with permission, from Ref. 18. Copyright 1979, Springer.)

38). Furthermore, based on earlier calculations (*39*) for the type 1 copper protein plastocyanin, ligand-field parameters for the blue copper in laccase have been derived. These reports (*37, 38*) also include a structural representation of the type 1 center composed of a flattened tetrahedron (D_{2d} symmetry) with two imidazole side-chains, a cysteine sulfur, and a fourth ligand (which probably is methionine sulfur), bound to the metal ion. Although no such low-temperature experiments have been performed with ascorbate oxidase, one might anticipate similar structural features for the blue type 1 centers.

Removal of the type 2 copper according to a reported procedure (*20*) leads to significant decreases of the absorbance at 330 and 750 nm. These decreases indicate that type 2 copper contributes to the absorbance in these regions. For fungal and tree laccase, structures based on tetragonal six, five, or square-planar four coordination, as found in several low-molecular-weight copper complexes, were proposed (*37*).

Fluorescence spectra of oxidized, partially reduced, and fully reduced ascorbate oxidase are shown in Figure 3. At pH 7.0 (phosphate buffer), the pure enzyme gives an excitation maximum at 295 nm, and an emission maximum at 330 nm. Earlier reported values (*15, 28*) differ slightly from our figures, that is, 325 and 335 nm are quoted for the emission maximum. Recently, a value of 328 nm for ascorbate oxidase from green squash was measured (*40*). This value, in contrast to all other values mentioned above, was obtained on a corrected fluorometer. From the optical data the A_{330}/A_{610} index was estimated to be greater than 1.0; furthermore, the absorption maximum was located at 605 nm. For our preparations the emission maximum was always at 330 nm, independent of whether we used the purest fraction, enzyme with a lower copper content, or enzyme that had been treated with Chelex 100 or subjected to lyophilization (*18*). Obviously, despite significant differences within

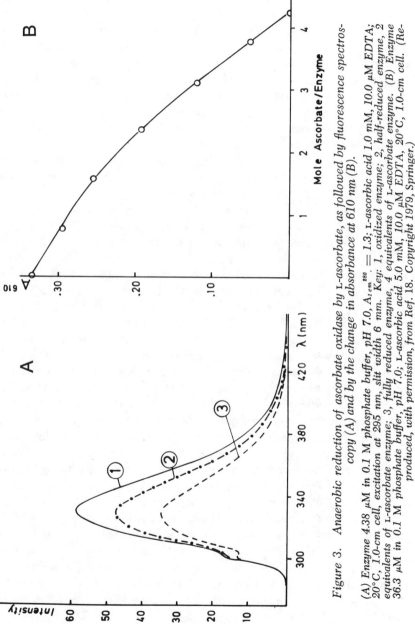

Figure 3. Anaerobic reduction of ascorbate oxidase by L-ascorbate, as followed by fluorescence spectroscopy (A) and by the change in absorbance at 610 nm (B).

(A) Enzyme 4.38 μM in 0.1 M phosphate buffer, pH 7.0, $A_{1 cm}^{280} = 1.3$; L-ascorbic acid 1.0 mM, 10.0 μM EDTA; 20°C, 1.0-cm cell, excitation at 295 nm, slit width 6 mm. Key: 1, oxidized enzyme; 2, half-reduced enzyme, 2 equivalents of L-ascorbate enzyme; 3, fully reduced enzyme, 4 equivalents of L-ascorbate enzyme. (B) Enzyme 36.3 μM in 0.1 M phosphate buffer, pH 7.0; L-ascorbic acid 5.0 mM, 10.0 μM EDTA, 20°C, 1.0-cm cell. (Reproduced, with permission, from Ref. 18. Copyright 1979, Springer.)

the optical or EPR properties of the individual preparations of ascorbate oxidase, the fluorescence emission maximum retains its 330-nm value.

Upon stepwise addition of stoichiometric amounts of reducing substrates under the rigorous exclusion of dioxygen (for technical details, see Ref. 18), the intrinsic fluorescence emission at 330 nm increases by 1.5–1.75 (Figure 3) without changes in peak shape or position. In comparison with tree laccase or fungal laccase (41, 42), ascorbate oxidase reacts rapidly with L-ascorbate, even after the acceptance of five to six electrons per molecule. For the identical experiment, a fluorescence enhancement factor of two for a sample of ascorbate oxidase prepared according to Reference 17 was observed (40). Furthermore, at intermediate reduction stages a time-dependent fluorescence decrease and increase parallel to changes in absorbance at 330 and 605 nm was detected, and was attributed to an intramolecular electron transfer between the type 1 and the type 3 copper sites.

A similar relationship between the intrinsic fluorescence and the redox state of the copper atoms in lacquer tree laccase was reported (43).

EPR Spectra and Stoichiometry of the Copper Classes. Among the physical methods that have contributed to our knowledge about structural and mechanistic aspects of copper enzymes and proteins, EPR spectroscopy has played a dominant role over the past two decades (5, 6). At pH 7.0 (phosphate buffer), pure ascorbate oxidase gives the EPR signal (recorded at X-band, $\sim$ 9.3 GHz) illustrated in Figure 4. The signal demonstrates the presence of the type 1 and type 2 copper, shown by the different hyperfine splittings in the $g_{||}$ region (Table I). The spectrum shown in Figure 4 is nearly identical with the spectra published earlier for the enzyme from cucumber (16), and for ascorbate oxidase isolated from green squash, cucumber, or marrow squash (28, 44).

Double integration of the area under the first derivative reveals that 48 ± 2% of the chemically determined copper (18) is EPR detectable in frozen solution. Table I summarizes the experimental g and A values measured from the recorded spectra. A best fit of the EPR spectrum of oxidized ascorbate oxidase is obtained by computer simulation, using the high-frequency measurements at 35 GHz (28). The ratio of type 1 to type 2 copper is estimated by double integration of the first low-field line, which arises from the type 2 copper, at approximately 0.270 T (18). Roughly 25% of the EPR-detectable copper in ascorbate oxidase is type 2, whereas 75% is blue type 1 copper. This ratio is confirmed by computer analysis (18) and agrees with earlier results (28) (Figure 4).

Addition of reducing equivalents causes complete loss of the EPR signal (Figure 2), which reappears rapidly and completely upon reoxidation with dioxygen or ferricyanide. Structural changes of the type 1 and type 2 copper sites can be conveniently monitored by the EPR technique. Thus, after lyophilization of the pure enzyme in phosphate buffer (pH 7.0) a second peak close to the $m = -3/2$ line of the type 2 center appears in the EPR signal (Figure 4). Furthermore, the type 1 to type 2 copper ratio becomes 1.5:1 or even 1:1, as shown by the changes in the purity index A_{330}/A_{610} from 0.65 to 0.9 and greater. Recently, similar observations were made following dialysis (aerobic or anaerobic) against acetate buffer (pH 5.0 or 4.5) (45). The amount of type 1 copper decreases significantly, yielding a new EPR spectrum with larger nuclear hyperfine splittings $A_{\parallel}$ (Figure 4; for further details, see Ref. 18).

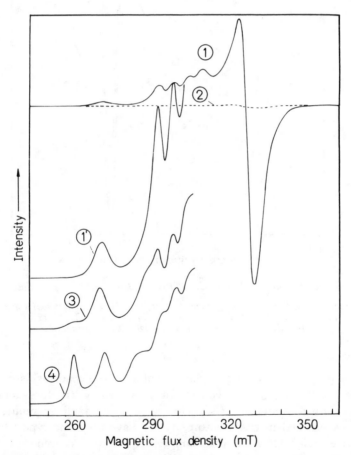

Figure 4A. Experimental X-band EPR spectra of ascorbate oxidase.

Enzyme 0.228 mM in 0.1 M phosphate buffer (pH 7.0), temperature 105 K, 100 kHz modulation frequency, 1.0 mT modulation amplitude, ~ 2 mW power (20 dB), 0.2 s time constant, 0.10 mT/s scan rate, 9.39148 GHz microwave frequency. Key: 1, oxidized enzyme; 1' as 1, but 5 × instrument sensitivity; 2, reduced enzyme, sensitivity as in 1'; 3, oxidized enzyme, lyophilized at 0°C, redissolved, $A_{330}/A_{610} = 1.1$; 4, oxidized enzyme, after treatment with Chelex 100, $A_{330}/A_{610} = 1.0$, sensitivity in 3 and 4 as in 1'. (Reproduced, with permission, from Ref. 18. Copyright 1979, Springer.)

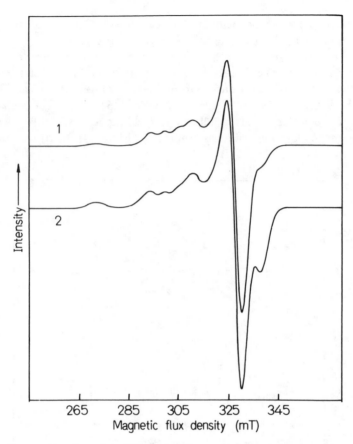

Figure 4B.   Simulated X-band EPR spectra of ascorbate oxidase.

Spectra were simulated with the parameters of Table III. Lorentzian lineshape (18). Key: 1, 3 type 1 Cu, 1 type 2 Cu; 2, 2 type 1 Cu, 2 type 2 Cu. (Reproduced, with permission, from Ref. 18. Copyright 1979, Springer.)

The presence of a single type 2 center in ascorbate oxidase is not consistent with the proposed concept of a quaternary structure composed of two identical subunits $\alpha\beta$ (25). On the other hand, all the multicopper oxidases described in the literature (5–8) have only one type 2 center per active molecule. Additional copper with type 2 characteristics can be bound by the macromolecule during isolation and purification (19). A close examination of the EPR spectra presented by Lee and Dawson (9) indicates the presence of so-called nonspecific copper with large hyperfine splittings at $g_{||}$. As expected, the ratio A_{330}/A_{610} is approximately 1.5–2 for these preparations (estimated from Figure 2 in Ref. 9).

Anaerobic Reduction of Ascorbate Oxidase–Number of Redox Equivalents and Midpoint Potentials of the Copper Sites

Reduction and reoxidation of the copper in ascorbate oxidase can be easily followed by spectrophotometry at 330 and 610 nm, fluorescence emission at 330 nm (described in the previous section), and EPR spectroscopy (Figure 4). Using the anaerobic titration techniques described in Reference *18*, complete reduction of the enzyme is achieved by four equivalents of L-ascorbate or reductate. With total reduction, the absorbance at 610 nm completely disappears, whereas some residual absorbance in the 330-nm region remains, caused by the absorbance of reduced protein and oxidized substrate. Potentiometric titrations of the type 1 copper with ferricyanide as a mediator (equal amounts or a tenfold excess/enzyme give a Nernst factor, n_{610}, of 1.1 and a midpoint potential, $E'_{o,610}$, of 344 mV [vs. standard hydrogen electrode (SHE), 25°C, phosphate buffer (pH 7.0) with $I = 0.1$ M] (Figure 5). For many titrations a relatively long lag phase of up to three electrons was observed before any decrease in absorbance at either 610 or 330 nm was

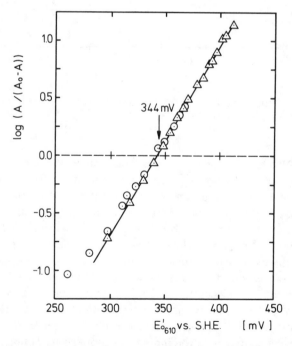

Figure 5A. Anaerobic potentiometric titration of the type-1 Cu centers in ascorbate oxidase using ferricyanide as mediator, phosphate buffer (pH 7.0), $I = 0.10$ M, 25.0°C, $K_3Fe(CN)_6$ 210 μM, enzyme 21 μM.

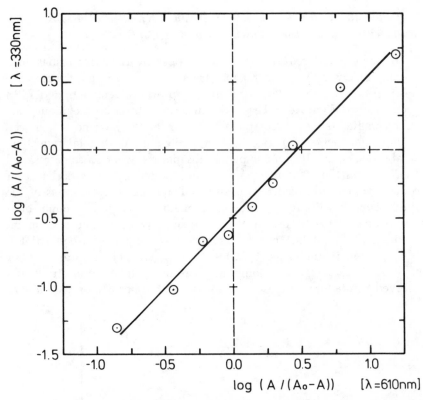

Figure 5B. Double Nernst plot of the reduction by L-*ascorbate at 610 and 330 nm, phosphate buffer (pH 7.0),* I = 0.20 M, 10.0°C, *enzyme* 28 μM. *Potentials are reported in mV vs. SHE.*

detected. This effect probably arises from traces of dioxygen left in the resting enzyme even after rigorous deoxygenation (*18*).

The results of a simultaneous spectrophotometric titration at 330 and 610 nm are depicted in a double Nernst plot in Figure 5, giving an $E'_{o,330}$ value for the type 3 center that is nearly identical to $E'_{o,610}$ of the type 1 copper. However, at lower temperatures (e.g., 10°C) a value of 30 ± 10 mV was measured for the difference $E'_{o,330} - E'_{o,610}$. A similar redox situation is found for tree laccase (E'_o for the type 1 copper, 394 mV; E'_o for the type 3 copper, 434 mV). However, at 25°C, where the difference $E'_{o,330} - E'_{o,610}$ is considerably diminished in ascorbate oxidase (in the presence of the redox mediator ferricyanide); thermodynamic control for the occupancy of the individual copper sites is less pronounced.

Interestingly, in the case of both the three type 1 centers and the four type 3 centers, a linear Nernst relationship exists in the 10–25°C temperature range, phosphate buffer (pH 7.0), indicating equivalence among the single members of the two copper classes. The Nernst coefficient ratio n_{330}/n_{610} (Figure 5), which here does not approach the expected number of 2, raises some controversial points regarding the mode of electron transfer between the two chromophores. Based largely on potentiometric evidence, and the complete lack of an EPR signal in either the fully oxidized or fully reduced state (8, 46), the type 3 copper pair probably functions as a cooperative two-electron acceptor (7). However, this is open to question; uncoupling of the type 3 copper pair was proposed to occur in the majority of cases (47). Double Nernst plots for spectrophotometric titrations of tree laccase (such as Figure 5) produced slopes of 1.0–2.0, depending on the titrant used. Titrants such as hydroquinone or ferrocyanide gave slopes of 2.0, whereas $Ru(NH_3)_6^{2+}$ gave a slope of 1.0. According to some reports strong reducing agents are capable of uncoupling the type 3 copper unit, turning it into a successive one-electron acceptor. An alternative interpretation is the existence of pseudocooperativity between the type 1 copper and the optically almost invisible type 2 center handling two-electron packages to the type 3 dimer. Because the type 2 copper in tree laccase has the lowest potential, its ability to become involved in a pseudocooperative electron-transfer mechanism would increase with the reducing power of the titrant, in agreement with experimental findings (47).

Mechanism of Action of Ascorbate Oxidase—Kinetics of the Anaerobic Reduction by Ascorbate and Reductate

Faced with the problem of elucidating the individual roles of the different copper centers in the blue oxidases, the researcher has naturally focused in recent years on the laccases (9). Being easier to isolate, better characterized, and containing fewer copper atoms than ceruloplasmin or ascorbate oxidase, the laccases from the Japanese lacquer tree *Rhus vernicifera* and the fungus *Polyporus versicolor* have been the subject of several transient kinetic studies in the millisecond range, that is, studies using stopped-flow spectrophotometry and rapid-freeze EPR spectroscopy (9, 49, 50).

Laccase, by analogy with ascorbate oxidase, catalyzes the oxidation of o- or p-aryldiamines and diphenols by dioxygen to produce water and the corresponding quinones. Steady state kinetics have established that a "ping-pong" mechanism is operative (51). This finding implies that the reduction of dioxygen and the oxidation of the organic substrate are separate events, requiring the enzyme to function as a multielectron mediator. During the catalytic cycle the organic substrate undergoes a rapid one-electron oxidation to a free radical, which probably decays by nonenzymatic dismutation (52), as found in various enzyme-catalyzed oxidation reactions (53). Kinetic experiments under anaerobic conditions have led to the conclusion that the type 1 copper is the entry site of electrons into the enzyme (49, 54). The type 3 copper pair is reduced in a process dependent upon the intramolecular transfer of one electron from the type 1 copper. Furthermore, the rate of electron transfer between the type 1 and the type 3 centers is controlled by the pH of the medium, possibly via a trigger mechanism involving the type 2 copper (49).

A complex mechanism for the four-electron reduction of dioxygen to water must complete the catalytic cycle. Any mechanism involving four consecutive single-electron transfers is unlikely (55). For laccase some experimental evidence indicates that at least two single electrons are exchanged, because during dioxygen reduction a paramagnetic intermediate, which decays slowly by the reaction with the reduced type 2 center, is formed (56, 57). This paramagnetic species, most likely the radical $O\cdot^-$, is trapped during simple oxidation reactions. Using oxygen-17-isotope-enriched dioxygen, only one product water molecule is rapidly released into the solution, whereas the second one remains coordinated to the type 2 copper site and exchanges slowly in comparison to the first (56, 57). From these results it appears that the type 2 copper plays an important role in both the reductive and oxidative functioning of the enzyme. (For further details, see Refs. 9 and 49).

Another interesting aspect of the reduction of dioxygen by laccase arises from the observation that the enzyme forms a stable intermediate with hydrogen peroxide (58, 59, 60). This peroxy compound of laccase is obtained either by oxidation of the reduced enzyme with hydrogen peroxide or by direct titration of the oxidized enzyme with hydrogen peroxide. Primarily on the basis of absorption and circular dichroism spectra it was proposed that the peroxide binds to the type 3 copper pair. Meanwhile, these investigations were extended to magnetic susceptibility measurements (60), which give further support for a peroxide-coordinated type 3 copper couple.

Some of these experiments have been repeated with ascorbate oxidase (two type 3 copper pairs), confirming the spectrophotometric data of Reference 58. Two equivalents of hydrogen peroxide, that is, 1 mol/type 3 copper pair (18), where specifically bound to ascorbate oxidase, produced an increase in the absorbance around 330 nm. These experimental results, although of rather preliminary nature, suggest that there might be some similarities between the laccases and ascorbate oxidase, with respect to the dioxygen-reducing sites of the enzyme.

The kinetic results of the anaerobic reduction of ascorbate oxidase by L-ascorbate or reductate presented in this chapter have been obtained by anaerobic stopped-flow spectrophotometry and rapid-freeze EPR spectroscopy. In view of the dioxygen sensitivity of the reduced enzyme, extreme care must be exercised to obtain reproducible and statistically meaningful data. For the anaerobicity of the instrument, both the mixing and the observation chamber including the syringe system were embedded into a thermostated, water circulating bath (normally maintained at 10–15°C), which was kept under a constant pressure of purified argon (*18*), as described in Reference *61*. A similar system was constructed for the rapid-freeze apparatus, allowing anaerobic mixing of the reactants prior to freeze-quenching of the reaction mixture in an isopentane cooling bath at approximately −145°C (*62*).

Stopped-Flow Spectrophotometry. The reduction of the type 1 copper [observed at 610 nm, phosphate buffer (pH 7.0), $I = 0.20$ M, 25°C] was very rapid and complex, by both L-ascorbate and reductate. Furthermore, trace amounts of dioxygen (less than 1 μM) produced significant plateau regions in the reduction profile. Addition of small amounts of reductant resulted first in the reduction of this plateau phase to zero and then in the partial reduction of the enzyme, judging from the total absorbance at 610 nm. To decrease the reduction rate, the temperature was lowered to 10°C with similar but slower optical changes.

Similar observations were made for the change in absorbance at 330 nm (Figure 6).

REDUCTION KINETICS OF THE TYPE-1 COPPER. There is an initial rapid phase during which plots of log $(A_t - A_\infty)$ vs. time are linear, yielding first-order rate constants, k_{init}^{610}. A linear dependence of k_{init}^{610} on reductate concentration is found within the limit of 5.2 mM reductate. The amplitude of the initial phase increases with reductate concentration, leveling off to approach a limit of approximately 50% of the total absorbance at 610 nm.

At 25°C, the initial reaction is much faster, indicating a considerable activation enthalpy, and the concentration range is limited to a value equal to or less than 1.35 mM for the time scale of our stopped-flow spectrophotometer. Again the rate is first order with respect to both enzyme and substrate. The amplitude of the initial phase at this higher temperature also increases with reductate concentration, but in a more pronounced manner. At the highest concentration used, this initial rapid phase represents 80% of the total reaction amplitude.

In the absence of dioxygen, the initial rapid step is followed directly by a slower reaction. This second rate, k_2^{610}, is again first order in enzyme concentration. From a plot which is linear, of $1/k_2^{610}$ vs. the

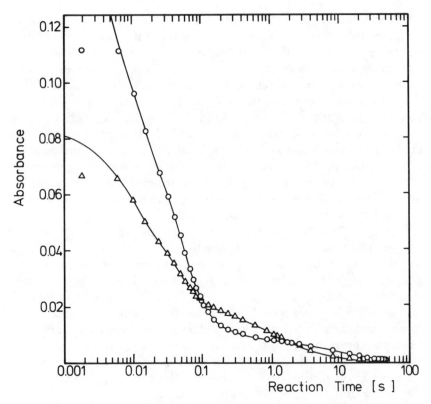

Figure 6. Anaerobic reduction of ascorbate oxidase by reductate; time course of the reaction at 610 (○) and 330 nm (△). Conditions: phosphate buffer (pH 7.0), I = 0.20 M, 10.0°C, enzyme 12 μM, substrate 2.4 mM. The solid line was obtained by computer simulation.

reciprocal concentration of reductate, a limiting rate of approximately 80 s⁻¹ can be estimated. The above-mentioned features were remarkably reproducible using separate ascorbate oxidase samples prepared and stored in liquid nitrogen over a 3-year period (*18*).

There is a very slow final stage, accounting for approximately 4–5% of the total reaction amplitude at 610 nm. The low amplitude makes quantitative evaluation of this stage very difficult, and the reproducibility was not very satisfactory. However, the rate is probably independent of the reductate concentration with a rate constant, k_3^{610}, of less than 1.0 s⁻¹.

In the presence of dioxygen, the initial rapid phase and the slower second phase are separated by a plateau on the stopped-flow trace, as also measured for the decay of the absorbance at 330 nm (Figure 7). The extent of the initial rapid phase decreases significantly with increasing dioxygen concentration. The effects of dioxygen removal by induced enzyme turnover, and of partial prereduction of the enzyme, are shown in Figure 7.

Variation of pH from 7.0 to 6.1 resulted in little change qualitatively, although measured k_{init}^{610} values were slightly higher. A single run at pH 7.8 confirmed this trend (Table II).

REDUCTION KINETICS OF THE TYPE 3 COPPER. Quantitative assessment of the complex kinetic behavior at 330 nm is difficult. This difficulty probably is partially caused by the small and varied contribution from the production and decay of the substrate radical species (63), a feature that is revealed when runs at at various wavelengths are compared. The decay rate of the radical, presumably decay by non-enzymatic dismutation, has a magnitude similar to the reduction rate of the type 3 copper. In the experiments with ascorbate as substrate,

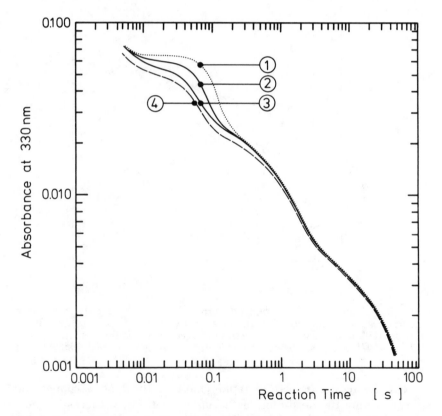

Figure 7. Anaerobic reduction of the type 3 Cu of ascorbate oxidase by reductate. Conditions as in Figure 6. Curves 1–4 show the effect of stepwise addition of reductate to the enzyme prior to kinetic stopped-flow runs. Curve 1 represents ~ 6 μM dioxygen, curves 2–4 demonstrate the successive removal of dioxygen and partial reduction of the enzyme.

Table II. Variation with pH of Second-Order Rate Constants, k_{init}^{610} and k_2^{610}

pH	k_{init}^{610}	k_2^{610}
6.1	2.23×10^4	1.2×10^4
7.0	1.69×10^4	1.0×10^4
7.8	1.43×10^4	0.8×10^4

Note: Data presented as M^{-1} s^{-1}, 10.0°C, reductate. Rate constants were obtained by plotting the observed rate constant, k_{obs}, against substrate concentration. k_2^{610} values were taken from the linear part of these plots, i.e., at low nonsaturating concentrations.

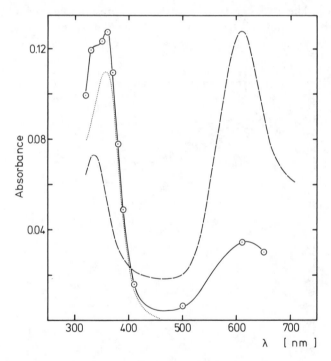

Figure 8.   Transient spectra obtained during the anaerobic reduction of ascorbate oxidase by L-ascorbate. Conditions as in Figure 6, except: enzyme 13 μM, substrate 0.97 mM. Key: – – –, spectrum of ascorbate oxidase prior to reaction; ——, transient observed after 5 ms, · · ·, difference spectrum.

the enzyme reduction was so rapid (most of the type 1 copper was reduced within the dead-time of the instrument, i.e., within ~ 3.5 ms) that there was initially a very rapid and strong increase of the absorbance around 330 nm, with a true absorption maximum at 360 nm (Figure 8), corresponding to the generation of the ascorbate free radical (63).

In the studies carried out with reductate as substrate (pH 7.0, 10.0°C), multiphasic behavior that is unaffected by varying amounts of EDTA [added to complex free Cu(II) ions in solution, or to remove nonspecifically bound Cu(II)] is observed. Again, as for the type 1 copper, a very slow phase of reduction is always present, corresponding to 10–30% of the total absorbance change at 330 nm. Correlation with rapid-freeze EPR experiments shows that this process cannot be associated with the free radical since the reaction is too slow. Furthermore, the effects of traces of dioxygen can be observed. As with the reduction of the type 1 copper at 610 nm, a lag phase that disappears after removal of dioxygen by prior addition of small amounts of reductant is seen (Figure 7). Subtraction of the slow phase (Figure 6) by extrapolation of primary semilogarithmic plots to zero time, and then plotting log $(A_t - A_\infty)$ vs. time leads to semilogarithmic plots corresponding to the fast stages of the reduction at 330 nm (Figure 6). The plots so obtained vary in linearity. In many cases there is no definite linearity, indicating that the absorbance change reflects a single first-order process. Assuming a generally linear, semilogarithmic relationship for this rapid first stage of reduction of the 330-nm chromophore, the dependence of this rate constant, k_{init}^{330}, on the concentration of reductant can be derived. A plot of k_{init}^{330} vs. concentration of reductate results in a curved line, indicating that a limit is being approached; this limit is estimated to be approximately 100 s^{-1}.

When reductate is replaced by L-ascorbate, the initial rate of reduction of the type 1 copper increases dramatically and is accompanied by the formation of the ascorbate radical (Figure 8). Therefore, some problems arise in evaluating the kinetic data at 330 nm for the reduction of the type 3 copper. However, as with reductate, a final slow reaction with similar absorbance changes and rate occurred at both 330 and 610 nm.

Rapid-Freeze EPR Spectroscopy.   EPR analysis of the rapid-freeze– quenched reaction with both L-ascorbate and reductate reveals a very rapid decrease in the signal intensity, due to the reduction of the type 1 copper (Figure 4). This observation is consistent with the independent observation from stopped-flow spectrophotometry that most of the 610-nm chromophore is reduced within the dead-time of the spectrophotometer. Reduction of the type 2 copper is much slower under the conditions used for the rapid mixing in the freeze–quench apparatus (pH 7.0, $I =$ 0.20 M, 5°C). A dominant feature of the EPR spectrum in the earliest stages of measurement (~ 5 ms) is a signal at $g = 2.005$, arising from the substrate radical, that is, the L-ascorbate or reductate radical. A similar signal is observed in many other biological oxidoreductions at both room temperature and 77 K (*64, 65*). No hyperfine splitting is displayed in the EPR spectrum of the L-ascorbate radical at 77 K, but at least four lines can be resolved for the reductate radical (Figure 9).

Discussion and Possible Mode of Electron Transfer. In view of the excellent reproducibility of the kinetic measurements, particularly regarding the reduction of the type 1 copper, we assigned certain sequences of redox events and electron movements within the multicopper enzyme to our observations.

The reduction of the blue chromophore is multiphasic, but not because of the effects associated with the possible kinetic behavior of three different type 1 copper sites. Initial rate constants, k_{init}^{330}, for the reduction by reductate show first-order dependence with respect to

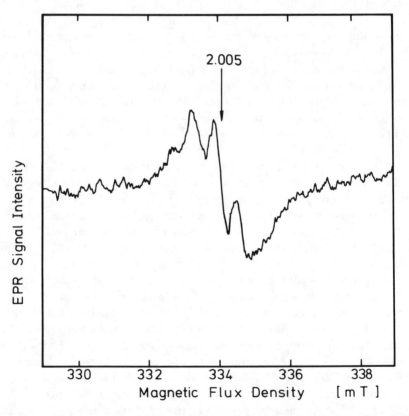

Figure 9.   EPR spectrum of the substrate radical formed during the rapid initial phase of the anaerobic reduction of ascorbate oxidase by reductate. Conditions as in Figure 6.   The spectrum was recorded at 77 K, ~ 9.4 GHz, 100 kHz modulation frequency, 0.05 mT modulation amplitude.

reductate over a wide concentration range at pH 7.0 and 6.1. This behavior is consistent with a one-electron transfer from reduced substrate to the type 1 copper(II) producing type 1 copper(I) and the substrate radical (Figure 9).

In studies on the anaerobic reduction of tree laccase by hydroquinone and ascorbate (49), the existence of a plateau phase at low substrate concentration was reported for the reaction of the type 1 copper. This observation was explained in terms of an intramolecular reoxidation by the type 3 copper pair. A similar plateau phase is a dominant feature of the reduction of both chromophores of ascorbate oxidase by reductate (Figure 7). However, the plateau phase is only observed in the presence of "contaminating" dioxygen; rigorous removal of these dioxygen traces removes the plateau phase at all wavelengths. The reaction of reduced ascorbate oxidase with dioxygen is very rapid, $k = 5 \times 10^6 \, M^{-1}s^{-1}$, at pH 5.8, 1.7°C (66). If electron transfer from type 1 to type 3 copper couples the two halves of the enzyme cycle, as proposed for laccase, then this intramolecular redox reaction must be extremely rapid to account for the effects of trace dioxygen on the reduction of the type 1 copper. Consequently, despite the fact that an ambiguous assignment of a type 1 to type 3 transfer is not possible in this example, facile intramolecular electron transfer processes probably ensure a rapid distribution of electrons among the type 1 and type 3 copper centers, at least in some of the enzyme molecules. The equilibrium distribution, and quite conceivably the relative rates of approach to this state, should be influenced by the oxidation–reduction potentials, which, as described earlier in this chapter (Figure 5), favor electron occupancy of the type 3 copper pairs at 10.0°C.

For the subsequent slower reductions of both the 610- and 330-nm chromophores, similar maximum rate constants were obtained. This result indicates that at high substrate concentrations the reduction of both copper types may be limited by a common rate-determining step.

The rapid initial reduction of the type 1 copper is very similar to that reported for tree laccase (49). The amplitude of this reduction increases with substrate concentration to a maximum value of approximately 50% of total absorbance change at 10°C. In laccase this effect is explained by the existence of two forms of the enzyme in an acid–base equilibrium. The active form allows rapid type 1 to type 3 electron transfer, whereas in the inactive form this process is inhibited. At higher substrate concentrations, the reduction of the type 1 copper is faster than the interconversion of inactive enzyme into its active form, leading to an increase in initial phase amplitude. Turnover-induced activation of ascorbate oxidase (67) could also be explained in terms of displacement of this inactive–active equilibrium.

The optical spectrum of the ascorbate radical extrapolated from the stopped-flow traces is in good agreement with a spectrum in the literature (68) with an absorption maximum at 360 nm ($3700\ M^{-1}cm^{-1}$). Analysis of the stopped-flow data reveals that little or no reduction of the type 3 copper has occurred during the initial rapid absorbance loss at 610 nm. This observation is consistent with the assumption that entry of electrons into the enzyme occurs at or near the type 1 copper atoms.

The finding from rapid-freeze–quench EPR experiments, that the reduction of the type 2 copper is slow compared with that of the type 1 copper, is analogous to the behavior noted for tree laccase at higher pH values (50). In this enzyme the slow reduction of the type 2 center is linked to the inhibition of the type 3 reduction. In ascorbate oxidase, however, reduction of the type 3 copper pairs proceeds despite the slow reduction of the type 2 copper, suggesting that the two electrons necessary for the proposed intramolecular reduction of the two type 3 copper pairs can be transferred from two of the three type 1 copper centers, without involving the type 2 center in any redox process.

Acknowledgments

The authors thank the Royal Society (fellowship, F. A. Armstrong) and the European Molecular Biology Organization (two short-term fellowships, A. Marchesini). This research was supported by Deutsche Forschungsgemeinschaft (Kr 451/4-7).

Literature Cited

1. Szent-Györgyi, A. *J. Biol. Chem.* **1931**, *90*, 385.
2. Stark, G. R.; Dawson, C. R. "The Enzymes"; Boyer, P. D.; Lardy, H.; Myrbäck, K., Eds.; Academic: New York, 1963; Vol. 8, p. 297.
3. Dawson, C. R.; Strothkamp, K. G.; Krul, K. G. *Ann. N.Y. Acad. Sci.* **1975**, *258*, 209.
4. Burstein, S. R.; Gerwin, B.; Taylor, H.; Westley, J. "Iron and Copper Proteins"; Yasunobu, K. T.; Mower, H. F.; Hayaishi, O., Eds.; Plenum: New York, 1976; p. 472.
5. Malkin, R.; Malmström, B. G. *Adv. Enzymol.* **1970**, *33*, 177.
6. Fee, J. *Struct. Bonding (Berlin)* **1975**, *23*, 1.
7. Malmström, B. G.; Andréasson, L.-E.; Reinhammar, B. "The Enzymes"; Boyer, P. D.; Lardy, H.; Myrbäck, K., Eds.; Academic: New York, **1975**; Vol. 12B, p. 507.
8. Reinhammar, B. "Advances in Inorganic Biochemistry"; Eichhorn, G. L.; Marzilli, L. G., Eds.; Elsevier: Amsterdam, 1979; Vol. 1, p. 91.
9. Lee, M. H.; Dawson, C. R. *Arch. Biochem. Biophys.* **1979**, *191*, 119.
10. Beutler, H. O.; Beinstingl, G. *Dtsch. Lebensm.–Rundsch.* **1980**, *76*, 69.
11. Marchesini, A.; Capelletti, P.; Canonica, L.; Danieli, B.; Tollari, S. *Biochim. Biophys. Acta* **1977**, *484*, 290.
12. Canonica, L.; Casagrande, C.; Marchesini, A.; Tollari, S. *Proc. 11th Congr. IUPAC, Gold Sand, Bulgaria, 1978.*

13. White, G. A.; Krupka, R. M. *Arch. Biochem. Biophys.* **1965,** *110,* 448.
14. Marchesini, A.; Bosi, I.; Dal Pero Berini, R.; Scagliarini, R. *Agrochimica* **1974,** *18,* 432.
15. Lee, M. H.; Dawson, C. R. *J. Biol. Chem.* **1973,** *248,* 6596.
16. Nakamura, T.; Makino, N.; Ogura, Y. *J. Biochem. (Tokyo)* **1968,** *64,* 189.
17. Avigliano, L.; Gerosa, P.; Rotilio, G.; Finazzi-Agrò, A.; Calabrese, L.; Mondovì, B. *Ital. J. Biochem.* **1972,** *21,* 248.
18. Marchesini, A.; Kroneck, P. M. H. *Eur. J. Biochem.* **1979,** *101,* 65.
19. Rydén, L.; Björk, J. *Biochemistry* **1976,** *15,* 3411.
20. Avigliano, L.; Desideri, A.; Urbanelli, S.; Mondovì, B.; Marchesini, A. *FEBS Lett.* **1979,** *100,* 318.
21. Joselow, M.; Dawson, C. R. *J. Biol. Chem.* **1951,** *191,* 1.
22. Ibid., 11.
23. Clark, E. E.; Poillon, W. N.; Dawson, C. R. *Biochim. Biophys. Acta* **1966,** *118,* 72.
24. Clark, E. E.; Poillon, W. N.; Dawson, C. R. *Biochim. Biophys. Acta* **1966,** *118,* 82.
25. Strothkamp, K. G.; Dawson, C. R. *Biochemistry* **1974,** *13,* 434.
25. Krul, K. G.; Dawson, C. R. *Bioinorg. Chem.* **1977,** *7,* 71.
26. Penton, Z. G.; Dawson, C. R. "Oxidases and Related Redox Systems"; King, T. E.; Mason, H. S.; Morrison, M., Eds.; John Wiley & Sons: New York, **1965;** p. 222.
27. Krul, K. G.; Dawson, C. R. *Bioinorg. Chem.* **1977,** *7,* 71.
28. Deinum, J.; Reinhammar, B.; Marchesini, A. *FEBS Lett.* **1974,** *42,* 241.
29. Malmström, B. G.; Reinhammar, B.; Vänngård, T. *Biochim. Biophys. Acta* **1970,** *205,* 48.
30. Pecht, I.; Faraggi, M. *Nature* **1971,** *233,* 116.
31. Faraggi, M.; Pecht, I. *J. Biol. Chem.* **1973,** *248,* 3146.
32. Pecht, I.; Goldberg, M. "Fast Processes in Radiation Chemistry and Biology"; Adams, G. E.; Fielden, E. M.; Michael, B. D., Eds.; John Wiley & Sons: New York, 1975; p. 277.
33. Byers, W.; Curzon, G.; Garbett, K.; Speyer, B. E.; Young, S. N.; Williams, R. J. P. *Biochim. Biophys. Acta* **1973,** *310,* 38.
34. Kroneck, P. M. H. *J. Am. Chem. Soc.* **1975,** *97,* 3839.
35. Stark, G. R.; Dawson, C. R. *J. Biol. Chem.* **1962,** *237,* 712.
36. Briving, C.; Deinum, J. *FEBS Lett.* **1975,** *51,* 43.
37. Dooley, D. M.; Rawlings, J.; Dawson, J. H.; Stephens, P. J.; Andréasson, L.-E.; Malmström, B. G.; Gray, H. B. *J. Am. Chem. Soc.* **1979,** *101,* 5038.
38. Solomon, E. I.; Hare, J. W.; Dooley, D. M.; Dawson, J. H.; Stephens, P. J.; Gray, H. B. *J. Am. Chem. Soc.* **1980,** *102,* 168.
39. Solomon, E. I.; Hare, J. W.; Gray, H. B. *Proc. Natl. Acad. Sci. U.S.A.* **1976,** *73,* 1389.
40. Avigliano, L.; Rotilio, G.; Urbanelli, S.; Mondovì, B.; Finazzi-Agrò, A. *Arch. Biochem. Biophys.* **1978,** *185,* 419.
41. Fee, J. A.; Malkin, R.; Malmström, B. G.; Vänngård, T. *J. Biol. Chem.* **1969,** *244,* 4200.
42. Malmström, B. G.; Finazzi-Agrò, A.; Antonini, E. *Eur. J. Biochem.* **1969,** *9,* 383.
43. Goldberg, M.; Pecht, I. *Proc. Natl. Acad. Sci. U.S.A.* **1974,** *71,* 4684.
44. Aikazyan, V. T.; Nalbandyan, R. M. *Biokhimiya* **1977,** *42,* 2027.
45. Jakob, W., private communication.
46. Reinhammar, B.; Malkin, R.; Jensen, P.; Karlsson, B.; Andréasson, L.-E.; Aasa, R.; Vänngård, T. *J. Biol. Chem.* **1980,** *255,* 5000.
47. Farver, O.; Goldberg, M.; Wherland, S.; Pecht, I. *Proc. Natl. Acad. Sci. U.S.A.* **1978,** *75,* 5245.
48. Tokuyama, K.; Clark, E. E.; Dawson, C. R. *Biochemistry* **1965,** *4,* 1362.

49. Andréasson, L.-E.; Reinhammar, B. *Biochim. Biophys. Acta* **1976**, *445*, 579.
50. Ibid., **1979**, *568*, 145.
51. Petersen, L. C.; Degn, H. *Biochim. Biophys. Acta* **1978**, *526*, 85.
52. Broman, L.; Malmström, B G..; Aasa, R.; Vänngård, T. *Biochim. Biophys. Acta* **1963**, *75*, 365.
53. Yamazaki, I.; Mason, H. S.; Piette, L. *J. Biol. Chem.* **1960**, *235*, 2444.
54. Andréasson, L.-E.; Malmström, B. G.; Strömberg, C.; Vänngård, T. *Eur. J. Biochem.* **1973**, *34*, 434.
55. Hill, H. A. O. "New Trends in Bio-Inorganic Chemistry"; Williams, R. J. P.; Da Silva, J. R. R. F., Eds.; Academic: London, New York, San Francisco, **1978**; p. 174.
56. Andréasson, L.-E.; Brändén, R.; Reinhammar, B. *Biochim. Biophys. Acta* **1976**, *438*, 370.
57. Brändén, R.; Deinum, J. *Biochim. Biophys. Acta* **1978**, *524*, 297.
58. Farver, O.; Goldberg, M.; Lancet, D.; Pecht, I. *Biochem. Biophys. Res. Commun.* **1976**, *73*, 494.
59. Farver, O.; Goldberg, M.; Pecht, I. *Eur. J. Biochem.* **1980**, *104*, 71.
60. Farver, O.; Pecht, I. *FEBS Lett.* **1979**, *108*, 436.
61. Ballou, D. P., Ph.D. Thesis, Univ. of Michigan, Ann Arbor, 1971.
62. Ballou, D. P.; Palmer, G. A. *Anal. Chem.* **1974**, *46*, 1248.
63. Bielski, B. H. J.; Allen, A. O. *J. Am. Chem. Soc.* **1970**, *92*, 3793.
64. Yamazaki, I.; Piette, L. H. *Biochim. Biophys. Acta* **1961**, *50*, 62.
65. Lohmann, W.; Schreiber, J.; Gerhardt, H.; Breithaupt, H.; Löffler, H.; Pralle, H. *Blut* **1979**, *39*, 147.
66. Nakamura, T.; Ogura, Y. *J. Biochem. (Tokyo)* **1968**, *64*, 267.
67. Gerwin, B.; Burstein, S. R.; Westley, J. *J. Biol. Chem.* **1974**, *249*, 2005.
68. Schöneshöfer, M. *Z. Naturforsch., Teil B* **1972**, *27*, 649.

RECEIVED for review January 22, 1981. ACCEPTED June 23, 1981.

Metabolism of L-Ascorbic Acid in Plants

FRANK A. LOEWUS and JOHANNES P. F. G. HELSPER

Institute of Biological Chemistry, Washington State University, Pullman, WA 99164

A detailed study of the catabolism of L-ascorbic acid in tartrate-accumulating and oxalate-accumulating plants has revealed a precursor–product relationship which, in the case of tartrate accumulators, involves two mutually exclusive pathways. In the Vitaceae, the carbon chain of ascorbic acid is cleaved at the C4–C5 bond to furnish a C_4 fragment that is converted to L-(+)-tartaric acid and a C_2 fragment that is recycled into products of hexose phosphate metabolism. In the Geraniaceae, cleavage occurs at the C2–C3 bond to produce oxalic acid from the C_2 fragment and L-(+)-tartaric acid from the C_4 fragment. Other oxalate accumulators that fail to accumulate tartaric acid also cleave ascorbic acid at the C2–C3 bond. The nature of the product(s) obtained from the C_4 fragment must still be determined. Conversion of D-glucose to ascorbic acid and its catabolic products has been studied in both types of plants with the aid of specifically labeled D-glucose. Results support a biosynthetic route that involves oxidation of C1 of D-glucose, epimerization at C5, and conservation of the hydroxymethyl function at C6.

K nowledge of metabolic events encompassing the formation and decomposition of ascorbic acid in plants is meager although L-ascorbic acid is a common constituent in actively growing tissues of higher plants. Despite a plethora of information on chemical, biomedical, and nutritional aspects of ascorbic acid, progress on plant-related processes has lagged. In part, the reason for this may lie in the generally accepted view that ascorbic acid is a secondary product of plant metabolism, a sugar acid outside the mainstream of carbohydrate interconversions. Again, it may rest in a paucity of well-established roles for ascorbic acid in plant

0065-2393/82/0200–0249$06.00/0

metabolism. For whatever reasons are behind this neglect, renewed efforts to discover the biochemical events that govern participation of ascorbic acid in cellular processes are in order.

Conversion of Ascorbate to Tartrate in the Grape

An important discovery in 1969 (1) linked the catabolism of L-ascorbic acid to tartaric acid biosynthesis. When immature grape berries were fed L-[1-14C]ascorbic acid over a 24-h period, 72% of the acid extractable 14C appeared in tartaric acid, virtually all of it in carboxyl carbon. When the metabolic period was extended another 24 h, only 48% of the 14C remained in tartaric acid, an indication that catabolic processes were removing a part of the labeled tartaric acid (2, 3, 4). Saito and Kasai (1) suggested that C1 through C4 of L-ascorbic acid was converted directly into tartaric acid (Figure 1). Indirect support of this was the failure of L-[6-14C]ascorbic acid to produce labeled tartaric acid (5). Subsequently, Wagner and Loewus (6) confirmed the observations of Saito and Kasai (1).

Williams and Loewus (7) prepared L-[4-14C]ascorbic acid by the method of Bakke and Theander (8) and showed that this form of specifically labeled ascorbic acid, like L-[1-14C]ascorbic acid, was an effective precursor of tartaric acid in grape berries and grape leaves (Table I) (9). Over 98% of the 14C was located in the carboxyl groups of labeled tartaric acid from L-[1-14C]- or L-[4-14C]ascorbic acid labeled leaves or berries. Only L-(+)-tartaric acid was formed (10). The C_2 fragment of this cleavage, as judged by studies with L-[6-14C]ascorbic acid, was recycled into products of hexose phosphate metabolism (5, 6, 11, 12).

Conversion of L-ascorbic acid to tartaric acid in the grape was limited to certain stages of development (Tables I and II). Leaves detached from the tip of the vine or the position opposite the flower cluster prior to anthesis (or at anthesis) readily utilized ascorbic acid for tartaric acid

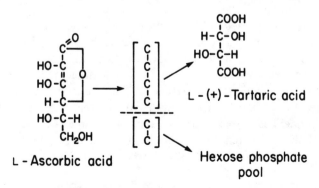

Figure 1.   Cleavage of L-ascorbic acid in plants of the Vitaceae.

Table I.   Conversion of L-Ascorbic Acid to Tartaric Acid in the Grape (Metabolic Period, 25 h)

Conditions		[1-^{14}C]	[4-^{14}C]	[6-^{14}C]
		Percent of Acid Extractable ^{14}C		
Berry (6, 9)	light	69	—	2
	dark	67	—	—
	light	66	60	—
Leaf (5, 9)	anthesis	81	81	< 1
	+ 14 days[a]	—	57	—
	+48 to 57 days[a]	0.1	3	< 1

[a] Days after anthesis.

Table II.   L-Ascorbic Acid Catabolism in Grape Leaves (Metabolic Period, 24 h)

	Days Before (—) or After (+) Anthesis					
	−28		−14		+15	
	Position of Label in Ascorbic Acid					
	[1-^{14}C]	[6-^{14}C]	[1-^{14}C]	[6-^{14}C]	[1-^{14}C]	[6-^{14}C]
Compound	Percent of Administered ^{14}C					
CO$_2$	2	8	2	4	4	2
Sugars	< 1	9	< 1	18	5	9
Dehydroascorbic acid	2	4	4	10	26	32
Tartaric acid	71	< 1	71	< 1	4	< 1
Other solubles	8	25	14	32	58	54
Residue	17	52	8	35	3	3

biosynthesis. Leaves removed from the still elongating tip of the vine or the position opposite the flower cluster after anthesis (during berry formation) slowly lost that capacity; 7–8 weeks later none of the ^{14}C from L-[1-^{14}C]- or L-[4-^{14}C]ascorbic acid was recovered in tartaric acid when leaves from the tip region were so labeled (9). Leaves located directly opposite to the developing berry cluster lost this quality within 2 weeks after anthesis (12), but grape berries continued to form some tartaric acid until 9 weeks after anthesis (13).

Tartaric acid production was accompanied by a process involving recycling of C6 of ascorbic acid into sugars and polysaccharides. When leaves were labeled with L-[6-^{14}C]ascorbic acid before anthesis, about 70% of the ^{14}C appeared in soluble (sugar) or residual (polysaccharide) fractions (Table II), a quantity comparable to that found in tartaric acid when the source of label was L-[1-^{14}C]ascorbic acid. The bulk of the label in the solution fraction was sucrose, glucose, and fructose while that in the residual fraction was starch and cell wall glycans (12). Minor differences in distribution of ^{14}C among these metabolic products from leaves taken 28 or 14 days before anthesis probably reflect changes in the utilization of labeled hexose as it was withdrawn from the hexose phosphate pool. Shortly after anthesis, cleavage of L-ascorbic acid diminished, eventually ceasing entirely, and the only labeled products of consequence were dehydroascorbic acid and an unidentified C_6 sugar acid (included in Table II with "other solubles").

Our results have led us to suggest a role for L-ascorbic acid in phloem transport (9) in which ascorbic acid is translocated from its biosynthetic site in the leaf to a catabolic site in the fruit cluster where C4–C5 cleavage of the carbon chain produces tartaric acid and a putative C_2 precursor of carbohydrate biosynthesis. The sugar/organic acid balance that influences grape quality in winemaking may well be determined by the role of ascorbic acid as the precursor of tartaric acid.

Conversion of Ascorbate to Tartrate in Virginia Creeper

The grape is a seasonal plant. Moreover, conversion of ascorbate to tartrate, as noted above, is limited to certain stages of growth and development. Efforts to find an alternative species of Vitaceae more amenable to research led us to Virginia Creeper (*Parthenocissus quinquefolia*). In a controlled environment, this plant retains its leaves and continues to lengthen its vines indefinitely, an ideal system for study of Vitaceae-type ascorbic acid metabolism on a year-around basis.

Virginia Creeper leaves were fed L-ascorbic acid with ^{14}C in C1, C4, C5, or C6 or ^3H on C6 (14). In each experiment, three compound leaves from the fifth position behind the tip of the vine were used. After a 24-h metabolic period, the distribution of radioisotope was determined (Table III). As in the grape, L-[1-^{14}C]- and L-[4-^{14}C]ascorbic acid produced carboxyl labeled tartaric acid. Virutally no radioisotope appeared in tartaric acid from the other L-[5-^{14}C]-, L-[6-^{14}C]-, or L-[6-^3H]ascorbic acid. The larger amount of $^{14}CO_2$ released by L-[1-^{14}C]ascorbic acid labeled leaves has been confirmed in subsequent studies.

Within experimental limits, leaves labeled with L-[5-^{14}C]- or L-[6-^{14}C]ascorbic acid gave comparable results (Table III). Additively, the ^{14}C in CO_2, sugars, and malic acid accounted to 62–63% of that present in the leaves. Another 7% appeared in the residue as glycans. The total amount of ^{14}C found in hexose or products of hexose metabolism of L-[5-^{14}C]- or L-[6-^{14}C]ascorbic acid labeled leaves was similar to that found in tartrate (and CO_2) after labeling with L-[1-^{14}C]- or L-[4-^{14}C]-ascorbic acid. Cleavage of the carbon chain of ascorbic acid at the C4–C5 bond accounts for these observations.

**Table III.   L-Ascorbic Acid Catabolism in Virginia Creeper
(Metabolic Period, 24 h)**

	Position of Label in Ascorbic Acid				
	[1-^{14}C]	[4-^{14}C]	[5-^{14}C]	[6-^{14}C]	[6-^{3}H]
	Date of Experiment				
	8/79	10/79	11/79	9/79	2/80
Compound	Percent of Administered Label				
CO_2	22	1	14	18	—
Sugars	< 1	< 1	34	27	8
Dehydroascorbic acid	6	10	7	5	19
Tartaric acid	54	69	2	2	< 1
Other solubles	14	18	36	41	29
Residue	4	1	7	7	2
H_2O	—	—	—	—	40

The identity of the C_2 fragment released during cleavage of L-ascorbic acid by grape or Virginia Creeper was initially thought to be glycolic acid (*12*) since this compound could be recycled into hexose by the glycolic acid pathway (*15*). A recent study in which 5 mM 2-pyridyl-hydroxymethanesulfonate, a glycolic pathway inhibitor, was given to leaves of Virginia Creeper along with L-[6-^{14}C]ascorbic acid had no inhibitor effect on incorporation of ^{14}C into sugars (*14*).

In a study of high L-(+)-tartrate excreting mutants of *Gluconobacter suboxydans*, Kotera et al. (*16, 17, 18*) proposed a scheme in which 5-keto-D-gluconic acid was cleaved between C4 and C5 to yield glyco-aldehyde as a C_2 intermediate. In their scheme, this C_2 fragment was oxidized to glycolic acid, which was recovered from the growth medium. We have explored the possible production of labeled glycolaldehyde after labeling Virginia Creeper leaves with L-[5-^{14}C]-1 or -[6-^{14}C]ascorbic acid (*14*). When a small amount of glycolaldehyde was supplied to the leaves along with the labeled ascorbic acid, a new radioactive, low molecular weight compound was recovered by high performance liquid chromatography from the neutral fraction. It had the same retention time as glycolaldehyde. Attempts to characterize it as glycolaldehyde by thin layer chromatography (*19*) were unsuccessful. However, recent experiments involving comparison of specific radioactivity of dimedon formaldehyde of the periodate-treated C_2 fragment and its sodium borohydride-reduced product indicate that glycolaldehyde is the C_2 fragment. Its entry into hexose metabolism may proceed through the carbon reduction cycle by condensing with ribose 5-phosphate to form sedoheptulose 7-phosphate and/or with erythrose 4-phosphate to form fructose 6-phos-

phate. In both reactions, the carbon from glycolaldehyde is swept
rapidly into products of hexose phosphate metabolism (20).

Conversion of Ascorbate to Oxalate and Tartrate in Geranium

Tartrate is found in plant families besides the Vitaceae (21, 22).
Its quantitative occurrence has been reported for 52 species of Geraniaceae (23). Using this list, *Pelargonium crispum* (lemon geranium)
was chosen to examine a possible relationship between L-ascorbic acid
metabolism and tartaric acid biosynthesis in a plant family other than
Vitaceae (24). L-[6-^{14}C]Ascorbic acid and its precursor, L-[6-^{14}C]galac-
tono-1,4-lactone (25), were converted to carboxyl labeled L-(+)-tartaric
acid (10) by leaves from the lemon geranium (Table IV). When
L-[1-^{14}C]ascorbic acid was the source of label, none of the ^{14}C appeared
in tartaric acid but 15% was recovered in oxalic acid. L-[U-^{14}C]Galac-
tono-1,4-lactone-fed leaves produced labeled ascorbic, tartaric, and oxalic
acids (24). The best explanation for these results was a process involving C2–C3 cleavage of L-ascorbic acid to produce a C_2 fragment destined
to become oxalic acid and a C_4 fragment to become tartaric acid (Figure
2). Since geranium leaves metabolize oxalic acid to CO_2, the amount of
[14]C recovered in oxalic acid relative to that in tartaric acid was low as
illustrated by a time course study of L-[U-^{14}C]ascorbic acid metabolism
in geranium (Figure 3) (11).

Further evidence that the tartaric acid arose from a C_4 fragment
of L-ascorbic acid corresponding to C3 through C6 was obtained from
studies with L-[4-^{14}C]- and L-[6-^{14}C]ascorbic acid (Table IV) (9). The
former was converted to carboxyl-labeled tartrate in grape and Virginia

Table IV.   L-Ascorbic Acid Catabolism in Geranium (Metabolic Period, 72 h)

	Position of ^{14}C in Ascorbic Acid		
	[1-^{14}C]	*[4-^{14}C]*	*[6-^{14}C]*
Compound	Percent of Acid Extractable [14]C		
Oxalic acid	15	1	1
Tartaric acid*	< 1	45	51
Other acids	—	47	36
Other compounds	—	7	12
*Location of ^{14}C in tartaric acid	Percent of Total ^{14}C in Tartrate		
C1 + C4		2	99
C2 + C3		98	1

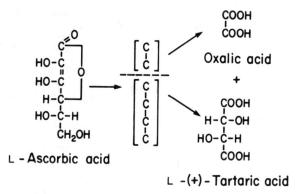

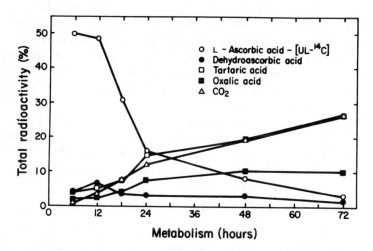

Figure 2.   *Cleavage of L-ascorbic acid in plants of the Geraniaceae. Oxalate accumulating plants also cleave L-ascorbic acid between C2 and C3 but the C_4 fragment does not accumulate as tartrate.*

Figure 3.   *Time course of L-[U-14C]ascorbic acid catabolism in the lemon geranium.*

Creeper. The latter, which failed to produce labeled tartaric acid in grape or Virginia Creeper, produced carboxyl labeled tartaric acid in geranium.

In geranium, the C2–C3 cleavage of L-ascorbic acid is enantiomerically specific (*11*). When L-[6-14C]ascorbic acid was replaced by D-[6-14C]ascorbic acid, labeled tartaric acid was not found in the acid extractable fraction (Table V). There was considerable decomposition of D-ascorbic acid. Only 17% of the D-ascorbic acid remained in the tissues at the end of the metabolic period. Some metabolism of these

Table V.   Dual Labeled Ascorbic Acid Catabolism in Geranium
(Metabolic Period, 72 h)

L-[4-³H]Ascorbic Acid   L-[4-³H]Ascorbic Acid
+   +
L-[6-¹⁴C]Ascorbic Acid   D-[6-¹⁴C]Ascorbic Acid

Percent of Incorporated Label

Compound	^3H	^{14}C	^3H	^{14}C
CO_2	—	4	—	16
H_2O	28	—	25	—
Oxalic acid	0	3	0	2
Tartaric acid	48	49	53	5
Other acids	19	22	15	48
Other compounds	5	22	7	29

breakdown products probably occurred since 16% of the radiolabel appeared as $^{14}CO_2$. In these experiments leaves were dual labeled with L-[4-³H]ascorbic acid to follow tartaric acid biosynthesis. As the data indicate (Table V), hydrogen attached to C4 of L-ascorbic acid was retained during tartaric acid biosynthesis. In a similar experiment involving grape leaves dual labeled with L-[4-³H]- and L-[U-¹⁴C]ascorbic acid, the ³H exchanged with the medium to exactly the same amount as ¹⁴C appeared in tartaric acid (11).

The enzymatic process responsible for C2–C3 cleavage of L-ascorbic acid is undetermined. One possibility, oxidation to dehydro-L-ascorbic acid followed by cleavage, has its chemical counterpart (26). Other processes, including cleavage of L-ascorbic acid, are not excluded.

Oxalate Formation from Ascorbate in Oxalate Accumulating Plants

Although oxalic acid is a well-recognized product of the chemical or biochemical decomposition of ascorbic acid in animal tissues (27), its formation from ascorbic acid in geranium leaves appears to be the first time that a metabolic relationship between these two compounds has been described in plants (24). Oxalic acid and its salts are widely distributed among plant species in both soluble and insoluble forms, the latter often occurring as calcium oxalate in discrete morphological structures that are formed from single crystals (styloids), or from bundles and clusters of crystals (druses and raphides). Some plants accumulate large amounts of oxalate, a notable example being *Halogeton glomeratus* with up to 35% of its dry weight as sodium oxalate (28). Other more familiar oxalate accumulators included in our study are *Spinacia oleracea* (spinach), *Beta vulgaris* (sugar beet), *Begonia evansiana* (begonia),

Oxalis stricta and *O. oregana* (woodsorrel), *Rheum rhabarbarum* (rhubarb), and numerous common weeds such as *Rumex crispus* (curly dock), *Chenopodium album* (lamb's-quarters), and *Amaranthus retroflexus* (red root pigweed).

S. oleracea utilized L-ascorbic acid and dehydro-L-ascorbic acid (but not diketo-L-gulonate) for oxalic acid biosynthesis (Table VI) (*29*). In these experiments, L-[1-^{14}C]ascorbic acid was converted to labeled oxalic acid. The fate of the C_4 fragment from L-ascorbic acid or dehydro-L-ascorbic acid was not determined. Similar results (Table VI) were obtained with *O. stricta* and *O. oregana*. Conversion to labeled oxalate proceeded in the dark as well as in the light when detached leaves were given L-[1-^{14}C]ascorbic acid. *Hordeum vulgare* (barley), a nonaccumulator of oxalate, converted only 2% of the ^{14}C in L-[1-^{14}C]ascorbic acid to oxalic acid under conditions identical to those used in studies with *Oxalis* species.

As noted earlier, geranium apices with newly unfolded leaves respire a substantial portion of L-[1-^{14}C]ascorbic acid as [^{14}C]CO_2. Older leaves from *O. oregana* and other oxalate formers (*29, 30*) produced less $^{14}CO_2$ from L-[1-^{14}C]ascorbic acid although conversion to [^{14}C]oxalate was as great as 55% of the administered label. Evidence to suggest that ascorbate-produced oxalate was further metabolized to CO_2 was obtained with seedlings from *H. glomeratus* and *R. crispus* (Table VII). If these seedlings were given [^{14}C]oxalic acid directly, 50–60% of the label appeared in CO_2 in 24 h (*30*). Clearly, rapidly respiring tissues of

Table VI. Formation of Oxalic Acid from L-[1-^{14}C]Ascorbic
Acid and Dehydro-L-[1-^{14}C]Ascorbic Acid in *Oxalis*
Species and *Spinacia oleracea*

Oxalis Species	Substrate	Metabolic Period	Oxalic Acid Formed	CO_2 Respired
		Hours	Percent of Administered ^{14}C	
O. stricta	ascorbic acid	48	37	12
	dehydroascorbic acid	24	18	2
O. oregana	ascorbic acid	48	36	8
	dehydroascorbic acid	24	26	3
O. oregana	ascorbic acid, dark	48	44	12
S. oleracea	ascorbic acid	28	29	24
	dehydroascorbic acid	24	25	14
	diketo L-gulonate	24	2	19

Table VII. L-[1-^{14}C]Ascorbic Acid Catabolism in Seedlings of
Plants Recognized as High Oxalate Accumulators
(Metabolic Period, 24 h)

Plant	Period of Germination Days	Oxalic Acid Formed	CO$_2$ Respired
		Percent of Administered ^{14}C	
Halogeton	3	15	55
	4	17	38
	4, dark	16	28
Rumex crispus	5	23	26
	7	shoot 5	34
		roots 15	

oxalate accumulating plants possess an enzymatic mechanism for disposing of ascorbate-produced oxalate as CO$_2$ while older tissues accumulate oxalate in a variety of ways in leaves and other organs.

To establish the common origin of oxalate as a C$_2$ fragment from
C1 plus C2 of ascorbate, paired experiments were performed with several
oxalate accumulating plants and a nominal oxalate former (30) using
L-[1-^{14}C]- or L-[U-^{14}C]ascorbic acid as the source of label. Theoretically,
the former will furnish three times as much ^{14}C to oxalic acid as the
latter if C1 plus C2 of ascorbic acid corresponds to the C$_2$ donor. All
seven oxalate accumulating plants tested had two to three times more
^{14}C in oxalate when L-[1-^{14}C]ascorbic acid rather than L-[U-^{14}C]ascorbic
acid was fed (Table VIII). A nominal oxalate former, tomato, produced
very little [^{14}C]oxalate from either source.

Ascorbic Acid Biosynthesis in Plants

Conversion of D-glucose to L-ascorbic acid in higher plants, a process
quite unlike that found in ascorbate-producing animals, involves oxidation of C1, a second oxidation internal to the carbon chain, presumably
at C2, and epimerization of C5. The hydroxymethyl group at C6 is
conserved (31). This process was studied in geranium with D-[1-^{14}C]-
and D-[6-^{14}C]glucose (32). The catabolic products of ascorbic acid
breakdown, oxalate and tartrate, were recovered along with ascorbic acid.
Ascorbic acid from [6-^{14}C]glucose-treated leaves had 86% of its ^{14}C in
C6. Nine times more ^{14}C appeared in oxalate from [1-^{14}C]glucose-treated
leaves. The labeling pattern in tartrate also supported the view that
ascorbic acid was formed by a process involving oxidation of C1 of
glucose.

Recently a study of the D-glucose to L-ascorbic acid conversion in
Virginia Creeper was completed in which C1, C6, H1, or H6 labeled

Table VIII.   **Comparative Production of Oxalic Acid from L-[1-^{14}C]-
and L-[U-^{14}C]Ascorbic Acid (Asa) in Oxalate Accumulating
Plants (Metabolic Period, 24 h)**

Plant	[1-^{14}C]Asa	[U-^{14}C]Asa	Ratio
	Percent of Administered ^{14}C		*[1]/[UL]*
C. album (lamb's quarters)	55	22	2.5
H. glomeratus (halogeton)	31	10	3.1
B. vulgaris (sugar beet)	32	13	2.5
A. retroflexus (pigweed)	18	8	2.2
R. rhabarbarum (rhubarb)	21	7	3.0
R. crispus (curlydock)			
cutting	36	12	3.0
seedling	22	7	3.1
L. esculentum (tomato)	3	2	—

D-glucose was used as tracer. Sucrose, as well as ascorbate and tartrate, was isolated from the labeled leaves to recover a source of D-glucose from the metabolic pool that could be used to measure redistribution of label (14). During the 6-h metabolic period, about 50 times more label was incorporated into tartrate from D-[1-^{14}C]glucose-treated leaves than from D-[6-^{14}C] glucose-treated ones (Table IX). The distribution of ^{14}C in ascorbic acid (Table X) was consistent with a process involving oxidation of C1 of hexose as found in earlier studies (31, 33–36). Ascorbate from D-[6-^{3}H]glucose-treated leaves contained 8.5 times more ^{3}H than that from D-[1-^{3}H]glucose-treated leaves. In both cases, all of the ^{3}H appeared on C6. The presence of ^{3}H on C6 of ascorbic acid after labeling with D-[1-^{3}H]glucose is not surprising since triose phosphate metabolism shifts some ^{3}H from C1 to C6 of hexose and this will eventually appear in C6 of ascorbic acid. No ^{3}H from either source was found in tartrate.

Although these tracer studies provide neither information on the nature of intermediates between D-glucose and L-ascorbic acid, nor the identity of the catalytic steps involved, we do see, once again, this time in a plant of the Vitaceae, the same overall pattern in which oxidation of hexose at C1 determines the carboxyl function of L-ascorbic acid.

Table IX. Metabolism of D-Glucose in Virginia Creeper
(Metabolic Period, 6 h)

| Compound | Position of Label in D-glucose | | | |
| | [1-^{14}C] | [6-^{14}C] | [1-^{3}H] | [6-^{3}H] |
	Percent of Administered Label			
CO$_2$	4	3	—	—
H$_2$O	—	—	36	24
Sugars	63	63	55	69
Ascorbic acid	1.7	2.0	0.2	1.7
Tartaric acid	1.0	0.02	—	—
Other compounds	30	32	9	5

Table X. Labeling Patterns in D-Glucose and L-Ascorbic Acid
after Glucose Metabolism in Virginia Creeper

| | D-[1-^{14}C]Glucose | | D-[6-^{14}C]Glucose | |
| | glucose from sucrose | ascorbic acid | glucose from sucrose | ascorbic acid |
Carbon	Percent of Total ^{14}C in Molecule			
C1	89	80	10	11
C6	10	12	90	83

Efforts must now be directed toward elucidation of intermediates on this pathway and the enzymology involved therein.

Acknowledgments

This work was supported in part by grants from the National Institutes of Health, GM-22427; The National Science Foundation, PCM-78-13254; and the Netherlands Organization for the Advancement of Pure Research (Z.W.O.).

Literature Cited

1. Saito, K.; Kasai, Z. *Phytochemistry* 1969, 8, 2177–2182.
2. Saito, K.; Kasai, Z. *Plant Cell Physiol.* 1968, 9, 529–537.
3. Takimoto, K.; Saito, K.; Kasai, Z. *Phytochemistry* 1976, 15, 927–930.
4. Ibid., 1977, 16, 1641–1645.
5. Loewus, F. A.; Stafford, H. A. *Plant Physiol.* 1958, 33, 155–156.
6. Wagner, G.; Loewus, F. A. *Plant Physiol.* 1974, 54, 784–787.
7. Williams, M.; Loewus, F. A. *Carbohydr. Res.* 1978, 63, 149–155.
8. Bakke, J.; Theander, O. *J. Chem. Soc. D* 1971, 175–176.
9. Williams, M.; Loewus, F. A. *Plant Physiol.* 1978, 61, 672–674.
10. Wagner, G.; Yang, J. C.; Loewus, F. A. *Plant Physiol.* 1975, 55, 1071–1073.

11. Williams, M.; Saito, K.; Loewus, F. A. *Phytochemistry* **1979**, *18*, 953–956.
12. Saito, K.; Loewus, F. A. *Plant Cell Physiol.* **1979**, *20*, 1481–1488.
13. Saito, K.; Kasai, Z. *Plant Physiol.* **1978**, *62*, 215–219.
14. Helsper, J. P. F. G.; Loewus, F. A. *Planta* **1981**, *152*, 171–176.
15. Zelitch, I. *Plant Physiol.* **1972**, *50*, 109–113.
16. Godama, T.; Kotera, U.; Yamada, K. *Agric. Biol. Chem.* **1972**, *36*, 1299–1305.
17. Kotera, U.; Umehara, K.; Kodama, T.; Yamada, K. *Agric. Biol. Chem.* **1972**, *36*, 1307–1313.
18. Kotera, U.; Kodama, T.; Minoda, Y.; Yamada, K. *Agric. Biol. Chem.* **1972**, *36*, 1315–1325.
19. Nakai, T.; Ota, T.; Wanaka, N.; Bepper, D. *J. Chromatogr.* **1974**, *88*, 356–360.
20. Nosticzius, Á. *Acta Agron. Acad. Sci. Hung.* **1976**, *25*, 183–208.
21. Buch, M. L. "A Bibliography of Organic Acids in High Plants", Agric. Handbook No. 164; U.S. Dept. Agric.: Washington, D. C., 1960.
22. Stafford, H. A. *Am. J. Bot.* **1959**, *46*, 347–352.
23. Ibid., **1961**, *48*, 699–701.
24. Wagner, G.; Loewus, F. A. *Plant Physiol.* **1973**, *52*, 651–654.
25. Baig, M. M.; Kelly, S.; Loewus, F. *Plant Physiol.* **1970**, *46*, 277–280.
26. Herbert, R. W.; Hirst, E. L.; Percival, G. V.; Renolds, R. J. W.; Smith, F. *J. Chem. Soc. (London)* **1933**, 1270–1290.
27. Hodgkinson, A. "Oxalic Acid in Biology and Medicine"; Academic: New York, 1977; p. 325.
28. Williams, M. C. *Plant Physiol.* **1960**, *35*, 500–505.
29. Yang, J. C.; Loewus, F. A. *Plant Physiol.* **1975**, *56*, 283–285.
30. Nuss, R. F.; Loewus, F. A. *Plant Physiol.* **1978**, *61*, 590–592.
31. Loewus, F. A. *Phytochemistry* **1963**, *2*, 109–128.
32. Loewus, F. A.; Wagner, G.; Yang, J. C. *Ann. N.Y. Acad. Sci.* **1975**, *258*, 7–23.
33. Loewus, F. A.; Jang, R.; Seegmiller, C. G. *J. Biol. Chem.* **1956**, *222*, 649–664.
34. Loewus, F. A.; Jang, R. *Biochim. Biophys. Acta* **1957**, *23*, 205–206.
35. Loewus, F. A.; Kelly, S. *Nature* **1961**, *191*, 1059–1061.
36. Loewus, F. A. *Fed. Proc. Fed. Am. Soc. Exp. Biol.* **1965**, *24*, 855–862.

RECEIVED for review January 22, 1981. ACCEPTED March 23, 1981.

Ascorbic Acid and the Illuminated Chloroplast

BARRY HALLIWELL

Department of Biochemistry, University of London King's College, Strand, London WC2R 2LS, England

The chloroplasts in the leaves of higher plants produce several damaging oxygen-derived species in the light, namely, hydrogen peroxide, singlet oxygen, lipid peroxides, superoxide, and the hydroxyl radical. The high concentration of ascorbic acid often present in the chloroplast helps to protect them against these species.

Toxic Effects of Oxygen on Illuminated Chloroplasts

Oxygen is, by definition, essential for the life of all aerobic organisms, including higher plants, but oxygen has long been known to be toxic to aerobic organisms at concentrations greater than those in normal air. High oxygen concentrations inhibit chloroplast development, decrease seed viability and root growth, damage the membranes of leaves and roots, stimulate leaf abscission, and increase the incidence of growth abnormalities (*1–3*). Exposure to oxygen at a pressure of 6 atm is lethal to a wide variety of plants (*4*).

Oxygen toxicity is seen not only in whole plants but also in cell cultures and even in isolated organelles. For example, high oxygen concentrations inhibit carbon dioxide fixation by isolated, intact chloroplast fractions (the so-called "Warburg effect"). Chloroplasts are especially prone to oxygen-toxicity effects because their internal oxygen concentration during photosynthesis is probably somewhat greater than that in the air surrounding the leaf (*5*). The effects of elevated oxygen concentrations on chloroplasts are attributable to a number of factors (*6*), two of which are considered in the next sections.

Generation of Superoxide Radicals and Hydrogen Peroxide in Chloroplasts. Isolated, illuminated chloroplast thylakoids slowly take up oxygen in the absence of added electron acceptors. This phenomenon was first observed by Mehler (*7*) and is often known as the "Mehler reaction." The reaction appears to result from the reduction of O_2 to the

0065-2393/82/0200–0263$06.00/0

superoxide free radical, $O_2^{\cdot-}$, by electron acceptors associated with photosystem I (8–12). Addition of ferredoxin increases the amount of oxygen uptake because ferredoxin is reduced by photosystem I much quicker than is oxygen and reduced ferredoxin rapidly reacts with oxygen (13).

$$\text{ferredoxin}_{red} + O_2 \rightarrow \text{ferredoxin}_{ox} + O_2^{\cdot-} \qquad (1)$$

Allen (14) suggested that reduced ferredoxin can also convert O_2^- into hydrogen peroxide (Equation 2) but this reaction has not yet been rigorously proved to occur.

$$\text{ferredoxin}_{red} + O_2^{\cdot-} + 2H^+ \rightarrow H_2O_2 + \text{ferredoxin}_{ox} \qquad (2)$$

In vivo, most electrons from reduced ferredoxin are passed onto nicotinamide adenine dinucleotide phosphate cation ($NADP^+$), via ferredoxin–$NADP^+$ reductase, to generate the NADPH needed to drive carbon dioxide fixation by the Calvin cycle. Thus electrons from photosystem I can pass through at least three routes (Figure 1), of which route C is preferred (11). However, if the supply of $NADP^+$ were limited, for example, because of a poor supply of carbon dioxide causing a slow turnover of the Calvin cycle, the electron flow rate along pathway C would be expected to be decreased and more O_2^- should be made by route B and, to a lesser extent, by route A (15–17). Some oxygen reduction takes place even when carbon dioxide is present in ample amounts (18).

The superoxide free radical in aqueous solution can act either as a reducing agent, giving up its extra electron, or as a weak oxidizing agent, becoming reduced to hydrogen peroxide. For example, O_2^- reduces cytochrome f and plastocyanin, which are components of the chloroplast electron transport chain, and oxidizes α-tocopherol and thiol compounds such as glutathione, although the rates of these latter reactions are slow (19–21). The protonated form of O_2^-, $HO_2\cdot$, is a much more powerful oxidant than is $O_2^{\cdot-}$ (22), but because the pK_a of the dissociation reaction

$$HO_2\cdot \rightleftarrows H^+ + O_2^- \qquad (3)$$

is 4.88 and the stromal pH of the illuminated chloroplast is greater than 7.0 (6) there is little $HO_2\cdot$ present in vivo.

Superoxide ions in aqueous solution can undergo a reaction known as "dismutation." The overall process may be represented by the equation

$$O_2^{\cdot-} + O_2^{\cdot-} + 2H^+ \rightarrow H_2O_2 + O_2 \qquad (4)$$

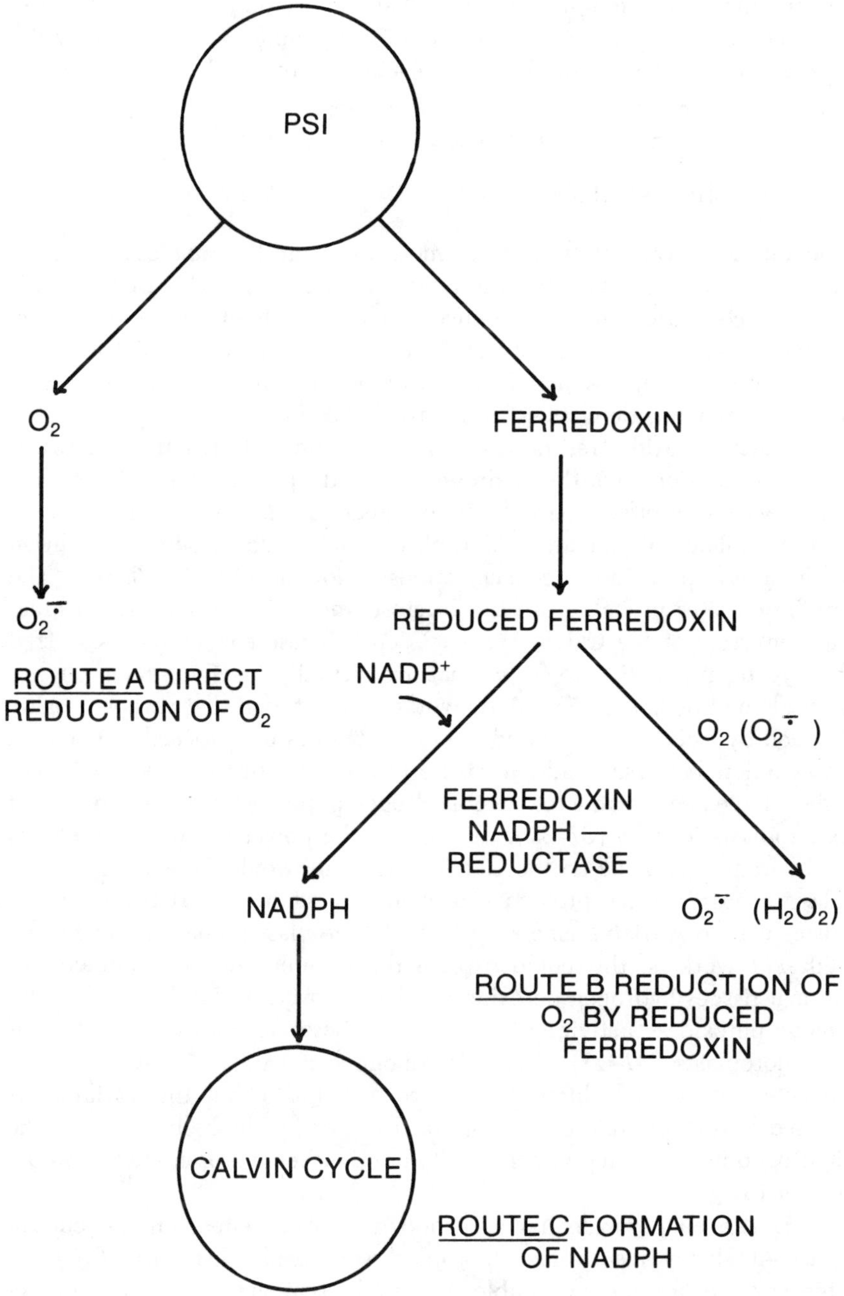

Figure 1.   Possible pathways of electron flow from reduced photosystem I.

but the direct reaction of two $O_2^{\cdot}$ radicals is very slow, probably because of electrostatic repulsion ($k < 0.2\ M^{-1}s^{-1}$). Dismutation can occur by the formation of $HO_2\cdot$ followed by the reactions shown below (22, 23):

$$HO_2\cdot + O_2^{\cdot} + H^+ \rightarrow H_2O_2 + O_2 \qquad k = 8.10^7\ M^{-1}s^{-1} \qquad (5)$$

$$HO_2\cdot + HO_2\cdot \rightarrow H_2O_2 + O_2 \qquad k = 8.10^5\ M^{-1}s^{-1} \qquad (6)$$

Spontaneous dismutation is thus most rapid at the acidic pH values needed to protonate $O_2^{\cdot}$, but the rate at neutral or alkaline pH values is greatly accelerated by the presence in chloroplasts of a superoxide dismutase enzyme, which catalyzes Reaction 4. Superoxide dismutase in the form of a copper–zinc enzyme is found both free in the stroma and bound to the outside of the chloroplast thylakoids (24–29).

The superoxide free radical is not a particularly reactive radical in aqueous solution, but the hydrogen peroxide produced by Reaction 4 has devastating effects on chloroplast metabolism. Carbon dioxide fixation by isolated, illuminated chloroplasts is inhibited by 50% on addition of hydrogen peroxide in concentrations as low as $10^{-5}\ M$ (30, 31). The inhibition sites probably are the fructose and sedoheptulose diphosphatase enzymes of the Calvin cycle (32, 33). These enzymes are oxidized by hydrogen peroxide to forms that are virtually inactive under physiological conditions (34, 35). Many workers have found that carbon dioxide fixation by isolated illuminated chloroplasts does not proceed at maximal rates unless catalase is added to the reaction mixture (18, 36), whereas others have been unable to detect hydrogen peroxide production by intact chloroplasts in vitro (37–39). In view of the powerful inhibitory effects of hydrogen peroxide on the Calvin cycle, one would expect the chloroplast to possess some protective mechanisms against it. If these mechanisms were of variable efficiency in the chloroplast preparations used by different workers, this could explain the different results obtained. In animal tissues hydrogen peroxide can be removed by catalase and glutathione peroxidase activities (23, 40), but these enzymes are not present in chloroplasts (41–43). Variable amounts of catalase activity can be detected in isolated chloroplast fractions (41, 44), but this variation is caused by cytoplasmic contamination (41) or by the feeble, nonspecific hydrogen-peroxide-degrading activity of other heme proteins in the preparation (45).

Hydrogen peroxide has a second deleterious effect on the chloroplast—it slowly inactivates chloroplast superoxide dismutase (46). If this enzyme becomes incapable of rapidly removing $O_2^{\cdot}$, then the remaining O_2^- can react with hydrogen peroxide to form the hydroxyl radical, $\cdot OH$ (23, 40). Hydroxyl radicals are the most reactive species known to chemistry: they will attack and damage almost every molecule found in living cells $(23, 40, 47)$. In particular, they can trigger the peroxidation and destruction of chloroplast membrane lipids (Figure 2). Pure hydrogen peroxide and $O_2^{\cdot-}$ will not react together at significant rates in vitro unless traces of iron salts are added, when the following reactions apparently occur, producing $\cdot OH$:

$$Fe^{3+} + O_2^{\cdot-} \rightarrow Fe^{2+} + O_2 \qquad (O_2^- \text{ acting as a reductant}) \qquad (7)$$

$$Fe^{2+} + H_2O_2 \rightarrow \cdot OH + Fe^{3+} + OH^- \qquad (\text{Fenton reaction}) \qquad (8)$$

Net $\qquad H_2O_2 + O_2^{\cdot-} \xrightarrow[\text{catalyst}]{\text{Fe salt}} O_2 + \cdot OH + OH^- \qquad (9)$

The overall reaction is sometimes called the iron-catalyzed Haber–Weiss reaction $(23, 40, 48)$. Of course, iron salts are abundant in extracts of plant tissues (49), so these reactions can readily occur in vivo. The iron component of reduced ferredoxin may be able to bring about Reaction 8 as well (50).

It is therefore imperative that the chloroplast has some mechanism for disposing of excess hydrogen peroxide.

Singlet Oxygen Formation, Lipid Peroxidation, and Chlorophyll Photobleaching. Absorption of light energy by chlorophyll molecules results in the formation of higher electronic excitation states. The energy of these excited states is mainly used to drive the movement of electrons in the chloroplast electron transport chain (for detailed reviews *see* Refs. $6, 51$–53). Any excited states not so dissipated can lose energy by fluorescence or, alternatively, they can pass energy onto adjacent O_2 molecules to form singlet O_2 $^1\Delta g$. This highly reactive form of oxygen can attack the chlorophyll molecule, causing loss of the characteristic green color (bleaching). Singlet oxygen will also react with polyunsaturated fatty acids to produce lipid peroxides, which can degrade to give aldehydes and other reactive products (Figure 2) $(54$–$56)$. The fatty acids in chloropast lipids are highly unsaturated (51) and therefore are very prone to such attack: formation of lipid peroxides causes increased leakiness of the membranes and an eventual loss of membrane integrity. Production of singlet oxygen by the illuminated chloroplast might be expected whenever there is excess excitation of the chlorophyll molecules, that is, when operation of the electron transport chain is restricted as, for example, when carbon dioxide is present in limiting amounts. Addition of inhibitors of electron transport, such as the herbicides chlorophenyldimethylurea or dichlorophenyldimethylurea to illuminated chloroplasts or cotyledons causes rapid chlorophyll bleaching and lipid peroxidation $(54, 55, 57, 58)$.

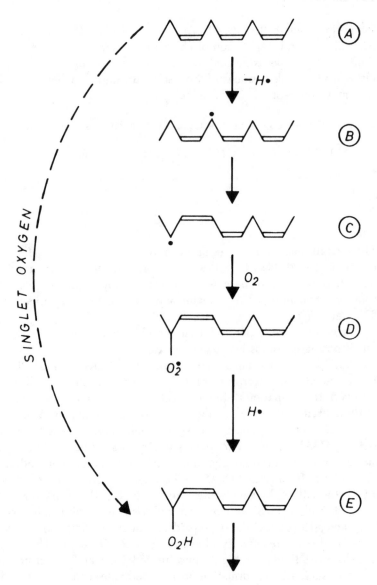

FRAGMENTATION PRODUCTS INCLUDING
ALDEHYDES
(ESPECIALLY MALONDIALDEHYDE)

Figure 2.   Mechanism of peroxidation of polyunsaturated fatty acids.

A, Hydrogen abstraction by a previously formed peroxide radical or by a
species such as OH· generated from O_2^-; B, rearrangement; C, conjugated diene
that can be detected by absorbance at 233 nm; D, peroxide radical that abstracts H· from another chain causing chain reaction; E, hydroperoxide.

There is a little evidence to suggest that part of the oxygen formed during reactions undergone by $O_2 \cdot^-$ radicals is singlet O_2 $^1\Delta g$. It is not clear whether singlet oxygen arises during Reaction 4 or 7. Experimental results are confusing, largely because of the lack of specificity of many of the compounds used as scavengers of singlet oxygen (*40*). Illuminated chlorophyll was also reported to directly generate hydroxyl radicals as well as singlet oxygen (*59*).

Therefore, illuminated chloroplasts must be protected against hydrogen peroxide and singlet oxygen. Ascorbic acid plays a key role in such protection, as summarized in the next section.

Ascorbic Acid in the Illuminated Chloroplast: A Key Protective Mechanism

Ascorbic acid is present in the chloroplast stroma at concentrations up to 50×10^{-3} M, although the concentration varies widely depending on the age and physiological state of the leaf (*60, 61*). The reasons for the high concentration of ascorbate in vivo have been unclear until recently; the concentration has usually been attributed to the need for "correct redox poiseing" of intermediates of the electron transport chain. Ascorbic acid is a cofactor for violaxanthin de-epoxidase (*62*), an enzyme involved in xanthophyll metabolism in chloroplasts, but the physiological function of this enzyme is unknown (*51, 63*). However, the principal role of ascorbic acid may be that of protecting the chloroplast against toxic oxygen-derived species.

Ascorbic Acid as a Scavenger of Superoxide, Hydroxyl Radical and Singlet Oxygen. The superoxide free radical reacts with ascorbic acid according to the equation:

$$2O_2 \cdot^- + 2H^+ + \text{ascorbate} \rightarrow \text{dehydroascorbate} + 2H_2O_2 \quad (10)$$

with a rate constant of 2.7×10^5 $M^{-1}s^{-1}$ at pH 7.4 (*64*). Although this rate constant is much smaller than that for the enzyme-catalyzed dismutation of $O_2 \cdot^-$ (2×10^9 $M^{-1}s^{-1}$), ascorbic acid is usually present in the chloroplast at much higher molar concentrations than is the superoxide dismutase enzyme. Therefore, ascorbic acid intercepts much of the $O_2 \cdot^-$ generated in vivo. Ascorbate's ability to react with $O_2 \cdot^-$ generated by illuminated chloroplasts in vitro was demonstrated (*26, 65*).

Ascorbic acid quenches singlet oxygen rapidly (*66*) and also reacts with hydroxyl radicals (*67*) at a fast rate ($k = 7 \times 10^9$ $M^{-1}s^{-1}$). Ascorbic acid can therefore protect against these species in vivo. However, the principal scavengers of singlet oxygen in illuminated chloroplasts are the carotenoids (*51, 68*) and α-tocopherol, which is present in large amounts. α-Tocopherol also helps protect against lipid peroxidation (Figure 2), reacting with lipid peroxide radicals to form relatively unreactive tocopheryl radicals (Equation 11) thus interrupting the chain reaction of lipid peroxidation (*48, 51*).

$$\text{lipid--}O_2^\intercal + \alpha\text{TH} \rightarrow \text{lipid--OOH} + \alpha\text{-T} \cdot \qquad (11)$$

The lipophilic nature of α-tocopherol enables it to react rapidly with singlet oxygen and lipid peroxide radicals generated within the thylakoid membranes. α-Tocopherol's radical form, αT· in Equation 11, can be reduced to α-tocopherol by ascorbic acid (*69*). Another function of ascorbic acid in vivo could therefore be that of interacting with tocopheryl radicals at the surface of the thylakoid membrane, regenerating α-tocopherol for further use in preventing lipid peroxidation.

Ascorbic Acid for Removing Hydrogen Peroxide in Chloroplasts. In 1976, it was suggested (*70*) that hydrogen peroxide could be removed in illuminated chloroplasts in vivo by a nonenzymic reaction with ascorbic acid:

$$\text{ascorbate} + H_2O_2 \rightarrow 2H_2O + \text{dehydroascorbate} \qquad (12)$$

This nonenzymatic reaction occurs at a significant rate in crude chloroplast or plant cell extracts (*71, 72*). At pH 8, the pH of the stroma in the illuminated chloroplast, dehydroascorbate is reduced to ascorbate by glutathione (GSH), which is present in the stroma of spinach chloroplasts at millimolar concentrations (*70*). Although nonenzymatic, the reaction is extremely swift at this pH (*73*).

$$\text{dehydroascorbate} + 2\text{GSH} \rightarrow \text{ascorbate} + \text{GSSG} \qquad (13)$$

Spinach leaves contain a dehydroascorbate reductase enzyme that catalyzes Reaction 13 at acidic and neutral pH values, but the enzyme is not, located within the chloroplast (*73–76*). GSSG produced by Reaction 13 can be re-converted to GSH by glutathione reductase, an enzyme located in the chloroplast (*77*).

$$\text{GSSG} + \text{NADPH} + H^+ \rightarrow 2\text{GSH} + \text{NADP}^+ \qquad (14)$$

Hence a cycle of reactions was postulated (*70*) (Figure 3), in which hydrogen peroxide and/or $O_2^\intercal$ are disposed of via ascorbate and glutathione at the eventual expense of oxidizing NADPH from the electron transport chain.

This postulated reaction cycle was greatly strengthened by the discovery of high activities of an ascorbate peroxidase enzyme in spinach chloroplasts (*71*), which catalyzes Reaction 12. Earlier attempts (*78, 79*)

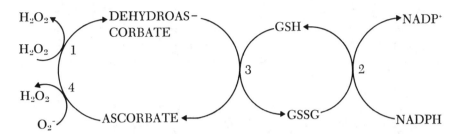

Figure 3. An ascorbate–glutathione cycle for removal of H_2O_2 in illuminated chloroplasts.

Enzymes involved: 1, ascorbate peroxidase; and 2, glutathione reductase. Reactions 3 and 4 are nonenzymatic. Reaction 3 proceeds rapidly at pH 8, the pH of the stroma in illuminated chloroplasts.

to detect this enzyme failed, presumably because its activity is low in chloroplasts at certain times of the year (71). Such variations in the ascorbate peroxidase activity, the ascorbate content, and possibly the glutathione content (80) of chloroplasts with leaf age, time of year, and probably other factors as well could account for some of the reported discrepancies in the experimental results of hydrogen peroxide generation by illuminated chloroplasts (see the section entitled, "Generation of Superoxide Radicals and Hydrogen Peroxide in Chloroplasts."). In chloroplasts with low ascorbate peroxidase, ascorbate, and/or glutathione contents, the reaction cycle shown in Figure 3 would be impaired. Hydrogen peroxide could accumulate during photosynthesis and catalase would have to be added to the reaction mixture to achieve maximum rates of carbon dioxide fixation. If the cycle works well, hydrogen peroxide is rapidly removed and catalase addition is not necessary. Indeed, addition of ascorbate can replace catalase in stimulating carbon dioxide fixation by certain chloroplast preparations (18, 81). Leaf tissues contain a soluble ascorbate peroxidase enzyme in addition to the chloroplast enzyme (82). The green alga *Euglena*, which contains no catalase activity, has all the enzymes needed to operate the ascorbate/glutathione cycle (83, 84). *Euglena* ascorbate peroxidase is capable of reducing artificial organic hydroperoxides as well as hydrogen peroxide. Therefore, that enzyme might be able to metabolize lipid peroxides in vivo, a point that requires further investigation.

Note Added in Proof

After this paper was submitted, further evidence for the operation of an ascorbate–glutathione cycle in spinach (85) and pea (86) chloroplasts was reported. The original failure to detect this cycle in pea chloroplasts (79) has been retracted (86) although in this plant there may be some dehydroascorbate reductase activity present within the chloroplast, in contrast to spinach. Exposure of cotton leaves to elevated oxygen concentrations increases their glutathione reductase activity (87).

Literature Cited

1. Poskuta, J.; Mikulska, M.; Faltynowicz, M.; Bielak, B.; Wroblewska, B. Z. Pflanzenphysiol. **1974**, 7, 387–393.
2. Marynick, M.; Addicott, F. T. Nature (London) **1976**, 264, 668–669.
3. Anderson, R. A.; Linney, T. L. Chem. Biol. Interact. **1977**, 19, 317–325.
4. Simon, E. W. New Phytol, **1974**, 73, 377–420.
5. Steiger, H. M.; Beck, E.; Beck R. Plant Physiol. **1977**, 60, 903–906.
6. Halliwell, B. Prog. Biophys. Mol. Biol. **1978**, 33, 1–54.
7. Mehler, A. H. Arch. Biochem. Biophys. **1951**, 33, 65–77.
8. Asada, K.; Kiso, K.; Yoshikawa, K. J. Biol. Chem. **1974**, 249, 2175–2181.
9. Harbour, J. R.; Bolton, J. R. Biochem. Biophys. Res. Commun. **1975**, 64, 803–807.
10. Miller, R. W.; Macdowall, F. D. H. Biochim. Biophys. Acta **1975**, 387, 176–187.
11. Lien, S.; San Pietro, A. FEBS Lett. **1979**, 99, 189–193.
12. Jursinic, P. A. FEBS Lett. **1978**, 90, 15–20.
13. Misra, H. P.; Fridovich, I. J. Biol. Chem. **1971**, 246, 6886–6890.
14. Allen, J. F. Biochem. Biophys. Res. Commun. **1975**, 66, 36–43.
15. Jennings, R. C.; Forti, G. Proc. Int. Congr. Photosynth., 3rd **1975**, 735–743.
16. Radmer, R. J.; Kok, B. Plant Physiol. **1976**, 58, 336–340.
17. Marsho, T. V.; Behrens, P. W.; Radmer, R. J. Plant Physiol. **1979**, 64, 656–659.
18. Egneus, H.; Heber, U.; Matthiesen, U.; Kirk, M. Biochim. Biophys. Acta **1975**, 408, 252–268.
19. Fridovich, I. Science **1978**, 201, 875–880.
20. Marchant, R. H. Proc. Int. Congr. Photosynth., 3rd **1975**, 637–643.
21. Nishikimi, M.; Yamada, H.; Yagi, K. Biochim. Biophys. Acta **1980**, 627, 101–108.
22. Sawyer, D. T.; Gibian, M. T. Tetrahedron **1979**, 35, 1471–1481.
23. Fridovich, I. Adv. Enzymol. Relat. Subj. Biochem. **1974**, 41, 35–97.
24. Jackson, C.; Dench, J.; Moore, A. L.; Halliwell, B.; Foyer, C. H.; Hall, D. O. Eur. J. Biochem. **1978**, 91, 339–344.
25. Asada, K.; Urano, M.; Takahashi, M. Eur. J. Biochem. **1973**, 36, 257–266.
26. Allen, J. F.; Hall, D. O. Biochem. Biophys. Res. Commun. **1973**, 52, 856–862.
27. Halliwell, B. Eur. J. Biochem. **1975**, 55, 355–360.
28. Elstner, E. F.; Heupel, A. Planta **1975**, 123, 145–154.
29. Doll, S.; Lutz, C.; Ruppel, H. Z. Pflanzenphysiol. **1976**, 80, 166–176.
30. Kaiser, W. Biochim. Biophys. Acta **1976**, 440, 476–482.
31. Robinson, J. M.; Smith, M. G.; Gibbs, M. Plant Physiol. **1980**, 65, 755–759.
32. Heldt, H. W.; Chon, C. J.; Lilley, R. Mc. C.; Portis, A. In "Photosynthesis '77"; Hall, D. O.; Coombs, J.; Goodwin, T. W., Eds.; Biochemical Soc.: London, 1978; pp. 469–478.
33. Kaiser, W. Planta **1979**, 145, 377–382.
34. Charles, S. A.; Halliwell, B. Biochem. J. **1980**, 189, 373–376.
35. Ibid., 185, 689–693.

36. Hind, G.; Mills, J. D.; Slovacek, R. E. In "Photosynthesis '77"; Hall, D. O.; Coombs, J.; Goodwin, T. W., Eds.; Biochemical Soc.: London, 1978; pp. 591–600.
37. Allen, J. F. *Plant Sci. Lett.* **1978**, *12*, 161–167.
38. Ibid., 151–159.
39. Allen, J. F.; Whatley, F. R. *Plant Physiol.* **1978**, *61*, 957–960.
40. Halliwell, B. In "Age Pigments"; Sohal, R. S., Ed.; Elsevier: Amsterdam, 1981; pp. 1–67.
41. Allen, J. F. *FEBS Lett.* **1977**, *84*, 221–224.
42. Flohe, L.; Menzel, H. *Plant Cell Physiol.* **1971**, *12*, 325–333.
43. Smith, J.; Shrift, A. *Comp. Biochem. Physiol. B* **1979**, *63*, 39–44.
44. Van Ginkel, G.; Brown, J. S. *FEBS Lett.* **1978**, *94*, 284–286.
45. Brown, R. H.; Collins, N.; Merrett, M. J. *Plant Physiol.* **1975**, *55*, 1123–1124.
46. Asada, K.; Yoshikawa, K.; Takahashi, M.; Maeda, Y.; Enmanji, K. *J. Biol. Chem.* **1975**, *250*, 2801–2807.
47. Walling, C. *Proc. Int. Symp. Oxidases Relat. Redox Systems*, in press.
48. Halliwell, B. In "Strategies of Microbial Life in Extreme Environments"; Shilo, M., Ed.; Verlag Chem.: Weinheim and New York, 1979; pp. 195–221.
49. Brown, R. C. *Plant Cell Envir.* **1978**, *1*, 249–257.
50. Elstner, E. F.; Saran, M.; Bors, W.; Lengfelder, E. *Eur. J. Biochem.* **1978**, *89*, 61–66.
51. Halliwell, B. "Chloroplast Metabolism: the Structure and Function of Chloroplasts in Green Leaf Cells"; Oxford Univ. Press: England, 1981.
52. Gregory, R. P. F. "Biochemistry of Photosynthesis," 2nd ed.; John Wiley & Sons: London, 1977.
53. Barber, J. *Rep. Prog. Phys.* **1978**, *41*, 1157–1199.
54. Rawls, R. R.; Van Santen, P. J. *Ann. N.Y. Acad. Sci.* **1970**, *171*, 135–137.
55. Heath, R. L.; Packer, L. *Arch. Biochem. Biophys.* **1968**, *125*, 850–857.
56. Ibid., 189–198.
57. Elstner, E. F.; Osswald, W. *Z, Naturforsch. Teil C* **1980**, *35*, 129–135.
58. Pallet, K. E.; Dodge, A. D. *Z. Naturforsch. Teil C* **1979**, *34*, 1058–1061.
59. Harbour, J. R.; Bolton, J. R. *Photochem. Photobiol.* **1978**, *28*, 231–234.
60. Gerhardt, B. *Planta* **1964**, *61*, 101–129.
61. Walker, D. A. *Methods Enzymol.* **1971**, 23A, 211–220.
62. Yamamoto, H. Y.; Higashi, R. M. *Arch. Biochem. Biophys.* **1978**, 514–522.
63. Ridley, S. M. *Plant Physiol.* **1977**, 59, 724–732.
64. Nishikimi, M. *Biochem. Biophys. Res. Commun.* **1975**, *63*, 463–468.
65. Allen, J. F.; Hall, D. O. *Biochem. Biophys. Res. Commun.* **1974**, *58*, 579–585.
66. Bodannes, R. S.; Chan, P. C. *FEBS Lett.* **1979**, *105*, 195–196.
67. Anbar, M.; Neta, P. *Int. J. Appl. Radiat. Isot.* **1967**, *18*, 495–523.
68. Foote, C. S. *Ann. N.Y. Acad. Sci.* **1970**, *171*, 139–148.
69. Packer, J. E.; Slater, T. F.; Willson, R. L. *Nature (London)* **1979**, *278*, 737–738.
70. Foyer, C. H. Halliwell, B. *Planta* **1976**, *133*, 21–25.
71. Groden, D.; Beck, E. *Biochim. Biophys. Acta* **1979**, *546*, 426–435.
72. Dilek Tozum, S. R.; Gallon, J. *J. Gen. Microbiol.* **1979**, *111*, 313–326.
73. Foyer, C. H.; Halliwell, B. *Phytochemistry* **1977**, *61*, 1347–1350.
74. Mapson, L. W.; Moustafa, E. M. *Biochem. J.* **1976**, *62*, 248–259.
75. Yamaguchi, M.; Joslyn, M. A. *Arch. Biochem. Biophys.* **1952**, *38*, 451–465.
76. Gero, E.; Candido, A. *Bull. Soc. Chim. Biol.* **1967**, *49*, 1895–1897.
77. Halliwell, B.; Foyer, C. H. *Planta* **1978**, *139*, 9–17.
78. Halliwell, B., unpublished data.

79. Jablonski, P. P.; Anderson, J. W. *Plant Physiol.* **1978**, *61*, 221–225.
80. Esterbauer, H.; Grill, D. *Plant Physiol.* **1978**, *61*, 119–121.
81. Ziegler, I.; Libera, W. *Z. Naturforsch. Teil C* **1975**, *30*, 634–637.
82. Kelly, G. J.; Latzko, E. *Naturwissenschaften* **1979**, *66*, 517–518.
83. Shigeoka, S.; Nakano, Y.; Kitaoka, S. *Biochem. J.* **1980**, *186*, 377–380.
84. Shigeoka, S.; Nakano, Y.; Kataoka, S. *Arch. Biochem. Biophys.* **1980**, **1980**, *201*, 121–127.
85. Nakano, Y.; Asada, K. *Plant Cell Physiol.* **1981**, *22*, 867–880.
86. Jablonski, P. P.; Anderson, J. W. *Plant Physiol.* **1981**, *67*, 1239–1244.
87. Foster, J. G.; Hess, J. L. *Plant Physiol.* **1980**, *66*, 482–487.

RECEIVED for review January 22, 1981. ACCEPTED March 31, 1981.

13

Ascorbic Acid and the Growth and Development of Insects

KARL J. KRAMER

U.S. Grain Marketing Research Laboratory, Agricultural Research, Science and Education Administration, U.S. Department of Agriculture, Manhattan, KS 66502 and Department of Biochemistry, Kansas State University, Manhattan, KS 66506

PAUL A. SEIB

Department of Grain Science, Kansas State University, Manhattan, KS 66506

The structural requirements for vitamin C activity in insects were comparable to those observed in guinea pigs. A dietary level of 0.5 mM L-ascorbic acid was necessary for normal development of the tobacco hornworm (Manduca sexta); magnesium 2-O-phosphono-L-ascorbate, sodium 6-O-myristoyl-L-ascorbate, and L-dehydroascorbic acid were equally potent. D-Ascorbic acid, 6-bromo-6-deoxy-L-ascorbic acid, and D-isoascorbic acid were approximately one-half, one-fifth, and one-tenth as effective, respectively. Tissues from M. sexta lacked L-gulono-γ-lactone oxidase, the biosynthetic enzyme usually absent from ascorbate-dependent species. Vitamin C was found in eggs, larval labial gland, hemolymph, gut, muscle, cuticle, adult nervous tissue, and gonads at concentrations ranging from < 10–170 mg/100 g of wet tissue. No ascorbate was detected in larval fat body, Malpighian tubules, or adult salivary gland. Insects reared on an L-ascorbate-deficient diet contained no detectable L-ascorbic acid. Some possible physiological actions of the vitamin in insects are discussed.

Considerable data are available on the insect's requirement for L-ascorbic acid. Dietary vitamin C is needed for normal growth, molting, and fertility of many insects, and vitamin C, or another compound with similar biological properties, is probably an essential growth

0065-2393/82/0200–0275$06.00/0
© 1982 American Chemical Society

factor for this class of animals. Although most insects subsisting on green plants need L-ascorbate to develop fully (1–6), it was proposed that some species may dispense with the vitamin or may synthesize it either de novo or rely on symbiotic organisms (7–10). However, the ability of certain insects (or their symbionts) to synthesize ascorbic acid has not been adequately demonstrated. This chapter reviews some of the previous work on the role of ascorbic acid in insects and includes results of efforts to develop a bioassay for vitamin C using an insect, measure the growth-promoting activity of compounds structurally related to L-ascorbic acid, determine diet and tissue levels of L-ascorbate in insects, and ascertain whether specific tissues in insects are capable of converting a putative precursor, L-gulono-γ-lactone, into vitamin C.

Experimental

Animals. *Manduca sexta* larvae were reared on an agar-based diet (11) at 28°C and 60% relative humidity with a 16-h photophase. The Indian meal moth, *Plodia interpunctella* Hubner, and American cockroach, *Periplaneta americana* L., were taken from laboratory cultures. Dissection was performed under anesthesia by cooling to 5°C (12).

Biological Assay. Prior to bioassay, the hot diet was cooled to 60°C, L-ascorbic acid or a related compound was added, and the mixture was thoroughly blended. Labile derivatives were applied to the surface of the gelled diet at room temperature. Neonate larvae were used in all tests and the growth of larvae on the control diet was compared with that of larvae on test diets. At 1–4-d intervals, up to 40 d, the mean weight of ten to twenty animals was determined. Fecal matter was removed at each observation. Test compounds were obtained or prepared as described previously (5).

Paper Chromatography. One-tenth of a gram of tissue was homogenized in 0.25 mL of 2% (w/v) metaphosphoric acid at 4°C. Descending paper chromatography was done on Whatman #1 paper using ethyl acetate:acetic acid: water (6:3:2) as developing solvent. Ascorbic acid was detected by dipping the chromatogram sequentially in 0.10 mL of saturated silver nitrate mixed with 20 mL of acetone containing 0.1 mL of concentrated ammonium hydroxide, 1 M NaOH in 95% ethanol, 0.2 M aqueous sodium thiosulfate, and water (13). The detection limit was 2 µg after chromatography.

High Performance Liquid Chromatography. Tissue extracts were analyzed with a Varian model 5020 liquid chromatograph equipped with a Rheodyne model 7120 loop injector valve, a Tracor 970 variable wavelength detector set at 257 nm, an automated Hewlett-Packard 3385A printer–plotter system for determining retention times and peak areas, and a Waters µ Bondapak column (3.9 mm i.d. × 300 mm) for carbohydrate analysis. The buffer was eluted isocratically at 1 mL/min with a 1:4 (v/v) mixture of 0.01 M monobasic sodium phosphate (pH 4.46) and methanol. The minimum amount detectable was 10 ng.

L-Gulonolactone Oxidase Assay. Tissues were assayed for L-gulonolactone oxidase by the method of Azaz et al. (14). Weighed portions of tissue (50–200 mg) were homogenized in 2 mL of 50 mM sodium phosphate (pH 7.4) containing 0.2% sodium deoxycholate. Homogenates were centrifuged at

5000 g for 10 min at 4°C, and 1-mL aliquots of the supernatant were incubated with 2 mM L-gulono-γ-lactone (Sigma Chemical Company) for 60 min at 35°C. Ascorbate was measured by the 2,4-dinitrophenylhydrazine method of Roe and Kuether (*15*) as modified by Geshwind et al. (*16*). Chicken kidney was assayed as a control tissue rich in L-gulonolactone oxidase.

Results

Bioassay.   The effect of L-ascorbic acid on the development rate of *M. sexta* is shown in Figure 1 (*5*). All neonate larvae developed into adults on the artificial diet that contained 0.5 mM L-ascorbic acid. Also, larvae raised on that diet exhibited a normal growth curve, and were robust and bright blue-green in color. Normal development occurred in 35 d with larval–pupal ecdysis occurring at day 15 and pupal–adult ecdysis at day 35. Higher levels of L-ascorbic acid were not more effective, but lower ones were inadequate for the hornworm. As the amount of L-ascorbic acid was decreased in the diet, pathological effects appeared after a feeding period that depended on the vitamin concentration. Animals reared on an ascorbate-deficient diet were reduced in size and colored a dull yellowish-green. Abnormalities in cuticle soon became apparent. Extremities such as mouth parts and tarsi exhibited premature darkening of cuticle. Navon (*6*) observed similar effects in the cotton leafworm, *Spodoptera littoralis*. In all tests, larvae appeared normal to the second instar, probably because of an amount of L-ascorbic acid derived from parent insects. In larvae on diets lacking in L-ascorbic acid, pathological consequences occurred at the third instar. At the beginning of the third molting period, the insects began to shrivel and 1 d later became moribund. Larvae fed medium containing 0.05 mM L-ascorbic acid were similarly affected, but at one stadium later. Fifty percent of the larvae fed diet supplemented with 0.25 mM vitamin C died in the prepupal stage; the other half underwent pupal and adult eclosion 3–6 d later than the control group.

We have used the growth effects and pathologies associated with L-ascorbic acid deficiency as a basis for the determination of the biological potency of related compounds (Table I). At a dietary concentration of 0.5 mM, L-ascorbic acid and dehydroascorbic acid were fully active, as well as some ester derivatives including the 6-myristate and 2-phosphate compounds. The insect may be metabolically like the guinea pig because both were able to utilize those esters (*17*). Carboxylesterases and phosphatases probably converted those derivatives to the free vitamin (*18*). The 6-bromo compound was less active and apparently cannot be metabolized to L-ascorbic acid or only poorly so.

One of the least active compounds in the insect bioassay was the 2-sulfate ester of L-ascorbic acid. To develop normally the hornworm

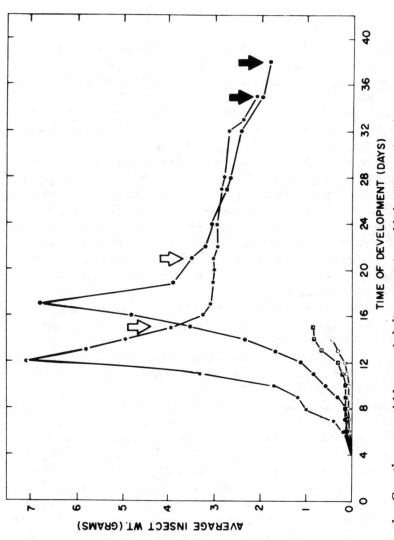

Figure 1. Growth curves of M. sexta fed diet containing added 0.50 mM (−−), 0.25 mM (−●−), 0.05 mM (−■−), or 0.00 mM (−○−) vitamin C. Open arrow and closed arrow denote the time of pupal and adult ecdysis, respectively (5).*

Table I. Effect of L-Ascorbic Acid and Related Compounds on Growth of *M. sexta* and *Cavia cobaya*

Compound	Relative Activity[a]	
	Hornworm	Guinea Pig
L-*threo*-Hex-2-enonic acid γ-lactone (L-ascorbic acid)	100	100
Sodium 6-O-myristoyl-L-ascorbate	100	100
Magnesium 2-O-phosphono-L-ascorbate	100	100
D-*threo*-Hex-2-enonic acid γ-lactone (D-ascorbic acid)	40 ± 10	0
6-Bromo-6-deoxy-L-ascorbic acid	20 ± 10	not available
D-*erythro*-Hex-2-enonic acid γ-lactone (D-isoascorbic acid)	10 ± 10	5
Potassium 2-O-sulfo-L-ascorbate	5	0
L-*erythro*-Hex-2-enonic acid γ-lactone (L-isoascorbic acid)	0	0
L-*threo*-Hex-2,3-diulosic acid γ-lactone (L-dehydroascorbic acid)	100	100

[a] Insect growth activity is expressed as the amount of compound relative to L-ascorbic acid (0.50 mM) required for >80% of the test animals to attain a weight of 1 g in 10 d (5).

required a twenty times greater concentration of this conjugate (10 mM). Apparently, *M. sexta* does not metabolize the sulfate ester back to L-ascorbic acid because it probably lacks a sulfohydrolase enzyme. Preliminary results indicated that the 2-sulfate derivative was about half as active as L-ascorbic acid in the southwestern corn borer, *Diatraea grandiosella* Dyar (19). That species required a dietary supplement of 21 mM L-ascorbic acid for optimal growth (20), approximately forty times higher than the level required by *M. sexta*. These differences may express the metabolic needs of individual species.

Three stereoisomers of L-ascorbic acid were also bioassayed using the tobacco hornworm (Table I). Configurational changes at C4 and C5 affected activity and indicated that the geometry of C5 was more critical for activity than that of C4. The enantiomer, D-ascorbic acid, had approximately 40% activity, while the C5 epimer, D-isoascorbic acid, had 10% activity. The relative potency of those isomers is reversed in vertebrate and invertebrate animals. With D-isoascorbic, 2–10% activity in other insects was reported (20–22), but this compound did not promote development of the cotton leafworm (23). L-Isoascorbic acid had no activity in the hornworm or guinea pig.

L-Dehydroascorbic acid, a derivative with potent vitamin activity in vertebrates, was inactive in our bioassay when it was mixed with hot diet prior to gelation. However, when we repeated the bioassay by applying dehydroascorbic acid to the surface of the gelled diet, the oxidized form proved to be as effective as L-ascorbic acid in promoting insect growth. Apparently, dehydroascorbic acid was destroyed at the elevated temperature (24).

The possibility that L-ascorbic acid was exerting its growth-promoting effect on the hornworm as a nonspecific reducing agent was tested. Organic and inorganic agents such as reductones, tocopherol, hydroquinone, pyrocatechol, thiols, ferrous sulfate, and sodium dithionite exhibited no activity. The carbon ring analog, reductic acid, was also inactive. Obviously, the tobacco hornworm displayed stereoselectivity for L-ascorbic acid and is a good model for the study of structure–activity relationships.

Ascorbate Levels in Tissues. Several tissues were dissected from *M. sexta* and analyzed for L-ascorbic acid by high performance liquid chromatography (HPLC) (Figure 2), paper chromatography, or the dinitrophenylhydrazine method (5). As anticipated, L-ascorbic acid was

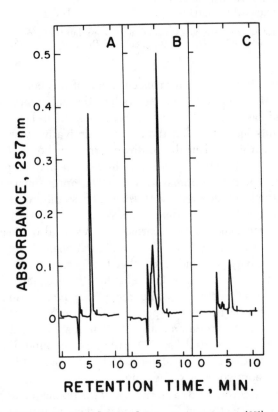

Figure 2. HPLC of L-ascorbic acid from insect tissues (65). A, L-ascorbic acid, 1.7 μg; B, M. sexta hemolymph (0.01 mL) extract; C, M. sexta labial gland extract, 1.4 mg wet weight.

present in nearly all tissues (Table II), although it was most abundant in larval labial gland and hemolymph, ranging from 1 to 10 mM. L-Ascorbic acid was also present at varying levels in eggs, larval gut, muscle, cuticle, adult nervous tissue, and gonads. For comparison, L-ascorbic acid was assayed in diet and fecal matter at 24 and 5 mg/100 g, respectively. This result indicated that approximately 80% of the vitamin was absorbed and/or metabolized by tissues. No ascorbate was detected in larval fat body, Malphigian tubule, or adult salivary gland. Thus, insects appear to be different from vertebrates, where the highest levels of L-ascorbic acid occur in the adrenals and nervous tissue (25).

L-Ascorbic acid was also analyzed in tissues from hornworms fed a vitamin-deficient diet. Without L-ascorbic acid neonate larvae grew into the third instar, but died before the next molt. These larvae retained little or no vitamin in tissues (Table II). A similar result was characteristic of fifth instar larvae reared on an ascorbate-deficient diet beginning at the mid fourth instar. These larvae failed to complete pupation. Apparently, the diet was the sole source of L-ascorbic acid and when tissues became depleted, major pathological consequences ensued.

Table II. L-Ascorbic Acid Content of Tissues from M. *sexta*

Tissue	Stage[a]	L-Ascorbate Content[b]
Labial gland	L5	86 ± 84 (24)
	L3	69 ± 10 (4)
Hemolymph	L5	48 ± 40 (24)
Brain and nerve cord	A	41 ± 30 (4)
Gonad	A	63 ± 8 (2)
	A	60 ± 14 (2)
Egg	—	43 ± 3 (4)
Gut	L5	39 ± 8 (6)
Muscle	L5	27 ± 11 (4)
Cuticle	L5	22 ± 15 (4)
Mouth exudate	L5	15 ± 4 (2)
Fat body	L5	< 1 (4)
Malphigian tubule	L5	< 1 (3)
Salivary gland	A	< 1 (2)
L-ascorbate deficient diet		
Labial gland	L5[c]	< 1 (6)
	L3[d]	< 1 (6)
Hemolymph	L5	< 1 (4)

[a] Key: L, larva; A, adult; 3, third instar; and 5, fifth instar.
[b] Units are mg of L-ascorbic acid/100 g of wet tissue or 100 mL hemolymph ± sd. Amounts of tissue or hemolymph analyzed were 20–300 mg or 0.3–0.5 mL, respectively. Number of determinations listed in parentheses.
[c] Hornworm reared on ascorbate deficient diet from middle of fourth larval instar.
[d] Hornworm reared on ascorbate deficient diet from neonate stage.

The titer of L-ascorbic acid in tissues was examined during development. During the fifth instar, L-ascorbate increased about eightyfold in the labial gland and ten-fold in the hemolymph, where millimolar levels were measured (Figure 3). Regression analysis of the tissue kinetics revealed that the labial gland accumulated L-ascorbic acid about twice

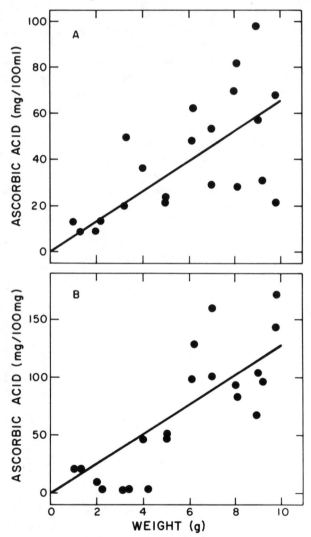

Figure 3.   Changes in the content of L-ascorbic acid in hemolymph and labial gland during larval development of M. sexta (65). A, Hemolymph: regression analysis yielded line defined as larval weight = 6.5 [ascorbic acid] at α = 0.01 level and R^2 = 0.83; B, labial gland: regression analysis yielded line defined as larval weight = 12.7 [ascorbic acid] at α = 0.01 level and R^2 = 0.87.

as fast as did hemolymph. Labial glands removed from a third instar larva also contained a high titer of L-ascorbate. Vitamin C may be depleted during the intermolt period, after which feeding recommenced and tissue accumulation occurred. Three other phytophagus species, *S. littoralis* (6); the silkworm, Bombyx mori (8); and the locust, *Schistocerca gregaria* (16) showed high ascorbic acid titers in various tissues during the instar and low titers at the molting stage.

Absence of L-Gulono-γ-lactone Oxidase in Insect Tissues. There is no conclusive evidence that any species of insect can synthesize L-ascorbic acid. As a first test to determine whether *M. sexta* could synthesize the vitamin, L-gulono-γ-lactone, a well-known precursor in animals, was tested in the bioassay (27). At 0.5 mM L-ascorbic acid in the diet or when injected into the hemocoel of larvae, no activity was observed. We also surveyed insect tissues for L-gulono-γ-lactone oxidase, the enzyme catalyzing the final step in animal biosynthesis of L-ascorbic acid from glucose. Chicken kidney and liver were control tissues; the former synthesized 10 μg L-ascorbate/mg/h, while the latter was inactive (28). Within the limits of the assay, no evidence for L-gulono-γ-lactone oxidase was detected in tissue homogenates from *M. sexta, P. interpunctella,* and *P. americana.* The latter two species were cultured on L-ascorbic-acid-deficient media. Apparently, certain insects may not require L-ascorbic acid for growth, may synthesize the vitamin or a similar factor at a rate too slow to measure, may use a synthetic pathway that the assay procedure (which was developed for vertebrate tissue) failed to detect, or may rely on a symbiotic organism to produce L-ascorbic acid. More work concerning biosynthesis needs to be done.

Discussion

Review of Literature. An obvious question is why use insects instead of vertebrate animals to study ascorbic acid biochemistry. Primarily, it is more convenient. Insects are relatively small and have a rapid generation time. Large numbers can be used to get valid statistical data. Biological effects can be analyzed using a synchronous population where stages of development can be timed with accuracy (29). Small amounts of test material (mg) can be used in most cases.

Although many insects nutritionally require ascorbic acid, numerous species have apparently been reared on artificial or synthetic diets without ascorbic acid or related nutrients. These include Diptera and assorted roaches, crickets, beetles, and moths, whose normal food comprises detritus, seeds, carrion, and dry stored products that are deficient in ascorbate for certain vertebrate animals. The general presumption has been that the diets lack vitamin C and that certain insects can biosynthesize it (Table III). Whether these diets are deficient for invertebrate animals is unknown. Thus, one must be careful about which insect is chosen as the experimental animal.

Insects and ascorbic acid have been studied for a relatively long time. A listing of such studies is presented in Table III. The earliest paper was that Girond et al. (30) who, over 40 years ago, detected L-ascorbic acid in the gonads and endocrine glands of a predaceous diving beetle, *Dytiscus marginalis*. A novel report concerned a patent obtained in Japan for preparing ascorbic acid from silkworm pupae (31). Dadd (32) first discovered a dietary requirement for vitamin C in insects using a grasshopper, *Locusta migratoria*. Overall, approximately seventy papers have been published concerning dietary requirements, tissue levels, biosynthesis, physiological effects, and structure–activity relationships involving one or more of fifty different species. In nearly all cases, L-ascorbic acid in the diet had a positive effect on growth and development. In two species, the ambrosia beetle, *Xyleborus ferrugineus* (33), and the sawtoothed grain beetle, *Oryzaephilus surinamensis* (34), L-ascorbic acid decreased the rate of development, survival, or progeny production. L-Ascorbic acid was proposed to cause browning of dietary protein that, in turn, led to amino acid deficiencies (33). Another study using *O. surinamensis* reported that L-ascorbic acid was beneficial in larval development (35). Since vitamin C is essentially nontoxic to other animals, it is most likely innocuous to insects as well.

Physiological Function. The mechanism by which L-ascorbic acid benefits an insect is unknown. The vitamin is found in many tissues where it probably plays a variety of roles related to its redox potential. Besides the possible general function of detoxifying superoxide and hydrogen peroxide, L-ascorbic acid may be involved in metabolic processes such as tyrosine metabolism, collagen formation, steroid synthesis, detoxification reactions, phagostimulation, or neuromodulation. At this time one can only speculate about the function of vitamin C in some specific tissues.

Table III.   Ascorbic Acid and Its Effects in Insects

Species	Comments	References
Alabama argillacea	levels in tissues decreased during development	41
Anthonomus grandis	dietary requirement	42
Apis indica	no biosynthesis detected	43
Apis mellifera	tissue levels at 5–600 µg/g	44
Argyrotaenia velutinana	no dietary requirement	45

Table III.   (Continued)

Species	Comments	References
Auripennis lepel	no biosynthesis detected	*43*
Bombyx mori	dietary requirement	*46–48*
	synthesis detected in pupal fat body from D-mannose	*8*
	detected in eggs	*49*
	patent for isolation from pupae	*49*
	phagostimulant	*50*
	D-isoascorbic acid slightly active, dehydroascorbic acid fully active	*21, 22*
	no biosynthesis detected	*43*
Chorthippus sp.	phagostimulant	*51*
Corcyra cephalonica	biosynthesis (?)	*52, 53*
	no biosynthesis	*43*
Culex molestus	beneficial in diet	*54*
Cutelia sedilotti	whole body levels at 1 mg/100 g	*38*
Dasycolletes hirtipes	whole body levels at 2 mg/100 g	*38*
Diatraea grandiosella	dietary requirement	*55*
	D-isoascorbic acid slightly active	*20*
Dichomeris marginalis	no vitamin detected in whole body	*56*
Dytiscus marginalis	~ 500 μg/g in gonads and endocrine glands	*30, 57, 58*
Ectomyelois ceratoniae	no dietary requirement	*59*
Ephestia (Caudra) cautella	beneficial effect due to prevention of oxidative rancidity in diet	*60*
Estigmene acrea	dietary requirement, vitamin accumulated in tissues during development	*41, 42*
Eurygoster integriceps	dietary requirement (0.4%)	*61*
Graphosoma lineatum	detrimental effect in diet	*61*
Heliothis zea	dietary requirement, vitamin accumulated in tissues during growth	*41*
Heliothis virescens	dietary requirement	*62*
Laspeyresia pomonella	dietary requirement	*63*
Leptinotarsa decemlimeata	dietary requirement	*64*

Continued on next page.

Table III.   (Continued)

Species	Comments	References
Leucophaea maderae	synthesis by fat body and by symbionts	9
Locusta migratoria	vitamin detected in tissues by histochemical staining	7
	dietary requirement, vitamin accumulated in hemolymph during development	26, 32
Lucilia sp.	vitamin detected in tissues by histochemical staining	7
Manduca sexta	dietary requirement (0.5 mM); dehydroascorbic acid, Mg 2-O-phosphonoascorbate, Na 6-O-myristoylascorbate fully active; D-ascorbic acid 50% active; 6-bromoascorbic acid 20% active; D-isoascorbic acid 10% active; K 2-O-sulfoascorbate, L-isoascorbic acid, L-gulonic acid γ-lactone inactive	5
	vitamin accumulated in hemolymph and larval labial gland (also present in eggs, gut, muscle, cuticle, nervous tissue and gonads), no L-gulonolactone oxidase detected	65
Melampsalata cingulata	whole body levels at 1 mg/100 g	38
Melanoplus biovittatus	dietary requirement	66
Musca domestica	whole body contained 1.5 mg/100 g, synthesis from hexose	38
Myzus persicae	dietary requirement, D-isoascorbic acid fully active	67
Neomyzus circumflexus	dietary requirement	68
Neotermes sp.	dietary requirement	69
Oryzaephilus surinamensis	detrimental effect in diet	34
	vitamin C replaced pantothentic acid requirement in diet	35
Ostrinia nubilalis	dietary requirement	70
Pectinophora gossypiella	no dietary requirement	71
	synthesized and accumulated vitamin C during development	41

Table III.   (Continued)

Species	Comments	References
Periplaneta americana	whole body at 10 mg/g, synthesis	72
	present in Malpighian tubules at 0.6–1.0 mg/g	73
	biosynthesis from hexose?	74
	synthesized by symbionts in fat body	75
	synthesized in gut (by symbionts?)	10
	no biosynthesis from hexose, glucuronate, L-gulono-γ-lactone, L-galactono-γ-lactone	43
Plebliogrylus guttiventri	no biosynthesis	43
Polistes herbraeus	no biosynthesis	43
Rhycacionia buoliana	dietary requirement	76
Schistocerca gregaria	hemolymph titer at 100–500 μg/mL, hemolymph titer increased during growth	26, 32
Sphingomorpha chlorae	no biosynthesis	43
Spodoptera littoralis	dietary requirement (0.5%) ; D-araboascorbic acid, D-glucurono-γ-lactone, L-glulono-γ-lactone inactive	77
	D-glucoascorbic acid (0.05–0.3%) in diet produced deformed spermatophores	78
	vitamin C present in hemolymph and molting fluid	6
	Na ascorbate, Ca ascorbate, L-dehydroascorbic acid active, D-isoascorbic acid inactive	23
Tenebrio molitor	none detected in whole body	56
Trichoplusia ni	dietary requirement, Na L-ascorbate and Ca L-ascorbate active	79
	dietary requirement	80
Tryporyza incertulas	no synthesis	43
Xyleborus ferrugineus	L-ascorbic acid, D-isoascorbic acid, and L-dehydroascorbic acid inhibited progeny by producing diet nutritionally deficient in protein (browning)	33

Ascorbic acid may be involved in molting because the titer decreased in the hemolymph and increased in the molting fluid during apolysis (6, 26). The old exoskeleton is digested by proteases and chitinases while the new exoskeleton is formed by tanning enzymes, chitin synthase, and protein synthase. The earliest pathology in vitamin-deficient insects was observed in the cuticle, which tanned abnormally and exhibited lesions (5, 6). In certain insects the absence of L-ascorbic acid may allow cuticle tanning reactions such as tyrosine hydroxylation and oxidation to occur prematurely. Reductants such as ascorbic acid have been implicated in enzymatic hydroxylation reactions (36, 37). However, evidence for this involvement is ambiguous. Navon (6) observed that catecholamine oxidation was inhibited in the cotton leafworm, while Briggs (38) reported that tyrosine oxidation in flies was stimulated by L-ascorbic acid. There may be a species dependence where oxidation of phenols is activated in Diptera and inhibited in Lepidoptera.

Another possible function of L-ascorbic acid in the cuticle is to promote collagen formation. No evidence for this has been obtained using insects, but L-ascorbic acid deficiency disease in penaeid shrimp, termed "black death," was related to collagen hypohydroxylation (39, 40). Melanized lesions of loose connective tissue occurred in endocuticle at intersegmental spaces. Perhaps insects also underhydroxylate collagen when deficient in ascorbic acid.

L-Ascorbic acid is plentiful in the larval labial gland of the tobacco hornworm. Whereas many lepidopterans use the gland for the production of silk fibroin, the hornworm uses the gland contents for "body wetting" (29). Prior to pupal apolysis, the larva wets itself all over with a proteinaceous fluid. This secretion may be used as an external lubricant for burrowing behavior or it may be involved in cuticle degradation. What role ascorbic acid plays in the labial gland is unknown.

The last tissue to be discussed is the hemolymph. Perhaps L-ascorbic acid has no particular function there, except to maintain a highly reducing environment that serves as a reservoir of L-ascorbic acid for other tissues.

Research Needs. Over the years L-ascorbic acid has been shown to be an essential nutrient for many insects including species of Lepidoptera, Orthoptera, Coleoptera, and Diptera. Others such as cockroaches, houseflies, and mealworms are reared on simple diets without added ascorbic acid. Perhaps those insects require very low levels of vitamin C in their diets. A sensitive analytical method is needed to measure levels of L-ascorbic acid and dehydroascorbic acid in insect tissue and food. Such a method, which is likely to be developed using HPLC with electrochemical detection, could be used to monitor vitamin C levels in feed ingredients as well as in tissues during an insect's life cycle. This information is needed to determine whether ascorbic acid is used to regulate the activity of enzymes, such as those involved in molting. Vitamin C appears to have a varied and almost ubiquitous role in insects. Much more research is required to determine whether ascorbic acid is an essential nutrient for all insects and to define its mechanism of action in insect development.

Acknowledgment

M. sexta eggs were obtained from J. P. Reinecke of the U.S. Department of Agriculture, Agricultural Research, Science and Education Administration, Fargo, North Dakota. We are grateful to Roy Speirs, Leon Hendricks, George Lookhart, and Doreen Liang for assistance with these studies and to Herbert Lipke and G. M. Chippendale for critical comments. This is contribution number 81-241-j from the Departments of Grain Science and Biochemistry, Kansas Agricultural Experiment Station, Manhatten, Kansas.

Literature Cited

1. Dadd, R. H. *Annu. Rev. Entomol.* **1973**, *18*, 381–420.
2. House, H. L. In "Physiology of Insecta," 2nd ed.; Rockstein, M., Ed.; Academic: New York, 1974; Vol. 5, pp. 1–62.
3. Chatterjee, I. G.; Majumder, A. K.; Nandi, B. K.; Subramanian, N. *Ann. N.Y. Acad. Sci.* **1975**, *258*, 24–47.
4. Chippendale, G. M. In "Biochemistry of Insects"; Rockstein, M., Ed.; Academic: New York, 1978; pp. 1–55.
5. Kramer, K. J.; Hendricks, L. H.; Liang, Y. T.; Seib, P. A. *J. Agric. Food Chem.* **1978**, *26*, 874–878.
6. Navon, A. *J. Insect Physiol.* **1978**, *24*, 39–44.
7. Day, M. F. *Aust. J. Sci. Res., Ser. B* **1949**, *2*, 19–30.
8. Gamo, T.; Seki, H. *Res. Rep. Fac. Text. Seri., Shinshu Univ.* **1954**, *4*(A), 29–38.
9. Pierre, L. L. *Nature* **1962**, *193*, 904–905.
10. Raychaudhuri, D. N.; Banerjee, M. *Sci. Cult.* **1968**, *34*, 461–463.
11. Bell, R. A.; Joachim, F. G. *Ann. Entomol. Soc. Am.* **1976**, *69*, 365–373.
12. Schneiderman, H. A. In "Methods in Developmental Biology"; Wessels, W. H., Ed.; Cromwell: New York, 1967; pp. 753–765.
13. Trevalyan, W. E.; Procter, D. P.; Harrison, J. S. *Nature* **1950**, *166*, 444–445.
14. Azaz, K. M.; Jenness, R.; Birney, B. C. *Anal. Biochem.* **1976**, *72*, 161–171.
15. Roe, J. H.; Kuether, C. A. *J. Biol. Chem.* **1943**, *147*, 299–407.
16. Geschwind, I. I.; Williams, B. S.; Li, C. H. *Acta Endocrinol.* **1951**, *8*, 247–250.
17. Tolbert, B. M.; Downing, M.; Carlson, R. W.; Knight, M. K.; Baker, E. M. *Ann. N.Y. Acad. Sci.* **1975**, *258*, 48–69.
18. House, H. L. "Physiology of Insecta," 2nd ed.; Rockstein, M., Ed.; Academic: New York, 1974; Vol. 5, pp. 63–117.
19. Chippendale, G. M., private communication, 1977.
20. Chippendale, G. M. *J. Nutr.* **1975**, *105*, 499–507.
21. Ito, T.; Arai, N. *Bull. Seric. Exp. Stn., Tokyo* **1965**, *20*, 1–19.

22. Mittler, T. E.; Tsitsipis, J. A.; Kleinjan, J. E. *J. Insect Physiol.* **1970,** *16,* 2315–2323.
23. Navon, A. *Entomol. Exp. Appl.* **1978,** *24,* 35–40.
24. Velisek, J. Davidek; Janicek, G. *Collect. Czech. Chem. Commun.* **1972,** *37,* 1465–1470.
25. Hornig, D. *World Rev. Nutr. Diet.* **1975,** *23,* 225–258.
26. Dadd, R. H. *Proc. R. Soc. London* **1960,** *153*(B), 128–143.
27. Touster, O. In "Comprehensive Biochemistry"; Florkin, M.; Stoltz, E. H., Ed.; Elsevier: Amsterdam, 1969; pp. 219–240.
28. Chadhuri, C. R.; Chatterjee, I. B. *Science* **1969,** *164,* 435–436.
29. Reinecke, J. P.; Buckner, J. S.; Grugel, S. R. *Biol. Bull.* **1980,** *158,* 129–140.
30. Girond, A.; Ratsimamanga, A. *Bull. Soc. Chim. Biol.* **1936,** *18,* 375–379.
31. Aizawa, D. Japanese Patent 179730, 1949.
32. Dadd, R. H. *Nature* **1957,***179,* 427–428.
33. Bridges, J. R.; Norris, D. M. *J. Insect Physiol.* **1977,** *23,* 497–501.
34. Davis, G. R. F. *Can. Entomol.* **1966,** *98,* 263–267.
35. Kaul, S.; Saxena, S. C. *Acta Entomol. Biochem.* **1975,** *72,* 236–238.
36. Lerner, P.; Hartman, P.; Ames, M.; Lovenberg, W. *Arch. Biochem. Biophys.* **1977,** *182,* 164–170.
37. Retnakaran, A. *Comp. Biochem. Physiol.* **1969,** *29,* 965–974.
38. Briggs, M. H. *Comp. Biochem. Physiol.* **1962,** *5,* 241–252.
39. Magarelli, P.; Hunter, B.; Lightner, D.; Colvin, B. *Comp. Biochem. Physiol.* **1979,** *63A,* 103–108.
40. Ibid., *64B,* 381–385.
41. Vanderzant, E. S.; Richardson, C. D. *Science* **1963,** *140,* 989–991.
42. Vanderzant, E. S.; Pool, M.; Richardson, C. *J. Insect Physiol.* **1962,** *8,* 287–297.
43. Gupta, D.: Gupta, S.; Chandhuri, R.; Chatterjee, I. B. *Anal. Biochem.* **1970,** *38,* 46–50.
44. Haydak, M. H.; Vivino, A. E. *Arch. Biochem. Biophys.* **1943,** *2,* 201–207.
45. Rock, G.; King, K. *J. Insect Physiol.* **1967,** *13,* 175–186.
46. Gamo, T. *Uyeda Bull. Seric. Ind.* **1941,** *13,* 63–69.
47. Gamo, T.; Nishiyama, C. *Res. Rep. Fac. Text. Seric. Shinshu Univ.* **1953,** *3,* 30–34.
48. Gamo, T.; Seki, H.; Takizawa, S. *J. Seric. Soc. Jpn.* **1952,** *20,* 106–110.
49. Sumiki, Y.; Yaita, M.; Okura, S.; Ito, C. *J. Agric. Chem. Soc. Jpn.* **1944,** *20,* 203–209.
50. Ito, T. *Bull. Seric. Exp. Stn., Tokyo* **1961,** *17,* 119–124.
51. Thorsteinson, A. *Entomol. Exp. Appl.* **1958,** *1,* 23–27.
52. Sarma, P.; Bhagvat, K. *Curr. Sci.* **1942,** *11,* 394–395.
53. Thangamani, A.; Sarma, P. S. *J. Sci. Ind. Res. Sect. C* **1960,** *19,* 40–42.
54. Lichtenstein, E. *Nature* **1948,** *162,* 227–228.
55. Reddy, G.; Chippendale, G. *Entomol. Exp. Appl.* **1972,** *15,* 51–60.
56. Nespor, E.; Wenig, K. *Biochem. Z.* **1939,** *302,* 73–78.
57. Girond, A.; Ratsimamanga, A.; Leblond, C.; Rabinowicz, M.; Drieux, N. *Bull. Soc. Chim. Biol.* **1937,** *19,* 1105–1109.
58. Girond, A.; Leblond, C.; Ratsimamanga, A.; Gero, E. *Bull. Soc. Chim. Biol.* **1938,** *20,* 1079–1083.
59. Levinson, H.; Gothilf, S. *Riv. Parassitol.* **1965,** *26,* 19–26.
60. Fraenkel, G.; Blewett, M. *J. Exp. Biol.* **1946,** *22,* 172–190.
61. Khlistovski, E. D.; Alfinov, V. A. *Entomol. Obozr.* **1979,** *58,* 233–239.
62. Vinson, S. *J. Econ. Entomol.* **1967,** *60,* 565–568.
63. Rock, G. *J. Econ. Entomol.* **1967,** *60,* 1002–1005.
64. Wardojo, S. *Meded. Landbouwhogesch* **1969,** *69*(16), 1–71.
65. Kramer, K.; Speirs, R.; Loookhart, G.; Seib, P. A.; Liang, Y. T. *Insect Biochem.* **1981,** *11,* 93–96.
66. Nayar, J. K. *Can. J. Zool.* **1964,** *42,* 11–22.

67. Dadd, R. H.; Krieger, D. L.; Mittler, T. E. *J. Insect Physiol.* **1967**, *13*, 249–272.
68. Ehrhardt, P. *Experientia* **1968**, *24*, 82–83.
69. Joly, P. *C. R. Seances Soc. Biol. Ses Fils.* **1940**, *134*, 408–410.
70. Chippendale, G. M.; Beck, S. D. *Entomol. Exp. Appl.* **1964**, *7*, 241–246.
71. Vanderzant, E. S. *J. Econ. Entomol.* **1957**, *50*, 219–221.
72. Wollman, E.; Girond, A.; Ratsimamanga, A. *C. R. Seances Soc. Biol. Ses Fils.* **1937**, *124*, 434–435.
73. Metcalf, R. L. *Arch. Biochem. Biophys.* **1943**, *2*, 55–62.
74. Rousell, G. *Trans. N.Y. Acad. Sci.* **1957**, *19*, 17–20.
75. Ludwig, D.; Gallagher, M. *J. N.Y. Entomol. Soc.* **1966**, *74*, 134–139.
76. Ross, R. H.; Monroe, R. E.; Butcher, J. W. *Can. Entomol.* **1971**, *103*, 1449–1454.
77. Levinson, H.; Navon, A. *J. Insect Physiol.* **1969**, *15*, 591–595.
78. Navon, A.; Levinson, H. *Bull. Entomol. Res.* **1976**, *66*, 437–442.
79. Toba, H.; Kishaba, A. *J. Econ. Entomol.* **1971**, *65*, 127–128.
80. Chippendale, G. M.; Beck, S. D.; Strong, F. M. *J. Insect Physiol.* **1965**, *11*, 211–218.

RECEIVED for review January 22, 1981. ACCEPTED March 19, 1981.

Kinetic Behavior of Ascorbic Acid in Guinea Pigs

DIETRICH HORNIG and DIETER HARTMANN

Department of Vitamin and Nutrition Research and Section for Mathematical Statistics, F. Hoffmann–La Roche & Company, Limited, CH-4002, Basle, Switzerland

The course of carbon-14-radioactivity derived from oral (1-¹⁴C)ascorbic acid in plasma and several tissues was studied in male guinea pigs up to 320 h after intake. The excretion of label was followed in respiratory carbon dioxide, urine, and feces. The evaluation by pharmacokinetic principles yielded an overall half-life of 61 h and a body pool of 21 mg with a total turnover of about 10 mg/d. The total turnover of ascorbate is lower than the daily intake (16 mg/d), indicating incomplete absorption. Ascorbic acid seemed to be bound in several tissues (adrenals, testes) to a higher percentage than in plasma. The maximum rate of excretion as carbon dioxide occurred at 0.5 h, whereas peak concentration of radioactivity in plasma was reached at 1.5 h. Therefore, presystemic metabolism must be considered.

In guinea pigs respiratory exhalation of carbon-14-labeled carbon dioxide after administration of (1-¹⁴C)ascorbic acid is the major route of catabolism, whereas urinary and fecal excretion of unchanged ascorbic acid and labeled metabolites contribute only to a minor part (*1*). From experiments in guinea pigs receiving (1-¹⁴C)ascorbic acid by intraperitoneal injection together with 5 mg ascorbic acid, the half-lives of the label in liver, heart, kidneys, adrenals, and spleen compared very well (2–3 d); in the brain this time period was about 5 d (*2*). This observation confirmed earlier findings on the overall biological half-life of ascorbic acid to be about 4 d in guinea pigs (*3*).

Many reports demonstrating the distribution of ascorbic acid in tissues of guinea pigs have appeared. Because this species is not able to

0065-2393/82/0200–0293$06.75/0

synthesize ascorbic acid, the concentration of ascorbic acid is dependent on intake. The highest concentrations were determined in the adrenal and pituitary glands; liver, brain, and spleen showed comparable levels. Less ascorbic acid was found in heart and skeletal muscles, bone marrow, and testes (4).

The distribution of labeled material following a single oral or intraperitoneal administration of (1-^{14}C)ascorbic acid has been studied in rats (5, 6), mice (6), and guinea pigs (7–10) employing either a tissue dissection method or whole body autoradiography. These investigations suggested that the various tissues might be classified into three groups according to uptake and retention of labeled material: a) tissues with a low retention capacity such as liver, lungs, kidneys, spleen, bone marrow, and lacrimal and parotid glands; b) tissues exhibiting a high retention capacity and also a comparable high and rapid accumulation of radioactivity such as adrenal and pituitary glands, submandibular glands, and pancreas; and c) tissues having a very strong retention capacity but with a long-lasting, continuing uptake of labeled material. To the last group belong cerebrum, cerebellum, bulbus olfactorius, and testes (7, 9, 10).

To achieve a more precise knowledge of the fate of ascorbic acid we have investigated in guinea pigs the kinetic behavior of the carbon-14-label derived from (1-^{14}C)ascorbic acid given as a single oral dose. In particular, the distribution of radioactivity in various tissues (tissue binding and turnover) and of elimination (respiration, urinary and fecal excretion) was aimed at. The obtained data were evaluated using pharmacokinetic principles.

Materials and Methods

Animals. Male guinea pigs (Himalayan spotted) were maintained prior to the experiment on a vitamin-C-free diet (Nutritional Biochemical Corporation) supplemented with 0.5 g of ascorbic acid/kg of diet and fortified with all other vitamins (11). The initial weight was 309 ± 22 (g ± sd), at the time of sacrifice of the animals 327 ± 37 (g ± sd). During the experiment the animals had free access to water and diet. Altogether twenty-eight animals were taken into the experiment. At each time point one animal was killed.

Radioacitvity and Dosage. L-(1-^{14}C)Ascorbic acid (New England Nuclear, NEC-146, spec. act. 8.44 mCi/mmol, purity at least 98.0%) was dissolved in water and given orally to each animal (50 μCi; 250 μL; 1.04 mg).

Respiratory Carbon Dioxide; Urine and Feces. After dosage of the labeled ascorbic acid, the animal was immediately placed in a closed, tight metabolic chamber equipped with a trap for the collection of urine and feces. The incoming air passed with a flow of 280 L/h through the metabolic chamber (volume ∼ 22 L) by suction from an electric pump. The respiratory carbon dioxide was absorbed by ethanol amine (Merck) contained in two flasks (50 mL) that were connected to the chamber by tubes. To determine the absorbed carbon dioxide, the two flasks could be removed after the outcoming airstream had been turned around into the new flasks. The samples were taken at predetermined time intervals. With this system, it was possible to change the flasks at any time without stopping the flow longer than a few seconds. From each withdrawn flask, an aliquot of 500 μL was added to a mixture of 10 mL of ethanol and 10 mL of scintillator solution [0.8% butyl-1,3,4-phenylbiphenylyloxadiazole (Ciba) in toluene].

During the experiment, urine and feces were collected every 24 h.

Dissection of Tissues. Guinea pigs were anaesthetized with Penthrane (Abbott Laboratories, Incorporated) at predetermined time intervals (15, 30, 45, and 90 min; 2, 4, 6, 8, and 12 h; 1, 1.5, 2, 2.5, 3, 4, 5, 7, 9, 10, 11, 12, and 13d). The abdomen was opened and the animals were sacrificed by bleeding caused by a cut through the vena cava. The blood was collected for determination of radioactivity. After centrifugation radioactivity and ascorbic acid concentration in plasma were determined. The tissues were dissected rapidly and kept frozen until processing for determination of radioactivity and ascorbic acid concentration.

Determination of Radioactivity. All samples were counted in a Nuclear Chicago Isocap 300 liquid scintillation counter equipped with a Teletype computerized for direct calculation of disintegrations per minute. Fifty microliters of blood were directly counted for radioactivity after solubilization (1 mL of 1 N NaOH). After incubation at room temperature for 15 min the sample was decolorized by adding 200 μL of hydrogen peroxide and incubating at 80°C for 30 min. The processed samples were mixed with 100 μL of 80% acetic acid and 15 mL of Insta-gel (Packard), and were counted. Approximately 60–100 mg of tissue were solubilized following the same method as for blood. From the collected urine an aliquot (2 mL) was counted directly with 15 mL Insta-gel. The feces were dried overnight at room temperature, and a 60–100-mg aliquot was combusted (12) and counted for radioactivity.

Determination of Ascorbic Acid. A 500-μL aliquot of plasma was mixed with 4.5 mL of 5% metaphosphoric acid followed by analysis in an autoanalyzer using a modified fluorometric method (13). Ascorbic acid content in tissues was determined according to a published method (14).

Results

Animals. From the food intake/24 h and an assumed 100% bioavailability of the ascorbic acid present in the diet, a turnover of 16 ± 3 mg ascorbic acid/d was calculated.

Radioactivity. The specific activity in plasma, defined as 10^6 dpm of ^{14}C-radioactivity/mg of unlabeled ascorbic acid, is plotted against dissection time in Figure 1. The time courses of ^{14}C-radioactivity for various tissues are presented in Figures 2–4.

The cumulative ^{14}C-radioactivity excreted with respiratory carbon dioxide up to 220 h is shown in Figure 5. In Figure 6 the rate of excretion (10^6 dpm/h) for the time period up to 30 h is presented; the peak appears after about 0.5 h.

The cumulative amount of radioactivity (10^6 dpm) excreted with urine is plotted in Figure 7; which also presents a plot of the accumulated radioactivity (10^6 dpm) excreted with the feces as a function of time.

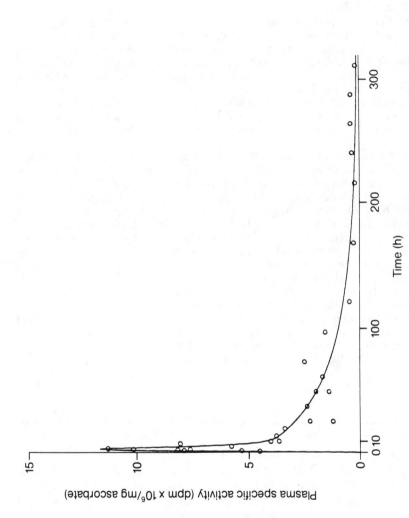

Figure 1. Specific activity (10⁶ dpm/mg ascorbic acid) vs. time. Circles represent the experimental data. The curve was calculated on the basis of a three-compartment system with first-order absorption.

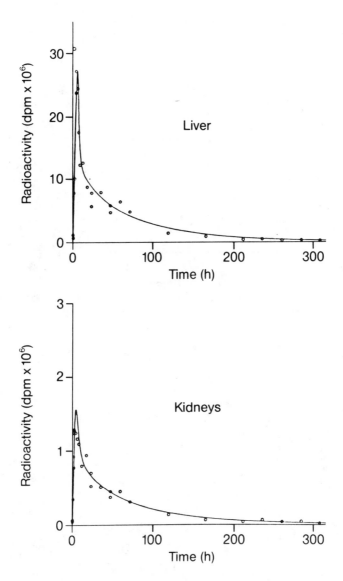

Figure 2. Time course of total radioactivity (dpm × 10⁶) derived from (1-¹⁴C)ascorbic acid in liver and kidneys. Continued on next page.

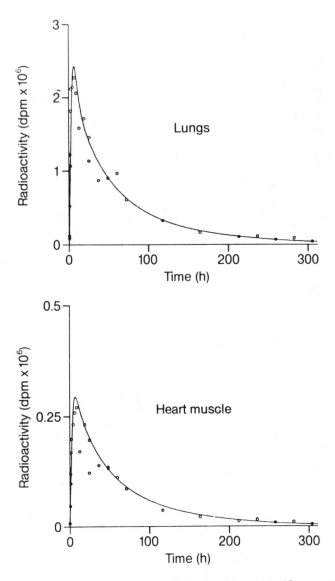

Figure 2 continued.   Time course of total radioactivity (dpm × 10⁶) derived from (1-¹⁴C)ascorbic acid in lungs and heart muscle.

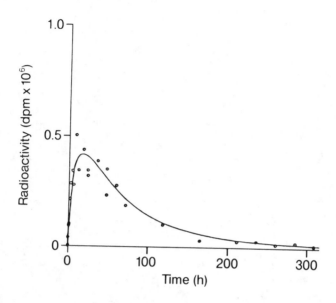

Figure 3. *Time course of total radioactivity (dpm × 10⁶) derived from (1-¹⁴C)ascorbic acid in adrenal glands.*

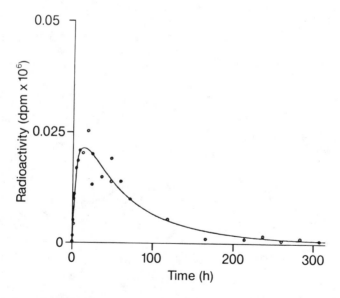

Figure 3 continued. *Time course of total radioactivity (dpm × 10⁶) derived from (1-¹⁴C)ascorbic acid in putuitary glands. Continued on next page.*

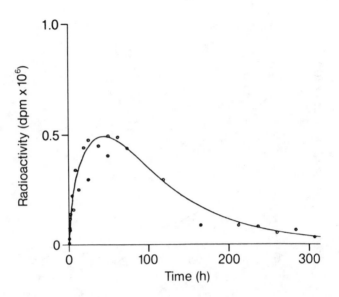

Figure 3 continued.   Time course of total radioactivity (dpm × 10⁶) derived from (1-¹⁴C)ascorbic acid in testes.

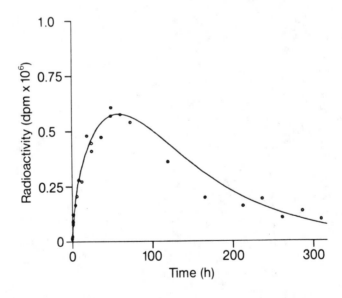

Figure 4.   Time course of total radioactivity (dpm × 10⁶) derived from (1-¹⁴C)ascorbic acid in cerebrum.

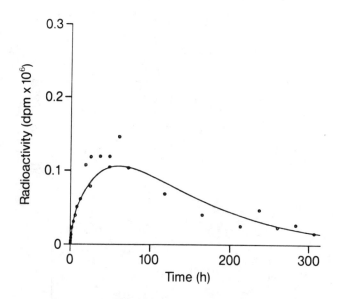

Figure 4 continued.   Time course of total radioactivity (dmp × 10⁶) de-rived from (1-¹⁴C)ascorbic acid in cerebellum.

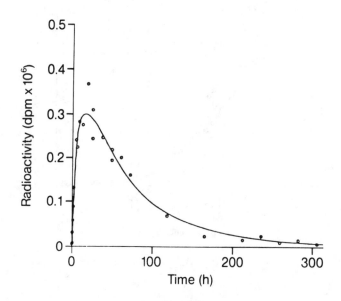

Figure 4 continued.   Time course of total radioactivity (dmp × 10⁶) de-rived from (1-¹⁴C)ascorbic acid in eyes.

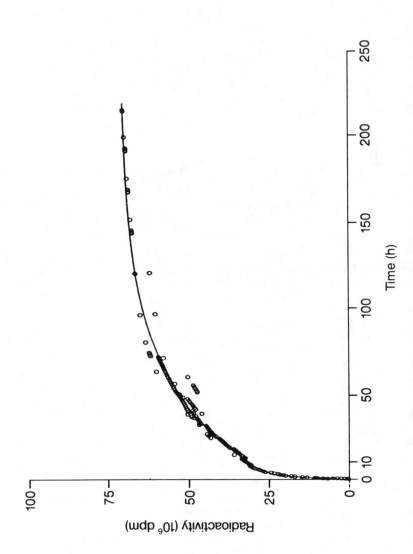

Figure 5. Cumulative ¹⁴C-radioactivity (10^6 dpm) excreted as CO_2. Plotted curve calculated using the empirical model given in Figure 8.

The percentage of administered ^{14}C-radioactivity excreted as respiratory carbon dioxide, with urine and feces, and the total percentage excreted are given in Table I.

The mean values ($\pm$ sd) of the steady state concentration (C_{ss}) of ascorbic acid in plasma and various organs are summarized in Table II.

Table I.   Percentage of Administered Carbon-14-Radioactivity Excreted with Respiratory Carbon Dioxide, with Urine and Feces, with Respect to Time after Oral Administration of 50 μCi (1-^{14}C) Ascorbic Acid to Guinea Pigs

Time (h)	CO_2	Urine	Feces	Total
1	9.9	0.2		
2	16.5	1.2		
6	25.7	1.6	0.3	27.6
12	30.3	2.6	0.8	33.7
24	36.9	2.8	1.3	41.0
48	47.2	4.7	2.0	53.9
96	58.7	6.5	2.5	67.7
144	60.8	6.4	2.7	69.9
192	62.5	6.6	2.8	71.9
216	63.3	6.8	2.8	72.9
264		6.8	2.8	
312		6.7	2.6	

Table II.   Mean $\pm$ sd of Organ Weight and Steady State Concentration (C_{ss}) of Ascorbic Acid (AA) in Tissues and Mean Content (XT) of Ascorbic Acid in Tissues

Organ	Organ Weight (g)	C_{ss} (mg AA/g of Tissue)	XT (mg)
Liver	12.30 $\pm$ 3.2	0.33 $\pm$ 0.07	4.1
Spleen	0.42 $\pm$ 0.1	0.45 $\pm$ 0.06	0.2
Testes	0.84 $\pm$ 0.3	0.47 $\pm$ 0.06	0.4
Cerebrum	2.43 $\pm$ 0.2	0.28 $\pm$ 0.06	0.7
Lungs	2.08 $\pm$ 0.3	0.28 $\pm$ 0.07	0.6
Adrenal glands	0.11 $\pm$ 0.02	1.46 $\pm$ 0.27	0.2
Parotid gland	0.56 $\pm$ 0.1	0.48 $\pm$ 0.02	0.3
Submandibular glands	0.50 $\pm$ 0.1	0.56 $\pm$ 0.13	0.3
Kidneys	2.57 $\pm$ 0.2	0.13 $\pm$ 0.04	0.3
Cerebellum	0.41 $\pm$ 0.05		
Heart muscle	0.93 $\pm$ 0.1		
Eyes	0.77 $\pm$ 0.05		
Pituitary gland	0.01 $\pm$ 0.002		
Sublingual glands	0.08 $\pm$ 0.03		
Plasma		0.0095 $\pm$ 0.004 [a]	

[a] Expressed in mg of ascorbate/mL.

Also given are the mean values ($\pm$ sd) of the organ weights as well as the content [XT (mg)] of ascorbic acid in the organs, which have been estimated by multiplying the mean steady state concentration by the mean organ weight.

Evaluation of Kinetic Parameters

Specific Activity. The time course of the specific activity of ascorbic acid in plasma has been fitted by an analog computer to a sum of four exponentials:

$$S_1 = 76.1e^{-0.65t} + 1.93e^{-0.032t} + 2.75e^{-0.0114t} - 80.8e^{-0.88t} \qquad (1)$$

The experimental data and the calculated curve are plotted in Figure 1. The type of Equation 1 implies a three-compartment system with first-order absorption, that is, at least three kinetically distinguishable pools for ascorbic acid are reflected in the plasma. From the data available it

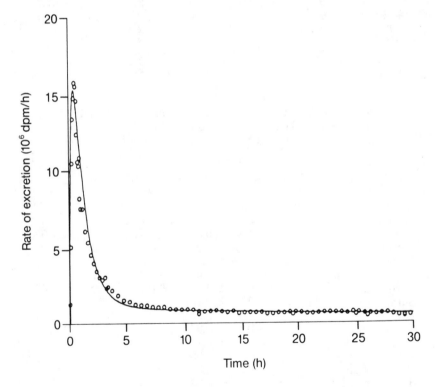

Figure 6.   Excretion rate (10^6 dpm/h) of ^{14}C-radioactivity as CO_2.

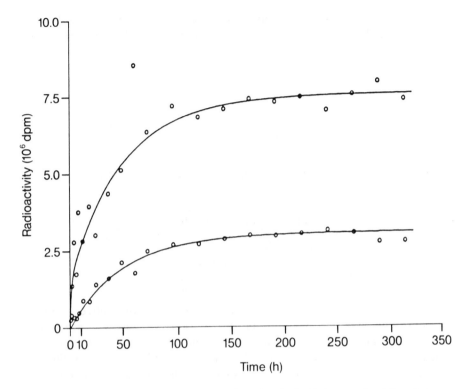

*Figure 7. Cumulative ^{14}C-radioactivity (10^6 dpm) excreted with urine
(upper) and feces (lower curve). The plotted curves were calculated using
the empirical model given in Figure 8.*

cannot be decided unambiguously which exponential in Equation 1
actually describes the absorption. In this case the exponential with the
largest rate constant is assumed to be the absorption term.

Despite the large scattering of the ratios of the specific activity in
plasma to the specific activity in several organs (values not given), it
appears that even after attainment of the pseudo steady state (distribution equilibrium) those ratios are higher than unity. This suggests the
specific activity in plasma to be higher than in tissues.

Binding of Ascorbic Acid in Tissues. Following Equation 1, the
apparent volume of distribution (V_1) of the rapidly accessible part of
the body (central compartment) was derived to be 0.47 L. Furthermore,
an apparent volume of distribution (V_{ss}) of 2.2 L has been estimated
(15). V_{ss} relates the amount of ascorbic acid in the body in the steady
state to the concentration in plasma. The value of V_1 and V_{ss} are calculated assuming 100% absorption of the administered labeled ascorbic

Table III.   Turnover Rates of Ascorbic Acid and Mean Transit Time

Organ	T_{rT} (mg/d)	$T_{rT}/Organ$ Weight (mg/d/g)	K_{T1} (1/d)	T_{T1}[a] (mg/d)	T_{T1}/T_{rT}	T_{tot}[b] (mg/d)	T_{mean} (h)
Liver	55.2	4.5	19.2	78.0	1.41	11.4	71
Spleen	0.31	0.74	2.16	0.41	1.32	10.6	81
Testes	0.13	1.5	0.58	0.23	1.77	14.2	111
Cerebrum	0.12	0.049	0.36	0.24	2.00	16.3	136
Lungs	2.16	1.0	5.04	2.92	1.35	11.0	75
Adrenal glands	0.21	1.9	1.68	0.27	1.29	10.5	84
Submandibular glands	0.14	0.28	0.84	0.24	1.71	13.7	99
Kidneys	1.92	0.75	8.88	2.93	1.53	12.5	73
Cerebellum	0.02	0.054	0.34	—	—	—	142
Heart muscle	0.23	0.25	3.84	—	—	—	77
Eyes	0.16	0.21	1.80	—	—	—	84
Pituitary gland	0.01	1.3	2.04	—	—	—	82
Plasma	—	—	—	—	—	8.05	—

[a] T_{1r} calculated according to Equation 5; $T_{T1} = K_{T1}$ (Equation 6).
[b] T_{tot} calculated according to Equation 9; T_{mean} calculated according to Equation 10.

In the pseudo steady state (distribution equilibrium), the ratio of the specific activities (S_{T1}/S_1) is independent with time, which leads to Equation 8.

$$\frac{S_1}{S_T} = \frac{T_{T1}}{T_{1T}} \tag{8}$$

This result suggests that the observed ratio of specific activities and the ratio of turnover rates (Table III) parallel each other according to Equation 8.

The total turnover of ascorbic acid (T_{tot}) in the body equals the intake of ascorbic acid (mg/d) under steady state conditions and assuming 100% bioavailability. T_{tot} can also be calculated by the occupancy priniciple (19) using the time course of radioactivity in organs:

$$T_{tot} = \frac{\text{dose} \cdot XT}{\int_0^\infty XT^* \, dt} = \frac{\text{dose}}{\int_0^\infty S_T \, dt} \tag{9}$$

with the following notations:

T_{tot} total turnover rate (mg of ascorbate/d) in the body
dose   administered ^{14}C-radioactivity (10^6 dpm)
XT amount (mg) of ascorbate in the respective organ in steady state
XT^* amount (10^6 dpm) of ^{14}C-radioactivity in the organ
S_T specific activity (10^6 dpm/mg of ascorbate) in tissues

Consequently the total turnover in plasma can be obtained by introducing the plasma specific activity (S_1, Equation 1) into Equation 9. The T_{tot} values calculated using Equation 9 are listed in Table III. These values may be compared with the daily intake of ascorbic acid present in the diet, which was determined to be 16 ± 3 mg.

The specific activity in plasma was found to be higher than that in tissues, therefore the total turnover derived from plasma is lower than the turnover derived from radioactivity in tissues.

Relevant kinetic parameters (half-life, body pool, and mean transit time in organs) can be calculated. According to Equation 1 the specific activity in plasma shows a triphasic decay with half-lives of $t_1 = 1.1$ h, $t_2 = 22$ h, and $t_3 = 61$ h. The half-lives t_1 and t_2 essentially describe the distribution of the compound into the system. The third half-life of 61 h (2.5 d) is valid for all tissues after attainment of the distribution equilibrium and represents the overall half-life of elimination from the body under the special conditions of the study (ascorbate status of the animals).

The amount of ascorbic acid in the body (body pool) can be obtained by multiplying the volume of distribution (V_{ss}) by the averaged steady state concentration [C_{ss} (Table II)] of ascorbic acid in plasma. This calculation yields a body pool of 21 mg. Unfortunately, the estimated body pool cannot be compared with an experimental value since the total pool was not accessible experimentally.

The mean transit time (t_{mean}) of ^{14}C-radioactivity in organs has formally been evaluated using Equation 10 with XT^* as the ^{14}C-radioactivity in the organs:

$$t_{mean} = \frac{\int_{o}^{\infty} t \cdot XT^* \, dt}{\int_{o}^{\infty} XT^* \, dt} \tag{10}$$

The resulting parameters are given in Table III.

The resulting mean transit time may be used as a measure of the residence time of a molecule in an organ compared with a second organ, regardless of possible recirculation.

Ranking the organs corresponding to these mean transit times (Table III) three groups may be distinguished: group 1 includes liver, kidney, lungs, and heart muscle with mean transit times of 71–75; group 2 includes spleen, pituitary gland, eyes, and adrenal glands with mean transit times of 81–84 h; and group 3 includes submandibular gland, testes, cerebrum, and cerebellum with mean transit times of 99–142 h. The classification agrees fairly well with the results of autoradiographic studies (7, 9, 10).

Excretion of ^{14}C-Radioactivity. The maximum rate of excretion (10^6 dpm/h) of ^{14}C-radioactivity as carbon dioxide is reached at about 0.5 h (Figure 6). However, the peak in activity vs. time curves of plasma and of the rapidly perfused organs like liver, lungs, kidney is at about 1.5 h (Figure 2). The excretion of ^{14}C-radioactivity as labeled carbon dioxide is not directly related to plasma in the first time period after administration of the label. An intermediate compartment X3 must be assumed.

In the second time period after administration it was not possible to describe the dependency of excreted radioactivity on time by relating it to the time course of specific activity in plasma or by relating it to the time course of radioactivity in organs. Therefore, a second intermediate compartment X2 must be introduced. The complicated excretion pattern was finally represented by an empirical model (Figure 8).

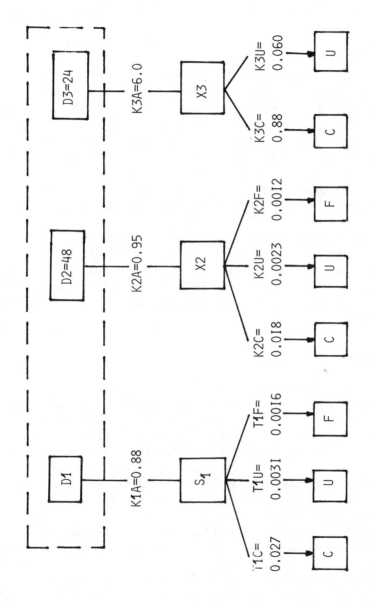

Figure 8. Empirical model for excretion of ^{14}C-radioactivity in guinea pigs. Key: D1, D2, D3, fractions of administered ^{14}C-radioactivity in the intermediate compartments 2 and 3; C, U, F, ^{14}C-radioactivity (10^6 dpm) excreted as CO_2 with urine and feces; T, turnover rates (mg/)h; K, rate constants (L/h).

The administered dose is subdivided into three parts. D1 denotes the fraction of the excretion that is linked to the time course of specific activity (S_1) in plasma. The amounts D2 and D3 are fractions appearing in the intermediate compartments X2 and X3, respectively.

The parameters of this empirical model have been evaluated by fitting the experimental data by using an analog computer. The model has been verified and the parameter estimates refined by simulations (program CSMP) on a digital computer. The resulting parameters are summarized in Figure 8. The calculated curves are compared with the experimental data in Figures 5 and 6. Because of the complexity of the system, the parameter set, and even the model itself, might not be unique; another model describing the data equally well might exist.

The excretion of ^{14}C-radioactivity with urine is also represented by the empirical model (Figure 8). The calculated curve of the cumulative ^{14}C-radioactivity in urine is shown in Figure 7 together with the experimental data.

According to the empirical model (Figure 8) the calculated curve of the cumulative ^{13}C-radioactivity in feces is plotted together with the data points in Figure 7 (lower curve). A fraction, which might be due to the large sampling intervals in the first period after intake of the label, was excreted from the intermediate compartment X3 but could not be detected.

Discussion

The fate of ascorbic acid administered orally as (1-^{14}C)ascorbic acid has been followed in the guinea pig. The data on the overall excretion of labeled material (Table I) confirm earlier reports demonstrating the respiratory pathway to be the major route of catabolism in the guinea pig (3, 20, 21). Ascorbic acid is rapidly and widely distributed throughout the body (4). We have attempted to determine the remaining part of the label in the tissues to obtain a balance using the total excreted radioactivity. It was not possible experimentally to determine the remaining label in stomach, intestine, and bone. In addition, only estimations of radioactivity in fat, skeletal muscle, and skin were possible, because the total mass was not available. Therefore, the total body pool of ascorbic acid in our investigation cannot be assessed and compared with the calculated value of 21 mg. However, figures from the literature suggest that, with daily intakes of 500 mg of ascorbic acid/kg of diet, a body pool of this size is achieved (22–24).

The ratio of the specific activities in plasma and tissues were larger than unity even after attainment of the steady state; this finding could be caused by tissue ascorbate not exchanging with the introduced, labeled ascorbic acid within the time period of the experiment. The failure to exchange suggests the existence of structures in tissues from which ascorbic acid is slowly released. If this supposition is valid the calculated value of the total body pool would be underestimated.

The fraction of unbound ascorbic acid in plasma was found in our study to be up to sixty times larger than that in tissues. The adrenals exhibit an extraordinarily high relative binding (170 times larger than plasma), which confirms the observation that several protein fractions can be isolated from adrenals by Sephadex chromatography; ascorbic acid was found to be bound to these fractions (25). The lower relative binding in cerebrum and lungs supports nonspecific binding of ascorbic acid to guinea pig brain homogenates (26) and to rat lung homogenates (27). The relative binding of ascorbic acid was also low in liver, in accordance with data reported earlier (28). However, a rather wide controversy exists on the binding of ascorbic acid to protein. Several authors have suggested that ascorbic acid is bound to protein in adrenals and in liver tissue (25, 29) whereas others found no evidence for any such binding (28). Also, no evidence for protein-bound ascorbic acid could be found in other tissues (brain, lung) (26, 27).

Different concentrations in compartments that can exchange ascorbic acid may also be achieved by nonlinear transfers such as active transport processes. Nonlinearity, however, cannot be determined by experimental designs using only one steady state level. The brain, adrenals, pituitary gland, and eyes take up ascorbic acid by an energy-dependent active transport mechanism (30, 31).

Our experimental design allowed the estimation of ascorbic acid turnover in various tissues (Figures 2–4). The amount of ascorbic acid per unit time (turnover) reaching the tissues was highest in the liver ($T_{1T} = 4.5$ mg/d/g of tissue, corresponding to a total turnover of 55 mg/d) followed by adrenals, testes, and pituitary gland (Table III). The rather high turnover in the liver exceeding the total turnover may be caused by a multiple recirculation of ascorbic acid to this organ.

The turnover rates of ascorbic acid from tissues (afflux T_{T1}) were larger than the afflux (*see* Table III, column headed "T_{T1}/T_{1T}"), suggesting either that the distribution equilibrium between labeled ascorbic acid and available tissue ascorbic acid has not been reached, or that part of the compartmental pool of ascorbic acid cannot be exchanged. Therefore, formal calculation of the total turnover of ascorbic acid using tissue data results in a turnover somewhat larger than that calculated using plasma data (mean value 12.5–8 mg/d). When calculated from the food intake, the turnover is 16 ± 3 mg/d; therefore, one must assume that the bioavailability of ascorbic acid present in the diet is not 100%. Studies on the absorption of ascorbic acid in humans have demonstrated ascorbic acid absorption of 80–90%, even with physiological doses up to 180 mg (*32*). The mechanisms for uptake in humans and guinea pigs are comparable (*33, 34*); therefore, ascorbic acid may not be absorbed completely by the guinea pig intestine.

Table III also lists the mean transit times for ascorbic acid in various tissues. Theoretically, this parameter may be used as a measure of the passage of a compound in tissues. The mean transit time might be used to classify the tissues with respect to retention capability for ascorbic acid. The finding that liver, kidneys, lungs, and heart muscle have the shortest transit times is physiologically important in case of existing body pool depletion, when these tissues preferentially lose their stores of ascorbic acid. On the other hand, brain submandibular glands and testes retain ascorbic acid in case of a depletion of this vitamin for a longer period of time. An enhanced retention capability for ascorbic acid was earlier reported for guinea pig eye lens and brain (*2, 35*). Also, autoradiographic studies with (1-^{14}C)ascorbic acid showed that brain, pituitary and adrenal glands, testes, and eye lens have a higher retention capability for ascorbic acid than do liver, lungs, and kidneys (*7, 9, 10*). No specific proteins for ascorbic acid binding in the brain are known (*26*); ascorbic acid is suggested to be retained in these tissues by binding to subcellular structures.

Under the experimental conditions, the overall half-life (biological half-life) of ascorbic acid elimination from the body was calculated at about 61 h (2.5 d). This value has been evaluated from the slope of the log linear phase (β-phase), indicating equilibration of the labeled ascorbic acid with the exchangeable body pool. The observed half-life compares well with data obtained in earlier studies—mainly calculated from the time dependence of the logarithm of radioactivity remaining in the body, and with the assumption that metabolites of ascorbic acid are rapidly eliminated. Thus, biological half-lives for ascorbic acid of 60–140 h (*3*), 85–115 h (*36*), 48–72 h (*2*), or 127 h (*22*) are reported. In one study (*22*) the half-life was determined from the plasma specific activity to be only 39 h.

The kinetic evaluation of our data revealed that in the guinea pig the time course of plasma radioactivity shows a rapid initial distribution in at least two distinguishable phases followed by a log linear phase. Distribution equilibrium was attained after 40 h (Figure 1). In one report (*22*) the kinetics of ascorbic acid were analyzed in guinea pigs following intraperitoneal administration of (1-^{14}C)ascorbic acid. The half-life of the initial rapid phase was calculated to be 5.9 h (from semilogarithmic plot of dose remaining vs. time) and 2.2 h (from plasma ascorbate specific activity). These values compare well with the half-life of 1.1 for the very early distribution phase obtained from our data. There are no data available in the literature for the second phase of distribution (~ 22 h).

In guinea pigs there is considerable conversion of ascorbic acid to respiratory carbon dioxide (3, 37). Further, the entire carbon chain of ascorbic acid is subjected to extensive oxidation to carbon dioxide (3, 21). Following injection of (1-^{14}C)ascorbic acid, 66% of the label was recovered as (^{14}C)carbon dioxide during 10 d; up to 30–40% of the dose was catabolized to carbon dioxide during the first 24 h (20). Our data indicate that in a time period of 216 h about 65% of the oral dose of (1-^{14}C)ascorbic acid is exhaled as labeled carbon dioxide (Table I). The maximum rate of excretion occurred at 0.5 h (Figure 6), and we derived from this radioactivity–time curve that within the first 12 h about 30% of the label was exhaled (36% after 24 h).

In comparing the peak (at 1.5 h, Figure 1) in radioactivity in plasma and in the strongly perfused tissues (liver, lungs, kidneys) with the peak in carbon dioxide excretion (0.5 h, Figure 6) one has to consider metabolism of ascorbic acid before it reaches the systemic circulation. In the guinea pig the contents move rapidly through the stomach and small intestine. Within a period of 2 h these organs are practically emptied (38). A breakdown of the carbon chain in the acid environment of the stomach is unlikely. It is more likely that ascorbic acid is metabolized on the first passage through the intestinal wall, suggesting the presence of structures in the intestinal wall capable of efficiently metabolizing ascorbic acid to carbon dioxide.

The physiological meaning of the intermediate compartment X2, which had to be introduced to describe the experimental data for carbon dioxide exhalation, is presently not understood. The transport of (^{14}C)-carbon dioxide by the erythrocytes might be connected with this compartment.

During the experiment (220 h) only 8% of the label was recovered from urine. This amount agrees satisfactorily with data published earlier (3, 20, 39) and confirms that the elimination with urine is not an important route for the elimination of ascorbic acid and its metabolites. Also, the fecal appearance of the label (Table I) was very limited (about 3% of the dose).

Literature Cited

1. Hornig, D. *World Rev. Nutr. Diet.* **1975**, *23*, 225–258.
2. Pelletier, O. *Can. J. Physiol. Pharmacol.* **1969**, *47*, 993–997.
3. Burns, J. J.; Dayton, P.; Schulenberg, S. *J. Biol. Chem.* **1956**, *218*, 15–21.
4. Hornig, D. *Ann. N.Y. Acad. Sci.* **1975**, *258*, 103–108.
5. Martin, G. R.; Mecca, C. E. *Arch. Biochem.* **1961**, *93*, 110–114.
6. Hammarstroem, L. *Acta Physiol. Scand., Suppl.* **1966**, *70*(289), 1–83.

7. Hornig, D.; Weber, F.; Wiss, O. *Int. J. Vitam. Nutr. Res.* **1972**, *42*, 223–241.
8. Hornig, D.; Gallo-Torres, H. E.; Weiser, H. *Int. J. Vitam. Nutr. Res.* **1972**, *42*, 487–496.
9. Hornig, D.; Weber, F.; Wiss, O. *Int. J. Vitam. Nutr. Res.* **1972**, *42*, 511–523.
10. Ibid., **1974**, *44*, 217–229.
11. Hanck, A. B.; Weiser, H. L. *Int. J. Vitam. Nutr. Res.* **1973**, *43*, 486–493.
12. Kalberer, F.; Rutschmann, J. *Helv. Chim. Acta* **1961**, *44*, 1956–1969.
13. Deutsch, M. J.; Weeks, C. E. J. *J. Assoc. Off. Agr. Chem.* **1965**, *48*, 1248–1256.
14. Zannoni, V.; Lynch, M.; Goldstein, S.; Sato, P. *Biochem. Med.* **1974**, *11*, 41–48.
15. Wagner, J. G. *J. Pharmacokinet. Biopharm.* **1976**, *4*, 443–467.
16. Gillette, J. R. *Ann. N.Y. Acad. Sci.* **1976**, *281*, 136–150.
17. Oie, S.; Tozer, T. N. *J. Pharm. Sci.* **1979**, *68*, 1203–1205.
18. Hornig, D., unpublished data.
19. Orr, J. S.; Gillepsie, F. C. *Science* **1968**, *162*, 138–139.
20. Burns, J. J.; Burch, H. B.; King, C. G. *J. Biol. Chem.* **1951**, *191*, 501–514.
21. Dayton, P. C.; Eisenberg, F., Jr.; Burns, J. J. *Arch. Biochem.* **1959**, *81*, 111–118.
22. Frecker, B. A.; Holloway, D. E.; Rivers, J. M. *Fed. Proc., Fed. Am. Soc. Exp. Biol.* **1979**, *38*, 451.
23. Salomon, L. L. *J .Biol. Chem.* **1957**, *228*, 163–170.
24. Ginter, E.; Zloch, Z.; Cerven, J.; Nemec, R.; Babala, J. *J. Nutr.* **1971**, *101*, 197–204.
25. Fiddick, R.; Heath, H. *Biochim. Biophys. Acta* **1967**, *136*, 206–213.
26. March, S. C.; Tolbert, B. M. *Fed. Proc., Fed. Am. Soc. Exp. Biol.* **1971**, *30*, 521.
27. Willis, R. J.; Kratzing, C. C. *Biochim. Biophys. Acta* **1976**, *444*, 108–117.
28. Lewis, W. H.; Chiang, J. L.; Gross, S. *Arch. Biochem.* **1960**, *89*, 21–26.
29. Roe, J. H.; Itscoitz, S. B. *Proc. Soc. Exp. Biol. Med.* **1963**, *113*, 648–650.
30. Nicola, A. F. DE; Clayman, M.; Johnstone, R. M. *Gen. Comp. Endocrinol.* **1968**, *11*, 332–337.
31. Sharma, S. K.; Johnstone, R. M.; Quastel, J. H. *Biochem. J.* **1964**, *92*, 564–573.
32. Kallner, A.; Hartmann, D.; Hornig, D. *Int. J. Vitam. Nutr. Res.* **1977**, *47*, 383–388.
33. Stevenson, N. R.; Brush, M. K. *Am. J. Clin. Nutr.* **1969**, *22*, 318–326.
34. Stevenson, N. R. *Gastroenterology* **1974**, *67*, 952–956.
35. Hughes, R. E.; Hurley, R. J.; Jones, P. R. *Br. J. Nutr.* **1971**, *26*, 433–438.
36. Salomon, L. L. *J. Nutr.* **1962**, *76*, 493–502.
37. Hornig, D.; Weiser, H.; Weber, F.; Wiss, O. *Int. J. Vitam. Nutr. Res.* **1973**, *43*, 28–33.
38. Reid, E. *Proc. Soc. Exp. Biol. Med.* **1948**, *68*, 403–406.
39. Dayton, P. G.; Snell, M. M.; Perel, J. M. *J. Nutr.* **1966**, *88*, 338–344.

RECEIVED for review January 22, 1981. ACCEPTED May 29, 1981.

Metabolism of L-Ascorbic Acid in the Monkey

STANLEY T. OMAYE—U.S. Department of Agriculture–ARS, Western Regional Research Center, Berkeley, CA 94710

JERRY A. TILLOTSON—Letterman Army Institute of Research, Presidio of San Francisco, CA 94129

HOWERDE E. SAUBERLICH—U.S. Department of Agriculture–ARS, Western Human Nutrition Research Center, Presidio of San Francisco, CA 94129

The functions and fate of L-ascorbic acid in humans and other primates are reviewed in this chapter. Topics included are use of subhuman primates for research in nutrition; evolution and subsequent loss of ascorbic acid biosynthesis; absorption, tissue transport, and distribution of ascorbic acid; and catabolism, functions, and requirements of ascorbic acid. In retrospect, the insight provided by this chapter suggests new work areas of emphasis for developing better understanding of the vitamin's role in human health.

Use of Subhuman Primates for Research in Nutrition

The concept that studies of subhuman primates might provide an insight into the mechanisms of human health and disease led to the initiation of a wide range of investigations. Tremendous advances have occurred through studies of subhuman primates in the fields of infectious and degenerative disorders, toxicology, neurophysiology, space biology, organ transplantations, and behavioral sciences. However, studies of subhuman primates can often be influenced by the same genetic, health, and age-related considerations that made humans unsatisfactory candidates for certain types of investigations. Therefore the value of data from studies of subhuman primates varied with the ability of the researcher to define the health and condition of his experimental animal. In this regard, all investigations that utilize subhuman primates, whether biological or behavioral, must consider the nutritional status of the experimental animal prior to evaluation of any resulting data. Nutrition is well recognized as affecting the rates of growth and maturation, the course of infectious disorders, and the efficiency of healing and repair mechanisms.

Reviews are available that consider the taxonomy of subhuman primates, the diet of selected species in their natural habitats, and some aspects of various nutrient requirements of the monkey (1, 2). Since the 1940s many reports have appeared in which monkeys were fed semipurified diets deficient in individual vitamins. Such reports have greatly clarified the pathophysiology and sequelae of vitamin-deficiency states in humans. However, most of the work associated with the search for essential growth factors was done with other animal species and without the use of subhuman primates. Certainly, relatively few studies have been done on the effects of different levels of various nutrients on any species of subhuman primates. There are reasons to suspect that the optimum diets and requirements of the various primates may differ substantially (3). Types of natural food eaten, size range, and gut morphology emphasize the diversity of primate order. A serious limitation to the establishment of nutrient requirements in primates is the lack of adequate data on growth and development, with the Rhesus monkey and the chimpanzee being the exceptions.

An important problem in determining nutrient requirements and optimum diet is the definition of the criteria of health that must be met. Often relatively short-term assays of requirements based on weight gain, morbidity, and mortality, or the incidences of morphological or biochemical lesions are used as indices to establish optimum nutrition. However, if the subhuman primates are to be used effectively as a model for human nutrition, then we should consider studies into optimum nutrition for a long and vigorous life.

This chapter considers one such nutrient, ascorbic acid; how that nutrient is necessary to the subhuman primate; and how experiments of vitamin C nutrition in the subhuman primate can be extrapolated to humans. We intend to summarize the information available on vitamin C nutrition in the subhuman primate so that now in retrospect we can establish where work should be emphasized in the future.

Evolution and Subsequent Loss of Ascorbic Acid Biosynthesis

Ascorbic acid is biosynthesized from carbohydrate precursors including glucose and galactose by a wide variety of plant and animal species. After scurvy was recognized as a nutritional deficiency disease, humans, other primates, and guinea pigs were thought to be the only animals that are subject to scurvy. It is now recognized that the ability to synthesize ascorbic acid is absent in insects, invertebrates, fishes, and certain bats and birds (4–6). Apparently the biosynthetic capacity started in the kidney of amphibians and reptiles, was transferred to the liver of mammals, and was then lost in guinea pigs, flying mammals, and primates (5). Chatterjee et al. (5) suggested that the early amphibians started ascorbic acid synthesis in the kidney because the vitamin could be produced at high rates. The transition of ascorbic acid synthesis from the kidney of reptiles to the liver of mammals corresponds to when the vertebrates were evolving temperature regulatory mechanisms; the new site would accommodate the problems of life on dry land and the necessities of ion regulation (5, 6). Two other explanations that have been offered for the transition of ascorbic acid synthesis to the liver are that the relatively small kidneys became too crowded with other demands (7), or that mammals needed more ascorbic acid on a total body weight basis than did the reptiles (8) for the detoxification of histamine.

A similar transition in the biosynthetic ability of ascorbic acid was speculated for the evolution of birds (5, 6, 9). Birds are believed to have evolved from a quite different line of reptiles (10). Primitive birds retained the biosynthetic capacity in the kidney, but with the progress of evolution, synthetic capacity is found in the liver of passeriform birds (4, 11). Highly evolved Passeres birds are incapable of producing the vitamin (4).

No requirement for ascorbic acid is known for microbes.

Failure to synthesize ascorbic acid is caused by a common defect, namely the absence of the enzyme L-gulono oxidase (EC 1.1.3.8) (12). This microsomal enzyme is necessary for the terminal step in the conversion of glucose to ascorbic acid (Scheme 1). The absence of the enzyme is caused by a mutation that resulted in the loss of the gene responsible for synthesizing the enzyme. Fortunately this mutation was not lethal because ascorbic acid was present in food of the affected species.

Researchers have questioned whether the one-enzyme-deficiency theory applies to scurvy-prone animals (13). Studies showed no evidence for more than a one enzyme defect in scurvy-prone animals (14). Based on immunologic evidence of purified L-gulono-λ-lactone oxidase, scurvy-prone animals do not contain immunologically cross-reacting material to gulono-λ-lactone oxidase (15, 16).

A few prosimians appear able to synthesize vitamin C from L-1,4-gulonolactone because their need for exogenous ascorbic acid has not been identified (17).

Absorption, Tissue Transport, and Distribution

Absorption of ascorbic acid in the gut is a passive process for the rat (18), while scurvy-prone animals require an active transport system with a Na^+-dependent, gradient-coupled carrier mechanism that is inhibited by ouabain (19, 20). A transport model is favored that fea-

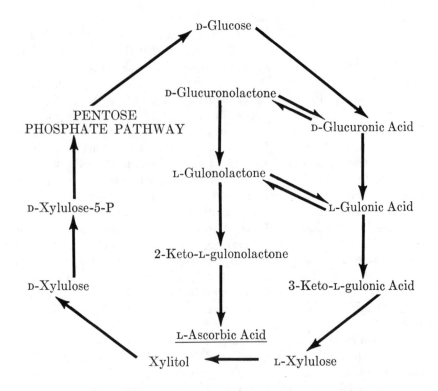

Scheme 1. Pathway for ascorbic acid biosynthesis in animals

tures a carrier-mediated mechanism for simultaneous entry of ascorbic acid and Na^+ across the brush border, similar to the Na^+-gradient mechanism postulated to effect sugar and amino acid transport in mammalian mucosa (21). This seems reasonable because ascorbate resembles sugar compounds in structure. Simple sugars are readily absorbed by active transport and diffusion in the duodenum, jejunum, and ileum depending upon their structure, the amounts of Na^+ and K^+ present, and the presence of other sugars and amino acids. However, despite contrary evidence (22, 23) the proposed minimum requirements for sugars actively transported across the gut wall seem to exclude ascorbic acid. An alternate model of ascorbic acid transport by diffusion would be that ascorbic acid in excess of tissue saturation would not be readily absorbed. Such a model is in line with the general hypothesis (24, 25) that ascorbic acid is readily absorbed when small quantities are ingested; however, there is a limited intestinal absorption when excess amounts of the vitamin are ingested. There is little information regarding the bioavailability of ascorbic acid from foods. The wide occurrence of the vitamin would suggest it would be a nutrient with little bioavailability problem; however, a recent study showed that diets high in hemicellulose enhanced the urinary excretion of ascorbic acid, and diets high in pectin decreased urinary excretion of ascorbic acid in humans (26). Increased urinary excretion of ascorbic acid at constant levels of intake is indicative of either enhanced absorption or decreased need.

The oxidative product of ascorbic acid, dehydroascorbic acid, is the preferred form of the vitamin for uptake by neutrophils, erythrocytes, and lymphocytes (27). Once within the erythrocyte, dehydroascorbic acid is reduced to ascorbic acid by a glutathione-dependent, dehydro-ascorbic-acid-reducing enzyme (20, 28). However, the reduced form of ascorbic acid is found in most other tissues, that is, liver, lungs, kidneys, skin, and pituitary and adrenal glands (20, 29). From these studies, ascorbic acid is taken up by several tissues by an energy-dependent and Na$^+$-sensitive process, but the transport of the oxidized vitamin form follows the principles of diffusion.

Adverse reactions might occur because of antagonism between sugars and ascorbate for transport mechanisms. Hyperglycemia could impair the intracellular availability of vitamin C; therefore, diabetics could suffer vitamin C deficiency with adequate vitamin intake (30–33). Also, ascorbic acid may inhibit glucose uptake by tissues, resulting in hyperglycemia and symptoms of diabetes following the ingestion of large doses of ascorbate. Related to this antagonism between sugars and ascorbate are the findings that diabetics often have elevated serum levels of dehydroascorbic acid (4) and that dehydroascorbic acid has an inhibitory effect on insulin secretion from mouse pancreatic islets (34). The implication from these studies is that the problems associated with diabetics may be related to an inability of the body to use dehydroascorbic acid or that excess dehydroascorbic acid may inhibit the release of insulin.

Ascorbic acid is widely distributed throughout the tissues of the body, both in animals in which synthesis occurs and in animals of the scurvy-prone groups provided an adequate amount of the vitamin in the diet. The largest concentration of the vitamin is in the adrenals and other glandular tissues (35). High levels are also found in the liver, spleen, and brain. Muscle content of ascorbate is relatively low with other tissues intermediate (29). Data on the ascorbic acid content of rodent organs are abundant, but very little data on the vitamin content of human or subhuman primate organs is reported. Recent compiled tables of ascorbic acid content of human organs (29) indicated that the concentration of the vitamin in brain and liver is low compared with glands and secretory organs, but their total combined organ content of ascorbic acid accounts for the major amount of the total body ascorbic acid.

Therefore, the brain and the liver appear to act as storehouses that the body could call upon in deficiency states.

Stress and various hormones markedly influence plasma and tissue levels of ascorbic acid. A decrease of ascorbic acid concentration in the adrenal gland, spleen, and brain of guinea pigs was demonstrated after subjecting the animals to physical stress caused by swimming (36). Cigarette smoke caused a significant reduction of ascorbic acid in guinea pig adrenal glands (37) and human blood (38). Changes in the ascorbic acid concentrations in rat tissues were also observed following hypophysectomy or thyroid treatment (20). The high concentration of ascorbic acid in adrenal glands was reduced by fatigue and stress-related changes. Injections of the pituitary hormone, adrenocorticotropin (ACTH), also deplete the adrenal cortex of ascorbic acid, which suggests that the vitamin plays a role in the synthesis of adrenal hormones as a response to stress. However, research indicates that ascorbate is not necessary for either the synthesis of adrenal hormones, or the mobilization of glucocorticoids or mineral-corticoids (39). Relationships between stress and ascorbate requirements or ascorbate metabolism are discussed elsewhere in this chapter.

More work is needed in this area with increased emphasis placed on the subhuman primate. Little information is available on the uptake, transport, and distribution of ascorbic acid in subhuman primates.

Turnover—Catabolism

In humans the urinary tract is the principal route for the elimination of metabolic products of ascorbic acid. Ascorbic acid is converted to oxalate from the C1 and C2 carbons; some of the vitamin is excreted unchanged. Aside from ascorbate-2-sulfate, little is known about the urinary ascorbic acid metabolites (40). Recently, authors reviewing ascorbic acid metabolism generalized that the catabolism of ascorbic acid to carbon dioxide occurs in the rat, guinea pig, and monkey, but not in humans (6, 20, 41). Such generalizations seem paradoxical because the guinea pig and the monkey, like humans, require ascorbic acid, but the rat does not. The current belief is that the guinea pig catabolizes ascorbic acid extensively to respiratory carbon dioxide. Others have shown that the oxidation of ascorbate to respiratory carbon dioxide is dependent on the dietary intake (42, 43) and stress (43). Ascorbic acid is first oxidized to dehydroascorbic acid by a variety of nonspecific enzymic and nonenzymic reactions. Dehydroascorbic acid is delactonized enzymatically to 2,3-diketogulonate, which is subsequently decarboxylated by a specific decarboxylase or nonenzymatically to carbon dioxide and pentonic acid (Scheme 2). The first reaction is reversible but the

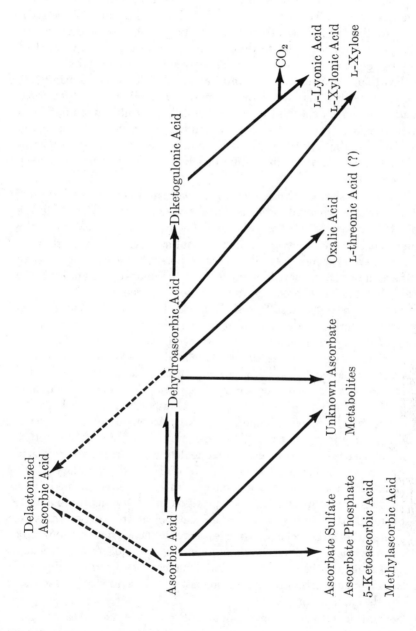

Scheme 2. Ascorbic acid metabolism in animals

other reactions are irreversible. However, this pathway of ascorbate catabolism in the guinea pig seems to be influenced by other factors.

When (1-^{14}C)-ascorbic acid is given orally to the monkey, 20–90% of the label is excreted as respiratory labeled carbon dioxide (20, 44, 45). Therefore, the monkey was thought to catabolize ascorbic acid to carbon dioxide in a manner similar to the guinea pig and that only humans had an alternate pathway. When the label is given to the monkey by iv injection, less than 1% is excreted as respiratory labeled carbon dioxide (20, 44, 45), suggesting that when the vitamin is not subjected to intestinal oxidation, either by the gut or by gut flora, there is little degradation to carbon dioxide. The results of these studies contrasted with an early report where labeled carbon dioxide could be detected after the parenteral (intramuscular) administration of labeled ascorbic acid to monkey (46).

One study showed that oxidation of ascorbate to carbon dioxide was to less than 3% when 20 mg or less of the vitamin was fed orally to the "trained" monkey (47). Trained was defined as, "familiarization of the monkey to all conditions, experimental routine, and personnel prior to the actual experimental period." The purpose of this training was to minimize any stress-related changes that the monkey might undergo because of sudden changes in the animal's environment. In general, stress-related changes result in decreased plasma and tissue concentrations of ascorbic acid and appear to increase the requirement for the vitamin (48–52). The monkey does not synthesize ascorbic acid; therefore, it is logical to presume the stress-related changes in ascorbic acid concentrations are caused at least in part by modification in the catabolism of the vitamin. The reduction of ascorbic degradation to carbon dioxide in the trained monkey suggests that ascorbic acid catabolism is influenced by the adrenal hypophysis axis. Among individual organs, ascorbic acid is found in the highest concentration in the adrenal cortex. Bodily injury or other stress results in a depletion of adrenal ascorbic acid in response to an increased secretion of ACTH by the pituitary gland. The mechanism remains to be defined, but may be explained by a spontaneous, rapid, hydrolytic decomposition of dehydroascorbic acid to 2,3-diketogulonate followed by rapid catabolism to carbon dioxide. Therefore, the stress-related changes may influence endogenous free dehydroascorbic acid tissue levels or reducing mechanisms (glutathione pools) that may be involved in the maintenance of reduced ascorbic acid levels. A similar relationship may also exist in the catabolism of ascorbic acid by the guinea pig (43).

Several investigators have suggested that the identification and quantitation of ascorbic acid metabolites will aid in our understanding the metabolic role of ascorbic acid (47, 53, 54). Ascorbic acid probably functions in more ways than as a hydroxylation cofactor and as a redox agent. Information from the vitamin's metabolites will enable us to understand what those functions might be. In humans, guinea pigs, and monkeys the ascorbic acid metabolites identified in the urine are dehydroascorbic acid (*48, 55, 56*), diketogulonic acid (*55, 56*), ascorbate sulfate (*40, 54*), oxalate (*55, 56*), methyl ascorbate (*57*), and 2-keto-ascorbitol (*58*). Twenty to forty percent of the compounds derived from ascorbic acid in urine have not been identified (*54*). Qualitative and quantitative reported differences in the amounts of metabolites in urine are likely caused by different preparatory and storage procedures, different dietary intake of ascorbate, and, perhaps, stress-related changes in the animals being studied.

The urinary ascorbic acid metabolites of primates were separated by ion exchange resins (*53, 59*). Urine collected from monkeys fed or injected with labeled ascorbic acid resulted in five to six fractions containing carbon-14 on diethylaminoethyl cellulose (*60*). Ascorbic acid, ascorbate sulfate, and oxalate were identified. The percentage of urinary carbon-14 recovered from chromatography was not reported. There was considerable variation in quantitation of the carbon-14 in the different fractions during the 48-h collection period. Others have found that 70–80% of the urinary carbon-14 was recovered in four chromatographic fractions (*59*). Extensive steps were taken to minimize the degradation of ascorbic acid and ascorbate metabolites during urine collection and analysis. Only slight variations were found in the percentages of carbon-14 measured in the four chromatographic fractions during the 30 d following the administration of the label. When 1 mg or less of ascorbic acid was fed to monkeys, ascorbate (17%) and oxalate (40%) were identified as the major carbon-14 urinary metabolites. When 10 mg or more of ascorbic acid was fed to monkeys, ascorbate (75%) was identified as the major carbon-14 urinary metabolite. Ascorbate 2-sulfate was not found as a metabolite using that procedure.

A significant role for ascorbate 2-sulfate seems questionable. Ascorbate 2-sulfate has been found in the urine and tissues of humans, rats, trout, brine shrimp cysts, and others. The sulfate can replace ascorbic acid in fish (*61*), but is not antiscorbutigenic in guinea pigs (*62*) or monkeys (*63*). Ascorbate 2-sulfate is found in high concentrations in brine shrimp cysts and certain tissues of fish, suggestive of some storage function, because in this form, ascorbate should be stable to oxidation. In other species ascorbate 2-sulfate is rapidly eliminated after parenteral administration and is poorly absorbed after oral ingestion. Ascorbate 2-sulfate does not appear to be a sulfating agent· and a biological role for the compound is not known.

2-O-Methylascorbic acid is present in the urine of rats and is likely a minor metabolite, formed by action of the enzyme catechol-O-methyl transferase (*57, 64*).

Functions—Biochemistry

Cholesterol and Triglyceride Metabolism. Hypercholesterolemia and hypertriglyceridemia in guinea pigs fed an ascorbate-free diet is well documented (65–67). In spite of subhuman primate studies, how the information can be extrapolated to humans is uncertain. Ginter et al. (68) concluded that the hypercholesterolemia effect was correlated to the duration of vitamin C deficiency, to the fat component of the diet, to the amount of cholesterol in the diet, and to various experimental parameters (66, 67). To reduce cholesterol values, an increased cholesterol intake must be accompanied by an elevated vitamin C intake (69), because exogenous cholesterol intake will stimulate ascorbate catabolism in the guinea pig (70). Vitamin C also affects cholesterol metabolism in monkeys (71, 72). The initial stress of captivity increased serum cholesterol in baboons (71); however, oral administration of vitamin C tended to lower serum cholesterol (52). These same investigators demonstrated that vitamin C repressed the production rate of cholesterol in vivo and increased the turnover rate of the fast miscible pool, but decreased the removal rate from the slow miscible pool (71). Withdrawal of all dietary vitamin C did not result in a concurrent increase in serum cholesterol. Ginter suggested that the less than dramatic effect of ascorbic on cholesterolemia is less pronounced in the monkey than in guinea pigs, because the lower rate of cholesterol catabolism is compensated in ascorbate-deficient baboons by a marked decrease in endogenous cholesterol synthesis (73). An inverse relationship between ascorbic acid and copper values in guinea pigs and monkeys was reported (74, 75). Further investigations with monkeys showed that the prolonged consumption of high levels of dietary ascorbic acid with marginal dietary copper produced small reductions in serum copper and serum ceruloplasmin, a copper-containing protein. Additional depletion of copper resulted in a gradual but significant ($p < 0.001$) increase in serum cholesterol. The level of ascorbic acid supplementation had no effect during this phase. When copper was added to the diet, serum cholesterol levels leveled off or declined in the monkeys receiving the low dose of ascorbic acid, and continued to increase in the monkeys receiving the higher ascorbic acid supplements. The data indicate that high levels of ascorbic acid supplementation may make dietary copper unavailable for regulating cholesterol metabolism. Such results support the observations of Klevay and suggest that high intakes of ascorbate may result in undesirable side effects (76).

High consumption of ascorbic acid causes the blood triglyceride levels to fall in weanling rats (77), cholesterol-fed rabbits and rats (78), hamsters, monkeys (63, 72, 79), and guinea pigs (67, 80). This hypotriglyceridemic effect of ascorbic acid may be associated with an increase in lipoprotein lipase activity in blood adipose tissues (78, 81, 82). In vitro, ascorbic acid at physiological concentrations strongly inhibits heart and adipose lipoprotein lipase activities (83, 74). Also, a large dose of ascorbate inhibits in vivo lipoprotein lipase (85) in the hearts of baboons and in the livers of guinea pigs (80, 82). However, baboons fed large amounts of vitamin C, when compared to ascorbate-deficient animals, had a higher plasma lipoprotein lipase activity response following the administration of heparin (83). Assuming that lipase is activated by adenosine 3',5'-cyclic monophosphate (cAMP) (86), then it is of interest that ascorbic acid raises the cAMP levels and reduces the guanosine cyclic monophosphate (cGMP) concentrations in baboon plasma (87), offering a possible mechanism of ascorbic acid participation in the regulation of plasma triglycerides in monkeys.

Electron Transport and Microsomal Drug Metabolism.   Ascorbic acid has been implicated in the control of oxido-reduction states of living cells (88–90). Numerous reports indicate that ascorbic acid deficiency decreases the in vitro activity of various drug-metabolizing enzymes in guinea pigs (91–94); however, the exact mechanism has not yet been detected. The assumption that ascorbate participates in the synthesis of the heme part of cytochrome P_{450} (95, 96) is not very feasible because vitamin C deficiency does not affect the activities of the key enzymes involved in heme synthesis (97, 98), and the original studies (95, 96) could not be confirmed by others (98, 100). Ascorbate deficiency was suggested to influence heme catabolism (101); however, the evidence seems contrary (100, 102, 103). The possibility remains that vitamin C deficiency interferes with the synthesis or catabolism of cytochrome P_{450} apoprotein (100, 104). Similar to human studies (105), the ascorbic acid status does not seem to influence the turnover rate of drugs in vivo in monkeys (106); however, ascorbate deficiency in monkeys and some unknown dietary factor impair the induction of o-demethylase and the stimulation of glucuronic acid system by dichlorodiphenyltrichloroethane in vitro (107).

Collagen Metabolism.   The participation of ascorbic acid in the hydroxylation of peptide-bound collagen proline is perhaps the most clearly understood function of vitamin C (108, 109). The work has been extensively studied in guinea pigs and awaits confirmation in primate studies. Addition of ascorbic acid to the granuloma tissue medium prior to incubation with labeled proline stimulates the incorporation of radioactivity into collagen hydroxyproline (110). Such incorporation does not occur when the medium lacks ascorbic acid (111). With purified preparations of the enzyme prolylhydroxylase, molecular oxygen, Fe^{2+}, α-ketoglutarate, and a reducing agent such as ascorbate were found for the hydroxylation of peptide-bound proline (112, 113). Ascorbic acid is also necessary for the activation of prolylhydroxylase, mediated through conformational changes of inactive subunits of the enzyme (114). Collagen extracts prepared from gingival and granulation tissues have a reduced hydroxyproline content in scorbutic Green monkeys (115). Hydroxyproline synthesis was almost totally impaired in the granulation tissue.

Many other biochemical changes that are related to ascorbate status have been observed in the guinea pig and other small animals. Such relationships are discussed elsewhere in this volume. However, these changes have not been considered in subhuman primate experiments.

Requirements

The prevention of scurvy has been accepted by many as the appropriate guideline and criterion for estimating the minimal vitamin C requirements (116). Others suggest that the vitamin C requirement should be an intake that provides optimal health in an organism (116). Since the precise biochemical functions of the vitamin remain obscure, the definition of optimal health remains, for the most part, subjective. Therefore, reported estimates of the ascorbic acid requirements for the monkey vary considerably. In early investigations, weight loss and the detection of clinical signs of scurvy (hemorrhages of the gums, loose teeth, exophthalmos, muscular tenderness, swelling and effusions) were used as indices to establish the ascorbic acid requirements in monkeys as well as humans and guinea pigs. Day (117) concluded that 1–3 mg of ascorbic acid/d was required by a 4-kg monkey, or 0.5–0.7 mg of ascorbic acid/kg of body weight, to prevent scurvy. Others proposed that the monkey required 0.5–0.9 mg of ascorbate/d (118), or 1 mg of ascorbic acid/kg of body weight/d. Chronic ascorbic acid deficiency in monkeys was maintained with 0.25 mg of ascorbate/d and the symptoms of scurvy were reversed with 7.5 mg of ascorbate/kg of body weight (119).

Recently, workers using serum ascorbic acid values as the reference of their estimation of ascorbic acid requirements in monkeys and baboons found that captivity and handling increased the ascorbic acid requirements (51, 52). They concluded that captive monkeys required 20 mg of ascorbic acid/d in addition to fruit supplements. No differences were measured in the response of serum ascorbic acid after supplementations of 5 or 10 mg of ascorbic acid/kg of body weight/d in the baboon.

Other investigators have found larger amounts of ascorbic acid were necessary to maintain normal concentrations of the vitamin in blood. For monkeys, 10 (63) and 25 (35) mg of ascorbic acid/kg of body weight were proposed as the minimum required amounts. Recent experiments showed that the trained monkey required only 3–6 mg of ascorbate/kg of body weight (120). Young monkeys (sexually immature) required twice the amount of dietary ascorbate than did older monkeys to maintain similar plasma ascorbate levels. This study (120) implied that untrained animals may metabolize more of the ascorbate to an alternate pathway under stress conditions.

Caution must be exercised in the use of blood ascorbic acid as an index to ascorbate status because of the well-documented influence of stress-related changes in ascorbic acid content of tissues especially plasma and serum (48, 51, 52). Generally, estimates of vitamin C status are obtained by measuring concentrations of the vitamin in serum, whole blood, leukocytes, or urine (121). These measurements are assumed to reflect the tissue levels and body pool size of the vitamin. Certain limitations are encountered in the use of each of these fluid parameters. Serum or plasma ascorbic acid concentrations are usually more reflective of recent intakes than of total body stores (120, 121) and could reflect the results of ascorbic acid redistribution after stress-related influences. Whole blood ascorbic acid concentrations reflect loss of body stores only until a certain degree of deficiency is reached. This was demonstrated by the work of Baker et al. (122), which showed that the relationship between whole blood levels of ascorbic acid and ascorbate body pool size exists only when the body pool was in excess of 300 mg (about 20% saturation). The use of urinary levels of ascorbic acid has limited value, and reflects the results of ascorbate degradation (59, 123). Urinary ascorbate values reflect recent dietary intakes of the vitamin. Leukocyte ascorbic acid levels are used rather infrequently because obtaining these values is more technically difficult and time-consuming than the other methods. However, it is generally considered that leukocyte ascorbic acid concentrations provide a better reflection of tissue stores than do other techniques. This belief is based largely on observations that leukocyte ascorbate levels drop slowly during ascorbate deficiency, reaching zero just before the onset of clinical symptoms of scurvy (124); that leukocyte ascorbate levels correlate well with ascorbic acid retention on diets with a fixed inadequate level of ascorbic acid (125); and that studies correlating plasma ascorbic acid levels with leukocyte ascorbate levels reflect the metabolic turnover rate of the vitamin (126–128). Conclusive evidence was obtained in the female Rhesus monkey that demonstrated a high correlation of leukocyte ascorbic acid levels with liver ascorbic acid levels and with the total body pool of ascorbic acid, especially at low plasma values of ascorbate (129).

The effectiveness of pharmacological levels of ascorbic acid remains controversial. The proponents base their argument on levels of ascorbate consumed in the wild by monkeys and the rate of ascorbate synthesized by nonrequiring species. Pauling pointed out that greenstuffs eaten by the gorilla provide about 4.5 g of ascorbic acid/d (130, 131). He extrapolates that if a rat synthesizes ascorbic acid at a rate of 26–58 mg/kg of body weight/d, this would correspond to 1.8–4.1 g/d for a 70-kg human. Arguments against the usefulness of high intakes of ascorbic acid point out the following.

1. In humans there is a Na^+-dependent active transport system with a K_m of about 1 mM. Absorption is very efficient at low intakes of ascorbic acid and becomes poor as stomach levels of ascorbic acid increase. The upper level of ascorbic acid in the blood is limited by kidney clearance with T_m of 1.5 mg/100 mL. Where intestinal absorption is excessive the efficiency of the kidney clearance improves. Transfer of ascorbic acid into the central nervous system and other tissues is a facilitated saturable process. Therefore, control at all levels appears to sharply limit maximum levels of ascorbate in tissues.
2. The direct extrapolations from animals that synthesize ascorbic acid to a 70-kg human ignores the observations that in large animals the synthesis of ascorbic acid only accounts for a small fraction of the L-gulonate oxidized (132). Also, extrapolation to 70 kg of body weight should first correct for differences in metabolic body size; the correction should include ($wt_{kg}^{3/4}$), which is appropriate in many instances (133).

When these two points were considered (134), values of 50–300 mg of ascorbic acid/d were calculated for a 70-kg human, but never were there calculated values exceeding 1 g of ascorbate/d/70 kg.

Comments

Many beneficial claims have been made for ascorbic acid, especially for the intake of ascorbic acid far in excess of that required to prevent scurvy. Whether vitamin C will increase resistance to disease, promote better health, or even cure certain diseases remains to be determined. The practical dietary advice offered depends upon how well the mode of action of this vitamin is understood, and understanding this mode of action in turn depends on how similar the model system used is to humans.

A major difficulty has been the selection of appropriate experimental models. All animals (species) do not respond in the same manner and in most instances doubt exists as to which species is the most appropriate. Long-term studies with nutritional modifications are next to impossible in humans, and epidemiologic conclusions will always be confused because there is no way to disregard the influence of modifications in lifestyle on the study of various dietary factors. Therefore, unless more attention is paid to the experimental animal used, the desired answers will be impossible to obtain. Questions about the etiology of diseases at the biochemical–physiological level and their prevention need answers. The subhuman primate physiology is different from human physiology; therefore, some comparative physiology and nutrition must be done to define the functional differences. At least then, the experimenter will be aware of the limitations of his experimental model.

Acknowledgments

The opinions or assertions contained herein are the private views of the authors and are not to be construed as official or as reflecting the views of the Department of the Army or the Department of Defense or U.S. Department of Agriculture.

Literature Cited

1. Kerr, G. R. *Physiol. Rev.* **1972**, *52*, 415.
2. Portman, O. W. *Nutr. Requir. Domest. Anim., n10, 2nd ed.* **1972**, 29.
3. Harris, R. S. "Feeding and Nutrition of Nonhuman Primates;" Academic: New York, 1970.
4. Chaudhuri, C. R.; Chatterjee, I. B. *Science* **1969**, *164*, 435.
5. Chatterjee, I. B.; Majumder, A. K.; Nandi, B. K.; Subramanian, N. *Ann. N.Y. Acad. Sci.* **1975**, *258*, 24.
6. Chatterjee, I. B. *World Rev. Nutr. Diet.* **1978**, *30*, 69.
7. Stone, I. *Am. J. Phys. Anthropol.* **1965**, *23*, 83.
8. Chatterjee, I. B. *Science* **1973**, *182*, 1271.
9. Halver, J. E.; Ashley, L. M.; Smith, R. R. *Trans. Am. Fish. Soc.* **1969**, 98, 762.
10. Romer, A. S. "The Procession of Life"; World: Cleveland, 1968; p. 1.
11. Roy, R. N.; Guha, B. C. *Nature* **1958**, *182*, 319.
12. Burns, J. J. *Nature* **1957**, *180*, 553.
13. Chatterjee, I. B.; Kar, N. C.; Ghosh, N. C.; Guha, B. C. *Nature* **1961**, *192*, 163.
14. Sato, P.; Nishikimi, M.; Udenfriend, S. *Biochem. Biophys. Res. Commun.* **1976**, *71*, 293.
15. Nishikimi, M.; Udenfriend, S. *Proc. Natl. Acad. Sci.* **1976**, *73*, 2066.
16. Sato, P.; Udenfriend, S. *Arch. Biochem. Biophys.* **1978**, *187*, 158.
17. Yess, N.; Hegsted, D. M. *Nature* **1966**, *212*, 739.
18. Spencer, R. P.; Purdy, S.; Hoeldtke, R.; Bow, T. M.; Markulis, M. A. *Gastroenterology* **1963**, *44*, 768.
19. Stevenson, N. R.; Brush, M. K. *Am. J. Clin. Nutr.* **1969**, *22*, 318.
20. Hornig, D. *World Rev. Nutr. Diet* **1975**, *23*, 225.
21. Mellors, A. L.; Nahrwold, D. L.; Rose, R. C. *Am. J. Physiol.* **1977**, *233*, E374.
22. Rose, R. C.; Nahrwold, D. L. *Int. J. Vitam. Nutr. Res.* **1978**, *48*, 382.
23. Stevenson, N. R. *Gastroenterology* **1974**, *67*, 952.
24. Nelson, E. W.; Lane, H.; Fabri, P. J.; Scott, B. *J. Clin. Pharmacol.* **1978**, *18*, 325.
25. Mayerson, M. *Eur. J. Pharmacol.* **1972**, *19*, 140.
26. Keltz, F. R.; Kies, C.; Fox, H. M. *Am. J. Clin. Nutr.* **1978**, *31*, 1167.
27. Bigley, R. H.; Stankova, L. *J. Exp. Med.* **1974**, *139*, 1084.
28. Hughes, R. E. *Nature* **1964**, *203*, 1068.
29. Hornig, D. *Ann. N.Y. Acad. Sci.* **1975**, *258*, 103.

30. Mann, G. V.; Newton, P. *Ann. N.Y. Acad. Sci.* **1975**, *285*, 243.
31. Mann, G. V. *Perspect. Biol. Med.* **1974**, *17*, 210.
32. Sherry, S.; Ralli, E. P. *J. Clin. Invest.* **1948**, *27*, 217.
33. Sarji, K. E.; Kleinfelder, J.; Brewington, P.; Gonzalez, J.; Hempling, H.; Colwell, J. A. *Thromb. Res.* **1979**, *15*, 639.
34. Pence, L. A.; Mennear, J. H. *Toxicol. Appl. Pharmacol.* **1979**, *50*, 57.
35. Kuether, C. A.; Telford, I. R.; Roe, J. H. *J. Nutr.* **1944**, *28*, 347.
36. Hughes, R. E.; Jones, P. R.; Williams, R. S.; Wright, P. F. *Life Sci.* **1971**, *10*, 661.
37. Hughes, R. E.; Jones, P. R.; Nicholas, P. *J. Pharm. Pharmacol.* **1970**, *22*, 823.
38. Pelletier, O. *Ann. N.Y. Acad. Sci.* **1975**, *258*, 156.
39. Kitubachi, A. E.; West, W. H. *Ann. N.Y. Acad. Sci.* **1975**, *258*, 922.
40. Baker, E. M.; Hammer, D. C.; March, S. C.; Tolbert, B. M.; Canham, J. E. *Science* **1971**, *173*, 826.
41. Hornig, D. "Vitamin C", Birch, G. G.; Parker, K. J., Eds.; John Wiley & Sons: New York, 1974; p. 91.
42. Salomon, L. L. *J. Nutr.* **1962**, *76*, 493.
43. Tillotson, J. A. *Nutr. Rep. Int.* **1980**, *22*, 555.
44. Johnson, D. O.; Joyce, B. E.; Bucci, T. J. *Fed. Proc., Fed. Am. Soc. Exp. Biol.* **1975**, *34*, 883.
45. Bucci, T. J.; Johnsen, D. O.; Baker, E.; Canham, J. E. *Fed. Proc., Fed. Am. Soc. Exp. Biol.* **1975**, *34*, 883.
46. Abt, A. F.; Von Schushing, S.; Enns, T. *Nature* **1962**, *193*, 1178.
47. Tillotson, J. A. *Int. J. Vitam. Nutr. Res.* **1978**, *48*, 374.
48. Baker, E. *Am. J. Clin. Nutr.* **1967**, *20*, 583.
49. Boddy, K.; Hume, R.; King, P. C.; Weyers, E.; Rowan, T. *Clin. Sci. Mol. Med.* **1974**, *46*, 449.
50. Irwin, M. S.; Hutchins, B. K. *J. Nutr.* **1976**, *106*, 823.
51. De Klerk, W. A.; DuPlessis, J. P.; Van Der Watt, J. J.; Dejager, A.; Lauhscher, N. F. *S. Afr. Med. J.* **1973**, *47*, 705.
52. De Klerk, W. A.; Kotze, J. P.; Weight, M. J.; Menne, I. V.; Matthews, M. J. A.; MacDonald, T. *S. Afr. Med. J.* **1973**, *47*, 1503.
53. Baker, E. M.; Halver, J. E.; Johnson, D. O.; Joyce, B. E.; Knight, M. K.; Tolbert, B. M. *Ann. N.Y. Acad. Sci.* **1975**, *258*, 72.
54. Tolbert, B. M.; Downing, M.; Carlson, R. W.; Knight, M. K.; Baker, E. M. *Ann. N.Y. Acad. Sci.* **1975**, *258*, 48.
55. Baker, E. M.; Saar, J. C.; Tolbert, B. M. *Am. J. Clin. Nutr.* **1966**, *19*, 371.
56. Hellman, L.; Burns, J. J. *J. Biol. Chem.* **1958**, *230*, 923
57. Blaschke, E.; Hetting, G. *Biochem. Pharmacol.* **1977**, *20*, 1363.
58. Tolbert, B. M.; Ward, J. B., Chap. 5 in this book.
59. Tillotson, J. A.; O'Connor, R. J.; McGown, E. L. *Fed Proc., Fed. Am. Soc. Exp. Biol.* **1980**, *39*, 1538.
60. Knight, M. K., M.S. thesis, University of Colorado, 1974.
61. Halver, J. E.; Smith, R. R.; Tolbert, B. M.; Baker, E. M. *Ann. N.Y. Acad. Sci.* **1975**, *258*, 81.
62. Kuenzig, W.; Avenia, R.; Kamm, J. *J. Nutr.* **1974**, *104*, 952.
63. Machlin, L. J.; Garcia, F.; Kuenzig, W.; Richter, C. B.; Spiegel, H. E.; Brin, M. *Am. J. Clin. Nutr.* **1976**, *29*, 825.
64. Tolbert, B. M.; Harkrader, R. J.; Johnsen, P. O.; Joyce, B. A. *Biochem. Biophysic. Res. Commun.* **1976**, *71*, 1004.
65. Hornig, D.; Weiser, H. *Experientia* **1976**, *32*, 687.
66. Ginter, E. *Adv. Lipid Res.* **1978**, *16*, 167.
67. Ginter, E. *World Rev. Nutr. Diet.* **1979**, *33*, 104.
68. Ginter, E.; Babala, J.; Cerven, J. *J. Atheroscler. Res.* **1969**, *10*, 341.
69. Weiser, H.; Hanck, A.; Hornig, D. *Nutr. Metab.* **1976**, *20*, 206.
70. Ginter, E.; Zloch, Z. *Int. J. Vitam. Nutr. Res.* **1972**, *42*, 72.

71. Kotze, J. P.; Weight, M. J.; de Klerk, W. A.; Menne, I. V.; Weight, M. J. A. *S. Afr. Med. J.* **1974**, *48*, 1182.
72. Kotze, J. P.; Menne, I. V.; Spies, J. H.; de Klerk, W. A. *S. Afr. Med. J.* **1975**, *49*, 906.
73. Weight, M. J.; Kotze, J. P.; de Klerk, W. A.; Weight, N. *Int. J. Biochem.* **1974**, *5*, 287.
74. Milne, D. B.; Omaye, S. T. *Int. J. Vitam. Nutr. Res.* **1980**, *50*, 301.
75. Milne, D. B.; Omaye, S. T.; Amos, W. H. *Fed. Proc., Fed. Am. Soc. Exp. Biol.* **1978**, *37*, 1256.
76. Klevay, L. M. *Proc. Soc. Exp. Biol. Med.* **1976**, *151*, 579.
77. Nambisan, B.; Kurup, P. A. *Atherosclerosis* **1974**, *19*, 191.
78. Sokoloff, B.; Hori, M.; Saelhof, C.; McConnel, B.; Imai, T. *J. Nutr.* **1967**, *91*, 107.
79. Ginter, E.; Cerna, O.; Ondreicka, R,; Roch, V.; Balez, V. *Food Chem.* **1976**, *1*, 23.
80. Nambisan, B.; Kurup, P. A. *Atherosclerosis* **1975**, *22*, 447.
81. Fujinami, T.; Okado, K.; Senda, K.; Sugimura, M.; Kishikawa, M. *Jpn. Circ. J.* **1971**, *35*, 1559.
82. Kamuth, S. K.; Tang, J. M.; Bramaute, P. O. *Fed. Proc., Fed. Am. Soc. Exp. Biol.* **1977**, *36*, 114.
83. Kotze, J. P.; Spies, J. H. *S. Afr. Med. J.* **1976**, *50*, 1760.
84. Tsai, S.; Fales, H. M.; Vaughan, M. *J. Biol. Chem.* **1973**, *248*, 5278.
85. Kotze, J. P.; Matthews, M. J. A.; De Klerk, W. A. *S. Afr. Med. J.* **1974**, *48*, 511.
86. Hynie, S.; Cernohorsky, M.; Cepelik, J. *Eur. J. Pharmacol.* **1970**, *10*, 111.
87. Van Wyk, C. P.; Kotze, J. P. *S. Afr. J. Sci.* **1975**, *71*, 28.
88. Staudinger, H.; Krisch, K.; Leonhauser, S. *Ann. N.Y. Acad. Sci.* **1961**, *92*, 195.
89. Weis, W. *Ann. N.Y. Acad. Sci.* **1975**, *258*, 190.
90. Bielski, B. H. J.; Richter, H. W.; Chan, P. C. *Ann. N.Y. Acad. Sci.* **1975**, *258*, 231.
91. Richards, R. K.; Keuter, K.; Klatt, T. J. *Proc. Soc. Exp. Biol. Med.* **1941**, *48*, 403.
92. Axelrod, J.; Udenfriend, S.; Brodie, B. B. *J. Pharmacol. Exp. Ther.* **1954**, *111*, 176.
93. Conney, A. H.; Bray, G. A.; Evans, G.; Burns, J. J. *Ann. N.Y. Acad. Sci.* **1961**, *92*, 115.
94. Degkwitz, E.; Staudinger, H. *Hoppe-Seyler's Z. Physiol. Chem.* **1965**, *342*, 62.
95. Degwitz, E.; Kim, K. S. *Hoppe-Seyler's Z. Physiol. Chem.* **1973**, *354*.
96. Luft, D.; Degkwitz, E.; Hochli-Kanfmann, L.; Staudinger, H. *Hoppe-Seyler's Z. Physiol. Chem.* **1972**, *353*, 1420.
97. Rikans, L. E.; Smith, C. R.; Zannoni, V. G. *Biochem. Pharmacol.* **1977**, *26*, 797.
98. Zannoni, V. G.; Smith, C. R.; Rikans, L. E. "Re-evaluation of Vitamin C", Hanck, A.; Ritzel, G., Eds.; Verlag Hans Huber Bern Stattgard Wien: Switzerland, 1977; p. 99.
99. Turnbull, J. D.; Omaye, S. T. *Biochem. Pharmacol.* **1980**, *29*, 1255.
100. Omaye, S. T.; Turnbull, J. D. *Life Sci.* **1980**, *27*, 441.
101. Walsch, S.; Degkwitz, E. *Hoppe-Seyler's Z. Physiol. Chem.* **1980**, *361*, 79.
102. Omaye, S. T.; Turnbull, J. D. *Biochem. Pharmacol.* **1979**, *28*, 1415.
103. Ibid., 3651.
104. Rikans, L. E.; Smith, C. R.; Zannoni, V. G. *J. Pharmacol. Exp. Ther.* **1978**, *204*, 702.
105. Wilson, J. T.; Van Boxtel, C. J.; Alvan, G.; Sjoqvist, F. *J. Clin. Pharmacol.* **1976**, *16*, 265.

106. Omaye, S. T.; Green, M. D.; Turnbull, J. D.; Amos, W. H.; Sauberlich, H. E. *J. Clin. Pharmacol.* **1980**, *20*, 172.
107. Chadwick, R. W.; Cranmer, M. F.; Peoples, A. J. *Toxicol. Appl. Pharmacol.* **1977**, *20*, 308.
108. Barnes, M. J. *Ann. N.Y. Acad. Sci.* **1975**, *258*, 264.
109. Myllyla, R., Kuiitti-Savolainen, E.-R.; Kivirikko, K. I. *Biochem. Biophys. Res. Commun.* **1978**, *83*, 441.
110. Manning, J. M.; Meister, A. *Biochemistry* **1966**, *5*, 1154.
111. Stone, N.; Meister, A. *Nature* **1962**, *194*, 555.
112. Cardinale, G. L.; Rhoads, R. E.; Udenfriend, S. *Biochem. Biophys. Res. Commun.* **1971**, *43*, 537.
113. Levene, C. I.; Aleo, J. J.; Prynne, C. J.; Bates, C. J. *Biochem. Biophys. Res. Commun.* **1971**, *43*, 537.
114. Berg, R. A.; Prockop, D. J. *J. Biol. Chem.* **1973**, *248*, 1175.
115. Ostergaard, E.; Loe, H. *J. Periodontal Res.* **1975**, *10*, 103.
116. "Recommended Dietary Allwances," *N.A.S.* **1974**.
117. Day, P. L. *Vitam. Horm. (N.Y.)* **1944**, *2*, 71.
118. Abt, A. F.; Van Schuching, S.; Enns, T. *Nature* **1962**, *193*, 1178.
119. Shaw, J. HJ.; Phillips, P. H.; Elvehjem, C. A. *J. Nutr.* **1945**, *29*, 356.
120. Tillotson, J. A.; O'Connor, R. J. *Int. J. Vitam. Nutr. Res.* **1980**, *50*, 171.
121. Sauberlich, H. E.; Dowdy, R. P.; Skala, J. H. "Laboratory Tests for the Assessment of Nutritional Status," CRC: Cleveland, 1974.
122. Baker, E. M.; Hodges, R. E.; Hood, J.; Sauberlich, H. E.; March, S. C.; Canham, J. E. *Am. J. Clin. Nutr.* **1971**, *24*, 444.
123. Hodges, R. E.; Baker, E. M.; Hood, J.; Sauberlich, H. E.; March, S. C. *Am. J. Clin. Nutr.* **1969**, *27*, 535.
124. Crandon, J. E.; Lund, C. C.; Dill, D. B. *N. Engl. J. Med.* **1960**, *223*, 353.
125. Lowry, O. H.; Bessey, O. A.; Brock, M. J.; Lopez, J. A. *J. Biol. Chem.* **1946**, *166*, 111.
126. Loh, H. S. *Int. J. Vitam. Nutr. Res.* **1972**, *42*, 80.
127. Ibid., *48*, 86.
128. Loh, H. S.; Wilson, C. W. M. *Br. Med. J.* **1971**, *3*, 733.
129. Omaye, S. T.; Turnbull, J. D.; Sudduth, J. H.; Sauberlich, H. E. *Fed. Proc., Fed. Am. Soc. Exp. Biol.* **1980**, *39*, 796.
130. Pauling, L. *Proc. Natl. Acad. Sci.* **1970**, *67*, 1643.
131. Ibid., **1974**, *61*, 4442.
132. Burns, J. J.; Conney, A. H. "Glucuronic Acid"; Dutton, G. J., Ed.; Academic: New York, 1966.
133. Klieber, M. "The Fire of Life"; John Wiley & Sons: New York, 1976.
134. Rucker, R. B.; Dubick, M. A.; Mouritsen, J. *Am. J. Clin. Nutr.* **1980**, *33*, 961.

RECEIVED for review January 22, 1981. ACCEPTED April 30, 1981.

Kinetics of Ascorbic Acid in Humans

A. KALLNER, D. HARTMANN,[1] and D. HORNIG[2]

Karolinska Institutet, Department of Clinical Chemistry,
S-104 01 Stockholm, Sweden

Kinetic parameters were estimated in nonsmokers and smokers to help elucidate the quantitative ascorbate metabolism in humans. This approach allows calculation of turnover rates at different levels of steady state intakes of ascorbate. Metabolic and renal turnovers were calculated separately. At plasma levels above about 0.7 mg/100 mL the renal elimination increased sharply and the metabolic turnover showed a saturation at a plasma level corresponding to a total turnover of about 60 mg/d. At the tested levels of intake of ascorbic acid the calculated total pool size increased to a level reached at a steady state plasma concentration achieved at an intake of about 90 mg/d. At intakes of this magnitude the absorption is substantially less than 100%. A daily intake of 100 mg of ascorbate for larger populations should be attained. Similar experiments with smokers showed an increase in the metabolic turnover corresponding to a demand of 140 mg/d to reach a similar stage.

Scurvy is the ultimate result of ascorbic acid deficiency. Untreated, this disease leads to a painful death with a multitude of symptoms, such as weakness, profuse bleeding from mucous membranes and infections, loss of teeth, and symptoms from joints and ligaments. In modern communities this condition should not be seen and even mild scurvy should be extremely rare. During recent years it has been questioned if ascorbate in very high doses might be beneficial to humans. Today, it is

[1] Current address: Biological Pharmaceutical Research Department, F. Hoffmann-La Roche & Co., Ltd., CH-4002, Basle, Switzerland.
[2] Current address: Department of Vitamin & Nutrition Research, F. Hoffmann-La Roche Co., Ltd., CH-4002, Basle, Switzerland.

relevant to discuss optimal instead of minimal intakes. The apparent nontoxicity of ascorbate makes it ethically and physiologically acceptable to argue for megadose intakes of this compound, although the benefits thereof may not yet be finally settled.

For several years the recommended dietary allowance (RDA) of vitamin C has varied from country to country. It was recently increased from 45 to 60 mg/d in the United States (1). Probably, healthy people in their active ages normally ingest this and even larger amounts through their dietary habits, whereas elderly people, diseased people, or people under special circumstances like alcoholics may be at an actual risk and need supplementation to meet the basal needs for the vitamin.

Transferring results of studies of the metabolic role and fate of ascorbate in animal experiments to humans is limited because most animals are able to synthesize their need of ascorbate endogenously and in those animals where ascorbate is a vitamin (e.g., the guinea pig), the metabolism of ascorbate differs from that in humans. Estimation of human needs will therefore have to be derived from experiments with humans.

Early Accounts of Scurvy

A large documentation on scurvy has been accumulated during the centuries. Some relevant reports, which contain kinetic information on the development of ascorbate deficiency, will be reviewed briefly. The first well-known, detailed, and comprehensive report on this disease, "Treatise on Scurvy," was published in 1757 by the Scottish naval physician James Lind (2). Some case reports are cited here. Thus, during the journey of H.M.S. *Salisbury* from August 10 to October 28, 1746 (i.e., 75 d), only one sailor was reported ill with the disease. In a report of four ships bound for the East Indies, 105 out of 424 sailors were reported dead from scurvy within 4 months. Other fragmentary notes are official reports by the Danish and Dutch East India Companies of regular outbreaks of the disease after 5–6 months at sea. This was in the seventeenth century.

Another interesting source of information is the famous report from the Danish dicoverer Jens Munk who had to stay the winter in Hudson Bay in the 1620s. In 9 months all but 3 out of about 400 sailors died, mainly from scurvy. Every case was reported by the captain (who was among those surviving) and the first case appeared around Christmas or about 3 months after the ships had been caught by the ice.

This information indicates that depletion of the ascorbate pools to a level causing scurvy takes 2–4 months, but some people may survive longer. In retrospect one may assume that the survivors had access to additional dietary sources.

Ascorbic Acid Kinetics in Humans

Experimental approaches to human requirements of ascorbate can be made using kinetic methods; the most obvious method is to perform depletion and repletion studies. Experimentation with depletion of a nutrient in human beings is difficult, but our fundamental knowledge about ascorbate kinetics in humans has been achieved through such studies.

In the late 1960s and early 1970s Baker and coworkers (3–5) found that an almost complete depletion of the ascorbate pools of their six participating subjects occurred in 100–130 d. At this time, signs and symptoms of scurvy also occurred. The decrease of ascorbate pools followed an exponential path and showed a relative decrease of about 3%/d, corresponding to a half-life of about 60 d. The signs and symptoms of scurvy occurred at a body pool of about 300 mg of ascorbate. On repletion, ingested ascorbate was excreted in urine when the pool had reached about 1500 mg. Baker and his group stated that a daily intake of 45 mg (3% of 1500 mg) would maintain this pool size. This amount also became the official RDA in the United States for several years. Retrospectively, the calculations were made on observations during a depleted stage, therefore the relative decrease of the ascorbate pool in comparison with a normal ascorbate status may have been underestimated. In agreement with this underestimation, the half-life would have been overestimated and the minimum dosage to retain balance consequently would have been underestimated.

Alternatively, studies based on steady state kinetics of physiological intakes can be performed. Such studies require that the subject be equilibrated on a certain level of intake of the compound to be studied. After equilibration, a radioactive tracer dose of the compound under consideration is given. The distribution of the labeled compound in the body is studied as well as its elimination.

Thus volunteers can be subjected to intakes of various magnitudes, and in our study (6) healthy, male, nonsmoking volunteers were equilibrated on four different levels of intakes of ascorbate. The levels studied were 30, 60, 90, and 180 mg/d. These amounts are below, at, and above the presently recommended dosages, but all may be regarded as physiological in the sense that the main part of the population probably has intakes of these magnitudes. The experiments were ended 2 weeks after administration of the ^{14}C-labeled ascorbate by giving large doses (2–4 $\times$ 500 mg) of ascorbate to "wash out" the label. This washout prevents an unnecessary exposure to radioactivity and improves the accuracy of the estimation of the absorbed amount of radioactivity.

The kinetic approach requires choosing a mathematical model that can be fitted to the experimental data. A properly chosen model will allow calculation of turnover of metabolic and excretional pools. Further, one can calculate the various pool sizes. However, the model is nothing but a model and does not necessarily have any resemblance to physiological or medical circumstances.

The decay pattern of plasma radioactivity (Figure 1) indicated that a three-compartment model could be chosen for calculation of the kinetic data. The chosen model consists of a central compartment (Figure 2) into which dietary ascorbate is absorbed and from which it is eliminated unchanged. Two other compartments are equilibrated with the central compartment. In compartment 2 the metabolism is assumed to take place and from this compartment metabolites are eliminated. Compartment 3 is a deep pool that acts as a storage compartment.

During the experiment the participants limited their dietary intake of ascorbate, particularly by avoiding fresh vegetables, canned food, and other nutrients known to have a high ascorbate content (e.g., potatoes). The participants were administered specially prepared capsules of ascorbate several times during the day to achieve an even administration of doses. The recommended diet undoubtedly limits the intake, but particularly at the lower dosages, relatively substantial amounts of ascorbate may be ingested. The nominal intakes (30, 60, 90, and 180 mg/d) therefore may not be the actual intakes; accordingly we have made all correlations to a total turnover estimated from the plasma decay curves rather than to the administered amounts. The relationship of total turnover to plasma level is shown in Figure 3. In this diagram we have also plotted literature data where plasma concentrations have been measured at well-controlled intakes. There is good agreement between the data of our study and that of the literature. In this range, the plasma level of ascorbate can be considered a good indicator of the total turnover.

The model used allows the calculation of the total body pool. As shown in Table I, the total body pool varies with ascorbate intake and ranges between about 10 and 20 mg/kg body weight.

The ascorbate is assumed to be filtered in the glomeruli and reabsorbed in the renal tubuli. The renal turnover suddenly increases at a certain plasma level (Figure 4), indicating a threshold value at which the tubular absorption is exceeded by the glomerular filtration. The renal

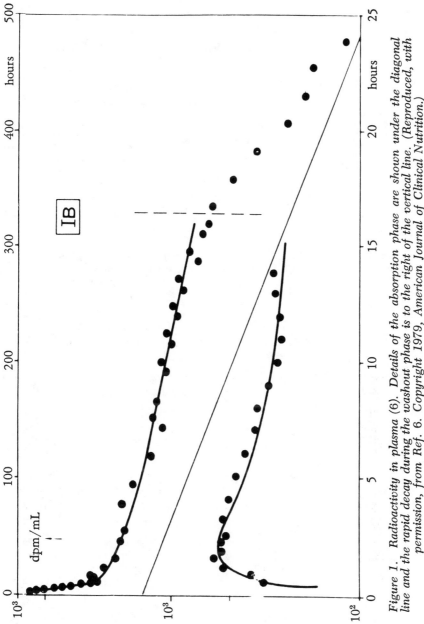

Figure 1. *Radioactivity in plasma (6). Details of the absorption phase are shown under the diagonal line and the rapid decay during the washout phase is to the right of the vertical line. (Reproduced, with permission, from Ref. 6. Copyright 1979, American Journal of Clinical Nutrition.)*

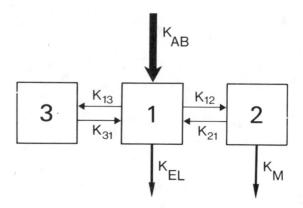

Figure 2. A schematic of the model (6). (Reproduced, with permission, from Ref. 6. Copyright 1979, American Journal of Clinical Nutrition.)

Table I. Concentration of Plasma Ascorbate, Calculated Total Pool, and Half-Lives in the Groups Given Different Amounts of Ascorbate

Dosage (mg/d)	Plasma Ascorbate (mg/100 mL)	Total Pool (mg/kg body weight)	$T_{1/2}$ (d)
1 × 30	0.24	11.4	40.1
1 × 30	0.52	—	16.5
1 × 30	0.41	13.7	28.9
1 × 30	0.72	19.6	26.5
2 × 30	0.78	20.7	27.0
2 × 30	0.73	17.0	23.1
2 × 30	0.79	15.2	25.8
2 × 45	0.83	14.7	9.1
2 × 45	0.80	16.4	12.6
2 × 45	0.98	12.6	17.0
4 × 45	1.12	21.6	12.8
4 × 45	1.15	—	12.7
4 × 45	0.95	19.3	7.9
4 × 45	1.16	20.0	10.5

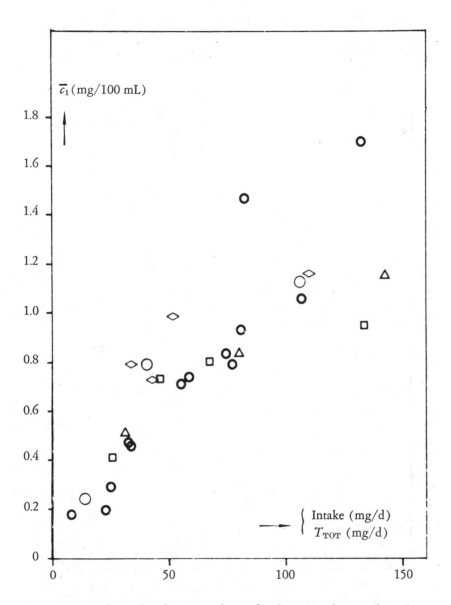

Figure 3. Relationship between plasma level of ascorbate and intake turnover (bold symbols), and plasma level of ascorbate and total turnover (fine symbols). Data on intakes are literature data (6).

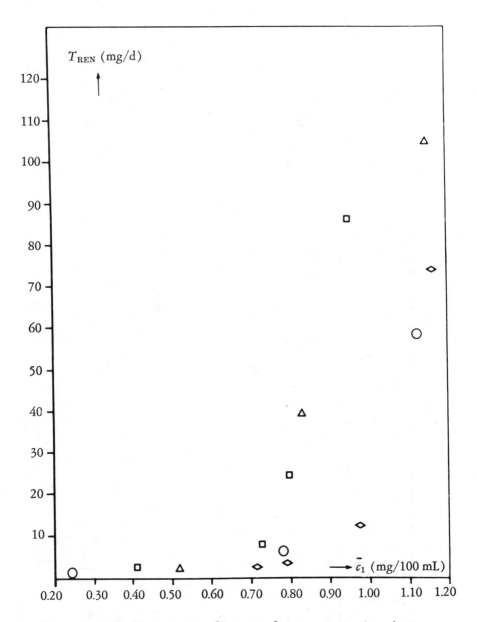

Figure 4.   Renal turnover in relation to plasma concentration of ascorbate (6). (Reproduced, with permission, from Ref. 6. Copyright 1979, American Journal of Clinical Nutrition.)

threshold occurs around a plasma concentration of about 0.7–0.8 mg/100 mL or a total turnover of about 60 mg/d. However, in subjects with low ascorbate intake (1×30 mg/d), a certain amount of unchanged ascorbate is already excreted in the urine (Table II).

Table II. Unchanged Ascorbate Recovered from Urine, in Relation to Total Amount of Radioactivity in the Urine, at Various Levels of Oral Intake

Dosage (mg/d)	n	^{14}C-Ascorbate (%)	SEM
1×30	4	6.6	1.1
2×30	4	20.3	7.2
2×45	3	34.1	6.3
4×45	4	61.7	2.5
4×250	4	82.4	1.8
4×500	3	87.9	3.8
2×1000	8	87.0	2.1

The total turnover is the sum of the renal turnover and the metabolic turnover. The metabolic turnover shows a saturation at about 40–50 mg/d (Figure 5), and this saturation occurs at a total turnover of about 60 mg/d. These values imply that up to this total turnover the metabolic rate of ascorbate increases; the asymptotic value could reflect the maximum physiological need for ascorbate.

The main metabolites of ascorbate in the human body are oxalate, dehydroascorbic acid, 2,3-diketogulonic acid, and ascorbic acid 2-sulfate. Of these, oxalate has attracted the most attention because of the potential hazard for renal complications by precipitation of oxalate stones. The above-mentioned metabolic turnover for ascorbate, which appears saturable, indicates that in normal humans the amount of oxalate that can be formed is limited. Therefore, the overall risk of inducing oxalate precipitation by increasing the intake of ascorbate probably is minute.

The kinetic model also allows the calculation of half-lives at various regimens of ascorbate intake. The half-lives range from 8 to 40 d (Table I). The half-lives in the literature or calculated from available information correspond to subjects on a comparatively low total turnover, 20–40 mg/d, consistent with the status of the subjects and the dietary regimens that could be assumed or were defined in the experimental set up. The range of half-lives also indicates that the kinetic behavior of ascorbate is very complicated and is related to the nutritional status; for example, the calculated half-lives are generally longer on low intakes than on higher (Table I). Although Baker and his group (3–5) reported that

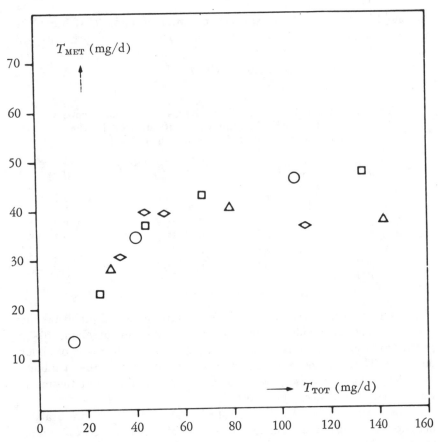

Figure 5. Metabolic turnover in relation to total turnover (6). (Reproduced, with permission, from Ref. 6. Copyright 1979, American Journal of Clinical Nutrition.)

the pools decreased exponentially, the course of the elimination seems to be related to the total pool and thus the elimination is not a simple first-order one.

Gastrointestinal Absorption of Ascorbate

The gastrointestinal absorption of ascorbate should be considered before summarizing this study. In no case did we achieve a complete recovery of the administered radioactively labeled ascorbic acid. In a separate set of experiments (7), the subjects were equilibrated on a limited intake of ascorbate and given a small oral dose of ^{14}C labeled ascorbate together with about 30 mg of carrier ascorbate (7). After a few hours this intake was followed by large intakes of unlabeled ascorbate and all urine was collected and analyzed until no label was found in the urine, usually during a 10-d period (Figure 6). The subjects absorbed between 80 and 90% of the administered label. The recovery in the kinetic experiments was generally lower, possibly because in the absorption study the distribution of the absorbed label was incomplete, which leads to a more efficient washout of the label within the period of the experiment. Thus a better estimation of the absorbed amount would be achieved by measuring recovery of label from the urine with this experimental design than in the kinetic experiment. However, in all cases the absorption is incomplete at low and physiological levels.

High Risk Groups

With reference to the literature, decreased plasma levels of ascorbate are found in some groups of people. One such group is the smokers, in which considerably lower plasma levels have been observed and documented in numerous publications since the 1940s. This prompted us to select smokers as a risk group on which a similar kinetic experiment should be performed and tested (8).

The same parameters as in the study on nonsmokers were measured and calculated. Thus, in the lower region, smokers require a higher total turnover (intake) to reach the same plasma concentration as the nonsmoking group. The smokers' renal handling of ascorbate was similar to that of the nonsmokers and the rate of gastrointestinal absorption was in the same order of magnitude, or about 75%. However, the smokers formed a group of their own when the metabolic turnover was related to the plasma steady state concentration (Figure 7), indicating an increased metabolic turnover at comparable steady state concentrations. No differences in the two groups were found in the relationship between the half-life and total turnover. Thus, the smoking habits seem to influence just one of the links in the chain of events from absorption to excretion of ascorbate and this link is the metabolism. The kinetic model does not allow any conclusions on the nature of the changed metabolism. Thus we cannot differentiate between a changed metabolism and an increase in the metabolic rate above that of the nonsmoker. However, the findings may indicate that ascorbate has functions in the body that have been difficult to prove, for example, in the protection against or detoxification of noxious substances.

A numerical treatment of the kinetic data obtained in the smokers study indicates that to compensate for the increased metabolic turnover, smokers have to increase their daily intake beyond that of nonsmokers. Based on the same assumptions as in the nonsmokers group, an intake value of about 140 mg/d seems appropriate.

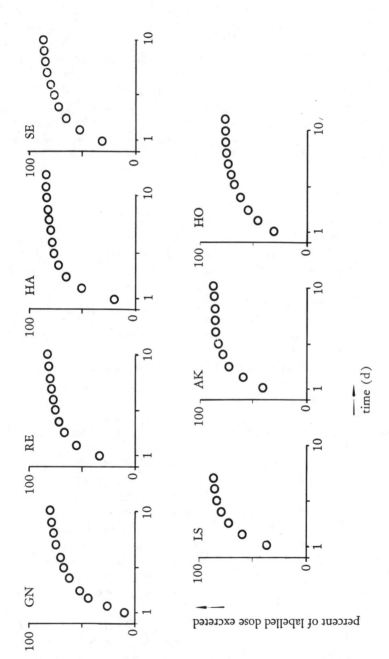

Figure 6. Cumulative recovery of label after administration of tracer dose of ^{14}C-labeled ascorbate. (Reproduced, with permission, from Ref. 9. Copyright 1977, Williams & Wilkins.)

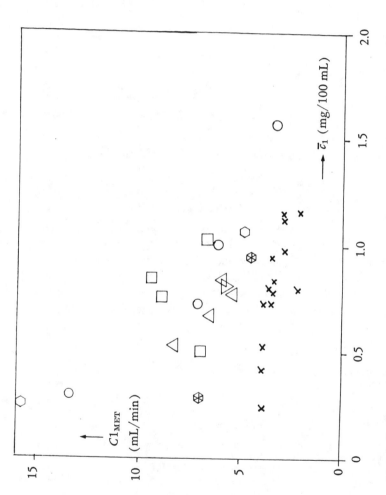

Figure 7. Metabolic clearance as a function of plasma concentration of ascorbate. Bold symbols refer to nonsmokers.

Other risk groups are various stress groups since ascorbate fulfills a function in the biosynthesis of corticosteroids and other hormones. Such studies are planned but because of the nature of the experimental setup, they are not easily carried out. Other groups of potential interest are alcoholics, obese people, and certain diseased or injured patients where the metabolic handling of ascorbate may be widely different from that of normal humans.

Conclusion

In conclusion:
- The bioavailability of ingested ascorbate in healthy non-smoking males is substantially less than 100%
- The elimination of unchanged ascorbic acid via the kidneys has a threshold value corresponding to a total turnover of about 60 mg/d
- The metabolic turnover levels at a total turnover of about 60 mg/d
- The total body pool can be increased, reaching about 20 mg/kg body weight at a steady state concentration in plasma of 0.90 mg/100 mL, corresponding to a total turnover of about 90 mg/d.

Taking all these observations into account, a total intake of about 70–80 mg/d should be the goal for nonsmoking healthy males. The statistical variation observed indicates that a daily intake of about 100 mg should be appropriate to cover the needs of 95% of the population. For smokers the daily ascorbate intake should be increased to 140 mg/d.

Literature Cited

1. "Recommended Dietary Allowances," 9th ed. National Academy of Sciences, 1980, p. 75.
2. Lind, J. "Treatise on the Scurvy," 2nd ed., London, 1757.
3. Baker, E. M.; Saari, J. C.; Tolbert, B. M. *Am. J. Clin. Nutr.* 1966, *19*, 371.
4. Baker, E. M.; Hodges, R. E.; Hood, J.; Sauberlich, H. E.; March, S. C. *Am. J. Clin. Nutr.* 1969, *22*, 549.
5. Baker, E. M.; Hodges, R. E.; Hood, J.; Sauberlich, H. E.; March, S. C.; Canham, J. E. *Am. J. Clin. Nutr.* 1971, *24*, 444.
6. Kallner, A.; Hartmann, D.; Hornig, D. *Am. J. Clin. Nutr.* 1979, *32*, 530.
7. Kallner, A.; Hartmann, D.; Hornig, D. *J. Vitam. Nutr. Res.* 1977, *47*, 383.
8. Kallner, A.; Hartmann, D.; Hornig, D. *Am. J. Clin. Nutr.* 1981, *32*, 1347.
9. Kallner, A.; Hartmann, D.; Hornig, D. *Int. J. Vitam. Nutr. Res.* 1977, *47*, 383.

RECEIVED for review January 22, 1981. ACCEPTED April 15, 1981.

Biochemical Functions of Ascorbic Acid in Drug Metabolism

V. G. ZANNONI, E. J. HOLSZTYNSKA, and S. S. LAU

Department of Pharmacology, University of Michigan Medical School, Ann Arbor, MI 48109

Ascorbic acid participates in the detoxification of a variety of pharmacological agents. The quantity of cytochrome P_{450} and drug-metabolizing activities are significantly reduced under deficiency. Studies indicate that de novo protein synthesis is operable and key enzymes involved in heme synthesis are not significantly reduced. In addition, no significant change in affinity for drug substrates in normal and ascorbic acid deficient animals was found. Also, there is no increase in microsomal lipid peroxidation or decrease in the quantity of phosphatidyl choline. In contrast, there is a marked decrease in the quantity of particular forms of cytochrome P_{450} in deficient guinea pigs; that is, polypeptides with molecular weight of 44,000, 52,000, and 57,000 daltons. These results indicate that ascorbic acid deficiency may have its effect on the apoprotein moiety of cytochrome P_{450}.

The metabolism of pharmacological agents can be markedly influenced by a variety of environmental and genetic factors. Some of these factors include age, sex, strain and species, stress, hormones, drugs, environmental chemicals, and the nutritional status of the animal (1–3). Our knowledge of the complicated hepatic microsomal electron transport system involved in the metabolism of xenobiotics and environmental chemicals is shown in Scheme 1. With regard to vitamin C, the effect of ascorbic acid in maintaining drug metabolism and steroid metabolism was established by several laboratories and is of current interest (4–9).

In 1941 pentobarbital sleeping time was shown to be prolonged in scorbutic guinea pigs compared with normal controls; this effect could be reversed by the administration of vitamin C (10). In 1954 a significant increase in the plasma half-life of acetanilide, aniline, and antipyrine

0065-2393/82/0200-0349$06.00/0

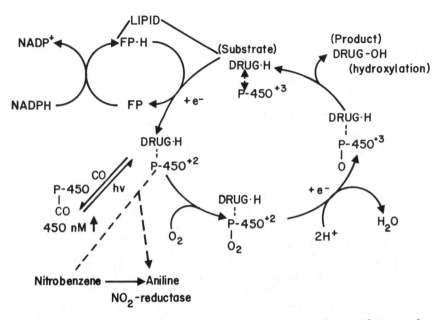

Scheme 1. *Hepatic microsomal electron transport for drug oxidation and reduction.*

in guinea pigs depleted of ascorbic acid was demonstrated (*11*). In the vitamin C deficient animals the half-life of acetanilide was increased about threefold and upon repletion of the animals with ascorbic acid the half-life of the drug returned to normal.

In 1961 vitamin C deficient guinea pigs with no obvious signs of scurvy were reported to be sensitive to the muscle relaxant, zoxazolamine, and the increased duration of this drug in vivo correlated with a decrease in its liver microsomal oxidation in vitro (*12*). In 1965 the *p*-hydroxylation of acetanilide was shown to be depressed up to 90% and the hydroxylation of coumarin also decreased in vitamin C deficient animals (*8*). In addition the decreased hydroxylation of coumarin could be reversed by the in vivo administration of ascorbic acid (*9*). In 1969 liver microsomes from scorbutic animals showed significant decreases in the demethylation of aminopyrine, hydroxylation of acetanilide, and quantity of cytochrome P_{450} (*13*). In addition, phenobarbital and 3-methylcholanthrene caused an increase in the mixed function oxygenase in the scorbutic animal, and the effect of these drug enzyme inducers could be blocked by the prior administration of ethionine.

The metabolism of a variety of compounds such as aniline, hexobarbital, zoxazolamine, aminopyrine, diphenhydramine, meperidine, *p*-nitrobenzoic acid, and *p*-dimethylaminoazobenzene in microsomes isolated from adult guinea pigs maintained on a vitamin C free diet for only 12 d was studied (*14*). In contrast to some of the earlier studies, these investigations showed that although the metabolism of aniline, hexobarbital, and zoxazolamine decreased, the metabolism of the other drugs was unchanged. These researchers concluded that the effect of vitamin C deficiency is rather specific on hydroxylation reactions and involved the "terminal oxidase" component of the electron transport system. The previous studies have shown decreased hepatic metabolism of a variety of drugs as well as steroids (*4–7*). However, the underlying biochemical mechanism for the action of the vitamin in drug metabolism needs to be elucidated.

Liver Microsomal Activity in Neonatal Guinea Pigs

Activity vs. Ascorbic Acid Concentration. Studies in our laboratory with liver microsomes prepared from vitamin C deficient guinea pigs maintained on a vitamin C free diet for 21 d showed marked decreases in electron transport components such as cytochrome P_{450} and NADPH cytochrome P_{450} reductase. In addition, overall drug oxidative reactions such as aniline hydroxylation, aminopyrine N-demethylation, and p-nitroanisole O-demethylation were significantly decreased (Table I). These studies were done mainly with mature guinea pigs (3–4 months old, 250–400 g); it was important to determine if drug-oxidizing systems in younger animals would be more dependent on ascorbic acid and if the liver microsomal system in these animals would be affected before the scorbutic state was approached. Furthermore, it was also important to establish what effect an increase in dietary ascorbic acid would have on drug-metabolizing systems. For these studies neonatal guinea pigs (1–2 weeks old, 90–100 g) were used. Neonatal guinea pigs were placed on an ascorbic acid deficient diet supplemented by amounts of ascorbic acid varying from 2 to 500 mg/d for 8 d. Other groups were maintained on a vitamin C deficient diet for 8–15 d without supplementary ascorbic acid.

Figure 1 shows a significant increase in the NADPH-dependent cytochrome P_{450} reductase activity in the neonatal guinea pigs with increasing liver ascorbic acid concentrations. The first point—3.2 μmol of cytochrome P_{450} reduced/h/100 mg of microsomal protein—is the activity in 15-d ascorbic acid deficient animals (liver ascorbic acid less than 1.0 mg%). The second point—5.7 μmol of cytochrome P_{450} reduced—is the activity in 8-d ascorbic acid deficient guinea pigs (liver ascorbic acid: 2.7 mg%), and is an 80% increase over the activity in 15-d deficient animals. The last point represents the activity of 10.3 μmol of cytochrome P_{450} reduced/100 mg of microsomal protein and is the

Table I. Effect of Deficiency on Electron Transport Components and Drug Enzymes in Guinea Pig Liver Microsomes

| | | Activity | |
Component	Normal	Vitamin C Deficient (21 days)	Decrease (%)
Cytochrome P_{450}[a]	0.05 ± 0.01	0.03 ± 0.003 $p < 0.01$	40
NADPH cytochrome P_{450} reductase[b]	0.80 ± 0.2	< 0.1	85
NADPH cytochrome c reductase[b]	124 ± 21	83 ± 11 $p < 0.05$	33
Cytochrome b_5[a]	0.03 ± 0.004	0.02 ± 0.006 $p < 0.05$	33
Aniline hydroxylase[c]	1.6 ± 0.2	0.8 ± 0.2 $p < 0.001$	50
Aminopyrine N-demethylase[c]	3.9 ± 0.1	1.7 ± 0.3 $p < 0.001$	56
p-Nitroanisole O-demethylase[c]	3.2 ± 0.4	1.1 ± 0.2 $p < 0.001$	66
Liver ascorbic acid supernatant fraction 15,000 × g (μg/g wet weight)	194 ± 29	25 ± 15	
microsomal fraction (μg/g wet weight)	11 ± 3.8	3.5 ± 2.0	

Note: Data given as mean ± se of 10 animals/group.
[a] Specific content equals μmol/100 mg microsomal protein.
[b] Specific activity equals μmol reduced/h/100 mg of microsomal protein at 27°C.
[c] Specific activity equals mol of product formed/h/100 mg of microsomal protein at 27°C.
Source: Reference 15.

amount found in animals with liver ascorbic acid levels of 27 mg%. This activity is more than 200% higher than the activity in 15-d deficient animals.

The data in Figure 2 show an increase in the liver microsomal activity of p-nitroanisole O-demethylation in neonatal guinea pigs with increasing concentrations of liver ascorbic acid. O-Demethylation increases significantly with increasing concentrations of liver ascorbic acid. When the liver ascorbic acid reached 27 mg%, O-demethylase activity was 300% higher than the level in the 15-d deficient animals and 70% higher than that of the 8-d deficient animals. Liver microsomal aminopyrine N-demethylase activity in neonatal guinea pigs also increased with increasing liver ascorbic acid concentration, although less than was found for O-demethylation. The activity in neonatal guinea pig microsomes with 21.0 mg% liver ascorbic acid was at least 50% higher than in 15-d deficient animals.

The correlation between the concentration of liver ascorbic acid and the quantity of cytochrome P_{450} is illustrated in Figure 3. Guinea pigs fed a normal chow diet supplemented with 1 mg/mL of ascorbic acid in their drinking water were divided into groups according to the quantity of their liver ascorbic acid and compared with guinea pigs fed chow diet alone or with animals fed an ascorbic acid deficient diet for 20 d. The group with the highest quantity of cytochrome P_{450} (24 nmol/100 mg of supernatant protein) had 2.5 times more of the heme protein than did the ascorbic acid deficient group (9.6 nmol) and 1.7 times more than did the group on chow diet alone (14 nmol).

Additional studies with fetal guinea pig livers indicated a marked variation in cytochrome P_{450} and O-demethylase activity in individual fetal livers; these findings correlated well with the concentration of liver

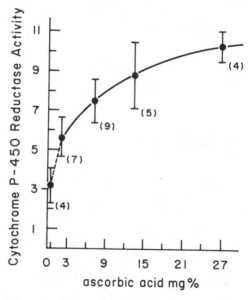

Figure 1. NADPH cytochrome P_{450} reductase activity in weanling guinea pigs given varying amounts of ascorbic acid (39).

Specific activity equals μmol of cytochrome P_{450} reduced/h/100 mg of microsomal protein at 27°C. The number of animals in each group is given in the figure. The diets of the various groups contained less than 1.0 mg ascorbic acid/100 g of liver, ascorbic acid deficient diet for 15 d (point 1), 2.3 mg of ascorbic acid/100 g of liver, ascorbic acid deficient diet for 8 d (point 2), 7.4 mg of ascorbic acid/100 g of liver, 25 mg of ascorbic acid/d for 3 d (point 3), 13.5 mg of ascorbic acid/100 g of liver, 75 mg of ascorbic acid/d for 8 d (point 4), 27.0 mg of ascorbic acid/100 g of liver, chow guinea pig diet plus greens for 8 d (point 5).

ascorbic acid (Table II). Fetal livers with an ascorbic acid concentration of below 5.0 mg/100 g of liver had no detectable cytochrome P_{450} or O-demethylase activity, but fetal livers with high ascorbic acid levels (> 17.0 mg/100 g of liver) had much higher drug metabolism activity (cytochrome P_{450} concentration, 84% of the dams'; and O-demethylase activity, 51% of the dams').

Specificity studies indicated that other reducing agents such as reduced 2,6-dichlorophenolindophenol dye, reduced glutathione, ascorbyl palmitate, and D-isoascorbic acid, when given to vitamin C deficient animals, were not as effective as the vitamin in maintaining drug-metabolism activity. Reduced 2,6-dichlorophenolindophenol dye did not significantly affect the liver microsomal levels of cytochrome P_{450} and NADPH cytochrome P_{450} reductase or the overall microsomal drug-oxidation reaction, p-nitroanisole O-demethylation. However, aminopyrine N-demethylation was somewhat increased compared with the deficient groups. Reduced glutathione did not significantly alter either

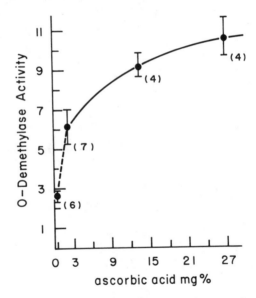

Figure 2. p-*Nitroanisole* O-*demethylase activity in weanling guinea pigs given varying amounts of ascorbic acid* (39).

Specific activity given in μmol of p-nitrophenol formed/h/100 mg of microsomal protein at 27°C. The number of animals in each group is shown in the figure. The diets of the various groups contained < 1.0 mg of ascorbic acid/100 g of liver, ascorbic acid deficient diet for 15 d (point 1), 2.7 mg of ascorbic acid/100 g of liver, ascorbic acid deficient diet for 8 d (point 2), 13.5 mg of ascorbic acid/100 g of liver, 75 mg of ascorbic acid/d for 8 d (point 3), 27.0 mg of ascorbic acid/100 g of liver, chow guinea pigs diet plus greens for 8 d (point 4).

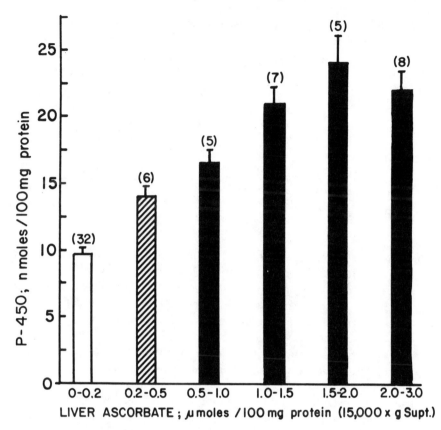

Figure 3. Correlation of hepatic cytochrome P_{450} and ascorbic acid concentration (32).

Cytochrome P_{450} and ascorbic acid were determined in the liver 15,000 × g supernatant fraction from guinea pigs (200–250 g) maintained on an ascorbic acid deficient diet for 20 d (open bar), normal chow diet (cross-hatched bar), or chow diet plus 1.0 mg/mL of ascorbic acid in the drinking water/d (solid bars). Animals were divided into groups according to their liver concentration of ascorbic acid; 1 μmol of ascorbic acid/100 mg of protein equals 19 mg/100 g wet weight of liver. Number in parentheses represents number of animals.

liver microsomal cytochrome P_{450} concentration or *p*-nitroanisole *O*-demethylase activity from those values in 8-d ascorbic acid deficient animals. However, aminopyrine *N*-demethylase activity and NADPH cytochrome P_{450} reductase activity increased (59%) over the activities in 8-d deficient animals. D-Isoascorbic acid was not effective in increasing either drug-metabolism activities or electron transport components. In comparison, ascorbyl palmitate increased the levels of electron transport components and overall drug-oxidation reactions. For example, the

Table II.   Cytochrome P_{450}, O-Demethylase Activity, and Quantity of Ascorbic Acid in Fetal Guinea Pig Livers

Source	Ascorbic Acid[a]	Cytochrome P_{450}[b]	O-Demethylase Activity[c]
Fetal (2)[d]	4.5	< 0.001	< 0.01
Fetal (3)[d]	11.2	0.004	0.11
Fetal (4)[d]	17.5	0.011	0.78
Dam (3)[d]	21.7	0.013	1.73

[a] mg/100 g of liver.
[b] μmol/100 mg of microsomal protein.
[c] μmol of p-nitrophenol formed/h/100 mg of microsomal protein at 27°C.
[d] Number in parentheses equals number of animals (64–66 d of gestation) individual values in groups did not differ by more than 12%.
Source: Reference 6.

administration of 50 mg/d (0.12 mM) led to a liver ascorbic acid concentration of 10.8 mg%; administration of 0.31 mM of ascorbic acid was required to obtain a comparable liver ascorbic acid concentration, that is, 13.5 mg%. The concentration of cytochrome P_{450} was as high as that found in the group of animals on a normal chow diet.

Kinetic studies on possible alterations in the affinities of drug enzymes for their substrates were carried out with microsomes prepared from vitamin C deficient guinea pigs and animals given extra supplements of the vitamin. Table III gives the K_m of liver microsomal aminopyrine N-demethylase for 8- and 15-d ascorbic acid deficient animals, and for animals given the normal diet. In contrast to the differences in aminopyrine N-demethylase activities found in these groups, the Michaelis–Menten affinity constants were not significantly altered. In addition, Table III lists the K_m of liver microsomal aminopyrine N-demethylase for weanling guinea pigs given 50 and 500 mg of ascorbic acid/d for 8 d, and for animals maintained on a normal chow diet. There was no significant difference in these values. Similar results were obtained in kinetic studies with O-demethylase in that there was no significant alteration in the K_m constants for this enzyme system in any of the groups.

In contrast to the K_m studies, a consistent alteration in the usual Type II aniline–cytochrome P_{450} binding spectrum was seen for vitamin C deficient guinea pig microsomes. The aniline–cytochrome P_{450} binding spectrum was atypical in that the trough of the spectrum appeared at 405 nm instead of at 390 nm, and the peak occurred at 440 nm instead of at 430 nm. A marked decrease in absorption intensity was also observed at these wavelengths (15). These findings cannot be explained by a concomitant decrease in the quantity of cytochrome P_{450} in the vitamin C deficient guinea pig microsomes because dilution of microsomes from normal guinea pigs to equivalent cytochrome P_{450} concentrations of vitamin C deficient guinea pigs still gave the usual aniline–cytochrome P_{450} binding spectra. The atypical binding spectrum observed in vitamin C deficient guinea pig microsomes may reflect an alteration in the integrity of the microsomal phospholipid membrane associated with cytochrome P_{450}, and ascorbic acid may be required for membrane maintenance. In vitro experiments in which ascorbic acid was added to vitamin C deficient liver microsomes did not restore drug-oxidation activities or substrate cytochrome P_{450} binding. Other reducing agents substituted for ascorbic acid, such as glutathione and reduced 2,6-dichlorophenolindophenol dye, were also ineffective. However, ascorbyl palmitate (2.3×10^{-3} M), a more lipophilic analogue of ascorbic acid, restored atypical aniline–cytochrome P_{450} binding spectra to the usual type in that the trough and peak of the spectrum were at 390 and 430 nm, respectively. The absorption intensity at these wavelengths was still depressed as was the drug-oxidation activity, which could reflect the lower quantity of cytochrome P_{450} that was not restored by ascorbyl palmitate.

Effect of Ascorbic Acid Replenishment. Reversal of decreased drug-metabolism activities in vitamin C deficient animals by the in vivo administration of ascorbic acid indicated that the quantity of liver ascorbic acid was restored to normal levels within 3 d but most of the drug enzyme activities such as N-demethylase, O-demethylase, and cytochrome P_{450} and P_{450} reductase required 6–10 d of vitamin administration to return to normal (Figures 4 and 5). Induction studies with phenobarbital indicated that overall drug oxidation activities (aniline hydroxylase, aminopyrine N-demethylase, and p-nitroanisole O-demethylase) and microsomal electron transport components increased in vitamin C deficient guinea pigs comparable with those found in normal animals. Aniline hydroxylase increased twofold in the vitamin C de-

Table III. Apparent Michaelis–Menten Affinity Constants of Aminopyrine N-Demethylation in Guinea Pig Microsomes under Varying Intakes of Ascorbic Acid

Diet	Liver Ascorbic Acid (mg/100 g of liver)	K_m (10^3 M)
Chow diet	27	1.67
Chow diet + 50 mg/d of ascorbic acid (8 d)	9.9	1.57
Chow diet + 500 mg/d of ascorbic acid (8 d)	23.3	1.85
Ascorbic acid deficient diet (8 d)	2	1.67
Ascorbic acid deficient diet (15 d)	< 1	1.82

Source: Reference 6.

ficient animal and p-nitroanisole O-demethylase increased sixfold. The difference between the level of activity after phenobarbital treatment and basal level (no treatment) in vitamin C deficient and normal guinea pigs was in the same order of magnitude for each enzyme activity. The individual electron transport components were also induced in vitamin C deficient guinea pigs and the increase was equivalent to, or in some cases better than that in the normal guinea pigs. These studies indicate that protein synthesis involved in the microsomal transport system is not compromised in the vitamin C deficient animal (15).

Mechanism of Reduced Metabolic Activity

Microsomal Phospholipids. It was of interest to determine if ascorbic acid, through its antioxidant property, protected drug enzyme activities by inhibiting lipid peroxidation. Lipid peroxidation was found to be on the order of 30% higher in microsomes isolated from normal guinea pigs compared with microsomes isolated from guinea pigs on the ascorbic acid deficient diet for 15 d (Table IV). The quantity of the phospholipid was slightly lower in the 15-d ascorbic acid deficient group

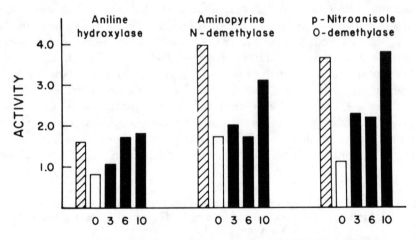

DAYS OF ASCORBIC ACID ADMINISTRATION

Figure 4. Reversal of decreased aniline hydroxylase, aminopyrine N-demethylase and p-nitroanisole O-demethylase activities in vitamin C deficient guinea pigs with ascorbic acid (15).

Groups of normal and vitamin C deficient guinea pigs (21 d) were given 50 mg of ascorbic acid in their drinking water for 3, 6, and 10 d. Enzyme activity measured as μmol of product formed/h/100 mg of liver microsomal protein at 27°C. Key: activity in normal animals, cross-hatched bar; activity in vitamin C deficient animals, open bar; vitamin C deficient animals given supplements of ascorbic acid for days indicated, solid bar.

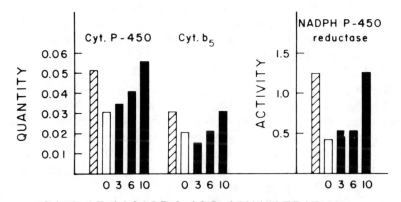

DAYS OF ASCORBIC ACID ADMINISTRATION

Figure 5. Reversal of decreased electron transport components in vitamin C deficient guinea pigs with ascorbic acid (15).

Groups of normal and vitamin C deficient guinea pigs (21 d) were given 50 mg of ascorbic acid in their drinking water for 3, 6, and 10 days. The quantity of cytochrome b_5 measured as μmol/100 mg of liver microsomal protein. NADPH cytochrome P_{450} reductase measured as μmol of cytochrome P_{450} reduced/h/ 100 mg of liver microsomal protein at 27°C. Key: activity in normal animals, cross-hatched bar; activity in vitamin C deficient animals, open bar; vitamin C deficient animals given supplements of ascorbic acid for days indicated, solid bar.

Table IV.   Lipid Peroxidation in Normal and Ascorbic Acid Deficient Microsomes

	Activity		
Microsomes	*Oxygen Uptake*[a]	*Malonaldehyde Formed*[b]	*NADPH Disappearance*[c]
Normal[d]	160	0.33	10.3
Ascorbic acid deficient[e]	118 (74%)[f]	0.23 (70%)	7.9 (77%)

Note: Lipid peroxidation was determined in microsomes from normal guinea pigs (23.7 mg of ascorbic acid/100 g of liver) and 15-d ascorbic acid deficient guinea pigs (4.3 mg of ascorbic acid/100 g of liver).
[a] μmol of oxygen consumed/h/100 mg of microsomal protein at 27°C.
[b] μmol of malonaldehyde formed/h/100 mg of microsomal protein at 27°C.
[c] μmol of NADPH disappeared/h/100 mg microsomal protein at 27°C.
[d] Phosphatidyl choline quantity, 27.2 μmol/100 mg of microsomal protein.
[e] Phosphatidyl choline quantity, 22.4 μmol/100 mg of microsomal protein.
[f] Number in parentheses is % of normal microsomes.
Source: Reference 6.

compared with the normal group (18%). This decrease is most likely not sufficient to impair drug metabolism because 3-d-starved, ascorbic acid-fed guinea pigs, which have increased drug metabolism activities (15), have an even greater decrease in the quantity of phosphatidyl choline than do the 15-d ascorbic acid deficient group (19.2 μmol/100 mg of microsomal protein compared with 22.4 μmol/mg). The starved animals lost 22% of their body weight and had 42.6 mg of ascorbic acid/100 g of liver.

Microsomal Cytochrome P$_{450}$. The properties of hepatic microsomal cytochrome P$_{450}$ prepared from normal and 15-d ascorbic acid deficient animals did not differ with respect to storage at 5°C, treatment with sodium cholate, treatment with glycerol, or microsomal protein concentration. The quantity of microsomal cytochrome P$_{420}$, the inactive form of cytochrome P$_{450}$, generated by these procedures was not significantly different for the two groups of animals. However, some physical chemical differences between normal and ascorbic acid deficient microsomes can be observed following sonication and following dialysis. For example, with sonication the time required to inactivate 50% of cytochrome P$_{450}$ prepared from normal animals was 180 s compared with 78 s for the 15-d ascorbic acid deficient guinea pigs.

Determination of the concentration of liver ascorbic acid and cytochrome P$_{450}$ indicated that a relatively consistent quantitative relationship of ascorbic acid to cytochrome P$_{450}$ existed in microsomal preparations. The ratio of liver ascorbic acid to cytochrome P$_{450}$ was 2.2 in the ascorbic acid deficient group and 2.3 in the normal group, and 1.7 and 1.6, respectively, when cytochrome P$_{420}$ was included. In adrenal tissue the ratio of microsomal ascorbic acid to cytochrome P$_{450}$ was on the order of 3:1, and 2:1 when cytochrome P$_{420}$ was included. However, in the kidney, the ratio of microsomal ascorbic acid to cytochrome P$_{450}$ was larger, on the order of 5:1 when cytochrome P$_{420}$ was included, considerably higher than in the liver and adrenal gland. This higher ratio may be caused, in part, by the capacity of the kidney to reabsorb the vitamin. The heme protein was partially purified from normal and ascorbic acid deficient guinea pig livers with ammonium sulfate fractionation, calcium phosphate gel adsorption, and elution; the quantity of ascorbic acid was determined in various fractions. The vitamin remained with cytochrome P$_{450}$ throughout the fractionation procedure; the ratio of the concentration of ascorbic acid to total carbon monoxide binding heme protein (cytochrome P$_{450}$ plus P$_{420}$) in the various fractions ranged from 1.3 to 3.7 in normal microsomes and from 1.2 to 3.0 in ascorbic acid deficient microsomes (16).

The correlation between the concentrations of liver ascorbic acid and cytochrome P$_{450}$ in microsomes prepared from normal and ascorbic acid deficient guinea pigs, after dialysis and partial purification of cytochrome P_{450}, suggested that ascorbic acid may be directly associated with the heme protein. Various metal chelators were used to investigate the possibility that ascorbic acid was involved with the reduced form of iron associated with cytochrome P_{450}, that is, ferrous iron. α,α'-Dipyridyl, a ferrous iron chelator, inhibits the carbon monoxide binding spectrum of cytochrome P_{450} resulting in a decrease in the cytochrome P_{450}–carbon monoxide absorption spectrum at 450 nm. The cytochrome P_{450}–carbon monoxide binding decreased by approximately 50% in the presence of 12.8 mM α,α'-dipyridyl. Importantly, the decrease of the cytochrome P_{450}–carbon monoxide spectrum by the chelator could be prevented by 22.7 mM ascorbic acid. o-Phenanthroline, another inhibitor with a high affinity for ferrous iron, inhibited the cytochrome P_{450}–carbon monoxide binding spectrum to the same extent as was found with α,α'-dipyridyl, and o-phenanthroline's action was also prevented by the vitamin. The decreased formation of the cytochrome P_{450}–carbon monoxide spectrum by α,α'-dipyridyl and o-phenanthroline can be accounted for because these metal chelators can bind to the reduced ferrous iron of cytochrome P_{450}, resulting in a spectrum that has an absorption maximum at the same wavelength as the absorption maximum of the carbon monoxide ligand, that is, at 450 nm (16). Of the chelators tested only ferrous iron chelators such as α,α'-dipyridyl and o-phenanthroline significantly inhibited the cytochrome P_{450}–carbon monoxide spectrum (55% inhibition). On the other hand, structurally related chelators with high affinity for copper, 8-hydroxyquinoline sulfonate, bathocuproine, and diethyldithiocarbamate were not significantly inhibitory (less than 5%). The metal chelators, in general, showed only slight inhibition of the microsomal heme protein cytochrome b_5 (8–20%). The apparent affinity constants of α,α'-dipyridyl for cytochrome P_{450} are 2.99×10^{-4} M for normal microsomes and 3.14×10^{-4} M for ascorbic acid deficient microsomes. The apparent affinity constants for protection by ascorbic acid are 4.98×10^{-4} M for normal microsomes and 4.83×10^{-4} M for ascorbic acid deficient microsomes (16).

The administration of a precursor of heme, d-aminolevulinic acid (ALA), to vitamin C deficient guinea pigs caused an increase in the quantity of cytochrome P_{450}, suggesting that ascorbic acid may be involved in the formation of this essential metabolite of heme synthesis (17). A general route for the synthesis of heme is given in Scheme 2. In view of these findings, it was important to determine if vitamin C deficiency affected the activity of ALA synthetase, the rate-limiting enzyme in heme synthesis, or other important enzymes in heme synthesis such as ALA dehydratase and ferrochelatase. Although cytochrome P_{450} is markedly reduced in vitamin C deficient microsomes, there is no sig-

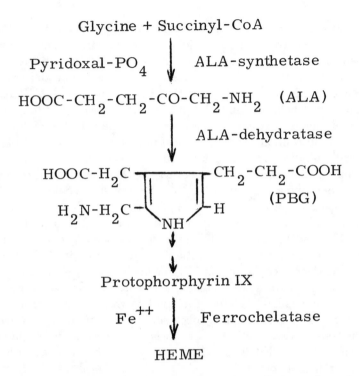

Scheme 2. *Pathway for the synthesis of heme from glycine and succinyl coenzyme A.*

nificant decrease in any of the key enzymes involved in heme synthesis (Table V). Similar results were recently obtained (*18*). In addition, recent evidence showed that the decrease in cytochrome P_{450} in ascorbic acid deficiency is not caused by increased heme catabolism, at least not by induction of microsomal heme oxygenase activity (*19–21*). However, the possibility that the vitamin is involved in the synthesis of the apoprotein of cytochrome P_{450} should be considered.

The effect of ascorbic acid deficiency on different forms of cytochrome P_{450} was investigated in view of previous findings of substantial depletion of the heme protein (*15, 16, 22, 23*) and substantial in vitro inhibition by metal chelators, which is prevented by ascorbic acid (*16*). Reports have described multiple forms of cytochrome P_{450} in rabbit, rat, and mouse microsomes (*24–29*); these forms can be separated by gel electrophoresis in the presence of SDS. Our studies indicate that microsomes from guinea pigs contain multiple forms of cytochrome P_{450} as evidenced by heme-staining electrophoretic bands in the 40,000–60,000-molecular-weight region. Guinea pigs have nine distinct polypeptide bands compared with eight for rabbits (*30*) and five for rats (*27, 28, 31*).

Induction with phenobarbital and 3-methylcholanthrene and purification of the cytochromes indicate that eight of the guinea pig polypeptide bands with molecular weights from 44,000 to 60,000 contain cytochrome P_{450}, and the changes observed in the relative staining intensity of the bands may reflect changes in the quantity of different forms of cytochrome P_{450}. Microsomes from ascorbic acid deficient guinea pigs consistently demonstrated decreases in three of the polypeptide bands (molecular weights 44,000, 52,000, and 57,000) and increases in two (54,000 and 55,000) (Figure 6). Importantly, these differences were maintained in partially purified fractions from normal and ascorbic acid deficient guinea pigs (32).

Experiments to identify the various polypeptides in normal and ascorbic acid deficient microsomes as heme proteins were carried out. In crude microsomes at least seven heme-staining bands were found in the 40,000–60,000-dalton region and the intensity of the heme stain corresponded to the amount of cytochrome P_{450} present. In addition, specific heme-staining polypeptides were identified using partially purified fractions of cytochrome P_{450}. Microsomes from untreated guinea pigs contained five polypeptide bands that correlated with heme-staining bands; their molecular weights were 44,000, 52,000, 55,000, 56,000, and 60,000. Also, a heme-staining polypeptide with a molecular weight of 46,500 was evident in microsomes from phenobarbital-treated guinea pigs (32).

Further identification of the guinea pig polypeptide bands was obtained with known inducers of microsomal cytochrome P_{450}. The induction of a 46,500-dalton polypeptide with phenobarbital is similar to the induction found in rat (26, 28), rabbit (33, 34), and mouse (35) microsomes. The phenobarbital-inducible polypeptide was present in negligible amounts in uninduced microsomes and no difference was discernible between normal and ascorbic acid deficient microsomes.

Table V. Cytochrome P_{450} and Heme Synthesis in Normal and Ascorbic Acid Deficient Guinea Pigs

Enzyme	*Normal*[a]	*Deficient*[b]
Cytochrome P_{450} (nmol/100 mg of protein)	19.2 ± 1.1	9.5 ± 0.7
ALA synthetase (nmol ALA/h/100 mg)	16.5 ± 2.3	18.1 ± 1.9
ALA dehydratase (nmol PGB/h/100 mg)	1056 ± 53	922 ± 33
Ferrochelatase (nmol ^{59}Fe/h/100 mg)	536 ± 33	589 ± 58

[a] Normal guinea pigs: 1 mg of ascorbic acid/mL in drinking water/d. Liver ascorbic acid was 1740 nmol/100 mg of protein.
[b] Ascorbic acid deficient guinea pigs: on ascorbic acid free diet for 20 d. Liver ascorbic acid was 99 nmol/100 mg of protein.
Source: Reference *38*.

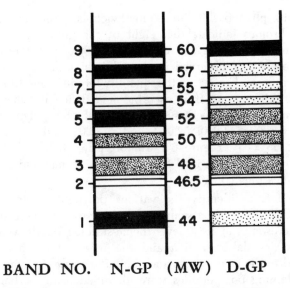

BAND NO.   N-GP   (MW)   D-GP

Figure 6.   Representation of SDS electrophoresis of liver microsomes prepared from normal and ascorbic acid deficient guinea pigs (32).

Administration of 3-methylcholanthrene, 40 h before sacrifice, yielded essentially no induction in guinea pigs, but a substantial increase in a form of cytochrome P_{450} with a molecular weight of 53,000–55,000 occurred in other species (25–27, 33, 35). On the other hand, treatment with 3-methylcholanthrene for 7 d resulted in induction in guinea pigs; the induced electrophoretic bands had molecular weights of 44,000, 48,000, 57,000, and 60,000. Two of these (molecular weights, 44,000 and 57,000) are polypeptide bands that are decreased in ascorbic acid deficient microsomes. No differences were noted between normal and ascorbic acid deficient guinea pigs in the polypeptide bands inducible by phenobarbital, 3-methylcholanthrene, or β-naphthoflavone. This finding is consistent with previous reports in which the degree of induction of cytochrome P_{450} in ascorbic acid deficient guinea pigs was equal to or greater than that in normal guinea pigs (9, 14, 15).

The results presented are in keeping with a selective action of ascorbic acid on specific forms of P_{450} apocytochromes. This selectivity is consistent with the overall effect of ascorbic acid deficiency on this important heme protein, which never decreases below 40–60% of normal–even in a severely deficient state (23, 36, 37). Ascorbic acid deficiency may selectively affect certain forms of cytochrome P_{450}; this possibly is important especially in light of the findings that benzo[a]-pyrene hydroxylase activity was unaltered in livers from deficient guinea pigs but 7-ethoxycoumarin dealkylase activity was less than 50% of normal (23). The correlation of decreases in the metabolism of various prototype drug substrates and environmental chemicals in various tissues with decreases in specific forms of cytochrome P_{450} will be important. We have recently found that ascorbic acid deficiency markedly affects particular MFO pathways of such environmental chemicals as bromobenzene and biphenyl. These compounds were interesting to study in that both of them are metabolized by specific forms of cytochrome P_{450} (31). For example, bromobenzene is metabolized to o-bromophenol via 2,3-epoxidation and to p-bromophenol via 3,4-epoxidation. Biphenyl is metabolized to either a 2-hydroxylated product or to a 4-hydroxylated product. The 2-hydroxy pathway is equivalent to o-hydroxylation and the 4-hydroxy pathway is equivalent to p-hydroxylation of bromobenzene. The p-bromophenol pathway of bromobenzene and 4-hydroxy pathway of biphenyl are markedly decreased in ascorbic acid deficiency, and the o-bromophenol and 2-hydroxylated biphenyl pathways are not statistically altered (*see* Table VI). These data are consistent with the hypothesis and the evidence that multiple forms of cytochrome P_{450}, some of which are depleted in ascorbic acid deficiency while others are not affected, exist and that specific forms of cytochrome P_{450} are responsible for the metabolism of a variety of xenobiotics and environmental chemicals.

Because heme synthesis is not altered in ascorbic acid deficiency, the determination of whether ascorbic acid is involved in the degradation of the cytochrome will be important (32, 38). Ascorbic acid in the MFO system does not affect the degradation of this heme protein (19–21). No difference in heme oxygenase activity, degradation of cytochrome P_{450} heme, or synthesis of cytochrome P_{450} heme was found in ascorbic acid deficient guinea pigs compared with normal animals (19–21).

Table VI. Bromobenzene and Biphenyl Hydroxylation via the Hepatic MFO System in Normal and Ascorbic Acid Deficient Guinea Pigs

Guinea Pigs[a]	Cytochrome P_{450}[b]	Bromobenzene[c]		Biphenyl[c]	
		o-Bromo-phenol	p-Bromo-phenol	2-OH biphenyl	4-OH biphenyl
Normal (15)[d]	0.19 ± 0.01	$9.3^e \pm 0.9$	122 ± 8	22 ± 1.0	164 ± 8
Deficient (11)[f]	0.07 ± 0.01	$6.3^e \pm 0.5$	$53^g \pm 9$	19 ± 2.0	86 ± 2

[a] Numbers in parentheses equal number of animals.
[b] nmol/mg of 15,000 × g supernatant protein.
[c] nmol product/min/100 mg of microsomal protein.
[d] 40 mg of ascorbic acid/100 g of liver.
[e] Difference not significant.
[f] 2 mg of ascorbic acid/100 g of liver.
[g] Significant difference from normal, $p < 0.01$.

It is well established that the MFO system metabolizes drugs to more hydrophilic products; in doing so, many drugs and environmental chemicals proceed via reactive epoxide intermediates, which in turn may bind covalently to tissue macromolecules resulting in necrosis, mutagenesis, or carcinogenesis. Alternatively, the organism has at its disposal enzymatic systems such as glutathione transferase or epoxide hydrase that divert the reactive intermediates into nontoxic metabolites or products (*see* Scheme 3). We have investigated the activity of these important enzymes in ascorbic acid deficient as well as normal guinea pig livers. Microsomal epoxide hydrase is not significantly lower in ascorbic acid deficiency (*see* Table VII). In addition to this, cytoplasmic epoxide hydrase was not significantly altered; also, cytoplasmic glutathione transferase was not significantly changed (Table VII). The determination of microsomal glutathione transferase in these animals will be interesting. The guinea pigs used in this study weighed around 250 g and were on ascorbic acid deficient diet for 19 d. These animals traditionally

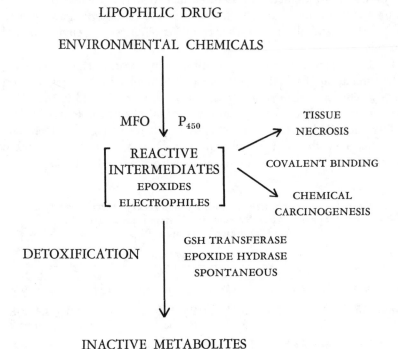

Scheme 3. *The metabolism and detoxification of drugs and environmental chemicals via the mixed function oxygenase, glutathione transferase, and epoxide hydrase pathways.*

Table VII. Hepatic Epoxide Hydrase and Glutathione Transferase in Normal and Ascorbate Deficient Guinea Pigs

Guinea pigs	Microsomal Epoxide Hydrase[a]		Cytoplasmic Glutathione Transferase[b]
	without THF	with THF	
Normal[c]	1527 (18)[d]	6215 (6)	38,400 (14)
Deficient[e]	1460 (13)	5930 (6)	42,000 (8)

Note: Ascorbate deficient diet, 19 d, guinea pig; 250 g.
[a] Activity in nmol of product/min/100 mg of protein, 37°C; THF, tetrahydrofuran (0.825 M); substrate, ^{3}H styrene oxide.
[b] Activity in nmol of product/min/100 mg of protein; 27°C; 15,000 × g supernatant fraction; substrate, p-nitrobenzyl chloride.
[c] 40 mg of ascorbate/100 g of liver.
[d] Numbers in parentheses equal number of animals.
[e] 2 mg of ascorbate/100 g of liver.

have shown the most significant decrease in cytochrome P_{450} under vitamin C deficiency. In contrast to these results, when older animals weighing 800 g were used, no significant difference in the cytochrome P_{450} and epoxide hydrase activity was noted. These findings are in agreement with those reported earlier (23).

Acknowledgment

This research was supported by grant 23007 from Hoffmann-La Roche, Incorporated.

Literature Cited

1. Conney, A. H.; Burns, J. J. *Adv. Pharmacol.* 1962, *1*, 31.
2. Conney, A. H. *Pharmacol. Rev.* 1967, *19*, 317.
3. Conney, A. H. In "Fundamentals of Drug Metabolism and Drug Disposition"; La Du, B. N.; Mandel, H. G.; Way, E. L., Eds.; Williams & Wilkins: Baltimore, 1971; Vol. 13, p. 253.
4. Zannoni, V. G.; Lynch, M. M. *Drug Metab. Rev.* 1973, *2*, 57.
5. Zannoni, V. G.; Sato, P. H. *Fed. Proc. Fed. Am. Soc. Exp. Biol.* 1976, *33*, 546.
6. Zannoni, V. G.; Sato, P. H. *Ann. N.Y. Acad. Sci.* 1975, *258*, 119.
7. Ginter, E. *Ann. N.Y. Acad. Sci.* 1975, *258*, 410.
8. Degkwitz, E.; Staundinger, H. *Hoppe-Seyler's Z. Physiol. Chem.* 1965, *342*, 63.
9. Degkwitz, E.; Luft, P.; Pfeiffer, U.; Staundinger, H. *Hoppe-Seyler's Z. Physiol. Chem.* 1968, *349*, 465.
10. Richards, R. K.; Jueter, K.; Klatt, T. I. *Proc. Soc. Exp. Biol. Med.* 1941, *48*, 403.
11. Axelrod, J.; Udenfriend, S.; Brodie, B. B. *J. Pharmacol. Exp. Ther.* 1954, *111*, 176.

12. Conney, A. H.; Bray, G. A.; Evans, C.; Burns, J. J. *Ann. N.Y. Acad. Sci.* **1961**, *92*, 115.
13. Leber, H.; Degkwitz, E.; Staudinger, H. *Hoppe-Seyler's Z. Physiol. Chem.* **1969**, *350*, 439.
14. Kato, R.; Takanaka, A.; Oshima, T. *Jpn. J. Pharmacol.* **1969**, *19*, 25.
15. Zannoni, V. G.; Flynn, E. J.; Lynch, M. M. *Biochem. Pharmacol.* **1972**, *21*, 1377.
16. Sato, P. H.; Zannoni, V. G. *J. Pharmacol. Exp. Ther.* **1976**, *198*, 295.
17. Luft, D.; Degkwitz, L.; Hochli-Kaufmann; Staudinger, H. *Hoppe-Seyler's Z. Physiol. Chem.* **1972**, *353*, 1420.
18. Walsch, S.; Degkwitz, E. *Hoppe-Seyler's Z. Physiol. Chem.* **1980**, *361*, 79.
19. Omaye, S. T.; Turnbull, J. D. *Biochem. Pharmacol.* **1979**, *28*, 1415.
20. Ibid., 365.
21. Ibid., **1980**, *29*, 1255.
22. Degkwitz, E.; Walsch, S.; Dubberstein, M. *Hoppe-Seyler's Z. Physiol. Chem.* **1974**, *355*, 1152.
23. Kuenzig, W.; Tkaczevski, V.; Kamm, J. J.; Conney, A. H.; Burns, J. J. *J. Pharmacol. Exp. Ther.* **1977**, *201*, 527.
24. van der Hoeven, T. A.; Coon, M. J. *J. Biol. Chem.* **1974**, *249*, 6302.
25. Hashimoto, C.; Imai, Y. *Biochem. Biophys. Res. Commun.* **1976**, *68*, 821.
26. Ryan, D.; Lu, A. Y. H.; Kawalek, J.; West, S. B.; Levin, W. *Biochem. Biophys. Res. Commun.* **1975**, *64*, 1134.
27. Welton, A. F.; Aust, S. D. *Biochem. Biophys. Res. Commun.* **1974**, *56*, 898.
28. Welton, A. F.; O'Neal, F.; Chaney, L. C.; Aust, S. D. *J. Biol. Chem.* **1975**, *250*, 5631.
29. Huang, M.; West, S. B.; Lu, A. Y. H. *J. Biol. Chem.* **1976**, *251*, 4659.
30. Haugen, D. A.; van der Hoeven, T. A.; Coon, M. J. *J. Biol. Chem.* **1975**, *250*, 3567.
31. Lau, S. S.; Zannoni, V. G. *Toxicol. Appl. Pharmacol.* **1979**, *50*, 309.
32. Rikans, L. E.; Smith, C. R.; Zannoni, V. G. *J. Pharmacol. Exp. Ther.* **1978**, *204*, 702.
33. Haugen, D. A.; Coon, M. J. *J. Biol. Chem.* **1976**, *251*, 7929.
34. Imai, Y.; Sato, R. *Biochem. Biophys. Res. Commun.* **1974**, *60*, 8.
35. Haugen, D. A.; Coon, M. J.; Nebert, D. W. *J. Biol. Chem.* **1976**, *251*, 1817.
36. Zannoni, V. G.; Lynch, M. M. *Drug Metab. Rev.* **1973**, *2*, 57.
37. Degkwitz, E.; Walsch, S.; Dubberstein, M.; Winter, J. *Ann. N.Y. Acad. Sci.* **1975**, *278*, 201.
38. Rikans, L. E.; Smith, C. R.; Zannoni, V. G. *Biochem. Pharmacol.* **1977**, *26*, 797.
39. Sato, P. H.; Zannoni, V. G. *Biochem. Pharmacol.* **1974**, *23*, 3121.

RECEIVED for review January 22, 1981. ACCEPTED April 13, 1981.

Nutritional and Health Aspects of Ascorbic Acid

MYRON BRIN

Department of Clinical Nutrition, Hoffmann-La Roche Incorporated, Nutley, NJ 07110

Ascorbic acid (AA) is not synthesized by humans, making it an essential dietary vitamin for this species. Although clinical deficiency (scurvy) is rare, marginal inadequacy results in behavioral changes, reduced drug metabolism, and reduced immunocompetence, thereby affecting social and work functions. AA is important in increasing iron absorption, in collagen synthesis, and as a biological blocking agent against nitrosamine formation; AA has also been used experimentally to reduce incidence of bladder tumors in mice. Heavy smoking increases the risk group fourfold. Blood levels are reduced in myocardial infarction and other conditions involving physical, infective, or traumatic insult. Scurvy still persists in certain parts of the world. The appropriate intake levels of vitamin C for each of its physiological functions have not yet been fully defined.

Humans require ascorbic acid as a vitamin. A recent report (*1*) established that the genetic basis of this need is a lack of L-gulonolactone dehydrogenase, the last enzyme in the synthetic sequence. This vitamin's function in, for example, preventing scurvy, and facilitating tyrosine and proline metabolism, is well documented and accepted. Virtually all other aspects of the health applications of vitamin C are controversial, including establishing a definitive daily requirement, which has varied over the years both within and between countries.

Perhaps it is more than happenstance that vitamin C is separated by name from the other water soluble "B" vitamins. Historically, this separation was the result of the normal procedure of labeling unknown dietary factors, as C was differentiated from B—which later was shown to be a complex group rather than an individual, water-soluble vitamin. It was

0065-2393/82/0200–0369$06.00/0

discovered that the B-vitamin group comprised a series of compounds, for which each individual compound could be assigned a highly specific vitamin–coenzyme structure, and which facilitated very specific enzyme reactions. Such was not the case for water-soluble vitamin C, for which a coenzyme structure has not yet been identified. The identification of the coenzyme forms of the B vitamins has lent credibility to their essentiality in human nutrition. So, water-soluble vitamin C must be evaluated at another level. That level is physiological function, rather than by specific reactions.

One could more readily explain the clinical signs of scurvy on the basis of the function of vitamin C in collagen formation, than one could explain the development of wet beriberi for thiamine, or of cheilosis for riboflavin function. For instance, why shouldn't riboflavin cause beriberi, and thiamine cause cheilosis—rather than the reverse? We cannot explain this. The situation exemplifies that we often cannot explain the clinical findings on the basis of what is known about the biochemical function of the vitamin. There is still much more to be learned about vitamin nutrition, and this is exemplified by vitamin C.

Bioactivity

The relative biopotency of synthetic vs. natural vitamin C is open to conjecture. By administering orange juice vs. synthetic vitamin C to adult males, and measuring levels of the vitamin in serum, leucocytes, and urine, the synthetic vitamin was but slightly more bioavailable (2). Using an intraluminal infusion technique of young male adults no differences in bioavailability were found (3). Presumably, the synthetic L-ascorbic acid is equally bioavailable to that found in nature.

Immunocompetence

Very provocative immunological work has been done with vitamin C during the last decade. White blood cell levels of vitamin C have been measured to evaluate nutritional status for this nutrient for almost forty years; therefore, it is not surprising that relationships to immunocompetence have emerged. Incubation of leucocytes with ascorbic acid at physiological pH augments the random migration and chemotaxis from onefold to threefold without affecting phagocytic capacity (4). This, as well as stimulation of hexose monophosphate shunt activity, was dose related, and could be reversed by washing the cells. The effect occurred at physiological concentrations of the vitamin. Glutathione also stimulated the shunt and the migration. This finding was considered significant because in polymorphonuclear lymphocytes (PMN), phagocytosis is accompanied by increased oxygen consumption, hexose monophosphate shunt activity, and hydrogen peroxide production (5). Vitamin C deficient guinea pigs yielded fewer macrophages (from peritoneal exudate), with reduced migration, but did not affect phagocytosis (6). The in vitro addition of vitamin C partially reversed the reduced migration. In the guinea pig, ascorbic acid depletion resulted in depressed immunological response (7), and high vitamin dosage supported elevated mitotic activity (8). PMN contain high levels of ascorbate (9); these levels are markedly reduced following viral infection (10, 11), and revert toward normal after recovery (11). Levels are also reduced in other leukemic and hematological conditions (12). Also, using the plaque inhibition method utilizing vesicular stomatitis virus, increased serum interferon following the subcutaneous injection of either ascorbic acid, sodium salicylate, or caffeine in mice was demonstrated (13). Similar findings of increased interferon induction were observed following exposure of human embryo skin in the presence of ascorbic acid to either Newcastle virus or poly I/poly C (14). Also, a threefold interferon increase in mouse cultures following poly I/poly C addition to mouse cell cultures containing vitamin C, and also in mice in vivo given 250 mg % ascorbic acid in drinking water, when exposed to murine leukemia virus was observed (13). A doubling of DNA synthesis by T-lymphocytes was remarked in spleens of mice on a high ascorbate diet following conconavalin A (con A) (15). In humans, the consumption of 1 g of ascorbic acid/d for 75 d resulted in increased serum levels of IgA, IgM, and C-3[1] complement (16). Increasing the weekly intake by human volunteers to 2 and 3 g/d enhanced neutrophil motility and lymphocyte transformation to phytohemagglutinin and con A (17, 18). In one study, however, hexose monophosphate shunt activity and serum levels of IgA, IgG, IgM, C′3, and C′4,[1] and total complement activity were not affected (18). Also, the numbers of leukemic cells in culture were reduced by 0.3 mM ascorbic acid (19). Normal myeloid cells were unaffected, and glutathione was ineffective. In summary, ascorbic acid probably influences various parameters of immunocompetence, and attention should be directed to studying effects of supplementation on these phenomena in the elderly, subjects on immunosuppressive drugs, pregnant women (20), and other risk groups.

Cancer

The relationship between ascorbic acid and cancer is of general interest. One of the first studies in this direction (21) demonstrated that vitamin C given to mice prevented the carcinogenicity in urinary bladders of implanted 3-hydroxyanthranilic acid. A few years later the ability of

---

[1] These factors are body proteins associated with immunocompetence.

ascorbate to block nitrosamine formation was demonstrated (22) using rat hepatotoxicity as a model. The ascorbate–nitrosamine relationship has been addressed in chapter 24 in this book. More recently, Pauling and coworkers have studied the usefulness of ascorbic acid in improving the quality of and lengthening the life of cancer patients (23), and in obtaining remission of reticulum cell sarcoma (24). Attempts to confirm these findings by others (25) have been unsuccessful, although different experimental designs, such as prior suppression of the immune system, were used (26). Current in vitro studies in conjunction with chemotherapy in neuroblastoma (27) and in malignant melanoma (28) demonstrated cell reversion to normal by vitamin C. The mechanism of action may be mediated through the enhanced production of hydrogen peroxide in tumor cells low in catalase and/or peroxidase. This mechanism may also apply to the enhancement by ascorbic acid of the toxicity of misonidazole as a radiosensitizing chemotherapeutic agent in the presence of radiation therapy in vitro (29).

Red Blood Cell

Ascorbic acid appears to be toxic to certain tumor tissues; however, it may increase the biological effectiveness of red blood cells by increasing the level of 2,3-diphosphoglycerate (30, 31). 2,3-Diphosphoglycerate is essential to maintaining the normal oxygen dissociation curve of hemoglobin. This increase has been shown in vitro (30) and in vivo, in human subjects (31).

Micronutrient Interactions

Certain interactions of vitamin C with other vitamins and minerals are of interest. There was little effect on encephalomalacia in chickens, but vitamin C reduced the incidence of exudative diathesis (32) probably because of an increased absorption of selenium. Also, it was suggested that ascorbic acid may regenerate reduced tocopherol from the oxidized phenoxy radical (33). Scorbutic megaloblastic anemia is associated with the excretion of 10-formylfolic acid, and following vitamin C administration, the major metabolite was 5-methyltetrahydrofolic acid (34). The allegation that vitamin B_{12} is destroyed in meals consumed with ascorbic acid (35) appears to have been overwhelmingly contradicted (36, 37). Another major interaction is that of ascorbic acid with iron. Excessive body iron, such as in hemosiderosis, results in accelerated, and somewhat modified oxidation of dehydroascorbic acid to carbon dioxide with a reduction of oxalate in urine (38). On the other hand, although it has been known for many years that iron absorption is enhanced by ascorbic acid, it is now recognized that greater enhancement is achieved if the ascorbic acid and iron are present in the gastrointestinal tract simultaneously. Furthermore, the twofold to tenfold increase in iron absorption at doses of 10–1000 mg of ascorbic acid was somewhat higher than anticipated (39). This unexpected increase was one of the factors that stimulated the Food and Nutrition Board to increase the recommended daily allowance (RDA) for vitamin C from 45 to 60 mg, in the 1980 edition (40).

Some Health Situations

The usefulness of vitamin C in preventing colds or ameliorating the symptoms remains controversial. Anderson, who initially found reduced winter illness as a result of supplementation (41), believes "that the weight of the evidence is in favor of there being some effect (at least on severity and duration) from supplementary vitamin C, but the magnitude of this effect has varied widely among the different studies." Chalmers also reviewed the "cold" literature and stated that "the data suggest that ascorbic acid does have some effect on the severity of cold symptoms, but the effects are quantitatively so small, and the possibility of suggestion as the primary mechanism so large, that it hardly seems worthwhile for anyone to take all these pills for such a long time" (42). In both of these studies, the ameliorating effects were acknowledged as statistically significant, with the judgment that they were not biologically important. Yet certain reports were very supportive of the usefulness of vitamin C in colds (43), just as others were less so (44). The usefulness of vitamin C in colds was related to an antihistamine effect of the vitamin (45) in guinea pigs, and, in human subjects blood histamine levels are elevated exponentially when plasma ascorbic acid falls below 1.0 mg %, and becomes highly significant at levels below 0.7 mg % (46). The scorbutic state is associated with levels below 0.2 mg %. Of course, the personal testimonials of usefulness of vitamin C in colds are manifold. This is a complex situation and requires further study.

The human need for ascorbic acid both in wound healing and in the postsurgical maintenance of strong scar tissue is well documented (47). These needs were restudied more recently in sixty-three surgical patients (48). There was a 42% reduction in circulating leucocyte vitamin C levels on the third postoperative day, regardless of the extent of surgical trauma, suggesting an increased need for the vitamin during surgery and the postoperative period.

More recently, some attention was experimentally directed to maintaining the integrity of the eye following induced alkali burns in rabbits. Ascorbate levels in rabbit aqueous humor remain depressed for 4 weeks following an alkali burn (49, 50). The incidence of corneal ulceration resulting from this trauma can be reduced from 60% in saline-treated controls to 22% by ascorbate injection (49) or from 47% to 6% by topical administration (50). Also, ascorbate prevents light-induced damage to the ocular lens cation pump in rat eyes, in vitro (51).

Because of current interest in atherosclerosis, we will mention some of the relationships between ascorbic acid and some of the associated phenomena. Vitamin C deficient guinea pigs have elevated cholesterol levels (52). More recently, a reduced rate of cholesterol catabolism was demonstrated in chronically deficient guinea pigs (53, 54). Similar observations were made in human subjects (55). Another factor of interest in atherosclerosis is platelet aggregation. In one report, platelet vitamin C levels were significantly lower in diabetics than in normal humans, and the addition of the vitamin in normal concentrations to platelet-rich plasma consistently reduced aggregation, as did the ingestion of 2 g of vitamin C/d for 7 d in vivo (56). Coupling these observations with those of decreased cholesterol catabolism suggests that vitamin C is a basic factor in atherogenesis.

In another medical situation, osteogenesis imperfecta, supplementation with vitamin C at a level of 1–2 g/d (to subjects with ascorbic acid levels in the normal range) resulted in increased physical activity and stamina, and in reduced fracture incidence (57). These findings remain to be confirmed.

Supplementation with vitamin C, 500–1000 mg/d, to forty-four pairs of monozygotic twins for 5 months resulted in shorter and less severe illness episodes in girls, and resulted in growth of an average of 1.3 cm more than untreated controls (58). The investigators are reinvestigating these findings.

Another observation in a double blind crossover trial on leg ulcers in individuals with β-thalassemia, showed a higher rate of either complete or partial healing with 3 g of ascorbic acid/d over an 8-week period (59).

The effects of stress on the depression of serum/leucocyte levels of vitamin C were recently summarized (60). Included were myocardial infarction, and other conditions involving physical, infective, or traumatic insult, including cold virus infection, and intravenous tetracosactrin. Associated with the reduced ascorbate level in myocardial infarction was an increased cortisol level over a period of 56 d. The authors recommended 1 g of ascorbic acid/d for 1 month following the traumatic event, with a comment concerning the need for additional study (60). Plasma ascorbate was also depressed following iv administration of adrenalin; this depression was prevented by prior administration of propranolol, a β-blocker (61). Smoking not only reduces blood levels of vitamin C (62, 63), but increases the proportion of the population in the scorbutic range of blood values fourfold (64). These effects are probably caused by increased rates of ascorbate metabolism, as discussed in chapter 16 of this book. Also, vitamin C or cysteine, when added to hamster lung cultures, protects against or reverses abnormal growth or malignant transformation after repeated exposure to smoke from tobacco or marijuana (65).

As of 1972, scurvy was still a pediatric problem in Australia (66), and in arctic and subarctic Canada (67), and of lesser, but continued concern in the Quebec area (68). In Australia the patients were primarily of Mediterranean origin, their symptoms appeared in the second 6 months of life, and they showed irritability and painful mobile legs (66). In the Canadian subarctic, scurvy was associated with hypertyrosinemia. In pregnant women, blood levels of less than 0.2 mg % were twenty times as common in the arctic as in French Canada (67). At the other end of the age spectrum, blood levels of vitamin C are lower in the elderly, in winter than summer, in smokers, and in males (69). The elderly with low vitamin C levels had a significantly higher mortality within 4 weeks of admission to a geriatric unit than did those with high levels (69). A later report suggested that the mortality of females with low vitamin C levels at 4 weeks after admission was not changed by 200 mg of vitamin C/d supplementation. The elderly females who responded with higher blood levels of vitamin C had a lower mortality, but leucocyte and plasma levels may not be the most reliable indication of vitamin C status (70). In a study in Wales, supplementation with 150 mg of vitamin C/d for 12 weeks followed by 50 mg/d for 2 years showed no advantage of supplementation except the higher mortality among those with lower leucocyte vitamin levels (71). The possible need for higher dosage was discussed. However, the possible simultaneous inadequacy of other vitamins and/or minerals was neither determined nor contemplated. Measurable behavioral changes, such as adverse Minnesota Multiphasic Personality Index (MMPI) scores of the neurotic triad (hypochondriasis, depression, and hysteria), result from vitamin C depletion before the onset of clinical signs (72).

Scurvy has virtually disappeared in the United States, except for in occasional severe alcoholics and/or neglected persons, as shown by two surveys (73, 74). Yet certain population groups appear "at risk" for vitamin C deficiency as shown by the two aforementioned surveys as well as a third survey (75). This means that these groups are depleted for vitamin C, as indicated by low intake level and/or low blood levels, in the absence of specific clinical signs for scurvy. We define this condition as "marginal deficiency," which comprises the first three of the five sequential stages shown in Table I (76). Stage three is the critical one because the depletion has progressed to the point that there are signs and symptoms of abnormal physiology, although the indications are

Table I. Five Stages in Development of Vitamin Deficiency

Deficiency Stage	Symptoms
1. Preliminary	Depletion of tissue stores (because of diet, malabsorption, abnormal metabolism, etc.). Urinary excretion depressed.
2. Biochemical	Enzyme activity reduced. Urinary excretion negligible.
3. Physiological and behavioral	Loss of appetite with reduced body weight, insomnia or somnolence, irritableness, adverse changes in MMPI scores. Reduced immunocompetence, impaired drug metabolism.
4. Clinical	Exacerbated nonspecific symptoms plus appearance of specific deficiency syndrome.
5. Anatomical	Clear specific syndromes with tissue pathology. Death ensues unless treated.

nonspecific for vitamin C, per se. For instance, aberrant behavioral changes were observed and measured at the University of Iowa, in a human depletion study in conjunction with the U.S. Army Medical Nutrition Laboratory (72). Work on drug metabolism is described in chapter 17 in this book. The effects on immunocompetence were described earlier in this chapter. These adverse effects of changes in behavior, drug metabolism, and immunocompetence were not so dramatic that a marginally deficient person would be recognized to have a vitamin problem. Rather, the effects are subliminal or preclinical, and probably impair the person's function in society. The latter is difficult to describe in cost/benefit numbers, but may affect other values such as self-esteem, social relationships, productivity on the job or at school, or the possibility of increased frequency of illness. However, after restoration of tissue levels, the RDA should theoretically maintain health in otherwise healthy persons (40).

In addition, RDA levels higher than those reported may be appropriate for some human conditions. Some such conditions are described in the RDA manual (40): "Infections, even mild ones, increase metabolic losses of nitrogen and of a number of vitamins and minerals." Also, "the period of recuperation following illness, trauma, burns, and surgical procedures, during which body stores are being replenished and tissues restored, is probably comparable to a period of growth."

Other conditions previously mentioned in this chapter, such as cancer, immunocompetence and interferon production, antihistamine effects in colds, increased iron absorption, effects on cholesterol metabolism, and nitrosamine blocking, were studied at higher than RDA dosage levels. These many situations require additional research study to determine what the minimum levels are to attain the optimal health condition.

Three cases that demonstrate the value of additional research are the effects of smoking on the rate of ascorbic acid metabolism, as described in chapter 16 in this book; the increase in the RDA for vitamin C in 1980 over that in 1974 on the basis of the significant improvement in iron absorption (40); and the blocking of nitrosamine production as described in chapter 24 in this book.

Conclusions

We tend to conceive of vitamin function in the context of its biochemical functions, without giving sufficient attention to the contributions to the whole body. It is clear now that vitamin C has functions beyond folacins, proline, and tyrosine metabolism; for example, vitamin C levels influence personality and immunocompetence—very distant from the enzyme level. The vitamin's reducing–antioxidizing functions in humans may be the basis for many of its nonenzymatic, less specific, although physiologically essential, effects. Perhaps, too, we should change our concept of vitamin C to one of a chemical conditioning vitamin—to aid the inner body environment ward off adverse external attacks such as by smoking pollution (lung differentiation), by drugs and environmental chemicals (mixed function oxidases), in cancer tissue culture (cell normalization), and so on. This concept should be defined not in terms of a therapeutic cure, but rather in terms of a nutritional supplement that when consumed in appropriate quantities will contribute to maintaining health. We do not feel that the appropriate quantities of vitamin C have been fully defined for all functions as yet, and we believe, therefore, that there is much research to be done.

Literature Cited

1. Sato, P.; Udenfriend, S. *Vitam. Horm.* **1978**, *36*, 33–52.
2. Pelletier, O.; Keith, M. O. *J. Am. Diet. Assoc.* **1974**, *64*, 271–275.
3. Nelson, E. W.; Streiff, R. R.; Cerda, J. J. *Am. J. Clin. Nutr.* **1975**, *28*, 1014–1019.
4. Goetzl, E. J.; Wasserman, S. I.; Gigli, I.; Austen, K. F. *J. Clin. Invest.* **1974**, *53*, 813–818.
5. Karnovsky, M. L. *Semin. Hematol.* **1968**, *5*, 156–165.
6. Ganguly, R.; Durieux, M. F.; Waldman, R. H. *Am. J. Clin. Nutr.* **1976**, *29*, 762–765.
7. Thurman, G. B.; Goldstein, A. L. *Fed. Proc., Fed. Am. Soc. Exp. Biol.* **1979**, *38*, 1173.
8. Fraser, R. C.; Pavlovic, S.; Kurahara ,C. G.; Murata, A.; Peterson, N. S.; Taylor, K. B.; Feigen, G. A. *Am. J. Clin. Nutr.* **1978**, *33*, 839–847.
9. DeChatelet, L. R.; McCall, C. E.; Cooper, M. R.; Shirley, P. S. *Proc. Soc. Exp. Biol. Med.* **1974**, *145*, 1170–1173.
10. Greene, M.; Wilson, C. W. M. *Br. J. Clin. Pharmacol.* **1975**, *2*, 369.
11. Hume, R.; Weyers, E. *Scott. Med. J.* **1973**, *18*, 3–7.

12. Barton, G. M. G.; Roath, O. S. *Int. J. Vitam. Nutr. Res.* **1976,** *46,* 271–274.
13. Geber, W. F.; Lefkowitz, S. S.; Huang, C. Y. *Pharmacology* **1975,** *13,* 228–233.
14. Dahl, H.; Degre, M. *Acta Pathol. Microbiol. Scand. Sect. B* **1976,** *84,* 280–284.
15. Siegel, B. V.; Morton, J. I. *Int. J. Vitam. Nutr. Res.* **1977,** *Suppl. 16,* 245–265.
16. Prinz, W.; Bortz, R.; Bregin, B.; Hersch, M. *Int. J. Vitam. Nutr. Res.* **1977,** *47,* 248–257.
17. Anderson, R.; Oosthuizen, R.; Moritz, R.; Theron, A.; Van Rensburg, A. J. *Am. J. Clin. Nutr.* **1980,** *33,* 71–76.
18. Delafuente, J. C.; Panush, R. S. *Int. J. Vitam. Nutr. Res.* **1980,** *50,* 44–51.
19. Park, C. H.; Amare, M.; Savin, M. A.; Hoogstraten, B. *Cancer Res.* **1980,** *40,* 1062–1068.
20. Thomas, W. R.; Holt, P. G. *Clin. Exp. Immunol.* **1978,** *32,* 370–379.
21. Schlegel, J. U.; Pipkin, P. E.; Mishimiera, R.; Schultz, G. N. *Trans. Am. Assoc. Genito-Urinary Surgeons* **1969,** *61,* 85–89.
22. Kamm, J. J.; Dashman, T.; Conney, A. H.; Burns, J. J. *Proc. Nat. Acad. Sci.* **1973,** *70,* 747–749.
23. Cameron, E.; Pauling, L. *Biol. Interact.* **1974,** *9,* 273–283.
24. Cameron, E.; Campbell, A.; Jack, T. *Biol. Interact.* **1975,** *11,* 387–393.
25. Creegan, E. T.; Moertel, C. G.; O'Fallon, J. R.; Schult, A. J.; O'Connel, J. J.; Rubin, J.; Frytak, S. *N. Engl. J. Med.* **1979,** *301,* 686–690.
26. Creagan, E. T.; Moertel, C. *N. Engl. J. Med.* **1979,** *301,* 1399.
27. Prasad, K. N. *Life Sci.* **1980,** *27,* 275–280.
28. Bram, S.; Froussard, P.; Guichard, M.; Jasmin, C.; Augery, Y.; Sinnousi-Barre, F.; Wray, W. *Nature* **1980,** *284,* 629–631.
29. Josephy, P. D.; Paleie, B.; Skarrssard, L. D. *Nature* **1978,** *271,* 370–372.
30. Wood, L. A.; Beutler, E. *Br. J. Hematol.* **1973,** *25,* 611–618.
31. Moore, L. G.; Brewer, G. J.; Oelshlegel, F. J.; Brewer, L. F.; Schoomaker, E. B. *J. Pharmacol. Exp. Ther.* **1977,** *203,* 722–728.
32. Combs, Jr., G. F.; Pesti, G. M. *J. Nutr.* **1976,** *106,* 958–966.
33. Packer, J. E.; Slater, T. F.; Wilson, R. L. *Nature,* **1979,** *278,* 737–738.
34. Stokes, P. L.; Melikian, V.; Leeming, R. L.; Portman-Graham, H.; Blair, J. A.; Cooke, W. T. *Am. J. Clin. Nutr.* **1975,** *28,* 126–129.
35. Herbert, V.; Jacob, E. *J. Am. Med. Assoc.* **1974,** *230,* 241–242.
36. Marcus, M.; Prabhudesai, M.; Wassef, S. *Am. J. Clin. Nutr.* **1980,** *33,* 137–143.
37. Ekvall, S.; Bozian, R. *Fed. Proc., Fed. Am. Soc. Exp. Biol.* **1979,** *39,* 452.
38. Hankes, L. V.; Jansen, C. R.; Schmaeler, M. *Biochem. Med.* **1974,** *9,* 244–255.
39. Cook, J. D.; Monsen, E. R. *Am. J. Clin. Nutr.* **1977,** *30,* 235–241.
40. "Recommended Daily Allowances," 9th ed. Food and Nutrition Board NAS/NRC: Washington, DC, 1980; p. 76.
41. Anderson, T. W., presented at the *West. Hemisphere Nutr. Cong., Proc., 4th, 1974–1975.*
42. Chalmers, T. C. *Am. J. Med.* **1975,** *58,* 532–536.
43. Sabiston, B. H.; Radomski, M. W., DCIEM Report #74R1012, Defense Research Board, **1974,** 1–10.
44. Pitt, H. A.; Costrini, A. M. *J. Am. Med. Assoc.* **1979,** *241,* 908–911.
45. Chatterjee, I. B.; Majumder, A. K.; Nandi, B. K.; Subramanian, N. *Ann. N.Y. Acad. Sci.* **1975,** *258,* 24–47.

46. Clemetson, C. A. B. *J. Nutr.* **1980**, *110*, 662–668.
47. Vitamin C, *Ann. N.Y. Acad. Sci.* **1961**, *92*, Art. 1.
48. Irvin, T. T.; Chattopadhyay, D. K.; Smythe, A. *Surg. Gynecol. Obstet.* **1978**, *147*, 49–55.
49. Pfister, R. R.; Paterson, C. A. *Invest. Ophthalmol. Visual Sci.* **1977**, *16*, 478–487.
50. Pfister, R. R.; Paterson, C. A.; Hayes, S. A. *Invest. Ophthalmol. Visual Sci.* **1978**, *17*, 1019–1024.
51. Varma, S. D.; Kumar, S.; Richards, R. D. *Proc. Nat. Acad. Sci.* **1979**, *76*, 3504–3506.
52. Bolker, H. I.; Fishman, S.; Heard, R. D. H.; O'Donnell, V. J.; Webb, J. L.; Willis, G. C. *J. Exp. Med.* **1956**, *103*, 199–205.
53. Ginter, E. *Science* **1973**, *179*, 702–704.
54. Ginter, E.; Nemec, R.; Cerven, J.; Mikus, L. *Lipids* **1973**, *8*, 135–   .
55. Ginter, E.; Bobek, P.; Babala, J.; Jakubovsky, J.; Zaviacic, M.; Lojda, Z. *Int. J. Vitam. Nutr. Res.* **1979**, *19*, 55–70.
56. Sarji, K. E.; Kleinfelder, J.; Brewington, P.; Gonzales, J.; Hempling, H.; Colwell, J. A. *Thromb. Res.* **1979**, *15*, 639–650.
57. Kurz, D.; Eyring, E. J. *Pediatrics* **1974**, *54*, 56–61.
58. Miller, J. Z.; Nance, W. E.; Norton, J. A.; Wolen, R. L.; Griffith, R. S.; Rose, R. J. *J. Am. Med. Assoc.* **1977**, *237*, 248–251.
59. Afifi, A. M.; Ellis, L.; Huntsman, R. G.; Said, A. I. *Br. J. Dermatol.* **1975**, *92*, 339–341.
60. Hume, R.; Vallence, B.; Weyers, E. *Int. J. Vitam. Nutr. Res.* **1977**, *16*, 89–98.
61. Cox, B. D.; Clarkson, A. R.; Whichelow, M. J.; Rutland, P. *Horm. Metab. Res.* **1974**, *6*, 234–237.
62. Pelletier, O. *Int. J. Vitam. Nutr. Res.* **1977**, *16*, 147–169.
63. Hoefel, O. S. *Int. J .Vitam. Nutr. Res.* **1977**, *16*, 127–137.
64. Ritzel, G.; Bruppacker, G. *Int. J. Vitamin. Nutr. Res.* **1977**, *16*, 171–183.
65. Leuchtenberger, C.; Leuchtenberger, R. *Br. J. Exp. Pathol. 1977*, *58*, 625–634.
66. Henderson-Smart, D. J. *Med. J. Aust.* **1972**, *14*, 876–878.
67. Clow, C. J.; Laberge, C.; Scriver, C. R. *CMA Journal*, **1975**, 624–626.
68. Vobecky, J. S.; Vobecky, J.; Blanchard, R. *Am. J. Clin. Nutr.* **1976**, *29*, 766–771.
69. Wilson, T. S.; Weeks, M. M.; Mukherjee, S. K.; Murrell, J. S.; Andrews, C. S.; *Gerontol. Clin.* **1972**, *14*, 17–24.
70. Wilson, T. S.; Datta, S. B.; Murrell, J. S.; Andrews, C. T. *Age Ageing* **1973**, *2*, 163–171.
71. Burr, M. L.; Hurley, R. J.; Sweetnam, P. M. *Gerontol. Clin.* **1975**, *17*, 236–243.
72. Kinsman, R. A.; Hood, J. *Am. J. Clin. Nutr.* **1971**, *24*, 455–464.
73. "Ten State Nutrition Survey Highlights," USDHEW **1968–1970**, Publ. # (HSM) 72-8134.
74. "HANES: Health and Nutrition Examination Survey," **1974**, USDHEW Publ. # (HRA) 74-1219-1.
75. "Household Food Consumption Survey," USDA **1965**.
76. Brin, M. *J. Am. Med. Assoc.* **1964**, *187*, 762–766.

RECEIVED for review January 22, 1981. ACCEPTED April 30, 1981.

Role of L-Ascorbic Acid in Lipid Metabolism

E. GINTER, P. BOBEK, and M. JURCOVICOVA

Institute of Human Nutrition Research, Bratislava, Czechoslovakia

The activity of the microsomal system containing cyto-chrome P_{450} that catalyzes 7α-hydroxylation of cholesterol is depressed in the livers of guinea pigs with marginal vitamin C deficiency. Slowing of the rate-limiting reaction of cholesterol transformation to bile acids causes cholesterol accumulation in the liver, plasma, and arteries; increase of plasma cholesterol half-life; decrease in the bile-acid body pool; atherosclerotic changes in coronary arteries; and cholesterol gallstone formation. In an ascorbate-deficient animal the plasma triglyceride level rises; the post-heparin plasma lipolytic activity decreases, and the half-life of plasma triglycerides increases, causing triglyceride accumulation in the liver and arteries. In hypercholesterolemic humans with low vitamin C status, L-ascorbic acid administration (500–1000 mg/d) lowers plasma cholesterol concentration. This effect may be reinforced through the simultaneous administration of agents that sequester bile acids.

The relationships among L-ascorbic acid, lipid metabolism, and athero-sclerosis were first studied at extreme L-ascorbate levels, which are unlike the intake levels prevailing in human nutrition. Those investigations were done on animals that either biosynthesize ascorbate, such as rabbits or rats (1, 2), or on acutely scorbutic guinea pigs (3, 4). Ascorbate levels in the tissues of animals synthesizing L-ascorbic acid are saturated, and they are only slightly influenced by exogenous vitamin C. Therefore the effect of ascorbate on cholesterol metabolism in such animals is small (5). Disorders of lipid metabolism in scorbutic animals are, for the most part, nonspecific, because such animals refuse food and lose body weight rapidly.

A more suitable model for our biochemical research is a guinea pig eating a diet marginally deficient in vitamin C (6). Guinea pigs are

0065-2393/82/0200–0381$06.00/0

given a vitamin-C-free diet for two weeks, which results in a rapid decline of their ascorbate body pool, although vitamin C deficiency does not appear outwardly. Then a maintenance dose of L-ascorbic acid (0.5–1.0 mg/24 h/animal) is initiated with the otherwise unaltered diet. Food consumption and weight curves of the deficient animals are similar to those of the controls, which receive the same diet but with a substantially higher intake of L-ascorbic acid. Vitamin-C-deficient animals appear to be in good health, but the ascorbate levels in their tissues are permanently very low.

Guinea pigs can be maintained in a state of marginal vitamin C deficiency for protracted periods, for example, for a whole year. This longevity is suitable for following up metabolic disorders of compounds with long biological half-lives and also for pursuing pathophysiological studies, such as research on atherogenesis. Moreover, the model of a marginal vitamin C deficiency comes close to the prevailing situation in many population groups, because the consumption of vitamin C in various parts of the world likewise reaches marginal limits, especially during the winter and spring.

L-*Ascorbic Acid and Cholesterol Metabolism*

If guinea pigs are kept in a state of marginal vitamin C deficiency for a protracted period, cholesterol accumulates in their livers and blood plasma, resulting in an elevated ratio of total cholesterol/high density lipoprotein (HDL) cholesterol (Table I). These data have been confirmed in vitamin-C-deficient guinea pigs (7–14). A different cholesterol turnover was found in vitamin-C-deficient baboons, but the plasma cholesterol level increased only with a concomitant stress (15). The effect of acute vitamin C deficiency on human plasma cholesterol is small (16). There are no data available on the effect of a chronically marginal vitamin C deficiency on plasma lipids in humans. However, hypercholesterolemia is more frequent in humans with a low vitamin C intake than in those adequately supplied with ascorbate (17–19). Even rainbow trout with chronic vitamin C deficiency are reported to develop a marked hypercholesterolemia (20).

Research on the mechanism of the onset of hypercholesterolemia during a state of marginal vitamin C deficiency (6, 21, 22) has led to the finding that ascorbate is necessary for cholesterol transformation to bile acids (23) at the rate-limiting reaction of bile-acid biosynthesis. That limiting step is the 7α-hydroxylation of cholesterol (6, 24–26). The action of ascorbate on 7α-hydroxylation is not a direct one because in vitro added L-ascorbic acid has no effect (24, 27). The effect is mediated by the intervention of ascorbate in the metabolism of cytochrome P_{450} in the endoplasmatic reticulum of the hepatal cell (6, 24). Through a

Table I.   Effect of a Chronic Marginal Vitamin C Deficiency
(19 Weeks on a Diet with 15% Predominantly Saturated
Fat and 0.03% Cholesterol) on Blood Serum Lipids
in Sated Male Guinea Pigs

Parameter	Control Group (0.5% L-ascorbic acid in diet)	Vitamin C Deficiency (0.5 mg of L-ascorbic acid/24 h/ animal)	Statistical Significance (student's t-test)
Body weight (g)	700 ± 14 (27)	681 ± 20 (27)	NS
Vitamin C in the liver (mmol/kg of fresh tissue)	1.86 ± 0.10 (27)	0.22 ± 0.03 (27)	$P < 0.001$
Total serum cholesterol (mmol/L)	1.78 ± 0.11 (27)	3.34 ± 0.19 (27)	$P < 0.001$
HDL cholesterol in serum[a]	0.52 ± 0.04 (15)	0.44 ± 0.03 (20)	NS
Ratio $\dfrac{\text{total}}{\text{HDL}}$ cholesterol	4.2 ± 0.5 (15)	9.0 ± 0.8 (20)	$P < 0.001$
Serum triglyceridesz (mmol/L)	1.76 ± 0.27	4.90 ± 0.43	$P < 0.001$

Note: Data presented as mean ± se. Figures in parentheses indicate numbers of animals analyzed. NS = not significant.
[a] HDL cholesterol was determined by the dextran sulfate precipitation method.

similar mechanism, ascorbate also affects the hydroxylation of xenobiotics (28). The exact mechanism of L-ascorbic acid on cytochrome
P_{450}, in spite of intensive research (28–31), is as yet unknown. The
hypocholesterolemic effect of L-ascorbate 2-sulfate (10) has been ascribed
to its capacity to transform cholesterol to the more water-soluble cholesterol sulfate (32). However, from a quantitative aspect, this process
is of minor significance in total cholesterol turnover (33, 34).

In guinea pigs with a marginal vitamin C deficiency, the decreased
transformation of cholesterol to bile acids provokes a series of pathological changes: hypercholesterolemia and cholesterol accumulation in
the liver, which has already been discussed; increase of plasma cholesterol half-life (6); increase in cholesterol concentration in gallbladder
bile (35); decrease in the bile-acid body pool and lowered excretion of
bile acids in the stool (26, 36); decrease of bile-acid concentration in
gallbladder bile with the resulting formation of cholesterol gallstones
(5, 35); cholesterol accumulation in the aorta; and atherosclerosis (7, 9,
37–41). Optimum prevention of these disorders may be achieved by

doses of L-ascorbic acid that are capable of ensuring a maximum steady state level (saturation) of ascorbate in the tissues (42).

L-Ascorbic Acid and Triglyceride Metabolism

Marked hypertriglyceridemia occurs in ascorbate-deficient guinea pigs (Table I) with triglycerides accumulating in the liver and the aorta (7, 8, 39, 42, 43). From a kinetic point of view, the reason for hypertriglyceridemia may be either an increased input or a decreased output of triglycerides from the plasma pool. A study of the secretion rate of endogenous triglycerides following a blockade of lipoprotein lipase with Triton WR 1339 has shown that the triglyceride input in guinea pigs with marginal vitamin C deficiency is lowered by 25% (44). Simultaneously, however, the rate of triglyceride output from the plasma pool, determined by a decline of radioactivity of endogenously labeled ^{3}H-triglycerides, is even more substantially reduced (Figure 1).

The rate of triglyceride output from the plasma is mainly controlled by the lipoprotein lipase activity of peripheral tissues. Post-heparin plasma lipolytic activity in vitamin-C-deficient guinea pigs decreases considerably. In addition, in some of the animals the response of the plasma lipolytic activity to intravenously administered heparin is also prolonged (45). Similar results have been reported in vitamin-C-deficient baboons (46).

Lipoprotein lipase activity determined in acetone powders from guinea pig tissues with a marginal vitamin C deficiency was not greatly altered (47). On the other hand, lipoprotein lipase activity in epididymal fat, following incubation of the tissue with heparin, dropped abruptly in vitamin-C-deficient guinea pigs, and this decrease was in good agreement with the enhanced triglyceride concentration in blood serum (Figure 2). Hence, vitamin C deficiency may affect lipoprotein lipase release from capillaries by influencing the heparin–lipoprotein lipase interaction. This assumption would agree with the fact that high doses of L-ascorbic acid depress hypertriglyceridemia in various animal species, the hypotriglyceridemic effect being associated with a stimulation of lipolytic systems (2, 7, 43, 45). However the inhibitory effect in vitro added L-ascorbic acid on lipoprotein lipase in the heart (46) and on hormone-sensitive lipase in the adipose tissue (48) is unexplained.

L-Ascorbic Acid and Hypercholesterolemia in Humans

In contrast to the unequivocal results obtained in guinea pigs, data on the effect of L-ascorbic acid on cholesterolemia in humans differ considerably (5, 22, 49). Some authors (2, 6, 11, 50–53) found a hypocholesterolemic effect, while others refute it (54–60). Those contradictions

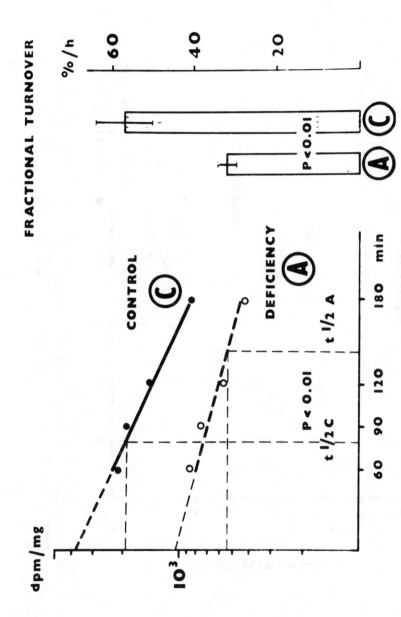

Figure 1. Removal of endogenously labeled ³H-triglycerides from blood plasma in control male guinea pigs (C, 0.5% L-ascorbic acid in diet) and in animals of equal weight with a marginal vitamin C deficiency (A, 0.5 mg of L-ascorbic acid/animal/d).

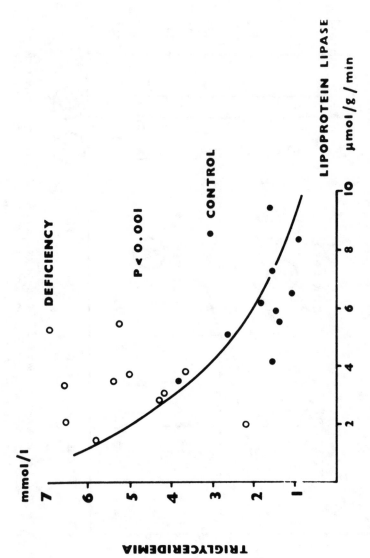

Figure 2. A negative correlation between lipoprotein lipase activity in epididymal fat tissue and tri-glyceride concentration in blood serum of conrtol male guinea pigs (0.5% L-ascorbic acid in diet) and in guinea pigs with a marginal vitamin C deficiency (0.5 mg of L-ascorbic acid/animal/d). Equation of the curve, $y = 7.91\,e^{-0.224x}$.

have partially been elucidated by the finding that the hypocholesterolemic effect of L-ascorbic acid depends on the initial level of cholesterol in blood serum (*61*) (*see* Table II and Figure 3). L-Ascorbic acid administration to humans with normal levels of cholesterol has no effect, but with elevated levels of cholesterol in serum, the hypocholesterolemic effect of ascorbate becomes evident. In light of this finding, reports of the inefficiency of vitamin C in depressing cholesterolemia in healthy humans with low cholesterolemia are irrelevant. If hypercholesterolemia occurs in humans with a permanently high vitamin C intake, its cause lies elsewhere than in vitamin C deficiency and therapy with L-ascorbic acid will be ineffective (*58, 60*). Genetically conditioned hypercholesterolemiae are caused by disorders in the receptors for plasma low-density lipoproteins (LDL) and it appears improbable that L-ascorbic acid could remedy this defect.

The hypocholesterolemic effect of L-ascorbic acid is most prevalent in humans with low levels of tissue ascorbate and in whom hypercholesterolemia results from a chronic imbalance between an enhanced input of exogenous or endogenous cholesterol and a reduced output in the form of bile acids. The most striking hypocholesterolemic effect of ascorbate has been observed in elderly hypercholesterolemic humans

Table II. Experimental Conditions for Determining Hypocholesterolemic Effect of L-Ascorbic Acid

Group	Number of Subjects	Dose (mg/d)	Duration
1. maturity-onset diabetics	35	500	1 year
2. pensioners with initial cholesterolemia > 230 mg %	19	1000	3 months
3. healthy people with mild hypercholesterolemia	24	300	7 weeks
4. pensioners with initial cholesterolemia > 200 mg %	46	1000	3 months
5. chronic inpatients	39	900	3 weeks
6. alcoholic inpatients	14	900	3 weeks
7. students	20	100	8 weeks
8. students	20	200	8 weeks
9. students	20	500	8 weeks
10. students	20	2000	8 weeks
11. pensioners with initial cholesterolemia < 200 mg %	36	1000	3 months
12. hyperlipemic outpatients	11	450[a]	6 weeks
13. healthy people with mild hypercholesterolemia	21	450[a]	6 weeks

Note: Regression line is obtained for mean values from the thirteen groups.
[a] Plus 15 g of citrus pectin/d.
Source: Reproduced with permission, from Ref. *61*.

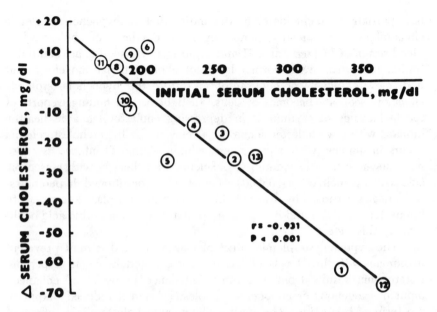

Figure 3. Mean change in total serum cholesterol concentration after L-ascorbic acid treatment vs. initial serum cholesterol levels. Experimental conditions are given in Table II.

with a marginal vitamin C deficiency and in hypercholesterolemic diabetics with very low vitamin C status (38). The decline of total cholesterol concentration after ascorbate treatment is caused by a decline of LDL cholesterol, for the amount of the protective HDL does not change or may even rise with an increased intake of vitamin C (53, 62, 63). However, the ascorbate-stimulated cholesterol transformation to bile acids leads to an increased bile-acid pool (26, 36), and the increased quantities of bile acids returning via the enterohepatal recirculation back to the liver may slow down the 7α-hydroxylation of cholesterol. Consequently this feedback effect must be eliminated if hypercholesterolemia is to be lowered.

Synergism Between L-Ascorbic Acid and Substances Capable of Binding Bile Acids

One possible method to interrupt the feedback effect of bile acids in the liver is to administer, along with vitamin C, cholestyramine (Questran), a synthetic resin that binds bile acids in the gastrointestinal tract. If a moderate hypercholesterolemia is provoked in guinea pigs through a marginal vitamin C deficiency and then 1.5% of Questran (i.e., 0.66% of cholestyramine) is added to their diet, the level of cholesterol in blood serum remains unaffected. The simultaneous administration of 1.5% Questran with 0.5% L-ascorbic acid in the diet, however, provokes a decline of cholesterolemia (Table III). If the addition of cholestyramine to the diet is increased to 1.0% (2.3% Questran), its hypocholesterolemic effect becomes evident even in guinea pigs with a marginal intake of vitamin C, and again the simultaneous addition of 0.5% L-ascorbic acid brings about a more substantial decline in cholesterolemia (Table IV). A synergetic effect is involved because the decline in cholesterolemia exceeds the sum of the hypocholesterolemic effect of cholestyramine and of L-ascorbic acid when administered separately. The ascorbate level in the tissues of these animals shows that cholestyramine does not affect ascorbate absorption from the gastrointestinal tract (Table IV).

Evidence has accumulated over the past few years that certain components of dietary fiber, for example, pectin, also have the ability to bind bile acids in the gastrointestinal tract (*64*). An addition of 5% citrus pectin and 0.5% L-ascorbic acid to a high-fat diet prevented cholesterol accumulation in the blood serum and liver of guinea pigs (*65*). A significant decline of total cholesterol level in the serum of a group of healthy subjects with mild hypercholesterolemia, and also in a group of hyperlipemic outpatients, was achieved through the administration of a granulated preparation containing 15 g of citrus pectin and 450 mg of L-ascorbic acid given daily for 6 weeks (*65*) (*see* Groups 12 and 13 in Table II). Since the HDL cholesterol level did not change, the decline noted was caused by the decline in the risk-constituting LDL cholesterol.

Table III. Effect of L-Ascorbic Acid and Questran on Total Cholesterol Concentration in Blood Serum of Male Guinea Pigs

Weeks	Type of Diet	Intake of L-Ascorbic Acid		Statistical Significance (student's t-test)
		Low (0.5 mg/24 h)	*High (0.5% in diet)*	
0	Starting values (cereal + vegetables)	1.58 ± 0.13[a] (10)		
9	Scorbutogenic diet	2.07 ± 0.13 (10)	1.55 ± 0.13 (10)	$P < 0.02$
13	Scorbutogenic diet + 1.5% Questran	2.10 ± 0.10 (9)	1.04 ± 0.08 (10)	$P < 0.001$
	Scorbutogenic diet + 1.5% Questran	2.02 ± 0.13 (9)	1.04 ± 0.05 (10)	$P < 0.001$

Note: Data presented as mean $\pm$ se (mmol/L). Figures in parentheses indicate numbers of animals analyzed.

Table IV. Synergism of Hypocholesterolemic Effect of L-Ascorbic Acid and Cholestyramine in Male Guinea Pigs (Duration of Experiment, 4 Weeks)

	Intake of L-Ascorbic Acid			
Intake of Cholestyramine	0.5 mg/24 h / 0	0.5% in Diet / 0	0.5 mg/24 h / 1.0% in Diet	0.5% in Diet / 1.0% in Diet
Total cholesterol in blood serum (mmol/L)	1.76 ± 0.21^a (9)	1.58 ± 0.21^a (10)	1.14 ± 0.08^b (22)	0.73 ± 0.05^c (26)
Vitamin C in tissues (mol/kg of fresh tissue)				
Liver	0.18 ± 0.02^a (9)	2.14 ± 0.17^b (10)	0.15 ± 0.01^a (22)	2.03 ± 0.13^b (26)
Spleen	0.37 ± 0.03^a (9)	2.94 ± 0.22^b (10)	0.33 ± 0.04^a (9)	3.19 ± 0.17^b (8)
Lungs	0.27 ± 0.02^a (9)	2.29 ± 0.12^b (10)	0.30 ± 0.05^a (9)	2.27 ± 0.12^b (8)
Testes	0.35 ± 0.05^a (9)	1.97 ± 0.11^b (10)	0.26 ± 0.01^a (9)	2.24 ± 0.11^b (8)

Mean ± se. Figures in parentheses indicate number of animals analyzed.
[a, b, c] Differential index indicates statistical significance of differences ($P < 0.05$ –0.001).

The probable mechanism of the synergetic effect of L-ascorbic acid and substances capable of binding bile acids in the gastrointestinal tract is shown in Scheme 1. An increased intake of L-ascorbic acid accelerates the formation of 7α-hydroxycholesterol and thereby also accelerates the overall rate of cholesterol transformation into bile acids. Bile acids excreted from the liver into the gastrointestinal tract become bound and thus are prevented from affecting 7α-hydroxylation of cholesterol through a feedback mechanism. In this way, a permanent disequilibrium occurs between cholesterol and bile acids with increased cholesterol transformation to bile acids and enhanced irreversible output of the products of this reaction, which results in a decline of cholesterol levels in the blood and tissues.

Conclusions

The results obtained underline the significance of vegetables and fruit—the most important sources of vitamin C and pectin—in human nutrition. It has been repeatedly demonstrated that population groups with a high consumption of these foodstuffs suffer less from hypercholesterolemia and have lower coronary mortality than is the case with the average population (66–68). An analysis of World Health Organization/ Food and Agriculture Organization data from thirty countries has shown a negative correlation between mortality rate due to ischemic heart disease and the consumption of vegetables and fruit (69). A significant decline in coronary mortality observed in the United States over the past decade was accompanied by an increase in the consumption of vegetables, fruits, and, particularly, synthetic L-ascorbic acid (70).

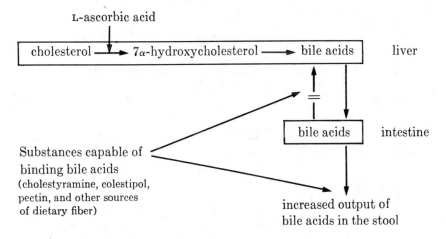

Scheme 1.

The data reviewed in this chapter may provide a promising point of departure leading toward the preparation of a natural hypocholesterolemic agent that, in contrast to synthetic hypolipemic drugs, will enable physiological control of certain types of hypercholesterolemia.

Literature Cited

1. Myasnikov, A. L. *Circulation* **1958**, *17*, 99.
2. Sokoloff, B.; Hori, M.; Saelhof, C.; McConnel, B.; Imai, T. *J. Nutr.* **1967**, *91*, 107.
3. Banerjee, S.; Singh, H. D. *J. Biol. Chem.* **1958**, *233*, 336.
4. Guchhait, R.; Guha, B. C.; Ganguli, N. C. *Biochem. J.* **1963**, *86*, 193.
5. Ginter, E. *Adv. Lipid Res.* **1978**, *16*, 167.
6. Ginter, E. *Ann. N.Y. Acad. Sci.* **1975**, *258*, 410.
7. Fujinami, T.; Okado, K.; Senda, K.; Sugimura, M.; Kishikawa, M. *Jpn. Cir. J.* **1971**, *35*, 1559.
8. Nambisan, B.; Kurup, P. A. *Atherosclerosis* **1975**, *22*, 447.
9. Higuchi, R.; Fujinami, T.; Nakano, S.; Nakayama, K.; Mayashi, K.; Sakuma, N.; Takada, K. *Jpn. J. Atheroscler.* **1975**, *3*, 303.
10. Hayashi, E.; Yamada, J.; Kunitomo, M.; Terada, M.; Watanabe, Y. *Jpn. J. Pharmacol.* **1978**, *28*, 133.
11. Hanck, A.; Weiser, H. *Int. J. Vitam. Nutr. Res.* **1977**, Suppl. *16*, 67.
12. Hanck, A.; Weiser, H. *Int. J. Vitam. Nutr. Res.* **1979**, Suppl. *19*, 83.
13. Sakuma, N. *Nagoya Med. J.* **1979**, *24*, 37.
14. Jenkins, S. A. *Br. J. Nutr.* **1980**, *43*, 95.
15. Kotzé, J. P. *South Afr. Med. J.* **1975**, *49*, 1651.
16. Hodges, R. E.; Baker, E. M.; Wood, J.; Sauberlich, H. E.; March, S. C. *Am. J. Clin. Nutr.* **1969**, *22*, 535.
17. Masek, J. *Nutr. Dieta* **1960**, *2*, 193.
18. Cheraskin, E.; Ringsdorf, W. M. *Int. J. Vit. Nutr. Res.* **1968**, *38*, 415.
19. Černá, O.; Ginter, E. *Lancet* **1978**, *1*, 1055.
20. John, T. M.; George, J. C.; Hilton, J. W.; Slinger, S. J. *Int. J. Vit. Nutr. Res.* **1979**, *49*, 400.
21. Hughes, R. E. *J. Hum. Nutr.* **1976**, *30*, 315.
22. Turley, S. D.; West, C. E.; Horton, B. J. *Atherosclerosis* **1976**, *24*, 1.
23. Ginter, E. *Science* **1973**, *179*, 702.
24. Björkhem, I.; Kallner, A. *J. Lipid Res.* **1976**, *17*, 360.
25. Holloway, D. E.; Rivers, J. M. *Fed. Proc.* **1978**, *37*, 589.
26. Harris, W. S.; Kottke, B. A.; Subbiah, M. T. R. *Am. J. Clin. Nutr.* **1979**, *32*, 1837.
27. Kritchevsky, D.; Tepper, S. A.; Story, J. A. *Lipids* **1973**, *8*, 482.
28. Zannoni, V. G.; Sato, P. H. *Ann. N.Y. Acad. Sci.* **1975**, *258*, 119.
29. Rikans, L. E.; Smith, C. R.; Zannoni, V. G. *Biochem. Pharmacol.* **1977**, *26*, 797.
30. Walsch, S.; Degkwitz, E. *Z. Physiol. Chem.* **1980**, *361*, 79.
31. Omaye, S. T.; Turnbull, J. D. *Biochem. Pharmacol.* **1979**, *28*, 3651.
32. Verlangieri, A. J.; Mumma, R. O. *Atherosclerosis* **1973**, *17*, 37.
33. Hornig, D.; Weber, F.; Wiss, O. *Z. Klin. Chem. Klin. Biochem.* **1974** *12*, 62.
34. Kunitomo, M.; Yamada, J.; Terada, M.; Hayashi, E. *Pharmacometrics* **1976**, *11*, 931.
35. Jenkins, S. A. *Biochem. Biophys. Res. Commun.* **1977**, *77*, 1030.
36. Hornig, D.; Weiser, H. *Experientia* **1976**, *32*, 687.
37. Ginter, E.; Babala, J.; Cerven, J. *J. Atheroscler. Res.* **1969**, *10*, 341.
38. Ginter, E.; Bobek, P.; Babala, J.; Jakubovský, J.; Zaviačič, M.; Lojda, Z. *Int. J. Vit. Nutr. Res.* **1979**, Suppl. *19*, 55.

39. Fujinami, T.; Okado, K.; Senda, K.; Nakano, S.; Higuchi, R.; Nakayama, K.; Hayashi, K.; Sakuma, N. *Jpn. J. Atheroscler.* **1975,** *3,* 117.
40. Sulkin, N. M.; Sulkin, D. F. *Ann. N.Y. Acad. Sci.* **1975,** *258,* 317.
41. Fujinami, T. *J. Jpn. Coll. Angiol.* **1980,** *20,* 91.
42. Ginter, E.; Bobek, P.; Vargová, D. *Nutr. Metab.* **1979,** *23,* 217.
43. Kamath, S. K.; Tang, J. M.; Bramante, P. O. *Fed. Proc.* **1977,** *36,* 1114.
44. Bobek, P.; Ginter, E.; Ozdín, L.; Mikuš, L. *Physiol. Bohemoslov.* **1980,** *29,* 337.
45. Bobek, P.; Ginter, E. *Experientia* **1978,** *34,* 1554.
46. Kotzé, J. P.; Spies, J. H. *South Afr. Med. J.* **1976,** *50,* 1760.
47. Ginter, E., unpublished data.
48. Tsai, S.; Fales, H. M.; Vaughan, M. *J. Biol. Chem.* **1973,** *248,* 5278.
49. Krumdieck, C.; Butterworth, C. E. *Am. J. Clin. Nutr.* **1974,** *27,* 866.
50. Myasnikova, I. A. *Trudy Voenno–Morskoi Med. Akad. Leiningrad* **1947,** *8,* 140.
51. Kothari, L. K.; Jain, K. *Acta Biol. Acad. Sci. Hung.* **1977,** *28,* 111.
52. Heine, H.; Norden, C. *Int. J. Vit. Nutr. Res.* **1979,** Suppl. *19,* 45.
53. Bordia, A. K. *Atherosclerosis* **1980,** *35,* 181.
54. Anderson, J.; Grande, F.; Keys, A. *Fed. Proc.* **1958,** *17,* 468.
55. Anderson, T. W.; Reid, D. B. W.; Beaton, G. H. *Lancet* **1972,** *2,* 876.
56. Samuel, P.; Shalchi, O. B. *Circulation* **1964,** *29,* 24.
57. Menne, I. V.; Grey, P. C.; Kotzé, J. P.; Sommers, De K.; Brown, J. M. M.; Spies, J. H. *South Afr. Med. J.* **1975,** *49,* 2225.
58. Naito, H. K.; De Wolfe, V. G.; Brown, H. B.; Wilcoxen, K.; Raulinaitis, I. *Fed. Proc.* **1977,** *36,* 1158.
59. Crawford, G. P. M.; Warlow, C. P.; Bennet, B.; Dawson, A. A.; Douglas, A. S.; Kerridge, D. F.; Ogston, D. *Atherosclerosis* **1975,** *21,* 451.
60. Peterson, V. E.; Crapo, P. A.; Weininger, J.; Ginsberg, H.; Olefsky, J. *Am. J. Clin. Nutr.* **1975,** *28,* 584.
61. Ginter, E. *Lancet* **1979,** *2,* 958.
62. Bates, C. J.; Mandal, A. R.; Cole, T. J. *Lancet* **1977,** *2,* 611.
63. Lopez-S, A.; Yates, B.; Hardon, C.; Mellert, H. *Am. J. Clin. Nutr.* **1978,** *31,* 712.
64. Kritchevsky, D. *Lipids* **1978,** *13,* 982.
65. Ginter, E.; Kubec, F. J.; Vozár, J.; Bobek, P. *Int. J. Vit. Nutr. Res.* **1979,** *49,* 406.
66. West, R. O.; Hayes, O. B. *Am. J. Clin. Nutr.* **1968,** *21,* 853.
67. Sacks, F. M.; Castelli, W. P.; Donner, A.; Kass, E. H. *New Engl. J. Med.* **1975,** *292,* 1148.
68. Phillips, R. L.; Lemon, F. R.; Beeson, W. L.; Kuzma, J. W. *Am. J. Clin. Nutr.* **1978,** *31,* S191.
69. Stamler, J. "Lipids and Coronary Heart Disease," Raven: New York, 1979; p. 25.
70. Ginter, E. *Am. J. Clin. Nutr.* **1979,** *32,* 511.

RECEIVED for review January 22, 1981. ACCEPTED September 1, 1981.

Ascorbic Acid Technology in Agricultural, Pharmaceutical, Food, and Industrial Applications

J. CHRISTOPHER BAUERNFEIND

Gainesville, FL 32605

Ascorbic acid, as well as its salts and esters, has many useful applications. In plants L-ascorbic acid has been reported to promote germination of seeds, growth of plants, and growth of roots on cuttings. Spraying of plants such as lettuce, celery, spinach, petunias, and roses with ascorbic acid or sodium ascorbate solutions enabled those plants to better withstand damage from ozone and smog exposure. Spraying tree or bush fruits with ascorbic acid solution synchronizes maturation and causes fruit to fall more easily in mechanical harvesting. In some instances ascorbic acid application has been cited to improve the defense mechanism of plants to attack by disease agents. Fish require a dietary source of vitamin C, without which they grow poorly and develop fracture dislocations of the spine, distortions of cartilage, and other deficiency signs. In some instances, ruminants and monogastric animals appear to benefit from administration of L-ascorbic acid under stress. Animals with viral disease, such as canine or feline distemper, have responded to treatment with high levels of ascorbic acid. Solid and liquid forms constitute a substantial pharmaceutical market for manufactured ascorbic acid. Tableting techniques have been devised to prepare a wide array of swallowable or chewable tablets with an assured vitamin C content after manufacture and prolonged storage. L-Ascorbic acid may be added to foods or food ingredients as a nutrient to fortify natural or fabricated foods having little or no vitamin C, to restore losses, and to standardize a given class of food products with a preselected quantity of

0065-2393/82/0200–0395$26.75/0
© 1982 American Chemical Society

the vitamin. Factors that must be considered with appropriate technology before adding ascorbic acid are the following: (i) cost of the specific food; (ii) convenience of use; (iii) relationship of the food in question to normal food selection or to replacement or supplemental food products; (iv) stability of the vitamin in the food during shelf life and home preparation; (v) public health considerations; and (vi) special food needs, such as infant, geriatric, and military. In addition to serving as an added nutrient in food, L-ascorbic acid is often used as a processing aid or as a preservative in certain foods or food ingredients. Examples include preventing enzymatic browning of cut fruit, scavenging oxygen in beer, fruit, or vegetable products, inhibiting oxidative rancidity in frozen fish, stabilizing the color and flavor in cured meats, maturing of wheat flour and improving of dough, and acting as a reducing agent in wine. An extensive list of patents and scientific papers exists on proposed industrial uses of ascorbic acid. The greatest interest appears to be in the synthetic polymer industry, in photoprocessing, and in metal technology. Miscellaneous uses have been proposed in cosmetics, tobacco, fibers, preservation of blood, preservation of cut plants, cleaning agents, and in assay reagents.

Approximately 50 years ago L-ascorbic acid had its beginning as a pure chemical compound. In the 1928–1931 period Szent-Györgyi (1, 2) extracted from adrenal glands, cabbage, oranges, and paprika, a substance he named hexuronic acid. In 1932 Waugh and King (3, 4) reported hexuronic acid was identical with vitamin C that they isolated from lemons and oranges. Subsequently Svirbely and Szent-Györgyi (5–8) in 1932–1933 demonstrated antiscorbutic activity for the substance. The structural formula (Figure 1) was determined in 1933 by several investigators (9–12).

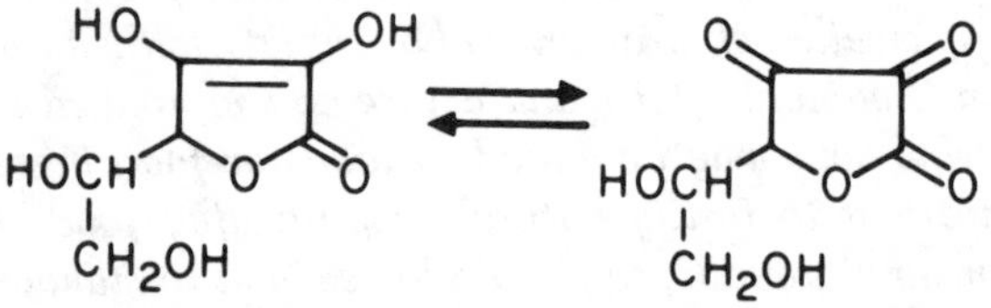

Figure 1. Structural formulas of L-ascorbic acid (reductant) (right) and L-dehydroascorbic acid (oxidant) (left).

L-Ascorbic acid was synthesized in 1933 by Reichstein and coworkers (*13*) in Switzerland and also independently by Ault et al. (*14*) in England. Industrial synthesis largely follows the L-sorbose process (Figure 2) of Reichstein. Continuous improvements in the various steps starting with D-glucose have made this approach the commercially feasible process. Commercial production has been continuous since 1933 and is currently practiced in several countries. In one large factory about 30 tons of pure L-ascorbic acid is produced daily, an amount equivalent to that contained in 1/2 billion (500,000,000) large oranges. Today, an increasing tonnage of this versatile substance is produced annually and a very wide range of applications has been found for it in the food industry. It occupies an established position as an essential nutrient and as a pharmaceutical agent in human nutrition (*915*) and medicine. Its use as an additive to animal feeds is growing. Applications on plants and crops as well as in various industries have been indicated.

L-Ascorbic acid, a six-carbon, water-soluble, white, crystalline compound is vitamin C (the antiscorbutic vitamin) and has also been called L-*xylo*-ascorbic acid, hexuronic acid, or cevitamic acid. L-Ascorbic acid ($C_6H_8O_6$) resembles the sugars in structure and reacts like sugars under some chemical conditions. The unusual properties of the molecule (mol. wt. 176.13) are due to the ene–diol grouping. Other properties are: melting point of 190°–192°C with decomposition; $[\alpha]_D^{20} + 23°$ in water; a pK_1 of 4.17 and a pK_2 of 11.57. It is a moderately strong reducing agent and is sufficiently acidic to form neutral salts with bases. L-Ascorbic acid (1 g) dissolves in about 3 mL of water, or 50 mL of absolute ethanol, or 100 mL of glycerol. The pH of a 10% aqueous solution is 2.1–2.5; for a 10% aqueous solution of sodium ascorbate it is 7.4–7.9.

Description, identification, specifications, and tests of L-ascorbic acid and sodium L-ascorbate are given in the U.S. Pharmacopoeia (*15*) and the Food Chemicals Codex (*16*). Similar information on palmitoyl L-ascorbic acid (ascorbyl palmitate) is contained in the Codex. Sodium ascorbate is twice as soluble in water as ascorbic acid. Ascorbyl palmitate is soluble in ethanol (25°C) at 12.5%, in hot (80°C) glycerin, propylene glycol, or decaglycerol octaoleate to 10%, in vegetable oils (25°C) at 0.01–0.1% and in water (70°C) at 0.2%.

Crystal structures of L-ascorbic acid varying from coarse to ultrafine powder constitute the major commercial product forms of the compound, followed by special coated and granulated forms. Sodium L-ascorbate is also produced in granular and powder forms. Limited production of other forms such as calcium ascorbate and ascorbyl palmitate depend on demand of these products in specialty use applications.

Hundreds of derivatives of L-ascorbic acid have been reported in the literature, some of which are as follows: metal complexes or salts of

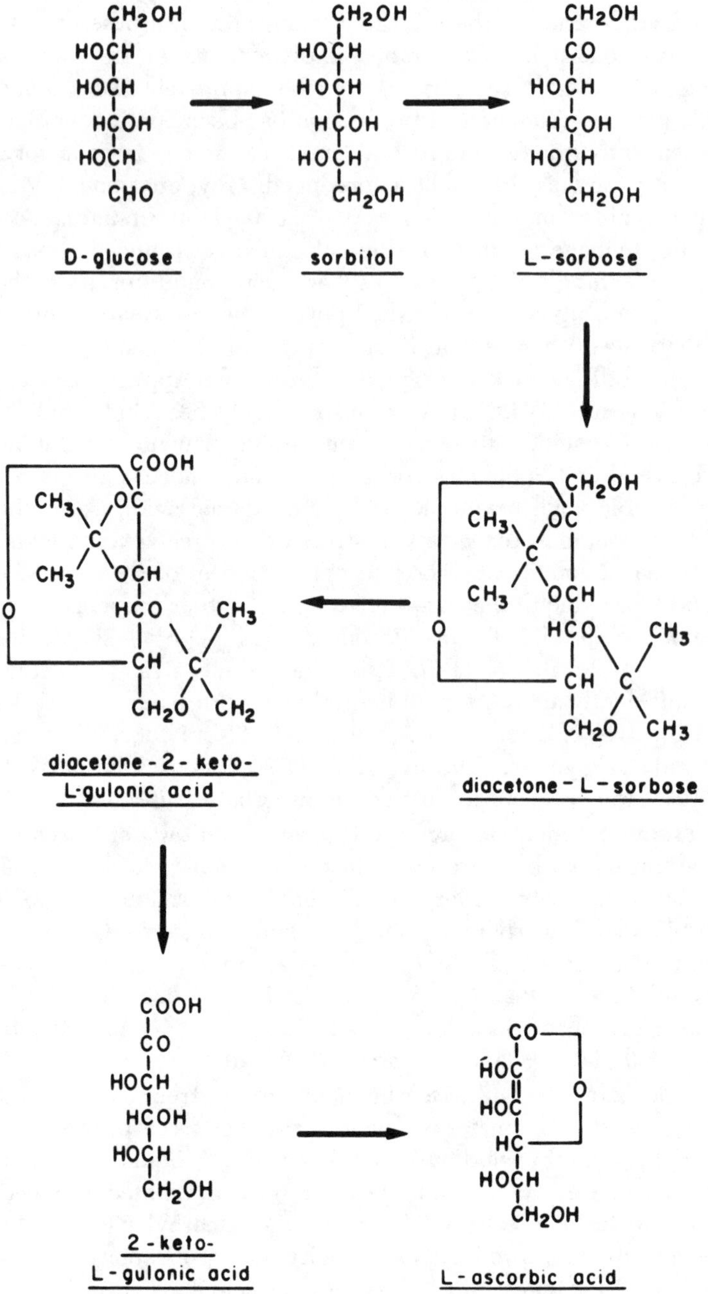

Figure 2.   The L-*sorbose synthesis of* L-*ascorbic acid.*

aluminum, copper, iron, and magnesium, inorganic esters, such as sulfates and phosphates, other esters, such as the acetate, diacetate, benzoate, dodecanoate, hexadecanoate, dihexadecanoate, octadecanoate, laurate, oleate, and stearate. Other structures include sulfamerazine ascorbate, sulfathiazole ascorbate, neomycin ascorbate, procaine ascorbate, erythromycin ascorbate, quinine ascorbate, tocopheryl ascorbate, nicotinamide ascorbate, pyridoxine ascorbic acid fatty acid esters, and thiamine bis ascorbate palmitate. In many reports synthesis only is cited for the compound; other reports include synthesis and indicate some declared merit for use of the derivative.

Plant Applications

The ubiquitous appearance of L-ascorbic acid in the plant world would imply that it must have some functional role or roles in the physiology of plant life of major value. Even leaves, stems, roots, and berries of native plants (17) of the Eastern Arctic have substantial levels of ascorbic acid (Table I). The occurrence and function of ascorbic acid in plants have been reviewed (see Reference 18). Several biosynthetic pathways have been envisaged in plants for the biosynthesis of L-ascorbic acid. General factors controlling ascorbic synthesis in plants include light and the quality of illumination, the presence of oxygen and trace minerals and favorable ranges of temperature and pH. Food production clearly involves aspects relating to preharvest and postharvest preservation, seed germination, bud and root growth, respiration, dormancy and its release, fruit ripening and its control, and storage performance. These life processes and others greatly influence the volume and quality of food produced. Plant growth regulators and/or harvesting aids, usually as organic compounds, added to the crop or food item in appropriate amounts, times, and manner, can help improve the yield, quality characteristics of the food, or economics of production. L-Ascorbic acid applications to plant foods have indicated some potential for meritorious use in the production of plant food; however, the economics of its use have not always permitted wide field usage of the developed application or technology at the present time. Some areas of plant use are detailed in the sections which follow.

Germinating, Growth, Rooting. Improvements of seed germination by treatment with ascorbic acid solutions alone or as synergist to other chemicals have been reported (19–23). Singh et al. (24) found soaking the seeds of *Datura innoxia* in an ascorbic acid solution (0.5–1.0%) to increase germination percentage and the rate of germination. Likewise, ascorbic acid solution (0.02%) treatment of *V. bipinnatifida* seed increased germination (25) and acted synergistically when combined with thiourea. Hardening of sweet pepper seeds was exhibited with subse-

Table I.   Ascorbic Acid and β-Carotene in

Latin Name	Common Name
Flowering plants	
Arctostaphylos alpina (L.) Spreng.	alpine bearberry
Arenaria peploides L. var. *diffusa* Hornem.	seabeach-sandwort
Cochlearia officianalis L.	scurvy grass
Draba glabella Pursh.	
Elymus mollis Trin. ssp. *mollis*	lyme grass
Empetrum nigrum L. var. *hermaphroditum* (Lange) Sor.	curlewberry
Epilobium angustifolium L. ssp. *angustifolium*	fireweed
Epilobium latifolium L.	dwarf fireweed
Hedysarum alpinum L. var. *americanum* Michx.	licorice root
Oxyria digyna (L.) Hill	mountain sorrel
Oxytropis campestris (L.) D.C. var. *terrae-novae* (Fern.) Barnaby	
Polygonum viviparum L.	bistort
Rubus arcticus L. var. *acaulis* (Michx.) Boivin	dwarf raspberry
Rubus chamaemorus L.	baked appleberry
Salix arctophila Cockerell	creeping willow
Salix ? planifolia Pursh	willow
Saxifraga tricuspidata Rottb.	prickly saxifrage
Sedum rosea (L.) Scop.	roseroot
Taraxacum sp.	dandelion
Vaccinium uliginosum L.	bilberry
Vaccinium vitis-idaea L. var. *minus* Lodd.	mountain cranberry
Seaweed	
Porphyra laciniata (Lightfoot) Agardh.	seaweed, laver
Rhodymenia palmata (L.) Greville	seaweed, dulse

Native Plants of the Eastern Artic

Col-lection Num-ber	Plant Part Analyzed	Ascorbic Acid		β-Carotene	
		Date of Analysis	mg/ 100 g	Date of Analysis	µg/g
	berries	15/9/64	52.5	23/9/64	1.80
8	leaves	6/8/65	42.5	6/8/65	34.52
7	seedpods and stems	6/8/65	111.0	6/8/65	27.28
10	leaves	6/8/65	180.3	6/8/65	47.69
18	stems	20/8/65	41.0		
		20/8/65	44.5		
	berries	15/9/64	24.0	23/9/64	1.12
		20/8/65	36.3		
16	leaves	11/8/65	220.0	11/8/65	112.25
		19/8/65	212.0	19/8/65	112.00
6	leaves	6/8/65	152.5	6/8/65	102.00
13	roots	30/7/65	28.2	30/7/65	nil
		30/7/65	30.4	30/7/65	nil
19	leaves and stems	6/8/65	40.0	6/8/65	53.40
12	roots	6/8/65	12.0	6/8/65	nil
9	leaves	6/8/65	158.8		
	berries	31/8/65	38.8	31/8/65	0.68
	berries	23/8/65	47.5	17/9/65	1.41
	leaves	4/8/64	308.8	30/7/64	104.34
		26/7/65	349.0	26/7/65	106.14
		29/7/65	340.0	29/7/65	110.88
	leaves	4/8/64	465.0	30/7/64	130.64
		26/7/65	415.0	26/7/65	143.84
		29/7/65	410.0	29/7/65	148.20
4	flowers and stems	6/8/65	135.5		
11	leaves	23/7/64	68.0	6/8/65	24.64
		6/8/65	45.3		
	leaves berries	23/8/65	66.0	23/9/64	1.21
	berries	15/9/64	22.5	23/9/64	0.79
	fronds	9/8/65	nil	9/8/65	28.00
	fronds	9/8/65	10.0	9/8/65	33.75

quent improved germination (26) when treated with an ascorbic acid solution (0.01%).

Spraying the plant, *Cucumis sativus*, with ascorbic acid solution (0.18%) 2–10 times during expanded growth of the first leaves increased production of male flower and at times the male/female flower ratio according to Severi and Laudi (27). When trees of the biennial-bearing mango (c.v. *Langra*) were sprayed (0.18%) twice, in August and September, increased flowering was observed by Maity et al. (28). Involvement of ascorbic acid in the control of petiole-longevity of two mango varieties has also been reported (29). Application of ascorbic acid influences growth and, at times, other properties of a variety of plants such as the cowpea (30), the onion (31), wheat (32), soybean (33), sugar cane cultivars (34), and *Cucumis sativus* (35). Ascorbic acid treatment was observed to retard leaf senescence of leaf discs of *Solanum melongena* (36). In combination with other chemicals, ascorbic acid treatment has been observed for growth or flowering influence on the soybean (37), cotton (38), and peas (39, 40). Treating cuttings of bearberry with a mixture of heteroauxin (0.015%) and ascorbic acid (0.15%) stimulated early rooting (41). Ascorbic acid treatment has been applied to grapevine cuttings (42) and grafts (43) prior to planting and for improved rooting of gram (44), *Phaseolus aureus* Roxb (45), and *Caesalpinia bonducella* seeds (46).

Ozone Protection. Air pollution has become an increasing problem of industrialized and urban centers, causing smog, a combination of nitrogen oxides, peroxides, sulfur dioxide, ozone, and other contaminants. In the Los Angeles atmosphere there has been evidence that ozone exists in sufficient concentration to damage plants (47). Middleton et al. (48) found that ozone at concentrations as low as 20 ppm produces visible leaf damage to pinto beans after a 2-h exposure. Small concentrations of ozone affect the respiration of plant cells (49). In laboratory trials, when ascorbic acid was added to ozone-treated plant mitochondrial suspensions reversal of the ozone inhibition was observed (47). Thus, a prophylactic or therapeutic role is suggested.

Freebairn and coworkers (50–54) were the early workers to apply ascorbic acid sprays (0.18–0.9%) to intact plants, such as lettuce, celery, pinto beans, spinach, endive, petunias, and roses to prevent the burning, bronzing, and stunting of leaves caused by airborne oxidants. Furthermore, the treatment increased the ascorbic content (53, 54) of the plant over control plants (Table II). Two to eight pounds per acre (2.25–9 kg/ha) were used with single or multiple applications. Too much ascorbic acid will burn the plant; hence salts of ascorbic acid or neutralized ascorbic acid have been favored for spray preparations having a more favorable pH range. A small scale trial on romaine lettuce as reported by Freebairn and Taylor (54) showed foliar application of ascorbic acid

Table II.   The Increase in Ascorbic Acid Content of Pinto
Bean Leaves Following Spray Treatment

Treatment	Molar Concentration	Increase (%) in Ascorbic Acid Content by Spray Treatment[a]
Water	—	36[b]
Calcium ascorbate	0.02	56
	0.05	46
Potassium ascorbate	0.02	54
	0.05	60[c]
Ammonium ascorbate	0.02	34
	0.05	65[c]

[a] Reduced ascorbic acid (average of that originally present) inside leaves; average of 12 determinations.
[b] Normal increase irrespective of treatment.
[c] Statistically different from the water spray at the 0.01 probability level.
Source: Reproduced, with permission, from Ref. *53.* Copyright 1960, Air Pollution Control Association.

to be effective against air pollution injury (Table III). Weaver et al. (*55*) confirmed that ascorbic acid treatment protects white bean plants from onset of bronzing associated with ozone exposure but questioned the practicality of the treatment as a field procedure. The tolerance of petunia plants to ozone exposure depending on the natural L-ascorbic acid content of the leaves was confirmed by Hanson et al. (*56*). Cathey and Heggestad (*57*) also found that the degree of damage by ozone exposure was related to ascorbic acid application to the plants. Foliar application of sodium ascorbate partially decreased ozone leaf damage in tobacco plants in studies in Japan (*58*). Ordin et al. (*59*) applied ascorbate dusts to plants as an alternate to aqueous sprays as a technological approach for protection against air pollutants.

Harvesting Aid. L-Ascorbic acid applied to the fruit or the plant has served as a harvesting aid or as a means of quality improvement. Spraying potato plants with ascorbic acid has influenced growth yield and yield components (*60*). Increased onion bulb size and yield have been reported by Saimbhi et al. (*61*) with ascorbic acid treatment (0.01–0.04%). Semiripe strawberries dipped in ascorbic acid solution (2%) and stored at 0°C in sealed plastic bags kept well for 13 days (*62*). Friction discoloration (skin browning) occurring in d'Anjou pears during shipment was reduced by prior spraying with ascorbic acid solution (5%) according to Wang and Mellenthin (*63*). The application of an ascorbic acid spray (1–2%) at the color break stage to fruit on the tree was effective as a degreening agent for harvested tangerine fruit (*64, 65*). Grapevine panicles at the prebloom stage dipped in a solution of ascorbic acid (0.005%) and sucrose (10%) enhanced bunch weight of

Table III.   Prevention of Air Pollution Injury to Romaine

Treatment	Molar Concentration	Number of Plants
Water	—	17
Potassium ascorbate	0.01	14
Potassium ascorbate	0.10	17

[a] µg/g fresh water.
[b] Statistically different from the water control at the 0.01 probability level.

fruit and reduced underdeveloped fruit (66). Chemical treatment of crops for improved performance has been reviewed by Schilling (67).

A major problem in the mechanical harvesting of tree or bush fruit is the ease of fruit fall at the proper ripening stage. Much effort has been put forth in the technology of induced fruit abscission. Cooper and Henry (68, 69) found that the application of ascorbic acid solution (2–5%) to the treed fruit effectively induced abscission in both Valencia and Pineapple oranges. As a beneficial side effect, the application increased the L-ascorbic acid content of the oranges by 4–8%. The ascorbic acid treatment can leave small reddish pits in the rind near the stem end if the residue is not washed off 3 d after the ascorbic acid application. Use of the sodium salt of ascorbic acid eliminates most of this problem. In other trials, ascorbic acid treatment aided mechanical harvesting of Hamlin, Pineapple, Jaffa, and Valencia oranges on a commercial scale (70). Wilson and coworkers (71, 72, 73) reported ascorbic acid application (1.5%) reduced the pull force of oranges from 14.5 to 7.0 lb and the percent plugs (a defect) from 90 to 5% within 6 d of application. About 1 lb of ascorbic acid is required per tree for Hamlin and Pineapple oranges under Florida conditions, making it a costly treatment. Other researchers (74–77) have studied the mode of action of ascorbic acid treatment in reducing selective abscission of citrus fruit. Citrus fruit treatments with ascorbic acid alone or with Fe EDTA or Cu EDTA were compared (78), and ascorbic acid (1%) plus Cu EDTA (0.1%) spray was found to be the most effective abscission treatment for calamondin fruit (79, 80). Edgerton (81, 84) observed ascorbic acid sprays to promote abscission on apple cultivars, but significant reductions in fruit removal force were usually associated with some leaf or fruit phytotoxicity and/or leaf drops. Trials with ascorbic acid as an abscission agent have been run on mango (82), olives (83), cherries (84), and raspberries (85). One different use (86–89) of ascorbic acid spray in abscission applications is in the removal of leaves of the cotton plant so the cotton can be more easily picked mechanically.

Lettuce Plants by the Foliar Application of Potassium Ascorbate

Total Number of Mature Leaves	Number of Leaves Damaged	Percent of Leaves Damaged	Average Ascorbic Acid Content[a] of Washed Leaves
131	60[b]	46	0.60
126	0[b]	0[b]	0.72
147	5[b]	3[b]	1.03

Source: Reproduced, with permission, from Ref. *54*. Copyright 1960, American Society for Horticultural Science.

To date, use of L-ascorbic acid as an abscission agent on any crop is not carried out on a commercial scale on a regular basis.

Disease Resistance.   Some varied reported uses of ascorbic acid applications include thinning of fruit trees (*90*), chemotherapy for control of young tree decline in Florida citrus (*91*), change in the vernalization rate in plants (*92, 93*), and relief of wilting of severed tomato plants (*94*). Plant resistance has been indicated to involve ascorbic acid. The role of L-ascorbic acid in the defense mechanism of plants to nematode attack has been studied by Arrigoni et al. (*95, 96*), including the relationship between ascorbic acid and resistance in tomato plants to *Meloidogyne incognita* (*97*), potato field resistance to phytophthorosis (*98*), resistance to bacterial black spot in mango (*99*), rust resistances of roses (*100, 101*), and inhibition of chemical tumorigenesis in *Nicotiana* hybrid (*102*).

Growth Regulator.   Intermediate compounds in the chemical synthesis of L-ascorbic acid such as sodium 2,3:4,6-di-*O*-isopropylidene-*α*-L-*xylo*-2-hexulofuranosonate, or commonly designated dikegulac-sodium, have plant growth regulatory activity (*103*). A series of monosaccharide derivatives, salts, and esters were examined; the finding was that the salts were generally more active than the esters. Growth retardation was observed in a wide range of plants, cereals, weed grasses, and woody plants. Induced abscission and stimulated ripening are other activities observed in some plant life. Dikegulac-sodium (trade name, **Atrinal**) applied as an aqueous spray is used for the post-shearing or chemical pinching of azaleas (*104–110*), also, of rhododendrons (*111*) and certain pot plants to promote lateral branching and compacting of the plants with abundant blooms. Worley (*112*) observed dikegulac-sodium, when applied in the fall of a dry year, to promote increased number of new shoots on young pecan trees the next spring (Table IV). It works on field-grown woody ornamental or landscape plants (*113, 114, 115*), reducing the need of trimming. Applied with proper timing, it can be used to eliminate bloom or fruit set.

Table IV. Number of New Living Shoots per Terminal $>$ 2.5 cm
in May 1979 from Young Pecan Trees Treated with Dikegulac
on October 4, 1978 in Three Georgia Orchards

New Living Shoots/Terminal Shoot[a]

Dosage (g Active/L)	Law Orchard[b] (Tifton)	Rigdon Orchard (Tifton)	Garrison Orchard (Ray City)
Control (no spray)	5.3 a	3.8 a	5.8 a
1.07	6.4 a	5.3 b	8.4 b
1.60	5.6 a	6.1 c	8.9 b
2.14	6.8 a	6.0 bc	9.5 b

[a] Mean separation by Duncan's multiple range test, 5% level.
[b] Cultivars in the Law orchard were "Cherokee" and "Chickasaw". The Rigdon orchard was "Desirable" and the Garrison orchard was "Stuart".
Source: Reproduced, with permission, from Ref. 112. Copyright 1980, American Society for Horticultural Science.

Animal Applications

As stated by Chatterjee et al. (116, 918), the ability to synthesize L-ascorbic acid is absent in insects, invertebrates, and fish. The biosynthetic capacity started phylogenetically in the kidney of amphibians, remained in that of reptiles, became transferred to the liver of mammals, and finally disappeared from the guinea pig, some flying mammals, the monkey, and humans. The overall pattern of ascorbic acid synthesis by different species of animals is correlated to their phylogeny (Figure 3). Traditionally, farm animals do not require ascorbic acid in their diets since this vitamin is produced within their bodies. However, it has long been thought that the capacity of the enzyme system involved could be overtaxed or impaired under stress conditions such as high temperature and disease. It is also conceivable that in breeding animals for high planes of productivity, the rate of synthesis could be inadequate. Depending upon circumstances and species, supplementary L-ascorbic acid in the diet of some animals has had a beneficial effect.

Fish.   Fish farming or aquaculture, as it is more likely to be called today, has been a time-honored practice going back over a thousand years. Until more recently, fish farming was practiced on a small scale basis as more or less a complement to other agricultural or marine pursuits. Little or no technology was involved; breeding stock was introduced into a suitable pond or fenced off estuary, and nature performed the rest. Harvesting was done by hooking, netting, or draining. Within the past two decades a new approach was introduced, namely the large-scale, environmentally controlled, research-guided aquaculture with an expectancy of large volume production of human food. Growing fish

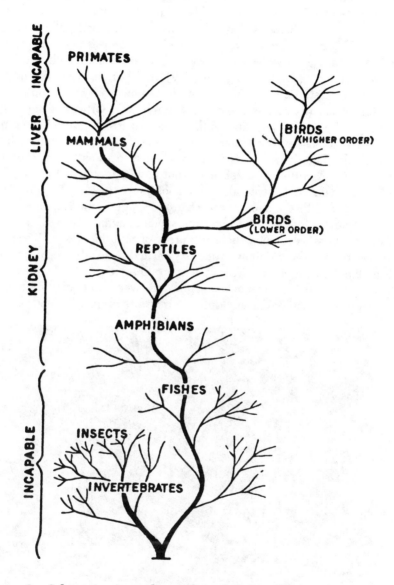

Figure 3. Schematic of ascorbic acid synthesizing abilities of various species of animals in relation to their phylogeny. (Reproduced, with permission, from Ref. 918. Copyright 1973, American Association for the Advancement of Science.)

confined in tanks with water temperature, acidity, and salinity controlled, fed artificially formulated diets, and treated with prophylactic drugs and pesticides brought forth problems absent in the old style practices.

As early as 1933, McCay and Tunison (117) had noted that brook trout fed formalin-preserved meat developed lordosis and scoliosis (Figure 4), but the causative agent was unknown until the mid-sixties when Kitamura et al. (118), Nakagawa (119), and Poston (120) demonstrated that these distortions of the vertebral column were the symptoms of a dietary deficiency of L-ascorbic acid (vitamin C). Other deficiency symptoms are fracture dislocation of the spine, bizarre distortion of cartilage, impaired collagen formation, depigmented areas, poor growth, and mortality. The deficiency is commonly referred to as the "broken back" syndrome. Ascorbic acid deficient trout have a low hematocrit and high plasma levels of triglycerides and cholesterol (121). By 1972 it was known (122) that salmon, trout, char, carp, aquarium fish, and probably many more kinds of fish develop specific avitaminosis C symptoms (Figure 4) when denied dietary sources of ascorbic acid. Hilton (123) reported that the rainbow trout has virtually no ability to synthesize ascorbic acid. While clinical aspects are dramatic, the subclinical manifestations of the deficiency may play an even more important role in resistance to bacterial or viral infections and the repair of tissue damaged

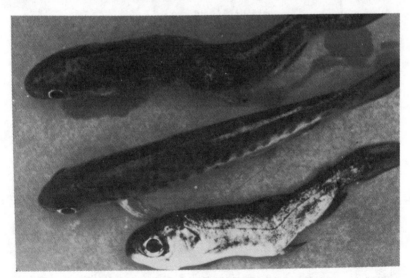

Figure 4. Ascorbic acid deficiency in fish. Coho salmon fed diet devoid of ascorbic acid and showing spinal curvatures typical of scoliosis (upper). Normal coho fed complete test diet containing 100 mg vitamin C/100 g dry ration (middle). Coho on same diet as upper fish and showing spinal curvature typical of lordosis (bottom). (Reproduced, with permission, from Ref. 130. Copyright 1969, American Fisheries Society.)

by parasitic invasion or by physical means. Black death is regarded as an ascorbic acid deficiency disease in penaeid shrimp (*124*). In large-scale aquacultural field practice, vitamin C deficiency was one of the unappreciated dietary aspects during the late sixties and the seventies.

Channel catfish from intensive cultures raised by local fish farmers and showing skeletal deformities stimulated Lovell (*125*) in 1973 to demonstrate experimentally that these symptoms were the result of a deficiency of L-ascorbic acid. In addition to the physical deformities, weight gains of the growing fish and feed conversion were adversely influenced. Wilson and Poe (*126*) in the same year induced the scorbutic condition in channel catfish reared in floating cages. The L-ascorbic acid requirement was determined to be about 50 mg/kg of diet (*127, 128*). While in the past catfish apparently were able to obtain a significant amount of ascorbic acid from organisms such as insects, larvae, and algae when raised in earthen ponds, Lovell and Lim (*129*) in 1978 showed that additional ascorbic acid was beneficial. Ascorbic acid supplemented diets are needed for trout (*118–121, 130, 131, 132*), salmon (*119, 130, 132*), carp (*133*), and eels (*134*).

Attempts have been made to develop more stable forms of vitamin C for fish feeds. Ascorbate-2-sulfate has been proposed as a stable form (*135*) of vitamin C. As a dietary component it has been reported to cure scorbutic signs in salmonoid fish (*136*), to prevent scurvy in catfish (*137*) but not to possess antiscorbutic activity for either the guinea pig (*138*) or the rhesus monkey (*139*).

An interesting pesticide–ascorbic acid interaction in fish has been studied by Mayer and coworkers (*140–143*). Several species of fish were continuously exposed to toxaphene on diets with and without ascorbic acid. The toxaphene reduced the ascorbic acid content of the vertebrae but not of the liver, leading the investigators to believe that this reduction unfavorably affects collagen formation. Diets containing the higher levels of L-ascorbic acid reduced toxaphene residues and increased the tolerance to the chronic effect of toxaphene on growth, bone development, and skin lesions.

Poultry. More than 100 papers have been published on the value of supplementing diets of farm animals with L-ascorbic acid. The overall results are at times controversial. Enhancement of poultry growth has been reported by several workers using purified (*144, 145*) and practical (*146, 147, 148*) rations and not by others (*149*), the general interpretation being that the ascorbic acid does not function directly but indirectly, involving a protective action or improved utilization of other nutrients. Added dietary ascorbic acid has been reported to stimulate synthesis or liberation of folic acid by intestinal bacteria, to aid in its conversion to folacin (*146, 150, 151, 152*), to reinforce antibiotics in high energy feeds and to improve iron absorption. High environmental temperatures reduce the thickness (153) of eggshells of hens, thus lowering the breaking strength of the eggs (154) as well as lowering egg production. High concentrations of ascorbic acid are found normally in the bird's tissues, especially in the kidneys and adrenals, gonads, and in the bursa (155). Near significant correlation has been found between the ascorbic acid content of the adrenal gland and egg production in the duck (156). Thorton and Deeb (157) noted that while ascorbic acid synthesis in the kidneys of laying hens was sufficient for physiological needs at normal environmental temperatures, it was not when temperatures were increased from 21° to 31°C as blood ascorbic acid levels decreased. Nestor et al. (158) demonstrated that ascorbic acid (330 mg/kg) added to the ration prevented a decline in blood ascorbic acid levels that occurred in turkeys consuming the unsupplemented ration during warm weather (30°C). In a trial during hot weather (35–40°C), Perek and Kendler (159) obtained significant improvement (Table V) in egg production and eggshell weight when ascorbic acid (25–400 mg/kg) was added to the ration of Leghorn laying hens. A subsequent report on ascorbic acid application (25–400 mg/kg) by the same workers (160) confirmed increases in egg production (11–24%), but egg weight differences were equivocal. Supplementation of diets with ascorbic acid counteracting high environmental temperatures for poultry were claimed by Ahmad et al. (161) and Pasual et al. (162). Under practical conditions of thermal stress (22.8–36.9°C) and humidity some benefit in egg production has been noted following the feeding of aspirin and ascorbic acid (163).

Since there is an abnormality of calcium metabolism in scurvy, it has been reasoned that supplementary ascorbic acid in the hen ration might help to resolve the problem of thin eggshell during summer heat. Some reports show improved shell soundness during high environmental temperatures; others do not. According to Thorton (164, 165) and Thorton

Table V. Effect of Feeding L-Ascorbic Acid to Hens

| | Ascorbic Acid in Feed (mg/kg) | | | |
Criteria	0	25	75	400
Culling and mortality (% of groups)	31.5	7.4	20.3	12.9
Egg production (total eggs/hen)	80.0	102.7	90.6	103.5
Feed efficiency (average g/egg)	232.2	210.4	206.7	202.8
Egg weights (average g/egg)	60.1	60.9	61.3	62.7
Eggshell weight (average % of whole egg)	9.05	9.87	9.25	9.47

and Moreng (*166*), ascorbic acid (22 mg/kg) added to the feed was of value during the hot summer months (29°C) for the maintenance of eggshell strength and thickness. It was believed that the added ascorbic acid in the feed increased feed consumption and oxygen consumption in hens during hot weather and that ascorbic acid counters the normal decline in thyroid activity during the hot summer months (*167*). Another explanation offered for the high temperature effect is a possible deformation in the structure of the inner layers of the shell upon which calcium is deposited during the egg laying process as well as the microstructure of the outer shell (*168, 169*). As noted by Lyle and Moreng (*153*), under increased temperatures, the addition of ascorbic acid (44 mg/kg) to the diet prevented the body temperature increase and the associated decrease in eggshell thickness. Sullivan and coworkers (*170, 171*) and El-Boushy and coworkers (*168, 172, 173*) published confirmatory results indicating significant improvement in egg quality under high environmental temperatures. For example (*168*), the shell percentage of the egg was significantly improved when ascorbic acid (50 mg/kg) was incorporated into the diet under a hot environmental temperature (Figure 5). In this report, the ascorbic acid added to the feed was shown to be present.

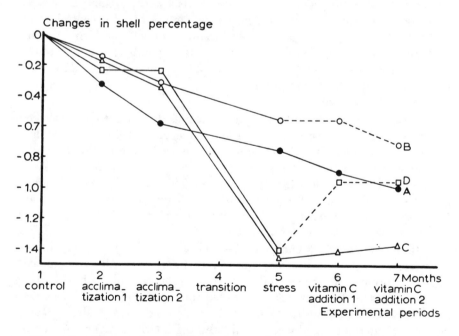

Figure 5. *Changes in eggshell percentage during the course of environmental temperature changes and vitamin C additions. Key:* ●, *control, cold;* ○, *treated, cold;* △, *control, hot;* □, *treated, hot;* - - -, *vitamin C addition. (Reproduced, with permission, from Ref. 168. Copyright 1966, H. Veenman & Zonen NV.)*

Kivimäe (*174*) obtained improvement in the quality of the eggshell with supplementary dietary ascorbic acid (100 mg/kg). Other workers (*160, 175–185*) have not been able to show improvement in shell thickness of eggs produced under the stress of high temperature environments. Some critics contend that past experimental studies did not involve currently used, high-producing genetic strains of poultry and the better formulated rations currently in commercial use. A general criticism leveled at many of the studies on ascorbic acid addition to the diet is that stability data are not reported and, due to the well-known lability of the compound, it may not have been always present in the feed at the time of consumption as declared.

Another index of egg quality, namely the thickness or viscosity of the albumen surrounding the yolk, measured in Haugh units, was found to be superior by Mostert (*186*), Herrick and Nockels (*187*), and Chen and Nockels (*188*) with ascorbic acid supplementation of the hen's diet, but Rauch (*189*) reported no effect. Stimulated spermatogenesis in cockerels was indicated by the early observations of Wawrzyniak (*190*) and Zanelli (*191*). These observations were confirmed by the studies of Perek and Snapir (*192*). When ascorbic acid (100–200 mg/kg) was fed in the diet over some months, the data showed a significant increase of spermatozoan production for the treated groups over the control group. Another type of stress, "laying cage fatigue," wherein the laying hen has difficulty in standing on the wire floor, has responded to administration of ascorbic acid by injections (100 mg) according to Polster (*193*). The role of vitamin C in the physiology and nutrition of poultry has been reviewed by Tagwerker (*194*).

Swine. It is generally accepted that pigs do not need a supplementary supply of L-ascorbic acid in their ration under field or pen confinement management practices. Some feeding trials where added ascorbic acid was tested resulted in negative reporting such as those of Barber et al. (*195*), Bowland (*196*), and Travnicek et al. (*197*). In others such as Cromwell et al. (*198*) a variable growth response was reported and Dvorak (*199*) reported equivocal data. Brown et al. (*200*) fed growing pigs supplementary ascorbic acid (0–1000 mg per head daily) in feed with different levels of energy (140–340 kcal $\times$ kg $W^{0.75}$ per head daily). Increases in growth observed were in an increasing order with increasing ascorbic acid intake and a decreasing increment with the rising energy intake. Burnside (*201*) reported some gain in feed efficiency with ascorbic acid (100 mg/kg), and Valdmauis (*202*) and Andresen (*203*) demonstrated increased viability in baby pigs. Others suggested L-ascorbic acid as a supplement for piglet feeds (*204*) or as protection against stress conditions (*205*). The state of ascorbic acid adequacy influences iron availability: Dvorak (*206*) reported iron deficiency anemic pigs to have lowered plasma levels of ascorbic acid, and Gipp et al. (*207*) observed increased plasma values of iron when ascorbic acid (0.5%) was added to feed of the piglets.

Ruminants. Treatment of ruminants with L-ascorbic acid has merit in unusual circumstances rather than any type of routine practice since these species synthesize their requirements in their normal life cycle pattern. The digestive system of the young calf or lamb functions similarly to that of monogastric animals for the early weeks of life until the ruminating process is initiated.

Phillips and coworkers (*208, 209, 210*) of the University of Wisconsin recommended L-ascorbic acid (250 mg), vitamin A (5000 IU), and niacin (50 mg) as a daily supplement for the first 10–21 days of life for the calf as prophylaxis and control of early calfhood diseases. Subsequent reports by Norton et al. (*211*) and Nevins et al. (*212*) did not confirm the declared benefits of supplementary vitamin feedings. In 1944 a strange eczematoid disease of calves with concomitant very low plasma ascorbic acid values occurring on dairy farms in Michigan was reported by Cole et al. (*213*). The condition responded to ascorbic acid therapy. Between 1951 and 1961 about 4% of the young calves in a Scottish large herd of Friesian cattle were noted with an inherited dermatological condition and other disorders with low liver, blood and urine ascorbic acid values. Calves treated with ascorbic acid produced a spectacular response (*214*) and relapsed after therapy ceased.

Olson and Tammeus (*215*) reported a syndrome of subperiosteal hemorrhages, progressive stiffness, and eventual immobility in a herd of Hereford cattle that responded to L-ascorbic acid treatment but relapsed when treatment ceased. Michigan workers (*216*) also observed a scurvy-like condition, a dermatitis, low hemoglobin and ascorbic acid blood values, and death (35 animals) in a herd of Shorthorn cattle.

Some decades ago it had been found that ascorbic acid injections improved a large percentage of sterile or partially sterile bulls (*217*). In very high producing milk cows, which have difficulty becoming pregnant, certain breeders have found, by practical experience, that ascorbic acid injected intravenously (2 g) and intramuscularly (2 g) before breeding with the bull on the same day or the following day improves conception, even though, in large herds, it is a burdensome procedure. Phillips et al. (*218*), as early as 1941, in observations and trials with "hard to settle" cows, indicated that certain cases (Table VI) were amenable to ascorbic acid therapy (0.5 g intravenously and 2 g subcutaneously). The vitamin A adequacy of these animals is not reported and, hence, could be an influencing factor as in vitamin A deficiency, synthesis of vitamin C is decreased (*219*).

Disease Therapy. Inactivation of viruses by L-ascorbic acid was reported in 1935 to occur rather quickly under in vitro conditions (*220*) and somewhat later by Jungeblut (*221*) with limited confirmation in vivo.

Table VI.   Data Showing the Effect of Ascorbic

Cow	Before Treatment (Number of Times Bred)	Type of Case
427	4	regular estrum—failed to settle
455	7	skips 1 or 2 periods after service
437	6	skips 1 or 2 periods after service
17	8	regular estrum—failed to settle
16	9	regular estrum—failed to settle
29	4	skips 1 or 2 periods after service
33	5	skips 1 or 2 periods after service
1W	6	regular estrum—failed to settle
9W	5	regular estrum—failed to settle
4W	4	regular estrum—failed to settle
1450	many	uterus—no tone
1479	many	uterus—no tone
B	4	
65	many	cystic ovary
404	many	cystic ovary
662	7	cystic ovary
D	many	regular estrum—failed to settle

In the chicken, the presence of increased ascorbic acid intake has been reported to lower the response to a T-independent antigen, *Brucella abortus*, and to raise the response in adults (*222*), and to inhibit replication and ineffectivity of the avian RNA tumor virus (*223*). Subsequent reports by others (*224–230*) showed encouraging results for ascorbic acid treatment in the inactivation or alleviation of certain viral and bacterial diseases. Nungester and Ames (*231*) noted that activity of phagocytes was significantly increased with higher ascorbic acid concentrations in the ambient medium. In 1971 a biochemical mechanism of action in phagocytosis was offered by DeChatelet et al. (*232, 919*) involving L-ascorbic acid.

Acid Therapy upon Hard to Settle Cows

After Treatment

Services	Result	Method of Treating
1	pregnancy	injections 8 weeks before breeding—weekly, subcutaneous
1	pregnancy	6 injections over 5 weeks, beginning with breeding
1	pregnancy	6 injections over 30 days prior to breeding
1	pregnancy	intravenous and subcutaneous injection at time of heat
1	pregnancy	4 doses over 10 days after breeding
1	pregnancy	4 doses over 10 days after breeding
1	pregnancy	4 doses over 10 days after breeding
1	pregnancy	3 doses over 12 days before breeding
1	pregnancy	3 doses over 12 days before breeding
1	pregnancy	3 doses over 12 days before breeding
many	no help	subcutaneous and intravenous
many	no help	subcutaneous and intravenous
3	?	subcutaneous
many	no help	subcutaneous
many	no help	subcutaneous
several	no help	subcutaneous
		subcutaneous and intravenous dosage too low

In 1967 Belfield (*233*) introduced a therapeutic program using L-ascorbic acid in the treatment against distemper of canines (2000 mg intravenously daily) and of felines (cats and toy breeds of dogs, 1000 mg) with supportive therapy with a resultant high degree of success. Confirmation of the treatment was reported by Edwards (*234*) in the treatment of cats with feline rhinotracheitis and by Brandt (*235*) in the treatment of feline distemper and pneumonitis in cats. Brandt was less successful with dogs. Leveque (*236*) treated dogs (67 animals) over a 22-month period with canine distemper with ascorbic acid and raised his recovery rate of animals to 72% (Table VII) from 5–10% previously experienced. Ward (*237*) indicated that he had success in ascorbic acid

Table VII. Recovery Rates Among Dogs Treated with Ascorbic Acid for Canine Distemper Complex

Patient Group	Number Treated	Number Recovered	Recovery Rate (%)
All dogs treated	67	48	71.6
Cases showing CNS disturbance	16	7	43.8
Atypical cases with CNS disturbance but no convulsions	4	3	75.0
Typical cases with convulsions	12	4	33.3
Cases without CNS disturbance	51	41	80.4
Typical cases with convulsions and given 3 or fewer doses of ascorbic acid	7	1	14.3
Typical cases with convulsions and given more than 3 doses of ascorbic acid	5	3	60.0
Typical cases without convulsions and given more than 3 doses of ascorbic acid	14	11	78.6

Source: Reproduced, with permission, from Ref. *236*. Copyright 1969, Veterinary Medicine Publishing Company.

treatment of canine and feline distemper over a period of years. Other viral diseases such as viral encephalitis (238), for which there is a lack of effective therapy, may respond to treatment with high levels of ascorbic acid.

Administration Methods. In administering L-ascorbic acid to animals, there are several feasible routes, depending on the size of the animal and its characteristics. For small animals such as chickens, it is possible to add the L-ascorbic acid to the automatic water supply, providing dissolved trace minerals such as copper and iron can be avoided or minimized, for example by incorporation of a chelating agent with the ascorbic acid. This route would only be considered for a short period or as an emergency measure since stability of aqueous solutions exposed to air is poor. For large animals, parenteral administration is the most rapid and effective route for short periods of need. For longer term administration the feed route is preferred, assuming adequate stability exists for the time period of intended use.

High moisture content in feeds or exposure of feed to high humidity, high temperature storage is detrimental to added ascorbic acid. Pelleting of feed, which includes exposure to steam or hot water and subsequent storage, also destroys (30–60%) ascorbic acid. Attempts to overcome this destructive action include the use of coated ascorbic acid product forms and the application of ascorbic acid to the pellet feed following the pelletizing process. L-Ascorbic acid coated with ethyl cellulose (4%) and finely powdered ascorbic acid uniformly blended into a warm edible hydrogenated fat (50%) and immediately sprayed in chilled air into small beadlet form are two methods that have improved stability in animal feeds (Table VIII). Even with these products, an excess over claim values must be added.

If solid fat is an ingredient of the feed as an energy source, one practical way of adding ascorbic acid is to uniformly suspend the finely powdered product into the liquified hydrogenated fat and spray the suspension onto the cooled pelleted feed in a tumbler or on a moving belt conveyor. Andrews and Davis (239) reported this method to be feasible for pelleted fish feed. Heat-expanded commercial catfish feed (32% protein) was sprayed with a warm fat suspension of ascorbic acid to 2, 5, and 10% fat coating on the feed. After drying, the water stability (water leaching of ascorbic acid) of the product was evaluated (Table IX) as fish feed is normally cast on water for fish consumption.

A problem arose as how to add L-ascorbic acid to baked monkey biscuits since baking is quite destructive to ascorbic acid. After some trial work it was discovered that ascorbic acid (10–20%) in concentrated

Table VIII. Ascorbic Acid Stability in Unpelleted Feed

	Storage Condition	
	3 Weeks/45°C 100% Humidity	6 Weeks/45°C Room Humidity
Type Product	(% Retention Ascorbic Acid)	
Ascorbic acid, crystalline	0	40–80
Ethocel coated, AA	0	84–87
Fat (50%) beadlets, AA	78–84	91–99

Table IX. Retention of Ascorbic Acid[a] in Fabricated Fish Feeds

Ascorbic Acid Level mg/kg Diet	Ascorbic Acid (%) Remaining in Feed Particles After Water Exposure		
	1 Minute	5 Minutes	10 Minutes
90	96	74	50
197	86	67	42
379	83	67	36

[a] Ascorbic acid in a warm fat suspension sprayed on feed after pelleting.

sucrose syrup (50–60%) could be brushed, sprayed, or dropped on to
the biscuits after baking with fairly good stability performance. Ascorbic
acid is quite stable in high sugar composition such as candy, added at
the last stage of processing because of the dense nature of the high
sucrose products and relative freedom from oxygen.

Miscellaneous. In miscellaneous animal applications relating to the
use of ascorbic acid, interactions with toxic levels of minerals have been
observed. Hill (240) found increased dietary ascorbic acid in chickens
was specific in counteracting metal toxicity in cases of selenium and
vanadium. This was also noted by Berg et al. (241). Cadmium toxicity
in the rat (242) and in Japanese quail (243, 244) has been reversed or
counteracted. Ascorbic acid (500 mg/kg) given intraperitoneally before
or simultaneously with an oral dose of paraquat altered the activity of
paraquat indicating ascorbic acid to be an effective detoxifying agent
(245). Kallistratos and Fasske (246) noted inhibition of benzo[a]pyrene
carcinogenesis in rats with ascorbic acid treatment. There is a decreased
level of ascorbic acid in lung tissue of mice following exposure to ozone,
and Kratzing and Willis (247) propose that one function of tissue ascorbic acid may be an extracellular antioxidant in the lungs. Use of ascorbic acid and mineral supplements in the detoxification of narcotic addicts
(248, 920) has been discussed. While not a practical approach, the
injection of young chickens with sodium ascorbate has been reported to
heal bruises at a faster rate than in nontreated animals (249).

Pharmaceutical Applications

L-Ascorbic acid (vitamin C) is an active ingredient in a variety of
pharmaceutical dosage forms such as: high-potency multivitamin supplement; high-potency multivitamin supplement with iron; high-potency
multivitamin supplement with minerals; vitamin B complex; vitamin B
complex with vitamin E; pediatric drops; tablets of a range of potencies;
injectables; and syrups and elixirs. An alternative list of pharmaceutical
dosage forms containing ascorbic acid would be: tablets with a wide
range of potencies, drops (especially for pediatric use), injectables, syrups
and elixirs, effervescent tablets, and multivitamin preparations.

Many vitamins are quite stable under normal processing conditions and present little or no stability problems in finished pharmaceutical products. These include biotin, niacin, niacinamide, pyridoxine,
riboflavin, and α-tocopheryl acetate. Others that can present problems
are ascorbic acid, calciferol, calcium pantothenate, cyanocobalamin, folacin, and retinyl esters. Overages above label claim are customarily
added to vitamin formulations as a means of maintaining the claimed
level of each vitamin for the expected shelf life of the products. The
percent overage for a particular vitamin such as L-ascorbic acid will vary

according to its performance pattern. In general, problems of instability of vitamins are much more acute in multivitamin liquids than in single vitamin formulations or in solid dosage forms.

Solid Dosage Forms. L-Ascorbic acid tablets constitute one of the major uses in pharmaceutical applications. Tablets may be of the coated or uncoated type, in various potencies and sizes, and also swallowable or chewable. These solid dosage forms are prepared either by double compression or slugging, by wet granulation, or by direct compression. In the usual process of tablet preparation ascorbic acid in powder or fine granular form together with suitable diluents of lactose, sucrose, or starch with lubricant is slugged and reduced to granules, then recompressed into tablets of the desired size. An alternate method consists of making a moist paste of lactose, starch, and sucrose, which is screened, dried, and reduced to granules, then mixed with ascorbic acid in coarse crystalline form and lubricant and compressed into tablets. Special L-ascorbic acid application forms are available that permit direct compression into tablet form. Chewable tablets contain sodium ascorbate in addition to ascorbic acid and flavoring agents to provide a more pleasant taste. Another special type of solid dosage form is the effervescent tablet, usually of higher potency (0.5–2.0 g) that is consumed when added water converts the tablet to a liquid preparation. There are a number of scientific papers and patents detailing the formulation and manufacture (250–257) of solid ascorbic acid dosage forms, their stability (258–266), in vitro release of nutrients (267, 268, 269), and bioavailability (270–275). Data (Table X) collected on commercial ascorbic acid tablets stored at room temperature (25°C) demonstrate full label potency over a shelf life period of many years. Under normal storage conditions, commercial type ascorbic acid tablets are stable for over 5 years (> 95% potency retention). The amount of three breakdown products (dehydroascorbic acid, diketogulonic acid, and oxalic acid) formed under various storage conditions constitutes a small percentage of the ascorbic acid content and poses no dietary hazard (276). In the application of sugar coating to multivitamin tablets, careful technique is required to prevent excessive penetration of moisture into the tablet core, which can lead to high losses of vitamins sensitive to moisture and pH influences.

Liquid Dosage Forms. In dry form and at very low moisture content, L-ascorbic acid is very stable, but in solution exposed to air or oxygen it is subject to oxidation accelerated by dissolved trace minerals (copper and iron) and light exposure. L-Ascorbic acid is a reducing agent and is subject to oxidative decomposition in solution. This proceeds first to dehydroascorbic acid, which has full vitamin C activity, but continues to diketogulonic acid and various other breakdown products. The degradation reactions are complex and vary with aerobic or anaerobic

Table X.   Stability of

Analysis of Ascorbic Acid, 100-mg Tablets,
After Long-Term Storage at 25°C

Lot Number	Storage Time (months)	Assay (% of claim)[a]	Initial Assay (% of claim)[a]
V-418	103	99	103
KRK-202-66I	103	104	107
KRK-202-65-III	103	106	110
KRK-202-65-IV	103	106	110
KRK-202-66-II	103	105	111
DMS-289-II	90	104	102
Lot 2082	120	111	—
Lot 2964B	240	101	—
Lot 002-0B097A	96	98	—

[a] Assay by iodometric and 2,6-dichloroindophenol titrations.

situations, the nature of the formulation, and the type of stress to which pharmaceutical solutions are subjected. Ascorbic acid degradation is also pH dependent. Under aerobic conditions, the rate of oxidation shows maxima at pH 5, corresponding to reaction with 1 equivalent of base, and at pH 11.5, corresponding to reaction with 2 equivalents of base. A pH–log rate profile (pH range of 3.5–7.2) for rate of aerobic oxidation of aqueous ascorbic acid solutions (67°C) was determined by Blaug and Hajratwala (277). A first-order degradation was observed. Rogers and Yacomeni (278) also studied the effect of pH on ascorbic acid solutions (25°C).

Under anaerobic conditions, the dependency of the stability of ascorbic acid in aqueous solutions on pH is relatively low, but there is a maximum rate of degradation, which is equal to the pK_{a1} of ascorbic acid, at a pH of about 4.1. Stability of ascorbic acid in multivitamin drops has been studied at various pH levels. Maximum losses occur in the pH range of 3.3 to 4.5 and smaller losses are found at higher pH (up to 5.5). Figure 6 shows stability data for ascorbic acid in multivitamin elixir preparations for teaspoon dosage for storage at 45°C. The pH of such solutions has a more pronounced effect than in multivitamin drops. Losses at pH 3.5 are as high as 40% in 6 weeks at 45°C. Rate studies on the anaerobic degradation of ascorbic acid as influenced by metal ions, Finholt et al. (279, 280), have indicated the involvement of salt–acid and metal complex formations.

During the past two decades ascorbic acid free radicals have become recognized and their kinetics studied (281–287) in the oxidation of ascorbic acid. Interactions between certain of the vitamins or ingredients

Vitamin C Tablets

Analysis of Ascorbic Acid, 100-mg Tablets,
After Long-Term Storage at 25°C

Loss in Potency (%)	Diketogulonic Acid (%)	Oxalic Acid (%)	Dehydroascorbic Acid (%)
4	1.0	0.5	0.5
3	2.0	0.5	0.2
4	1.0	0.5	0.2
4	1.0	0.5	0.4
6	2.0	1.0	2.4
—	0.5	0.5	0.3
—	—	0.2	0.4
—	—	0.4	2.3
—	—	—	1.3

Source: Reproduced, with permission, from Ref. *276*. Copyright 1976, American Pharmaceutical Association.

are of great interest to the pharmaceutical chemist both from the theoretical and the practical viewpoints.

1. Hand, Guthrie, and Sharp (*288*) reported that riboflavin catalyzes the photochemical oxidation of ascorbic acid that occurs in the presence of oxygen on exposure to light. Conversely, ascorbic acid exerts a reducing effect on riboflavin, which is very likely involved in the formation of chloroflavin in B-complex solutions containing ascorbic acid.

2. A yellow complex of 1 molecule of niacinamide with 1 molecule of ascorbic acid also forms readily in solution by what appears to be a charge-transfer reaction. The complex has been prepared in solid form. It has been claimed that the preforming of this complex presents difficulties with thickening and hardening of mixtures employed in soft gelatin capsules. Guttman and Brooke (*289*) found the extent of association between niacinamide and ascorbic acid to be pH dependent with maximum adsorbance at pH 3.8.

3. In acid medium the folic acid molecule is cleaved by reducing agents such as ascorbic acid. This reaction occurs in two stages: (i) cleavage to the pteridine moiety plus *p*-aminobenzoylglutamic acid, and (ii) destruction of the free amino group of the *p*-aminobenzoylglutamic acid. The decomposition of folic acid is more rapid at pH 3 than at pH 6.5.

4. Stabilization of vitamin B_{12} solutions in the presence of thiamine, niacinamide, and ascorbic acid has been the subject of a number of patents. Newmark (*290*) has described

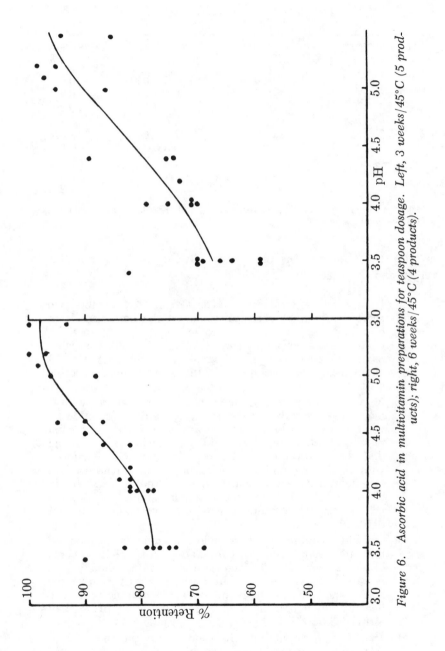

Figure 6. Ascorbic acid in multivitamin preparations for teaspoon dosage. Left, 3 weeks/45°C (5 products); right, 6 weeks/45°C (4 products).

the effective stabilization of B_{12} in such solutions by various iron compounds and salts.

5. Ascorbic acid will destroy many of the FD&C azo colors in solution, so stable colorants must be chosen.

6. The decomposition of ascorbic acid is catalyzed by trace metal ions in solution, hence the addition of sequestering agents such as EDTA and its salts has been shown to enhance the stability of ascorbic acid (*291, 292, 293*).

A review of such interactions was published by Scheindlin (*294*) in 1958. Porikh and Lofgren (*295*) demonstrated increased stability of ascorbic acid, confirmed by Kato (*296*), when glycerin and/or propylene glycol type products were substituted for part of the water in an oral multivitamin liquid. Baudelin and Tuschhoff (*297*) reported similar findings on ascorbic acid and, in addition, found that ethanol or sugars such as sucrose, corn syrup, and dextrose also provide a stabilizing effect on ascorbic acid. Paust and Coliazzi (*298*) and Fabrizi et al. (*299*) found that the first-order rate constants for oxidative decomposition of ascorbic acid decrease as a function of polysorbate 80 concentration up to 30% at 30°C. Similar findings were observed by Nixon and Chawla (*300*) with polysorbate 20. Other reports (*301–309*) deal with factors influencing formulation and stability of liquid dosage forms of ascorbic acid.

Sterile aqueous solutions prepared with high purity ascorbic acid and pyrogen-free distilled water in glass-lined equipment under absolute sanitary operations and filled into ampules are necessary for injectable solutions for parenteral use in humans and animals. For all injectable products, it is important to select container, stopper, preservative, and other ingredients that are compatible.

The formulator of liquid multivitamin pharmaceutical products such as baby drops, syrups, elixirs, and injectables encounters numerous problems in attempting to develop products having adequate physical and chemical stability as well as suitable taste, odor, color, and freedom from bacterial contamination. Many of these problems arise from the differing solubility and stability characteristics of the individual vitamins, particularly as these relate to the pH of the solutions and potential interactions. Despite these numerous problems, various ways have been devised for producing multivitamin combinations in liquid form containing L-ascorbic acid that have acceptable stability characteristics. Successful development of such products requires a knowledge of: (i) the fundamental aspects of the physical and chemical properties of the vitamin forms available; (ii) the use of adequate techniques of manufacture; and (iii) the employment of suitable overages based on critical stability studies.

Food Applications

L-Ascorbic acid may be added to foods or food ingredients as a nutrient to fortify natural foods having little or no vitamin C, to restore losses, to standardize a given class of food products to having a pre-selected quantity, and to endow or enrich synthetic foods with nutritional value. The term nutrification is used to cover all the above situations for adding a nutrient to a food product. To nutrify a food or to make it a nutrified food implies an act to make the food more nutritious. Adding micronutrients such as vitamins, minerals, amino acids, and vitamin A active carotenoid colorants to a food at low cost for nutritional improvement is not a new concept. Iodine was added to salt in the 19th century in South America. Nutrification is a most rapid, most economical, most flexible, and most socially acceptable method of changing the nutrient intake of a given population (310).

New technological advances enable the food processing industry to market many more food products than decades past. Factors that must be considered in conjunction with appropriate technology before added ascorbic acid is considered are: cost of the specific food; convenience of use; relationship of the nutrient to the usual food selection pattern or other replacement or supplemental food products; stability of the nutrient in the food during market shelf life and home preparation; special food needs, for example, infant, geriatric, or military; public health considerations.

L-Ascorbic acid is also added to food in essentially a non-nutrient capacity such as a preservative or oxygen acceptor, as an acidulant, as a stabilizer of cured meat color, or as a flour improver. Because of the ene–diol group, it has a marked inhibitory influence on the oxidation–reduction reactions responsible for undesirable color, flavor, and odor development. Its mechanism of action is dependent upon the characteristics of the food or food ingredient, the associated environments, the processing technology, and the storage expectancy of the product.

The food processing industry can obtain L-ascorbic acid and sodium ascorbate commercially in a variety of mesh sizes to meet the requirements of various kinds of food products. These crystalline compounds are stable for years when stored under cool, dry conditions in closed containers. Esters of ascorbic acid such as ascorbyl palmitate are also available.

Addition Methods. The four basic technologies developed for adding ascorbic acid to foods are:

1. *Tablets or wafers.* Compressed soluble discs containing inert, edible carriers and sufficient ascorbic acid to meet the ascorbic acid regulatory and (or) processing requirements of a given quantity of food. The tablet added to

the container prior to filling and sealing of liquid foods dissolves immediately, or may be dissolved and added to semisolid foods or dry foods at a late stage of food preparation.

2. *Dry premixes.* A uniform mixture of a known amount of ascorbic acid and a dry carrier, usually a constituent of the food. The premix blended with a prescribed quantity of dry food product gives a greater assurance of product uniformity since the quantity of the pure vitamin may be small.

3. *Liquid sprays.* Sprays of ascorbic acid solutions or suspensions that may be considered liquid premixes. The sprays are directed onto the surface of a food or injected into liquid food products to circumvent difficult or continuous processing conditions. For example, toasted ready-to-eat cereals are fortified by spraying a solution onto flakes still warm from the toasting process.

4. *Pure compound.* Crystalline ascorbic acid, sodium ascorbate or special coated product forms are widely added directly to food or predetermined quantities often in the form of preweighed packets for convenience. Addition is accompanied by mixing to ensure uniformity.

Hundreds, if not thousands, of reports have been published on the application of ascorbic acid to food products for either nutritional objectives or improvement in food quality. Bauernfeind reviewed the use of ascorbic acid (*311, 312*) in processing food in 1953 (406 references) and again in 1970 (520 references); other reviews (*313–332*) on food applications of ascorbic acid have appeared prior to and following these dates.

The stability of ascorbic acid is influenced by atmospheric oxygen, water activity, oxidative enzymes, pasteurization methods, metal contamination, and sulfur dioxide content.

The degradation of ascorbic acid in foods has been widely studied. It is complex in nature and depends on specific conditions and the presence of other substances. While degradation is not a topic of this review a few food related references are included as an introduction to the literature on this subject. Ascorbic acid has the ability to scavenge superoxide and hydroxyl radicals as well as singlet oxygen (*333*). In a 1975 report on the destruction of ascorbic acid as a function of water activity by Lee and Labuza (*334*), the half-life of ascorbic acid (Figure 7) is well illustrated as a function of moisture content. Degradation compounds formed by heating ascorbic acid in solution were identified by Tatum et al. (*335*) and Kamiya (*336*). Thompson and Fennema (*337*) observed differences in the effect of freezing on the rate of oxidation of ascorbic acid in foods as compared with dilute simple solutions. Timberlake (*338*) found the oxidation of ascorbic acid in the presence of metals was significant and could be influenced by metal chelating

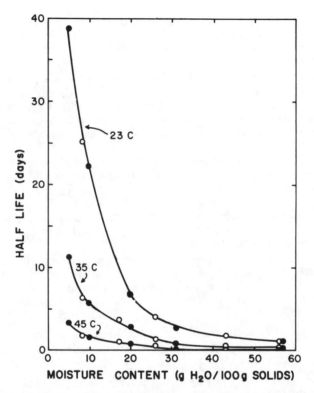

Figure 7. Half-life for ascorbic acid as a function of moisture content. Key: ●, *DM;* ○, *DH. (Reproduced, with permission, from Ref. 334. Copyright 1975, Institute of Food Technologists.)*

agents in black currant juice. In the last decade more attention has been given to kinetics of quality degradation including ascorbic acid oxidation in food products or model systems. Examples are moisture-sensitive products (339), ascorbic acid oxidation in infant formula during storage (340), ascorbic acid stability of tomato juice as functions of temperature, pH, and metal catalyst (341), the degradation of ascorbic acid in a dehydrated food system (342), and the oxygen effect on the degradation of ascorbic acid in a dehydrated food system (343).

The point in the food manufacturing process at which ascorbic acid is introduced is important. Ideally, it is added as close to the terminal process stage as possible, when conditions allow. To maximize the stability and efficacy of ascorbic acid added to foodstuffs, the following precautions are recommended for practical success according to Klaeui (317):

1. Direct contact of the food product or its ingredients with brass, bronze, monel, steel, and iron must be avoided.

2. The equipment used should be of stainless steel, aluminum, enamel, glass, china, or approved plastic.
3. Wherever possible, deaeration should precede processing, which should be carried out under inert gas or in a vacuum.
4. During mixing, emulsification, homogenization, and the like, oxygen or air should not be introduced into the product.
5. Where possible, food product should be protected from light and other radiant energy.
6. Containers should be filled to maximum capacity, that is, the headspace should be kept as small as possible.
7. After heat processing of sealed containers, rapid cooling should follow and the products should be stored at cool temperatures.
8. If practicable, sequestering agents such as phosphates, citrates, EDTA, or cysteine may be added.
9. All autoxidizable ingredients, such as flavoring oils, added to the food product should have a low peroxide value.
10. Whenever feasible, a short-time heat treatment of fresh food products should be employed to inactivate enzymes before adding ascorbic acid.
11. Where feasible, microorganisms may be removed by filtration or inactivated by heat treatment and, if possible, processing may be continued under aseptic conditions.
12. Preferably, some ascorbic acid should be present prior to bottling or canning (1 mL of residual air reacts, theoretically, with 3.3 mg of ascorbic acid).

L-Ascorbic acid is found in all living tissues, both animal and plant matter, and as such has been consumed by humans for thousands of years, thus giving encouragement that the compound is physiologically acceptable and safe. Furthermore, extensive testing of L-ascorbic acid prepared by chemical synthesis confirms its relative safety. Large-scale manufacture, coupled with high standards of purity and relatively low cost, makes application to food products economically feasible.

Use as a Nutrient. Processing never makes a food product more complete than the original fresh product nor can it compensate for nature's idiosyncrasies in content of original nutrients. However, the preservation, processing, and storage of food are necessary to provide palatability, safety to health, variety of selection, and provision for future use. In the production, handling, preserving, processing, and storage of food, some nutrients are lost or significantly lowered. Not only does the nutrient content vary in the natural whole-plant food—because of variety, climate, harvesting methods, storage—but processing (because of exposure to heat, oxygen, metals, and so forth, and food-fractionation processes) modifies the nutrient content. One nutrient especially sensitive to some of the factors mentioned is L-ascorbic acid. Furthermore, not only are the traditional natural and processed or refined foods sold today, but also new "convenience," "semblance," "fabricated," "novel," and "dietetic or low-calorie" foods. Some of these products simulate known foods. Others have no past counterpart and may have low levels of micronutrients such as L-ascorbic acid, which can be corrected by nutrification. Many countries (344) have established a recommended daily allowance or intake of ascorbic acid for humans (Table XI).

FRUIT BEVERAGE PRODUCTS. L-Ascorbic acid has been associated with fruit and fruit juices since 1753 when Captain James Lind, physician to the British Fleet, demonstrated the successful treatment of scurvy by incorporating citrus juices in the diet. The pattern of fruit products consumption has undergone a gradual change over the years. The decline of whole fresh fruit and vegetable consumption is correlated with increased use of frozen or canned fruits, vegetables, and juices and, more recently, reconstituted fruit-flavored beverages. Fruit and vegetable products are the primary sources of L-ascorbic acid in this diet. Apple, grape, pineapple, prune, and cranberry juices and peach and apricot nectars contain little or no ascorbic acid unless nutrified. Other juices may be variable sources. Fruit juices low in ascorbic acid are used interchangeably with those of high ascorbic acid content. It is the

Table XI. International Dietary Allowances for Vitamin C

Country	Adult Male	Pregnancy	Lactation
Australia	30	60	60
Canada	30	40	50
Columbia	50	65	65
Finland	30	50	90
East Germany	70	100	100
West Germany	75	100	120
INCAP	55 (50) [a]	60	60
India	50	50	80
Indonesia	60	90	90
Japan	60 (50) [a]	60	90
Malaysia	30	60	60
Netherlands	50	75	75
Philippines	75 (70) [a]	100	150
Thailand	30	50	50
Turkey	50	70	80
United Kingdom	30	60	60
United States [b]	60	80	100

Note: Values are given in milligrams per day.
[a] Female.
[b] NRC-1980 allowance.
Source. Reproduced, with permission, from Ref. 344. Copyright 1975, Common Agricultural Bureaux.

contention of some groups that it is desirable to nutrify those juices to make them more comparable with the latter from a standpoint of nutritive value, hence, leaving choice of selection based on flavor preferences.

Ascorbic acid levels of 30–60 mg/100–200 mL are meaningful concentrations. For example, Del Monte (345) began adding L-ascorbic acid to tomato juice (60 mg/180 mL) on a commercial basis in 1974. This conforms to U.S. FDA regulations. The effect of processing variables and product storage in ascorbic nutrified tomato juice has been studied by Flinn (346) and by Pope and Gould (347). In addition to the straight fruit juices, different beverage-based products have been studied as ascorbic acid nutrified foods; such products include a chocolate-flavored powder (348), a whey–soy drink mix (349), malt lemonades (350), and fruit juice carbonated beverages (351, 352). L-Ascorbic acid stability, its influence on quality during storage, and its influence on processing fruit juices and beverages remain a subject of active study (353–359).

The acid-type fruit and vegetable juices are good carriers of ascorbic acid, thus providing a relatively stable environment. Gresswell (322) and others in the past (311, 312, 318) have reviewed the use of L-ascorbic acid in beverages and fruit juices. In adding ascorbic acid to juices and beverages, a decision must be made about the nutrient level to be claimed for the product in the market place plus that expected to be destroyed in processing and during shelf life. It must be recognized that oxidative enzymes (ascorbic acid oxidase, peroxidases) exist in fruit and need to be heat inactivated. Removal of oxygen or air by vacuum deaeration and replacement by nitrogen or carbon dioxide or flushing headspace with inert gas will reduce ascorbic acid destruction. In some instances the addition of glucose oxidase and catalase is useful in removing dissolved and headspace oxygen, which minimizes required ascorbic acid addition. Use of minimum amounts of sulfur dioxide (insufficient to cause flavor changes) can be helpful in some products for better ascorbic acid retention values.

Exposure of ascorbic acid nutrified juices and beverages to direct sunlight, depending on the liquid formulation, can accelerate destruction of ascorbic acid and bring about flavor changes. If the product will be exposed, choice of packaging may minimize light influences. Oxygen permeability of packaging material should not be overlooked. In any new product to be nutrified, pilot-size production batches (Table XII) should be run with the best selected variants and storage data obtained before commercial production is commenced. Added L-ascorbic acid in dry, fruit-flavored powdered products to be reconstituted is quite stable if moisture levels are kept low and if they are packed in laminated, moisture-resistant packets.

It has been recognized that the elderly (360) do not always consume sufficient L-ascorbic acid due, in part, to lack of selection of appropriate

Table XII. Stability of Added

Product	Packaging	Goal	After Processing	
			Ascor- bic Acid	Vita- min C^a
Apple juice	glass, 1 qt	30 mg/4 fl oz	40	44
Apple juice	glass, 1 qt	30 mg/4 fl oz	38	41
Apple juice	glass, 1 qt	30 mg/10 fl oz	38	49
Apple juice	glass, 1 qt	30 mg/4 fl oz	38	43
Apple juice	glass, 24 oz	30 mg/8 fl oz	35	47
Apple juice	can, 20 oz	35 mg/100 mL	35	41
Apple juice	can, 18 oz	30 mg/4 fl oz	38	45
Apple juice	glass, 1 qt	30 mg/4 fl oz	42	49
Apple cherry	glass, 1 qt	30 mg/4 fl oz	53	54
Apple orange	glass, 4 oz	30 mg/4 fl oz	66	—
Apple orange	glass, amber	40 mg/100 mL	62	63
Apple orange	can	40 mg/100 mL	61	62
Applesauce	can, 1 lb	30 mg/100 g	69	74
Apricot nectar	can, 4 oz	30 mg/4 fl oz	57	59
Apricot nectar	can, 18 oz	30 mg/4 fl oz	35	40
Apricot nectar	—	30 mg/4 fl oz	39	—
Apricot pineapple	can, 4 oz	30 mg/4 fl oz	69	70
Apricot drink	can, 6 oz	30 mg/6 fl oz	47	48
Apricot drink	can, 12 oz	30 mg/4 fl oz	49	53
Apricot orange	can, 12 oz	30 mg/4 fl oz	47	49
Cereals, dry	box, liner	10 mg/oz	10.3	—
Cereals, dry	box, liner	10 mg/oz	11.4	—
Cereals, dry	box, liner	10 mg/oz	10.5	—
Cocoa powders	envelope	25 mg/100 g	34	48
Cocoa powders	foil bags	120 mg/lb	180	214
Cocoa powders	box, 1 lb	75 mg/20 g	78	80
Cocoa powders	can, 0.5 lb	15 mg/0.75 oz	14.1	—
Cocoa powders	package	15 mg/oz	18	—
Cranberry juice	glass, 16 oz	30 mg/4 fl oz	39	39
Cranberry juice	glass, 16 oz	30 mg/4 fl oz	60	61
Cranberry juice	glass, 16 oz	30 mg/4 fl oz	42	49
Cranberry juice	glass, 16 oz	30 mg/6 fl oz	38	41
Cranberry orange	glass, 1 qt	30 mg/6 fl oz	59	61
Cranberry apricot	glass, 1 qt	30 mg/6 fl oz	38	49
Fruit punch	can, 46 oz	30 mg/8 fl oz	44	48
Fruit punch	glass, 0.5 gal	30 mg/10 fl oz	67	68
Fruit carbonated beverages				
grape	can, 12 oz	30 mg/12 fl oz	42	46
orange	can, 12 oz	30 mg/12 fl oz	44	46
root beer	can, 12 oz	30 mg/12 fl oz	40	50
Fruit powder mixes				
orange	package, 3 oz	30 mg/3 oz	82	87
orange	envelope	30 mg/4 fl oz	78	79

Ascorbic Acid in Food Products

Storage, 70–75°F (23°C)

6 Months		12 Months	
Ascorbic Acid	Vitamin C	Ascorbic Acid	Vitamin C
31	40 (80) [b]	—	—
29	33 (80)	—	—
—	—	25	37 (76)
29	33 (77)	—	—
31	34 (72)	28	32 (68)
35	—	26	31 (76)
31	33 (73)	26	26 (58)
28	30 (61)	25	31 (63)
35	44 (81)	31	34 (63)
56 (85)	—	54 (82)	—
46	48 (76)	37	40 (64)
49	53 (85)	39	48 (77)
59	62 (84)	56	56 (76)
61	62 (100)	45	50 (84)
31	46 (100)	29	32 (80)
37 (95)	—	32 (82)	—
53	56 (80)	52	59 (84)
40	46 (95)	29	40 (83)
48	49 (92)	37	41 (77)
43	43 (88)	—	—
8.3 (80)	9.7	7.2 (70)	9.9
—	12.5	9.9 (87)	10.3
8.0 (76)	10.7	7.0 (67)	9.1
34	45 (94)	28	39 (81)
166	194 (90)	137	171 (80)
76	87 (100)	77	82 (100)
13.0 (92)	14.0	11.4 (81)	12.9
15.8 (88)	—	16.5 (91)	—
30	35 (90)	—	—
51	57 (94)	—	—
−7	39 (80)	32	38 (78)
33	35 (86)	32	34 (83)
47	53 (87)	—	—
35	40 (82)	38	40 (82)
31	35 (73)	—	—
54	58 (85)	—	—
30	35 (76)	26	28 (61)
30	35 (76)	22	25 (54)
31	41 (82)	28	32 (64)
75	80 (92)	73	79 (91)
71	77 (97)	68	76 (96)

Continued on next page.

Table XII.

Product	Packaging	Goal	After Processing	
			Ascorbic Acid	Vitamin C [a]
Fruit powder mixes				
orange	glass, 7 oz	136 mg/oz	136	—
orange	can, 4 oz	75 mg/4 fl oz	144	122
lemon	glass, 7 oz	60 mg/25 g	75	—
fruit gelatin	can, 24 oz	15 mg/3 oz	17.5	18.2
fruit gelatin	can, 24 oz	15 mg/4 oz	63	68
Fruit lollipops				
lemon		30 mg/pop	29	—
pineapple		30 mg/pop	30	—
Grape juice C [c]	can, 6 oz	15 mg/1 oz	13 [d]	14 [d]
Grape drink	can	30 mg/8 fl oz	31	33
Grape drink	can, 12 oz	30 mg/6 fl oz	44	48
Grape drink	can, 46 oz.	30 mg/6 fl oz	43	46
Grape drink	can, 1 qt	30 mg/6 fl oz	36	40
Grape drink	glass, 0.5 gal	30 mg/8 fl oz	26	35
Grape drink	glass, 0.5 gal	30 mg/8 fl oz	30	41
Grapefruit juice	glass, 17 oz	30 mg/4 fl oz	68	71
Grapefruit juice	can, 18 oz	30 mg/4 fl oz	56	58
Grapefruit juice	can, 18 oz	30 mg/4 fl oz	63	69
Grapefruit juice	can, 18 oz	30 mg/4 fl oz	57	57
Grapefruit juice	can, 6 oz	30 mg/4 fl oz	74	76
Grapefruit juice C [c]	can, 6 oz	30 mg/4 fl oz	44 [d]	47 [d]
Lemonade drink	can, 46 oz	30 mg/8 fl oz	76	78
Low-calorie drink powders				
vanilla	can, 8 oz	100 mg/qt	148	188
chocolate	can, 8 oz	100 mg/qt	140	180
Milk products				
liquid formula	can, 13 oz	50 mg/can	54	56
liquid formula	can, 13 oz	50 mg/can	99	—
evaporated milk	can, 13 oz		94	—
dry formula	can/g gas	60 mg/112 g	57	63
dry formula	can/g vacuum	60 mg/112 g	63	79
dry milk, whole	can, air	100 mg/lb	136	200
dry milk, whole	can, air	100 mg/lb	157	188
dry milk, whole	can, gas	100 mg/lb	184	200
Orange drink	can, 46 oz	30 mg/8 fl oz	47	50
Orange drink	can, 12 oz	30 mg/6 fl oz	33	39
Orange drink	can, 12 oz	60 mg/12 fl oz	67	88
Orange drink	glass, 1 qt	15 mg/4 fl oz	28	28
Orange drink	glass, 1 qt	30 mg/8 fl oz	53	56
Orange drink	glass, 1 qt	30 mg/8 fl oz	40	44
Orange drink	can, 46 oz	30 mg/8 fl oz	37	44
Orange drink	glass, 0.5 gal	30 mg/10 fl oz	79	82

Continued

Storage, 70–75°F (23°C)

6 Months		12 Months	
Ascorbic Acid	Vitamin C	Ascorbic Acid	Vitamin C
139 (100)	—	166 (85)	—
144	121 (99)	106	119 (97)
71 (95)	—	71 (95)	—
16.8	17.9 (98)	15.5	16.6 (91)
62	68 (100)	61	66 (97)
—	—	30 (100)	—
—	—	30 (100)	—
12^d	14^d (100)	11^d	12^d (86)
31	34 (100)	18	31 (94)
33	39 (81)	—	—
37	39 (85)	26	32 (70)
35	41 (100)	24	26 (65)
23	27 (80)	—	—
28	31 (76)	—	—
—	—	51	52 (73)
48	51 (88)	46	48 (83)
56	61 (90)	53	57 (83)
50 (88)	—	49	49 (86)
68	69 (90)	60	63 (83)
43^d	48^d (100)	—	—
69	77 (99)	60	67 (86)
141	168 (90)	100	121 (64)
136	160 (90)	129	143 (80)
27	34 (60)	—	—
49 (50)	—	49 (50)	—
62 (64)	—	—	—
—	—	58	61 (97)
—	—	63	76 (96)
147	195 (98)	138	168 (84)
115	158 (84)	133	122 (65)
184	189 (95)	188	186 (93)
37	41 (82)	—	—
27	30 (77)	—	—
62	81 (92)	—	—
25	27 (99)	16	23 (82)
50	54 (96)	32	46 (82)
36	40 (91)	31	33 (75)
31	37 (84)	27	34 (77)
71	73 (89)	66	68 (83)

Continued on next page.

Table XII.

After Processing

Product	Packaging	Goal	Ascorbic Acid	Vitamin C [a]
Orange drink C [c]	can, 6 oz	30 mg/4 fl oz	53 [d]	57 [d]
Orange drink C [c]	can, 6 oz	30 mg/4 fl oz	68 [d]	71 [d]
Orange drink C [c]	can, 6 oz	30 mg/8 fl oz	39 [d]	51 [d]
Pineapple juice	can, 11 oz	30 mg/4 fl oz	47	48
Pineapple juice	can, 18 oz	30 mg/4 fl oz	44	44
Pineapple juice	can, 46 oz	30 mg/4 fl oz	43	47
Pineapple juice	can, 46 oz	30 mg/4 fl oz	39	39
Pineapple juice		30 mg/4 fl oz	69	—
Pineapple juice C [c]	can, 6 oz	30 mg/4 fl oz	79 [d]	88 [d]
Pineapple grapefruit	can, 12 oz	30 mg/6 fl oz	40	42
Pineapple grapefruit	can, 46 oz	30 mg/6 fl oz	59	60
Pineapple grapefruit	can, 46 oz	30 mg/8 fl oz	39	40
Pineapple orange	can, 46 oz	30 mg/8 fl oz	36	37
Pineapple orange	can, 46 oz	30 mg/6 fl oz	43	45
Pineapple orange	can, 12 oz	30 mg/6 fl oz	42	49
Potato flakes	can	60 mg/3 oz	48	59
Potato flakes	can, air	60 mg/100 g	51	65
Potato flakes	can, gas	60 mg/100 g	70	79
Soybean products				
liquid formula	can, 13 oz	50 mg/can	45	—
dry powder	can, 1 lb	60 mg/4 oz	62	62
Tomato juice	can, 18 oz	30 mg/100 mL	52	54
Tomato juice	can, 46 oz	30 mg/100 mL	39	—
Tomato juice	can, 18 oz	30 mg/4 fl oz	40	41
Tomato juice	can, 46 oz	30 mg/4 fl oz	41	44
Tomato juice	glass jar	30 mg/6 fl oz	55	59
Tomato juice	can, 46 oz	30 mg/6 fl oz	72	75
Vegetable juice	can, 46 oz	30 mg/6 fl oz	53	58
Vegetable juice	can, 6 oz	30 mg/4 fl oz	36	42
Vegetable juice	glass jar	30 mg/4 fl oz	45	—

[a] Vitamin C equals ascorbic acid plus dehydroascorbic acid.
[b] Values in parentheses are percent retention during storage.
[c] Concentrate.
[d] 0°F.

Source: Reproduced, with permission, from Ref. *312*. Copyright 1970, Academic Press, Incorporated.

Continued

Storage, 70–75°F (23°C)

6 Months		12 Months	
Ascorbic Acid	Vitamin C	Ascorbic Acid	Vitamin C
55[d]	57[d] (100)	—	—
62[d]	66[d] (94)	61[d]	65[d] (91)
40[d]	47[d] (92)	41[d]	46[d] (90)
43	43 (90)	38 (81)	—
38	45 (100)	35	36 (82)
42	42 (89)	35	35 (74)
36	36 (92)	—	—
63 (91)	—	55 (80)	—
78[d]	82[d] (93)	—	—
35	39 (93)	—	—
50	54 (90)	38	46 (92)
36	38 (95)	—	—
32	32 (82)	—	—
38	41 (91)	—	—
36	41 (84)	—	—
30	43 (73)	—	—
40	60 (92)	—	—
68	71 (90)	—	—
47 (100)	—	43 (95)	—
49	60 (97)	48	61 (98)
45	45 (83)	44	44 (81)
35 (90)	—	27 (70)	30
37 (93)	—	34	37 (93)
41	50 (100)	32	35 (80)
51	56 (95)	39	47 (80)
57	63 (84)	45	48 (64)
40	43 (74)	32	38 (66)
32	34 (81)	29	29 (69)
42 (93)	—	41 (91)	—

foods because of dentition problems. Fruit purees such as apple sauce (361) have been overlooked products. Liked by the elderly as a breakfast fruit, as a dinner dessert, as a topping for ice cream, these would be one way of getting more ascorbic acid to the elderly if they were nutrified. Ascorbic acid (Table XII) can feasibly and economically be added to apple sauce. Cancel et al. (362) reported favorable retention of L-ascorbic acid added to citron slices packed in syrup and to citron bars.

ACID-FERMENTED PRODUCTS. Acid fermentation is a very ancient art of preserving and storing foods such as cabbage and pickles while retaining their nutritive value. Although cabbage has been known for centuries as a valuable antiscorbutic vegetable, sauerkraut manufacturing, packaging, and storage can affect ascorbic acid levels. During active acid fermentation, there is little loss, but in tank storage and the canning process losses of vitamin C can occur. In a study of 217 samples of canned kraut, variations of 1–25 mg/100 g were found. The canned product could be modified to contain a given amount of added ascorbic acid, producing a more uniform product (363).

POTATO PRODUCTS. In some countries, potatoes contribute an appreciable proportion of the daily L-ascorbic acid needs. During the last decade and foreshadowing the trend in the decade ahead, more of the annual potato crop is being converted to processed potato products, particularly in the developed countries. Average ascorbic acid values for varieties of potatoes that are commercially important range from about 10 to 33 mg per 100 g of the freshly dug tubers, with an overall value of 26 mg. Losses during storage approximate one-fourth of the ascorbic acid content after 1 month, one-half after 3 months and three-fourths after 9 months (364). A further degradation of about 40% occurs during washing and cooking, a loss that may increase if the cooked product is held on steamtables before serving. For french fries, a loss of 65% ascorbic acid has been observed (365). An ever-increasing percentage of the potato crop is processed into products such as dehydrated potato flakes, granules, chips or crisps, and frozen sticks. Dehydration of potatoes to flakes, granules, or slices induces losses of 30–89% of the natural ascorbic acid content (365–373). Interest continues in the L-ascorbic acid content of the potato and potato products (365–377) with attention given to assay methods that specifically measure ascorbic acid in processed potato products (365).

Concern has been shown for the restoration of L-ascorbic acid losses in potato products or its addition for product improvement (317, 366, 367, 371, 372, 373, 378). Restoration may not be a simple process, depending on the specific product. Mechanical mixing of the potato product, granules, or flakes with crystalline L-ascorbic acid will not yield a uniform product, and mechanical mixing breaks down the potato particle.

Powdered ascorbic acid suspended in an antioxidant-treated, saturated vegetable oil may be sprayed on the dried flakes, if the physical appearance of the nutrified product is not influenced. With potato chips, ascorbic acid can be added in a salt premix. Addition of ascorbic acid to the liquid potato mash may be practical if significant recycling of the heated product through the drying process is not excessive. In one study (367), ascorbic acid has been added to cooked potato mash, which was then drum-dried into flakes, packaged into cans, and sealed in air or nitrogen gas. Storage retention values in the product after 7 months at 70°F approximated 75% for air-packed containers and 90% for the nitrogen-packed. In another study (372), extrusion variables in the manufacturing of potato flakes were noted to significantly alter the ascorbic acid level of the extruded product (Table XIII).

Klaeui (317) indicates some success has been attained if sulfur dioxide at levels within legal limits and a small amount of sodium pyrophosphate acting as a sequestrant are added with ascorbic acid to potato

Table XIII. Percent Vitamin C Retention in Potato Flakes as Influenced by Extrusion Variables in Their Production

Extrusion Temperature (°C)	RPM	1/1 Screw		3/1 Screw	
		Small Die	Large Die	Small Die	Large Die
135	40	94.3	96.5	90.2	91.5
	80	90.1	95.1	84.7	90.2
	120	85.2	91.9	80.5	85.8
	160	81.9	86.8	80.1	82.8
	200	80.7	82.9	76.1	79.4
149	40	90.4	92.4	87.2	90.5
	80	82.5	91.0	80.1	86.2
	120	80.6	87.3	75.2	83.3
	160	77.1	82.5	70.7	74.0
	200	76.5	80.6	64.2	70.1
163	40	88.9	91.1	83.1	87.2
	80	83.5	88.2	80.8	83.3
	120	77.6	80.3	75.2	76.2
	160	70.2	75.6	68.3	72.4
	200	63.5	72.1	60.2	67.9
177	40	87.2	90.2	83.0	85.0
	80	81.5	89.4	77.2	80.8
	120	67.4	73.2	65.1	68.9
	160	50.7	60.0	48.3	52.4
	200	46.2	53.7	42.6	44.5

Source: Reproduced, with permission, from Ref. *372*. Copyright, 1978, Forster-Verlag AG.

mash, to aid in good ascorbic acid retention and uniformity of color. Using sodium ascorbate (400 $\mu g/g$) and ascorbyl palmitate (300 $\mu g/g$) in place of ascorbic acid provided antioxidant value and improved texture during the reconstitution of the dry product in addition to improved vitamin value. If nitrogen packing is not used to delay deterioration in dry potato products during packaging and storage, antioxidants may be incorporated to retard oxidative rancidity. Moisture content of the product should be kept as low as is technically feasible (preferably less than 6–8%).

CEREAL-GRAIN PRODUCTS. Cereal grain products contribute immeasurably to the human dietary state (379, 380) around the world. However, baked goods such as bread, buns, and rolls are not good carriers for added ascorbic acid when the expectancy of a specific nutritional claim is to be made. Ascorbic acid functions as a wheat flour improver, decomposing to a large extent in its improving action during the baking process; therefore little remains to meet a claimed ascorbic acid value in the baked product. If situations develop whereby it is desirable to have ascorbic acid in a baked item, it should be a product of the fast heat type such as donuts (381) or a cake or cookie formulation where added ascorbic acid is put in a cream filling or in an icing (382). Stable derivatives (383, 384) of ascorbic acid that will survive the baking process are known but have not been demonstrated as biologically available to humans.

A blend of corn, soy, and milk in a dry meal nutrified with mineral and vitamins, termed CSM, has been designed as a nutritious food for human consumption. One of the added vitamins is L-ascorbic acid. Vojnovich and Pfeifer (385) conducted some trials with ascorbic acid nutrified CSM and precooked dry infant cereals. Stability data revealed that destruction of the added ascorbic acid was a first-order reaction and that moisture content was a critical issue in ascorbic acid retention (Figure 8). Not more than 9% moisture was shown to provide good storage retention values. Ethyl cellulose coated ascorbic acid was preferred over regular crystalline ascorbic acid in this cereal product application. Linko (386) noted stability of ascorbic acid added to Finnish dry rolled oats was excellent during storage (88–96%) and during cooking (92%, 5 min boil in water). In the U.S., vitamins have been added to dry breakfast cereals (387, 388, 389) for some time, and technologies for adding them have been developed. The effects of processing and storage of cereals with added micronutrients, including L-ascorbic acid, were investigated by Anderson et al. (390), and a slight loss at 40°C was experienced for ascorbic acid in some cereals but not in others. The low moisture content of this class of products and use of moisture resistant packaging make them a good carrier. Klaeui (314) conducted

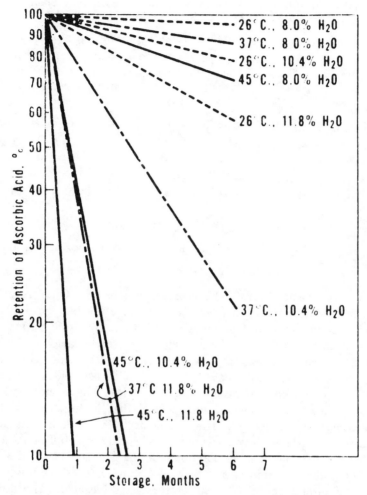

Figure 8.   Storage of CSM containing brand a: effect of moisture content and temperature on retention of ascorbic acid. (Reproduced, with permission, from Ref. 385. Copyright 1970, American Association of Cereal Chemists, Incorporated.)

a study including ascorbic acid, sodium ascorbate, and ascorbyl palmitate in various mixtures that illustrates the significant influence of the type of carrier on stability performances (Table XIV). Gage (*391*) has examined snack foods including those that may be suitable for nutrification with ascorbic acid.

IRON UTILIZATION. Iron deficiency, a major cause of anemia in humans, is a world-wide problem (*392, 393, 394*) and the search for

Table XIV. Stability of Various Vitamin C Forms in Some Edible Carriers (After 1 Year Storage in Closed Bottles)

Vitamin C-Retention in Percent of Initial Value

Vitamin Added	Temperature	Wheat Starch	Wheat Flour	Skimmed Milk Powder	Glucose Mono-hydrate	Glucose Anhy-drous
Ascorbic	RT	97.8	71.2	70.7	76.8	97.2
acid	45°C	83.7	68.5	70.2	74.2	75.8
Sodium	RT	97.5	70.4	81.3	84.5	94.8
ascorbate	45°C	81.4	70.2	72.1	74.5	74.2
Ascorbyl	RT	95.8	69.3	86.0	90.1	85.9
palmitate	45°C	85.4	43.4	81.8	55.3	80.4
Water content of carrier material		12.0%	12.5%	3.5%	9.1%	0.1%

Source: Reproduced, with permission, from Ref. *314*. Copyright 1974, Applied Science Publishers Limited.

effective supplements (*392, 394*) is a never ending one. One prevailing approach gaining momentum (*392*) is to improve the biological availability of existing dietary iron supplies or added iron by also incorporating some facilitating substance in the diet such as L-ascorbic acid (*395–404*). Cereal grain meals (*395, 398*), soy bean meal (*395*), salt (*396, 397*), sugar (*399, 407, 408*), MSG, coffee, tea, and milk (*401–404*) are some potential food carriers. In instances, both an iron source and ascorbic acid are added. Some investigators believe that in high cereal diets ascorbic acid may be needed. The enhancing by ascorbic acid is dose-dependent. As little as 25 mg, as a meal intake, may be significant (*400*), but intakes of 100 mg or more daily may be the goal sought. Coffee has been proposed as an iron carrier (*405, 406*) and Lee (*409*) raises the prospect of instant coffee as a carrier for L-ascorbic acid. The use of sodium ascorbate would prevent curdling of added cream or coffee whitener. Beverages nutrified with added ascorbic acid and containing iron are claimed to be stabilized by the addition of cysteine according to Morse and Hammes (*410*).

INFANT MILKS. The effect of preparation, technology, and storage conditions of ascorbic acid nutrified evaporated milk infant formulations has been studied by several investigators (*411, 412, 413*) and in the past has been reviewed by others. It is economically and nutritionally sound to nutrify evaporated milk with 50–100 mg of ascorbic acid per 13 fl oz (384.5 mL), for future reconstitution to a quart or liter, in vacuum-sealed containers according to Pennsylvania State University researchers. The sodium salt is preferred to avoid a potential destabilization effect on the milk proteins during the sterilization process. When 50 and 100 mg was added, 35 and 71 mg of ascorbic acid per liter, respectively, were present on a reconstituted basis after processing and 12 months' storage at room temperature (25°C). In the U.S. evaporated milk-base infant foods are marketed containing 50 mg of added ascorbic acid per 13-fl-oz can, which is diluted to a quart before consumption. Some dry-formulated infant foods are likewise fortified with ascorbic acid. Dry, low-calorie diet foods intended for the older adult market also contain added ascorbic acid; these products are to be reconstituted in water or milk before use. Many cereals and milk powders for infants are routinely nutrified with one of the various acceptable forms of iron. The bioavailability of such iron is strikingly improved when ascorbic acid is also present (414). A ratio by weight of at least 1:5 iron to ascorbic acid is recommended.

Head and Hansen (415) added L-ascorbic acid (42.3 mg/L) to whole, chocolate, and low fat (1%) fluid milks to increase the ascorbic acid intake of school children. Three milk treatments were examined (C) pasteurized milk, (E) pasteurization (74°C for 16 s) after ascorbic acid addition, and (F) ascorbic acid addition after pasteurization. Storage (4°C) retention of ascorbic acid (Figure 9) was good, and the taste reactions of children were favorable. Previously Weinstein et al. (416) and Anderson et al. (417) had reported on ascorbic acid nutrified fluid milk to which ascorbic acid was added at 50 and 200 mg/L, respectively. Infant milks nutrified with ascorbic acid were investigated by Cameron (418) during the preparatory procedures prior to infant feeding.

Use as a Processing Aid. In addition to serving as an added nutrient in food, L-ascorbic acid has the unusual property, because of its structure and chemical nature, to act as a processing aid for certain foods or food ingredients. In this role it is added for an intended purpose, usually foregoing nutritional considerations since much of the added ascorbic acid undergoes degradation to protect the quality of the food product. Only small amounts in some applications may remain of unreacted ascorbic acid. Examples of its improving agent role are: an oxygen scavenging agent in bottled and canned food products; an inhibitor of oxidative rancidity in frozen fish; a stabilizer of color and flavor in cured meats; a maturing agent for flour; an oxygen acceptor in beer production; and a reducing agent in wine.

FRUIT AND VEGETABLES. Fruits can be divided into two classes: those that show discoloration on cutting or injury, such as the apple, apricot, banana, cherry, nectarine, peach, and pear; and others that do not, such as citrus fruit. For this type of discoloration or browning to occur in cut fruit, three components—substrate, oxygen, and enzymes— are brought together. If one of the three is removed or prevented from reacting, browning does not take place. Heating would destroy the

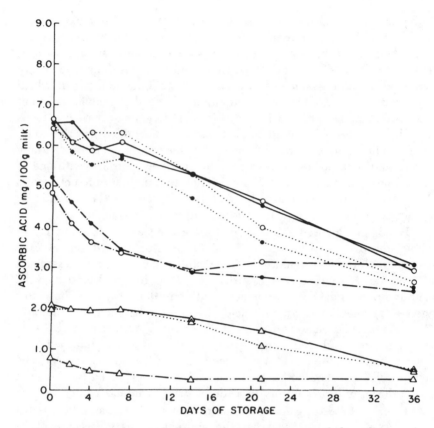

Figure 9. Ascorbic acid changes during storage of whole milk (——), chocolate-flavored whole milk (· – · –), and 1% fat milk (· · ·) with three treatments (△, C; ○, E; ●, F). (Reproduced, with permission, from Ref. 415. Copyright 1979, American Dairy Science Association.)

enzyme but would result in a cooked fruit flavor and a texture change. Fruit tissues that discolor have a combination of low concentration of ascorbic acid and highly active phenolases, acting on orthophenolic substrates to form the colored or the quinone compounds. L-Ascorbic acid inhibits the phenolase action or the enzymatic browning sequence by reducing orthoquinone products of the enzyme reaction back to the respective orthophenols. If the ascorbic acid content becomes exhausted, browning again commences. Use of ascorbic acid in this application has been previously reviewed (*311, 312, 321, 323, 332, 419*).

Selected graded fruit is peeled and sliced or diced, **and sugar is** added either as sugar syrup containing ascorbic acid or dry sugar previously blended with crystalline ascorbic acid, after which the fruit is compactly packaged, quickly frozen, and held in a frozen state until thawed by the consumer. The addition of 300–500 mg of L-ascorbic acid per kg of fruit sugar pack is adequate for the protection of the pack during processing, storage, and thawing. While a high percentage of ascorbic acid is converted to the reversible oxidation product, dehydroascorbic acid (*420*), during the thawing of the fruit (Table XV), the latter is fully biologically active (*915*) and is also considered as vitamin C. Since fresh apple tissue contains extracellular oxygen, slices must be cut thinly (6 mm) or a vacuum syrup step must be used on conventional slices to get ascorbic acid penetration (*421*). Certain additives with ascorbic acid such as NaCl (*421*), cysteine (*422*), sulfur dioxide (*423*), and citric acid (*424*) have been declared to have some merit. In a study of sliced apple treatment before freezing, Ponting and Jackson (*425*) favored soaking slices in a 20–30% sugar solution containing 0.2–1% ascorbic acid, 0.2–4% calcium, and 0.02% sulfur dioxide, following by rapid freezing.

The ascorbic acid treatment process has been used for holding cut fruit at refrigerated temperatures (*426, 427, 428, 432, 434*), for fruit to be frozen (*426, 429, 430*), and in some instances to reverse initial browning of cut fruit (*431*). Heaton et al. (*427*) reported sliced peaches treated with ascorbic acid (0.15%) and sodium benzoate (0.066% for microbial control) to hold up well stored for 12 months at 0°C. Eid and Holfelder (*432*) immersed (20 s) peeled, cored apples in ascorbic acid solutions (5–15%) and stored (9 d) them at cool temperatures (4–6°C) packaged in polyethylene bags, with some variation in performance based on apple variety. The ascorbic acid dipping approach has also been used (*433*) prior to drying apple slices. Other reports dealing with ascorbic acid application involve pineapples (*434*), avocado puree (*435*), pears (*436*), strawberries (*437*), and apricot juice (*438*).

Table XV. **Vitamin C Content of Thawed Frozen Sliced Peaches Packed with Sugar Syrup**[a]

Pack Number	Percent Sugar in Syrup	Added Ascorbic Acid	Assayed Immediately After Thawing		Assayed After Holding 24 Hours at 22°C (72°F) Thawed	
			Ascorbic Acid Content	Total Vitamin C Content	Ascorbic Acid Content	Total Vitamin C Content
1	65	0	9	11	2	9
2	65	150	140	146	76	154
3	65	200	178	188	88	190
4	35	0	4	7	1	11
5	35	150	36	141	79	156

[a] Hale Haven, yellow-fleshed, freestone sliced peaches (3 parts) packed in sugar syrup (1 part by weight).

In heat processing, the oxidases (ascorbic acid oxidase, polyphenol oxidase, peroxidase) naturally present in the product are destroyed, either during the blanching stage or finally during sterilization of the sealed containers. Color and flavor changes of fruits and vegetables during heat processing and storage, in part, result from oxidation by oxygen within the product and headspace. The addition of ascorbic acid helps to protect aromatic components and phenolic substrates from undergoing flavor and color changes. Combined with deaerating, filling, and scaling techniques, ascorbic acid addition efficiently helps to create and maintain an anaerobic atmosphere within the container. In the past this general subject has been reviewed (311, 319, 323, 419, 439) as it involves heat processed fruits and vegetables. As an example of one of the earlier trials (440), added ascorbic acid appreciably improved the appearance and flavor of home-canned sliced applies (Table XVI). In a subsequent study by Hope (441) the addition of ascorbic acid (500–600 mg/kg of fruit) to apple halves (canned without deaeration, the headspace containing 10–12 volumes percent oxygen) controlled browning, reduced headspace oxygen, protected the container from corrosion, protected flavor, and increased the residual ascorbic acid content.

A light colored pear juice was prepared by the use of ascorbic acid to retard browning while the pulp or juice was heated to inactivate the polyphenol oxidase (442). Birch et al. (319) have examined flavor changes during fruit juice processing both from a mechanism concept and from practical finding. They conclude that ascorbic acid addition and deoxygenation prior to pasteurization helps to reduce "processed flavor." The amount of ascorbic acid required to eliminate flavor change

Table XVI. Effect of Added Ascorbic Acid on
Canned Sliced Apples[a]

| Pack Number | Added Ascorbic Acid[b] | After Canning | | After 6 Months' Storage at 24°C (75°F) | | Appearance of Pack |
		Ascorbic Acid	Total Vitamin C	Ascorbic Acid	Total Vitamin C	
				mg/pt Jar		
1	0	0.1	3	—	5	dark throughout
2	67	15	18	5	15	slightly dark
3	135	57	59	22	33	normal
4	200	118	118	74	82	normal

[a] McIntosh apples peeled and sliced, cooked 3 to 4 min to soften, hot-packed with 50% syrup in Ball Ideal pint jars, 5/16-in. headspace, processed 10 min in boiling water.
[b] Ascorbic acid added in aqueous solution before sealing jar.
Source: Reproduced, with permission, from Ref. 440. Copyright 1947, Ogden Publishing Company.

is proportional to the glucose concentration. These workers find that grapefruit, lemon, and orange juice appear to contain sufficient ascorbic acid to exert the necessary protective effect. Apple, pineapple, and tomato juice may require ascorbic acid addition. Added ascorbic acid may also improve juice color, but this depends on the product and processing methods studied (*443–448*). Based upon practical experience and supported by theory, a sufficient level of ascorbic acid must be present, if the product is subject to oxidative deterioration, to survive processing, storage, and home preparation for consumption as an aid to maintenance of product characteristics. Even with oxygen exhaustion, subsequent loss of ascorbic acid may occur due to anaerobic decomposition (*449*). Ascorbic acid will not prevent the non-oxidative type browning (sugars and nitrogeneous compounds) and may even promote this type of reaction. In any new commercial production venture, pilot-scale studies (Table XII) are advisable to determine results based on the specific project detail to be encountered. As in fruit juices and canned fruit, similar beneficial effects can result when ascorbic acid is used as a processing aid for certain vegetables, for example, olives in brine (*450*), sauerkraut in brine (*311*), pickled cauliflower (*456*), canned (*457*) or glass-packed (*451*) and freeze dried (*452*) carrots, mushrooms (*453, 454, 455*), horseradish powder (*458*), and coleslaw (*459*).

FISH. Fish fillets, steaks, and some shellfish having a fatty component undergoing oxidative rancidity in frozen storage may benefit from ascorbic acid application (*311, 312*). Tarr and coworkers (*460, 461*) were the early investigative team that researched this subject. Ascorbic acid (0.5–3.0%) may be applied by either a dipping or a spraying technique. To ensure an even and a sufficiently thick coating, thickening agents may be added to the solution. The frozen storage shelf life of the fish may be extended several months by the ascorbic acid treatment. As an example, newly caught herring were filleted, dipped in a solution of ascorbic acid (0.5%) with a thickening agent, packed in a waxed cardboard box, frozen (−40°C), and stored (−20°C). Samples were thawed monthly and evaluated (*462*). Untreated samples became rancid after 2 months of storage, whereas treated samples remained palatable for 11 months judged by taste panel (Figure 10) and TBA values (Figure 11).

Jadhav and Magar (*463*) applied an ascorbic acid glaze, which delayed the yellow discoloration and allied organoleptic changes, to frozen white pomfret, surmai, and mackerel fish. Use of phosphates in combination with ascorbate esters has been declared to improve the color and flavor of fish products (*464*). Shellfish (*465, 466, 467*) including prawns and breaded shrimp, have been ascorbic acid treated, the latter in combination with citric acid. Formation of dimethylnitrosamine in Alaskan pollack roe (*468*) was inhibited when ascorbic acid was in-

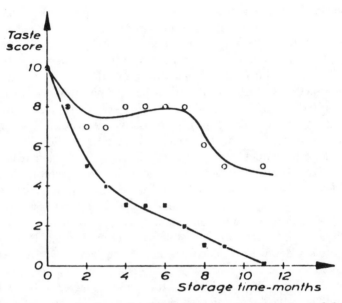

Figure 10. *Results from organoleptic evaluation of untreated herring samples (■) and samples treated with ascorbic acid (○) after different times of storage. (Reproduced, with permission, from Ref. 462. Copyright 1961, Institute of Food Technolgists.)*

cluded with a nitrite treatment. Alaskan pollack muscle treated with ascorbic acid was investigated by Yoshnaka et al. (*469*). Moledina et al. (*470*), working with mechanically deboned flounder meat, observed an improvement in color and flavor (Figure 12) when treated with a combination of ascorbic acid (0.5%), citric acid (0.5%), Na$_2$EDTA (0.2%) and phosphates (KENA, 0.2%). A number of papers (*468–474*) have recently discussed the processing of mullet including ascorbic acid application. The treatment appears more effective for fish in the round and in fillets then in minced tissue.

MEAT. For preservation purposes, meat has been cured with added salt (NaCl) and nitrates (saltpeter) since ancient times. With the recognition that nitrate was reduced by microbial action, about 60 years ago, added nitrite began to replace nitrate. The typical red color of cured meat results from the reaction of nitric oxide with myoglobin to form nitrogen monoxide myoglobin, more frequently referred to as nitrosomyoglobin, and with heat, nitrosomyochrome.

For nearly 30 years (*327, 475, 478*) it has been known that color fixation, flavor, and odor were greatly improved when ascorbic acid was included in the formulation of cooked, nitrited, ground pork products and that frankfurters containing ascorbate had a more desirable and

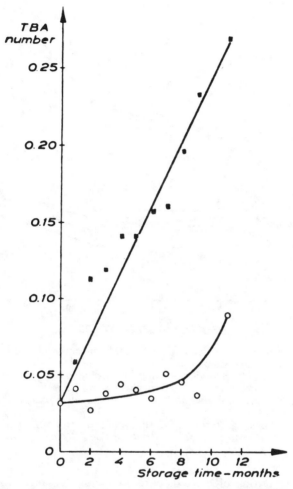

Figure 11.   TBA value as a function of time of storage in frozen herring, in untreated samples (■) and in the samples treated with ascorbic acid (○). (Reproduced, with permission, from Ref. 462. Copyright 1961, Institute of Food Technologists.)

uniform internal color and less tendency to fade under exposure to light than frankfurters without ascorbate. It was soon shown that ascorbate treatment hastens color development and, where desirable, lowers the amount of nitrite needed. More recently, greater interest in use of ascorbate, either alone or in combination with α-tocopherol, in meat curing has been exhibited as a nitrosation preventive. Reviews involving the ascorbic acid treatment of meat have appeared over a period of time (*311, 312, 321, 324, 326, 327, 479–486*).

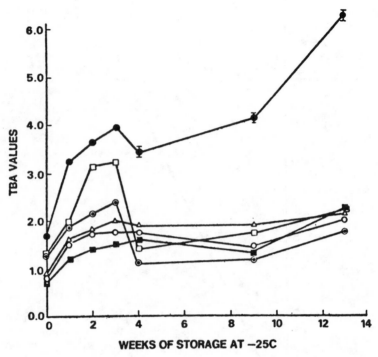

Figure 12.   Effect of ascorbic and citric acid concentration (added post-deboning) and frozen storage on TBA values of MDFM (Series III). Key: ●, *control;* □, *dip treatment only, no postdeboning additions (dip consists of 0.5% ascorbic acid, 0.5% citric acid, 0.2% KENA, 0.05% Na₂EDTA);* ■, *0.1% ascorbic acid, 0.1% citric acid + others;* ○, *0.3% ascorbic acid, 0.3% citric acid + others;* △, *0.5% ascorbic acid, 0.5% citric acid + others;* ◉, *Freez-Gard. (Reproduced, with permission, from Ref. 470. Copyright 1977, Institute of Food Technologists.)*

In the preparation of cooked, cured, comminuted meat food prod-ucts prepared from fresh meat and fat, 0.25 (7.1 g) to 0.33 oz (9.5 g) of nitrite is added per 100 pounds (45.5 kg) of meat. Legally in the U.S. either a maximum of 0.75 oz (21.3 g) of ascorbic acid or 0.88 oz (24.8 g) of sodium ascorbate per 100 pounds of meat can be used. Dissolved in cold water (25 mL water), it is added slowly near the end of the chop. Then the meat is stuffed, linked, and pasteurized in the smoke house. Hams and bacon are cured with a maximum level of 87.5 oz (2.48 kg) sodium ascorbate per 100 U.S. gallons (378.5 L) of pickling solution, pumping to a level of 10% meat weight prior to smoking. Nitrites and ascorbic acid ordinarily react quite vigorously with each other and should not be mixed together in water: either (*a*) introduce the curing salts early in the meat chop and add ascorbic acid alone or as part of the spice mix late in the meat chop, or (*b*) introduce the curing salts with sodium ascorbate dry or as a freshly prepared cool solution. Sodium ascorbate reacts much more slowly with nitrites than does ascorbic acid. The sodium salt is always used with nitrites in the curing pickle for pumping, injecting, or covering. Curing pickle containing sodium ascorbate and nitrites shows a higher rate of reaction at pH 5.2 as against 7.0. Sodium nitrite and sodium ascorbate curing salt mixtures (low moisture) are reasonably stable during dry, cool storage in moisture-resistant liners in closed drums.

Advantages cited in more recent reports with the ascorbate treatment include reduced curing time (480, 483, 485, 487, 488) better, more stable, and more uniform color (480, 482, 483, 485, 489–495), less nitrite required or lower nitrite levels (480, 482, 496–500), better flavor, and less rancidity. To emphasize the importance of the ascorbic acid application in lowering the residual nitrite levels in cured meat, the data of Brown et al. (497) may be examined (Table XVII). Other additives to accompany the ascorbic acid treatment of meat have been suggested. Borenstein and Smith (501, 502) reported the use of ethylenediaminetetraacetic acid (EDTA) or its salt (preferably Fe) in combination with ascorbate and with nitrite or nitric oxide to accelerate the formation of cured meat color. Other additives (503–506) cited with ascorbic acid were cysteine (505), glutamate (504), histidine (506), niacin, niacinamide (504, 505, 506), phosphates (503), and succinate (504).

Since one attribute of the use of nitrite in cured meats is its inhibition of the *C. botulinum* microorganism, concern developed whether added ascorbate would alter this action. From the various studies conducted (484, 507–511) it appears that added ascorbic acid (up to 1000 mg/kg) does not influence the antimicrobial action of nitrite against *C. botulinum*

Table XVII. Residual Nitrite Levels in the Semimembranous Muscle of Cured Ham as Influenced by Ascorbate and Days of Refrigerated Storage

Residual Nitrite (ppm) for Ascorbate Levels (Hams Pumped to 182 ppm Nitrite)

Days of Storage	0 ppm Ascorbate	227 ppm Ascorbate	455 ppm Ascorbate	568 ppm Ascorbate
0	49.7[b]	43.0[d]	18.0[h]	14.0[i,j]
2	49.7[b]	45.6[c]	19.7[g,h]	18.0[h]
5	58.7[a]	30.0[e]	21.0[g]	19.0[h]
8	32.0[e]	24.7[f]	15.7[i]	8.0[k]
16	12.3[j]	12.0[j]	8.3[k]	8.7[k]

[a,b,c,d,e,f,g,h,i,j,k] Means within the same row or column bearing different superscripts are different ($P < 0.05$).

Source: Reproduced, with permission, from Ref. 497. Copyright 1974, Institute of Food Technologists.

(Table XVIII). Baldini et al. (512) reported that the inhibitory power of nitrite against *C. sporogenes* was increased by the addition of ascorbic acid and salt.

The addition of ascorbic acid (200–2000 mg/kg) to fresh meat may improve the color of fresh meat (324, 475, 515, 517) as it aids in keeping myoglobin in the oxymyoglobin state while refrigerated, unwrapped or wrapped in oxygen-permeable transparent film. It also aids (475, 513, 514) in retarding rancidity. It does not significantly extend the shelf life of refrigerated fresh meat products (324, 514, 519). Harbers et al. (516) reported that bovine muscle dipped in ascorbic acid solutions (0.5–5.0%) then exposed to radiant energy retarded pigment and lipid oxidation and protected meat color. Improved flavor was found with ascorbate and polyphosphate treatment of fresh pork (518). Preslaughter intra-venous injection of sodium ascorbate (520–523) has been observed to inhibit metmyoglobin formation and to extend color appearances in the meat. A few studies have been conducted on stability improvement on poultry meat (524, 525). A study by Kilgore et al. (526) indicates that it is technically feasible to nutrify hamburger with added calcium, vitamin A, and L-ascorbic acid.

Nitrosated compounds have become of high interest since the dem-onstration of hepatoxicity of dimethylnitrosamine (527). Recognition of nitrosamines, a class of compounds (528–535) that might be associated with cured meat products, smoked fish products, tobacco products, cer-

Table XVIII. Effect of L-Ascorbic Acid on *Clostridium botulinum* in Vacuum Packed Bacon

Cure[a] Additive	Number of Days[b]	
	14	28
0 mg/kg ascorbic acid 0 mg/kg NaNO$_2$	9[c]	9
0 mg/kg ascorbic acid 100 mg/kg NaNO$_2$	0	1[d]
1000 mg/kg ascorbic acid 100 mg/kg NaNO$_2$	0	0
0 mg/kg ascorbic acid 200 mg/kg NaNO$_2$	0	0
1000 mg/kg ascorbic acid 200 mg/kg NaNO$_2$	1[d]	0

[a] Bacon contained an average of 4.4% salt on water phase (range 3.0–5.8%) and an initial level of 500 mg/kg sodium nitrate (pH of bacon 5.6–5.8).
[b] Stored at 25°C.
[c] Number of toxic packs out of 10 tested (5 inoculated with proteolytic and 5 with nonproteolytic strains of *C. botulinum*).
[d] Contained type B toxin (nonproteolytic inoculum).
Source: Reproduced, with permission, from Ref. 507. Copyright 1974, Centre for Agricultural Publishing and Documentation.

tain drugs and cosmetics, alcoholic beverages, and pesticides as carcinogens at low levels of intake in animals has accelerated scientific studies to learn of their significance in humans (536–540) and how they may be avoided by further technology. An ever widening examination is being made in the environment, industry, home products, and water supplies for the presence of nitrosamines to determine what is the degree of exposure to humans by ingestion, inhalation, dermal contact, and by in vivo formation. A review of amines in foods has been made by Maga (541) and of nitrosamines in foods by Scanlan (542). In addition to proprietary and ethical drug products (543, 544), cosmetics (545, 546, 547) are being examined to determine whether possible amine or amide ingredients represent a hazard.

Since nitrosamines, once formed, are quite stable compounds, the approach is not to consider therapeutic or treatment measures but to prevent their formation whenever possible. Nitrosated compounds result from chemical modification of amines (usually secondary and tertiary, but sometimes primary amines) or certain amides by contact with nitrites, nitrous acid, and possibly other nitrogen compounds. The nitrosating species is N_2O_3, which is formed by $2HNO_2 \rightarrow H_2O + N_2O_3$. To prevent the formation of the nitrosated compound a technology must be developed whereby the action of the nitrosating agent can be blocked by a more quickly reacting compound.

Two effective blocking agents are L-ascorbic acid (548–553) and α-tocopherol (554), both used singularly or combined (555, 556) in plant and animal tissues. Both possess biological activity as vitamin C and vitamin E, respectively, and both are produced in pure form by chemical synthesis in almost unlimited quantities and hence can be added to products as a prophylactic technology. Johnson (557) has recently reviewed the biological significance of these two antioxidant vitamins and a close interrelationship has been pointed up by Packer et al. (558). Ascorbic acid, while having no action on nitrosamines once formed, reacts strongly and preferentially with the nitrosating agents such as nitrite in aqueous solution, nullifying nitrosating action. It inhibits nitrosation by reaction with HNO_2 to form NO, thus inhibiting N_2O_3 production (548). In 1975 Kamm et al. (554) demonstrated α-tocopherol to be a useful agent for in vivo protection from nitrosamine formation and subsequent effects. α-Tocopherol in an emulsion form rapidly deactivates the nitrosating agent in lipophylic and hydrophobic environments. Under the latter conditions a combination prophylactic approach using α-tocopherol with either ascorbic acid or sodium ascorbate may be, a preferred approach (326, 546, 559). The prophylactic compounds must be present in the food or in the meal before and during the introduction of the troublesome amine or amide compound, not after the fact. Reviews on reactions (560) and technology (561) of nitrites in meat are available.

Bacon, a nitrite cured pork product highly preferred by the American public, has received more concern about its nitrosated compound content than other nitrite cured meats. Several workers (562, 563, 564) have tried ascorbic acid application in the processing of bacon to determine whether nitrosated compounds, typified by nitrosopyrrolidine, could be eliminated or reduced in concentration. Ascorbate levels of 0–2000 mg/kg have been tried, and nitrosopyrrolidine formation was inhibited or very significantly reduced at 1000 or more mg/kg in the fried bacon. Greenberg (565) describes a large commercial scale bacon processing test (20,000 lb test lots) using four bacon pickling formulations, the variables being two levels of sodium ascorbate (300 and 1000 mg/kg) with and without sodium tripolyphosphate (0.4%) followed by smoking and packing. Reduced nitrosopyrrolidine formation was found at the higher level of ascorbate treatment (Table XIX). Other reports (566–569, 917) attest to the effectiveness of added ascorbate in bacon or simulated model systems in inhibiting formation of nitrosated compounds and to its merits in associated product improvement.

Several ascorbic acid derivatives were examined by Pensabene et al. (570) for their ability to inhibit nitrosation of pyrrolidine in a model system developed to simulate the lipid–aqueous-protein composition of bacon. While sodium ascorbate was quite effective in the aqueous phase, a combination of an ascorbyl ester with sodium ascorbate gave a better effect in the lipid phase (Table XX). The use of ascorbates and tocopherol as inhibitors of nitrosamine formation and oxidation in foods of the aqueous and lipid type has been reviewed by Newmark and Mergens (326). These compounds in combination could be markedly useful in preventing food contamination with nitrosamines and/or nitrosamides in cured meats such as bacon.

Since nitrosamine formation can possibly occur in vivo after eating bacon cured with nitrite, as well as in vitro before consumption, it is

Table XIX.   U.S. Commercial Plant Bacon Study[a]

NPP[b] (in µg/kg) Assays of Fried Bacon
(170 mg/kg NO₂)

Added Ascorbate	With 0.4% TPP[c]		Without TPP	
	Fried by Packer	Fried by ARS	Fried by Packer	Fried by ARS
330 mg/kg	4	11	15	3
1000 mg/kg	3	0	3	0

[a] Analyses by USDA-ARS.
[b] Nitrosopyrrolidine precursors.
[c] Sodium tripolyphosphate.
Source: Reproduced, with permission, from Ref. 565. Copyright 1974, Centre for Agricultural Publishing and Documentation.

Table XX. Ascorbyl Monoesters as Inhibitors of the Nitrosation of Pyrrolidine in a Model System (570)

		Nitrosopyrrolidine[c,d]			
	Ascor-byl[b] Ester	Aqueous		Lipid	
Compound[a]	(ppm)	ppb	Percent Reduction	ppb	Percent Reduction
None	—	167	—	10.5	—
NaAsc (1000 ppm)	—	24.2	85.5	11.4	(+8.6)
NaAsc (500 ppm)	—	95.2	43.0	14.8	(+41.0)
NaAsc (500 ppm) +					
Asc palmitate	1046	63.5	62.0	5.4	48.6
Asc laurate	905	72.6	56.5	6.3	40.0
Asc oleate	1110	62.4	62.6	6.6	37.2
Ery palmitate	1046	56.3	66.3	6.8	35.2
Ery laurate	905	123	26.3	7.7	26.7
K_2 Asc-2-sulfate	880	50.4	69.8	5.8	44.8
Mg Asc-2-phosphate	731	82.4	50.7	9.5	9.5

[a] Plus pyrrolidine and $NaNO_2$.
[b] Equimolar with NaAsc, 2.52×10^{-4} mole.
[c] Confirmed by MS.
[d] All values are the average of three experiments.

desirable to have an adequate level of ascorbate present in the bacon as eaten to prevent the reaction of nitrite with proline in the intestinal tract. It was important to determine the stability (571) of sodium ascorbate added (0–2000 mg/kg) in bacon through the entire cycle of processing, storage, and preparation for eating (571). Retention of ascorbate in processing averaged 58%, 71%, 66%, and 83%, respectively, at the four levels of addition (overall average of 70%). Stability of ascorbate during storage in the freezer was good, with little or no difference between the intact vacuum packages and the opened packages. Residual sodium ascorbate levels after frying of the test bacons were determined after the various storage tests. The comparatively small losses of ascorbate during frying averaged 26% (Table XXI). Overall retentions after storage in the freezer for as long as 24 weeks followed by frying were about 30% of the 500 mg/kg level and increased with increasing levels of sodium ascorbate added to almost 50% of the 2000-mg/kg level. The stability of added α-tocopherol (0–1000 mg/kg) was also examined (572) in bacon processed with nitrite (125 mg/kg) and sodium ascorbate (550 mg/kg). After processing the average tocopherol recovery is 85%. After frying the overall recovery is edible portion (28%) and drippings (40%) approximated 70%. Refrigerator storage losses averaged 3% per week.

Inhibition of nitrosated products by ascorbates has also been reported in frankfurters. Fiddler et al. (573) observed that frankfurters formu-

Table XXI.   Retention of Sodium Ascorbate in
Bacon After Frying

Added Level of Sodium Ascorbate (µg/g)	Percent Retention After Frying (mean ± standard error)
500	67 ± 3.6
1000	73 ± 2.8
1500	81 ± 3.3
2000	75 ± 2.4

Source: Reproduced, with permission, from Ref. 571. Copyright 1974, Institute of Food Technologists.

lated with 550 or 5500 mg of ascorbate per kg did not develop nitrosamines as measured by dimethylnitrosamine formation, whereas as the control frankfurters did, when both were prepared with moderate thermal processing. Other investigators (574, 575, 576) have also reported on the effectiveness of ascorbates in reducing formation of nitrosamines in cured meat products. Walters (577) reviewed the role of ascorbic acid in nitrosamine formation in 1974.

FLOUR AND DOUGH IMPROVEMENT.   Thewlis (325), in his review of L-ascorbic acid in breadmaking, historically mentions that since the discovery by Jorgensen (578) in 1935 of the flour improving properties of L-ascorbic acid, it has become widely accepted as a flour additive in the EEC countries where in most cases, it is the only improver permitted. In the United Kingdom it is commonly used in conjunction with potassium bromate. In the U.S. Grain Marketing Research Center, Manhattan, Kansas, (579) where new flour samples are regularly monitored, the bread formulation includes ascorbic acid (80 mg/kg) and bromate (10 mg/kg) even though ascorbic acid is currently used to a limited extent in American breads. As of 1979, ascorbic acid is the only permitted flour improver in Austria, Belgium, Brazil, Denmark, Finland, France, Germany, Italy, Norway, Portugal, Spain, and Switzerland.

Flour improving agents, with the exception of ascorbic acid, are oxidizing agents. L-Ascorbic acid is the only one that is a component of natural food and that is also a dietary nutrient required by humans. In the most recent studies of Elkassabany et al. (580), practically all of the added ascorbic acid was converted to dehydroascorbic acid in optimally mixed flour–yeast–water blends during the dough mixing operation. Dehydroascorbic acid was observed to be relatively stable in flour–water doughs and extremely stable in flour–yeast–water doughs (Figure 13). Many investigators believe that the oxidation of ascorbic acid to dehydroascorbic acid or the rate of reaction does not solely determine the activity of ascorbic acid as an effective bread improver.

The precise mode of action of ascorbic acid as a dough improver continues to challenge cereal chemists. The early postulation of Maltha

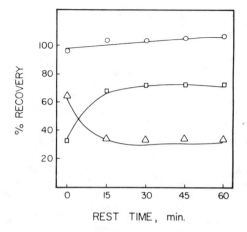

Figure 13. Effects of mixing (1 min) and rest time on ascorbic acid oxidation in yeasted doughs. Key: ○, total; □, dehydro-L-ascorbic acid; △, ascorbic acid. (Reproduced, with permission, from Ref. 580. Copyright 1980, American Association of Cereal Chemists, Incorporated.)

(581) proposed that ascorbic acid is converted, in the dough, in two consecutive steps. First, the ascorbic acid is slowly changed in the presences of oxygen or hydrogen acceptors into dehydroascorbic acid. In the second phase, the dehydroascorbic acid reacts rapidly with glutathione in its sulfhydryl state to form glutathione disulfide and ascorbic acid. The presence of glutathione in wheat flour and dough has been investigated by Grosch et al. (582). Flours from 11 varieties of wheat contained 0.27–0.72 μmol/g glutathione and 0.19–0.38 μmol/g oxidized glutathione. In dough, kneading for 5 min decreased the glutathione to the nondetectable range and oxidized glutathione increased. Addition of ascorbic acid accelerated the oxidation of glutathione. Glutathione dehydrogenase, present in wheat, is specific for glutathione as a hydrogen donor and reduces L-dehydroascorbic acid (583). In a 1979 study (584), GSH was rapidly oxidized to the sulfide during dough mixing, without a change in total glutathione content. The flour improvers, $KBrO_3$ and ascorbic acid, enhanced GSH oxidation. GSH oxidation by improvers may compete with an SH–SS interchange reaction of GSH with the gluten proteins. The extent and velocity of the SH–SS interchange depends on the flour variety. Thus Mair and Grosch (584) believe that the competition of the SH–SS interchange with the oxidation of GSH to GSSG is a valid explanation for ascorbic acid action (Figure 14).

Lillard et al. (585) do not find data on dough that suggest preferential oxidation of dehydroascorbic acid of glutathione or all combined sulfhydryl compounds to be very convincing. Using a spread-ratio test L-ascorbic acid retarded the flow of a nonyeasted dough soon after mixing

Action of Ascorbic Acid

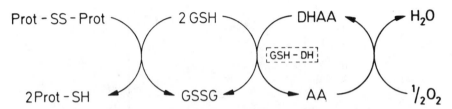

Figure 14.   Reactions of glutathione in dough in the presence of ascorbic acid. GSH-DH, glutathione dehydrogenase; Prot, protein. (Reproduced, with permission, from Ref. 584. Copyright 1979, Blackwell Scientific Publications Limited.)

and even more after a 60-min holding period. Other related chemical structures, not possessing good improver characteristics, increased dough flow out of the mixer and no retardation with time. Thus L-ascorbic acid's contribution to the first stage action is believed to be due to oxidation of thiol compounds in the water-soluble fraction of wheat flour. A suggested second stage action to explain how dehydroascorbic acid stops flow and makes the dough stronger needs further study. Ascorbic acid addition has been reported to have an insignificant effect (586) on the oxidation of linoleic acid in dough and in another report a short term protection effect (587) on the oxidation of unsaturated free fatty acids.

When ascorbic acid is the sole improving agent added to flour, it has no tendency to overoxidize or overtreat the flour proteins, which can be detrimental to loaf volume and texture. The level of added ascorbic acid necessarily depends on the flour quality and the type of breadmaking process. A range of 20–80 mg/kg is used in the bulk fermentation process, and 50–200 mg/kg in the continuous dough process. One has to clearly distinguish between continuous breadmaking processes and related processes where oxygen is mainly excluded and where added ascorbic acts as a reducing agent versus processes where oxygen is present as in the usual batch process where, in some fashion, added ascorbic acid functions as an oxidizing agent.

The practical advantages of added L-ascorbic acid in breadmaking are as follows: (a) enhanced bread texture and loaf volume; (b) greater elasticity and gas retention to the dough; (c) improved water absorption; (d) no danger of overimprovement or overtreatment; (e) reduced power, or minimal time, or lowered consistency in continuous dough making; and (f) storage period of unimproved flour eliminated (593). Freshly milled flour plus ascorbic acid can be used in place of time-matured flour (no improver added); hence, storage space is reduced. The ultimate fate of L-ascorbic acid (325) appears to be a mixture of carbon dioxide,

L-threonic acid, and 2,3-diketo-L-gulonic acid. No oxalic acid can be detected in bread.

L-Ascorbic acid as a flour improver has been reviewed (*321, 325, 588, 589, 590*) in the past. Papers involving discussions or studies of flour improvers, including ascorbic acid, are relatively numerous (*591–604*). Other publications (*584, 590, 605–611*) deal with mechanism of action. Some investigations deal with ascorbic acid in combination with other additives such as cysteine (*590, 611–617*) and bromate (*584, 613, 614, 618–625*). The combination of ascorbic acid and bromate or ascorbic acid and cysteine or ascorbic acid, bromate, and cysteine are favored by some researchers as each component is declared to function in a different manner or phase of the breadmaking cycle, giving a better overall result than each used singularly as flour improvers. High interest continues in the short-time or no-time breadmaking processes in which ascorbic acid with or without other additives has a functional role (*589, 590, 606, 612, 613, 614, 618, 621, 625–634*). The various short-time processes are based either on mechanical dough development, such as the Chorleywood, with high input of energy and the use of an oxidizing agent or on chemical dough development, such as the Delquik, with low input of energy and the combined use of oxidizing agent and reducing agent. The Chorleywood continuous breadmaking process, developed about 1961 and one of the first to specify ascorbic acid as an improver at a higher level than usual, has been a successful process and was a significant advance in breadmaking technology. It has been used successfully in England and other parts of Europe. Other short-time bread processes are the Brimec process, the formulation including ascorbic acid and potassium bromate, and the Delquik process involving ascorbic acid and cysteine (*590*).

Hoseney et al. (*635*) studied the salts of 6-acyl esters of L-ascorbic acid in the production of yeast-leavened baked products and noted them to have pronounced dough conditioning effects, namely doughs made up easier and antistaling and crumb softening properties were present. Ascorbyl palmitate can serve as a shortening replacer, a dough strengthener, and a crumb softener in commercially produced buns (*636*).

Abrol et al. (*637*), reporting on the darkening of whole wheat meal, due to the action of tyrosinase in bran, found added ascorbic acid (0.5–2.0 mg/kg) to retard the darkening effect. In another context, durum and other wheat granular flours (semolina) require retention of their natural yellow carotenoid content for the manufacture of pasta products which Dahle (*638*) and Walsh et al. (*639*) observed were stabilized by added L-ascorbic acid.

FATS AND OILS. Foods are complex structures of proteins, carbohydrates, fats, enzymes, vitamins and minerals. Fatty components or lipids are responsible in many foods for deteriorative changes during storage. These include phospholipids, lipoproteins, fatty acids, esters, fatty alcohols, and sterols. Fatty components occur in most food products in various amounts. Even minute amounts, if altered, may influence flavor quality during food storage. Deteriorative changes of fatty components may be caused by enzyme action, microbial growth, and/or oxygen, leading to oxidative and hydrolytic chemical action. If this action is not prevented or inhibited, valuable food products can become unpalatable to the consumer, causing serious economic loss to the producer. Antioxidants and synergists, substances that in minute quantities added to oxidizable foods, inhibit or suppress undesirable action of oxygen, exist in nature, and have been produced by chemical synthesis. Reviews (312, 316, 321, 329, 640) on the utility of ascorbic acid and ascorbic acid derivatives as antioxidants reveal the longtime recognition of their practical value and the interest in an understanding of their mechanism of action. For a fatty type food to be successfully stabilized, the antioxidant (and synergist) should be added before the initiation of oxidation. Compounds acting as antioxidants and also possessing some vitamin value (557) are α-tocopherol, γ-tocopherol, L-ascorbic acid, sodium ascorbate, and L-ascorbyl palmitate.

For antioxidant formulation for fats and oil products, the number of additives and the ratio of the additives depends in a large part on the food product to be treated. For example, one can examine the results of Pongracz (641) wherein ascorbyl palmitate and α-tocopherol were added singularly and combined to six different fats and oils, and the differences in response were noted. The combination antioxidant was most effective in animal fats, butter fat, and lard, and ascorbyl ascorbate was quite effective alone in vegetable and peanut oils, soybean, palm oil, and sunflower oil (Table XXII). The procedure for adding ascorbyl palmitate to an oil product is as follows: ascorbyl palmitate (20–50 g) is dissolved in heated (100°C) oil or fat (5 kg), and the resulting warm

Table XXII.   Stability of Various

| Antioxidants Added (µg/g) | Peroxide Value | |
	Peanut Oil (4 days)	Soybean Oil (4 days)
Control	58.1	> 400
500 AP[a]	31.2	26.1
200 α-TL[b]	61.4	> 400
500 AP + 100 α-TL	24.8	20.6
500 AP + 200 γ-TL	17.3	16.7

[a] Ascorbyl palmitate.
[b] Tocopherol.

liquid premix is then immediately added to the batch of oil or melted fat (95 kg) to be treated. Pongracz reported on a combination of ascorbyl palmitate, α-tocopherol (or γ-tocopherol), and lecithin as combination formulas with good antioxidant properties and as compositions widely approved for human consumption. Cort (642) has studied the anti-oxidant activity of L-ascorbic acid, L-ascorbyl palmitate, and the toco-pherols in some detail. Using the thin layer exposure technique she measured days to reach a level of peroxide formation. Tocopherol–ascorbyl palmitate combinations were very effective (Table XXIII) when applied to beef, chicken, and pork fat, giving results better than BHA and BHT. In another trial, Cort compared antioxidants in soybean oil and confirmed activity of ascorbyl palmitates when added to vege-table oil (Table XXIV). Not only is it effective alone, but offers extra stabilizing value when added to commonly considered antioxidants. An antioxidant combination of tocopherol, partially hydrolyzed gelatin, and ascorbic acid was reported by Kawashima et al. (643). Combinations of ascorbyl stearate and α-tocopherol have also been tried as an anti-oxidant combination (644).

When there is an appreciable aqueous phase in the food product it is advisable to consider ascorbic acid or sodium ascorbate and α- or γ-tocopherol in an emulsion form. The removal of traces of peroxide from food has been suggested (645) by the addition of ascorbic acid or sodium ascorbate during the cooking process. There are situations where powdered or fine crystalline ascorbic acid in a salt premix with an anti-oxidant such as tocopherol or BHA may be applied to oil cooked potato chips (646) as a method of maintaining freshness.

MILK PRODUCTS. "Cardboardy" or "metallic" or "tallowy" flavors resulting from oxidative changes in the cream fraction of cows' milk are distasteful in fluid milk and dairy products. These flavors develop more intensely in certain lots of fluid milk when the cows are fed dry rations.

Oils and Fats at 80°C

	Peroxide Value		
Palm Oil (*4 days*)	*Sunflower Oil* (*2 days*)	*Butterfat* (*3 days*)	*Lard* (*7 days*)
38.1	140	265	> 400
21.5	70.8	74.0	> 400
47.2	200	9.9	28.5
26.3	83.3	2.8	4.3
26.6	71.5	1.8	2.4

Source: Reproduced, with permission, from Ref. 641. Copyright 1973, Verlag Hans Huber.

Table XXIII. Comparative Antioxidant Activity[a]

Antioxidant	Concentration (%)	Chicken Fat	Pork Fat	Beef Fat
None		8	3	10
DL-α-Tocopherol	0.02	13	15	24
DL-α-Tocopherol	0.05	13	15	—
DL-α-Tocopherol	0.2	10	15	—
DL-α-Tocopherol	0.02	13	15	—
DL-α-Tocopherol	0.05	13	15	—
DL-α-Tocopherol	0.2	11	15	—
DL-γ-Tocopherol	0.02	29	37	40
DL-γ-Tocopherol	0.05	40	58	—
DL-γ-Tocopherol	0.2	46	61	—
Butylated hydroxyanisole	0.02	20	28	36
DL-α-Tocopherol Ascorbyl palmitate	0.02 each	28	28	38
DL-γ-Tocopherol Ascorbyl palmitate	0.02 each	53	67	70
Ascorbyl palmitate	0.02	10	9	12

Days to Reach 20 meq/kg PV[b] (column span header over Chicken Fat, Pork Fat, Beef Fat)

[a] Schaal oven, thin layer, 45°C.
[b] Peroxide value.
Source: Reproduced, with permission, from Ref. 642. Copyright 1974, American Oil Chemists Society.

The development is influenced, among other things, by oxygen content of the milk, oxidative enzyme activity, oxidation–reduction potential, exposure of the milk to light, presence of dissolved copper, tocopherol content, and ascorbic acid content of the milk. When milk is taken from the cow it contains little or no oxygen; however, when it comes in contact with the air it absorbs more oxygen. Freshly drawn cows' milk may contain as much as 30 mg of ascorbic acid in the reduced form per liter or per quart. Customary handling methods, pasteurization, and the long time interval necessary for shipment, storage, and delivery between milking and consumption can destroy 70–80% of the natural ascorbic acid originally present. Keeping milk deaerated and from light exposure delays flavor changes.

The practical use of added ascorbic acid has proved to be of benefit to the dairy industry (311, 321). The amounts of ascorbic acid or sodium ascorbate used vary between twenty and several hundred milligrams per liter, 30–50 mg usually being sufficient for fresh fluid milk. Discrepancies in the results of some workers attempting to elucidate the value of ascorbic acid in the development of off-flavor may be due to their examination of an incomplete system of oxidative reactions. It has been dem-

Table XXIV. Oxidation of Soybean Oil

Antioxidant	Days to Reach 72 meq/kg PV
None	7
0.01% AP	16
0.02% AP	19
0.05% AP	21
0.2% AP	25
0.02% BHA	9
0.02% BHT	10
0.02% TDPA	15
0.01% PG	20
0.02% PG	20
0.02% NDGA	21
0.02% TBHQ	26
0.02% Ascorbic Acid	12
0.2% Ascorbic Acid	17
0.01% AP + 0.01% PG	27
0.01% AP + 0.01% TDPA	21
0.01% AP + 0.01% BHA	18
0.01% AP + 0.01% BHT	17
0.01% AP + 0.01% NDGA	28
0.01% AP + 0.01% Tocopherol	16
AP at 0.05%, PG, TDPA at 0.01%	42
AP at 0.05%, BHA, TDPA at 0.01%	30
AP at 0.05%, BHA, PG at 0.01%	31
AP at 0.05%, BHT, TDPA at 0.01%	31

[a] Heated at 45°C.
[b] AP = ascorbyl palmitate, BHA = butylated hydroxyanisole, BHT = butylated hydroxytoluene, TDPA = thiodipropionic acid, PG = propyl gallate, NDGA = nordihydroguaiaretic acid, TBHQ = 2-*tert*-butylhydroquinone.
Source: Reproduced, with permission, from Ref. *642*. Copyright 1974, American Oil Chemists Society.

onstrated that the tocopherol content of milk also plays a role in the oxidative processes. Reports claim a synergistic effect of tocopherol and ascorbic acid to be beneficial in preventing oxidative off-flavor in dairy products. The α-tocopherol content of cows milk, as recently reviewed (*647*), varies with season and feeding practices, ranging from 4–30 $\mu g/g$ fat. Tocopherol is in the fat and removal of fat from milk obviously removes the tocopherol. Hence, both tocopherol and ascorbic acid should be considered equally important in milk and dairy product flavor stabilization. These observations confirm the data on butter reported in any earlier section.

Literature reports since the 1970 review (*312*) continue to show interest in stabilization of dairy products such as use of ascorbic acid and tocopherol in controlling oxidized flavor in sterilized cream (*648*).

Use of added ascorbic acid delayed flavor development in packaged milk concentrates (649), in milk fat (650), in goat milk curd (651), in butter from buffalo milk (652), in γ-irradiated skim-milk powder (653), in low-fat dairy spreads (654), and in khoa products (655). Experience in yogurt, cheese, and ice cream has been previously reviewed (311, 312).

BEER. For nearly 30 years added ascorbic acid has been recognized (312, 656, 657, 658) in beer processing as an oxygen scavenger, thus preventing changes in flavor and color, reducing chill and oxidation haze, and, thereby, extending shelf life. To achieve optimum stability in beer, dissolved and container headspace air should be kept as low as possible, and levels of trace metals should be kept as low as possible. It has been observed that the amount of ascorbic acid required to take up 1 mL of oxygen from bottled beer varies between 8 and 15 mg. The amount of added ascorbic acid found to be effective under most practical conditions is 20–40 mg/L, 2–4 g/hL, 2.4–4.8 g/barrel, or 0.54–1.08 lb/100 barrels. More may be helpful only when there is poor air control. Where brews have been previously treated with sulfites that have contributed to a special taste character, it is not necessary to remove all the sulfite when ascorbates are added since ascorbates are compatible with sulfite. Ascorbic acid may be added as a freshly prepared solution at any brewing stage after fermentation in room temperature water or beer [100 g per 1 (or more) L]. A proportioning device can be used to introduce the ascorbic acid solution while the beer is transferred during processing for uniform distribution without incorporation of air.

Reports continue in the 1970s on the ascorbic acid treatment of beer (658–669). Use of ascorbic acid with sulfites shows favorable results on beer quality as described by Scriban and Stienne (662) and Mastor et al. (669). Analyses of imported beer indicate addition of ascorbates even if not so labeled (665). Kormornicka (667) reported 3 g/hL addition of ascorbic acid extended beer quality 89 days; 5 g/hL, 108 days. Baetsle (666), on an industrial scale, found 2 g/hL preserved color and flavor of beer during storage for 66 days.

WINE. In 1948 Franzy (670) published his observations, in processing of grapes into sweet wines, on added L-ascorbic acid (100 mg/L) as a replacement compound for sulfurous acid in protecting the color of wine from oxidative changes and promoting fresh aroma. About a decade later ascorbic acid became quite widely understood to be a valuable processing aid in wine production: (a) to preserve taste and flavor; (b) to promote clarity by preventing ferric phosphate precipitation or by clarifying turbid wines; (c) to remove excess sulfur dioxides; and (d) to reduce the amount of required sulfurous acid when ascorbic sulfurous acid application is chosen in wine treatment. Today the use of ascorbic acid alone or combined with sulfurous acid treatment is legally permitted or tolerated in many countries. Reviews, wherein ascorbic acid application to wine are discussed, can be consulted for past publications on this subject (*312, 321, 671, 672, 673, 921*).

The quantity of L-ascorbic acid naturally present in grapes is relatively low and is mostly destroyed during fermentation. More frequently than not ascorbic acid and sulfurous acid (sulfur dioxide) are used together (*671, 674, 675–678*) since both compounds contribute unique advantages. Sulfur dioxide has antiseptic, fungicidal, antidiastase, and antioxidant properties. Ascorbic acid is a stronger reducing agent and potentiates the low reducing capacity of sulfur dioxide and, thereby, makes it possible to minimize the concentration of this necessary but headache-related sulfur additive (*673, 674*). A low value of the redox potential in wine is more favorable for full flavor development, and it would take a prolonged time to achieve this without ascorbic acid (*672*). In Swiss practice, it has been found that 50–100 mg/L of ascorbic acid in wine containing 15–20 mg SO_2/L, when added at the stage when the wine was ready for bottling, generally resulted in a fruitier bouquet and lighter color (*673*). Peynaud (*679*), in reporting on 3 years use of ascorbic acid in wine, suggests addition be made immediately before or after aeration or, best, just before bottling. Maximum addition allowed in France is 10 g/100 L; in Italy, 12 g/100 L.

More recent studies confirm the value of added ascorbic acid in wine for improvement of quality (*680–683*), in champagne production (*684*), in converting ordinary wine into sherry wine (*685*), in eliminating the need for heat sterilization of sulfur dioxide (*686*), and in the production of hot bottled Moselle wine (*687*). Reports on combined use of ascorbic acid and sulfur dioxide indicate its continued practical significance (*688–691*).

COLORS. The majority of the FDA certified food colors display instability (*692*) when brought into contact with reducing agents, hence these azo and triphenylmethane colorants may fade or become colorless by the reducing action of ascorbic acid (*692–695*). Decolorization of these coal tar dyes can occur in carbonated and still beverages in the presence of ascorbic acid (*696*) depending on: (*a*) the specific color's reaction to reducing agents; (*b*) the amount of ascorbic acid added; (*c*) the oxygen and dissolved metal content; and (*d*) the exposure of the bottled beverages to sunlight. Some control over this aspect can be exercised by reducing metal content with the use of ETDA and limited exposure of bottled products to light, such as with the use of cans or opaque containers (*692*). Another possibility to avoid color fading is the use of nonabsorbable, polymeric coal tar dyes as color additives since these are reported to be more stable to reducing agents (*697*) than the unbound dye.

Anthocyanins (*698, 699, 700*) are somewhat more stable to ascorbic acid, but beverages naturally colored with anthocyanins or with added anthocyanins should still be deaerated to bring oxygen levels to a minimum (701). Starr and Francis have investigated the influencing factors, oxygen (702) and trace minerals (703), on the anthocyanin–ascorbic acid interrelationship. The effect of heat, light, and storage conditions were observed by Segal and Dima (704) on five fruit juices with added ascorbic acid. Ikawa (705), in his investigation of the natural colors and the influence of antioxidants, reported that ascorbic acid (50–100 mg/ 100 g) stabilized betanine, and had no effect on canthaxanthin, cochineal, laccaic, and paprika. Other reports confirm the betanine observation (706, 707, 708).

The naturally occurring carotenoids, some of which are commercially available in pure form, are not only resistant to color fading but are stabilized by ascorbic acid (709, 710, 711). The added carotenoid food colors are stable when retorted with protein material and are stable when combined with reducing agents. Added β-carotene emulsions provide the orange juice color hue; β-apocarotenal, the deep orange color hue associated with orange beverages. By preliminary trials, the beverage manufacturer can choose an added color source, among the colors discussed and associated conditions, that will allow proper color hue and stability of L-ascorbic acid in the liquid product.

MISCELLANEOUS. Dried coffee extracts are stabilized if added ascorbic acid is incorporated during their processing (712, 713). Ascorbic acid has also been studied in the tea fermentation process (714). Confectionaries (715–721) can be a good vehicle for ascorbic acid, particularly, hard candy (311) because of the presence of fruit acids and low oxygen permeability. Also, ascorbic acid has been added successfully to caramels (312, 721), chocolates (312), marron glaces (715), and ice candies (716). A synthetic caviar has been developed and patented, the formulation of which calls for added ascorbic acid (722).

Patents have also been obtained on ascorbic acid as the active principle for the removal of chlorine from water, making the water palatable for drinking (723, 724, 725). The addition of ascorbic acid (1 g) and sodium bicarbonate (0.5 g) to chlorinated water (15 L) will result in a palatable water according to a U.S. patent (723). City tap water treated with chlorine–ammonia (726) was observed to cause hemolytic anemia in patients in dialysis units of a hospital. Confirmation of this condition was obtained in in vitro tests in which the suspected water damaged red blood cells. Ascorbic acid addition to the treated water reduced the anemia problem in the patients in subsequent time periods.

L-Ascorbic acid is not normally considered a bacteriostat, yet in aqueous solution at the higher concentrations used in the aqueous phase of ascorbic acid treated foods, it appears that it can confer some limited antimicrobial activity. Arafa and Chen (727), increased refrigerated shelf life of cut-up broiler parts previously dipped in ascorbic acid solution over water dipped controls without adverse effects in the consumed product. Svorcova (728), investigating ascorbic acid, potassium sorbate, and pH levels in carbonated beverages, noted some influence of ascorbic acid for control of nonspore-forming bacteria. Other instances have been cited for limited antimicrobial activity (729–732) of ascorbic acid.

Legal Aspects. The use of ascorbic acid as a nutrient or as a food processing aid is subject to government regulation in many countries. The status of ascorbic acid addition in each instance of desired use should be determined by consulting the pertinent regulations or pertinent governmental agency of the country.

THE UNITED STATES. Ascorbic acid is "generally regarded as safe," GRAS, for use in food as a nutrient or food processing aid provided that a standard has not been established by the Food and Drug Administration for the food wherein the use of ascorbic acid is excluded or permitted within the limitations specified by the standard.

Under GRAS conditions, the quantity added "does not exceed the amount reasonably required to accomplish its intended physical, nutritional, or other technical effect on food," and the quantity of ascorbic acid "becomes a component of food as a result of its use in the manufacturing, processing, or packaging of food, and which is not intended to accomplish any physical or other technical effect on the food itself, shall be reduced to the extent reasonably possible"; and the ascorbic acid "is of appropriate food grade and is prepared and handled as a food ingredient"; and the inclusion of ascorbic acid "in the list of nutrients does not constitute a finding on the part of the Department that 'ascorbic acid' is useful as a supplement to the diet for humans."

When a standard for a food product has been established wherein the use of ascorbic acid is permitted, the standard should be consulted to ensure that the labeling of the food product conforms with the labeling specifications of the standard.

In addition to the regulations established by the Food and Drug Administration, the United States Department of Agriculture has promulgated regulations pertaining to the use of ascorbic acid in meat processing and the Alcohol and Tobacco Tax Division of the United States Department of the Treasury has established a regulation pertaining to the use of ascorbic acid in wine. The standards established by these regulatory agencies as they exist are described in Tables XXV, XXVI, and XXVII. There are also Federal and Military Specifications in the United States for food procured by Federal agencies (Table XXVIII). Regulations change and must be monitored frequently.

OTHER COUNTRIES. Many countries have regulations concerning the addition of L-ascorbic acid to foods, some of which are general and others

**Table XXV. U.S. Standards or Regulations of Foods to
Which Ascorbic Acid May Be Added**[a]

Food	Purpose of Ascorbic Acid	Quantity Permitted
Artificially sweetened fruit jelly	preservative	not more than 0.1% by weight of finished food
Artificially sweetened fruit preserves and jams	preservative	not more than 0.1% by weight of finished food
Canned applesauce	preservative, nutrient	not more than 150 ppm, an amount to provide 60 mg/4 oz (113 g)
Canned apricots	preservative	an amount no greater than necessary to preserve color
Canned artichokes (packed in glass)	preservative	not more than 32 mg/100 g of finished food
Canned fruit cocktail	preservative	amount no greater than necessary to preserve color
Canned fruit nectars	preservative, nutrient	not more than 150 ppm, amounts to provide not less than 30 mg or more than 60 mg/4 fl oz
Canned mushrooms	preservative	not more than 37.5 mg/oz of drained weight of mushrooms
Canned peaches	preservative	amount not greater than necessary to preserve color
Canned pineapple juice	nutrient	amounts to provide not less than 30 mg or more than 60 mg/4 fl oz
Canned pineapple grapefruit juice drink	nutrient	amounts to provide not less than 30 mg or more than 60 mg/4 fl oz
Canned prune juice	nutrient	amounts to provide not less than 30 mg or more than 60 mg/4 fl oz
Cranberry juice cocktail	nutrient	amounts to provide not less than 30 mg or more than 60 mg/4 fl oz
Flour (white, whole wheat, plain)	dough conditioner	not to exceed 200 ppm
Frozen raw breaded shrimp	preservative	sufficient to retard development of dark spots

Table XXV. Continued

Food	Purpose of Ascorbic Acid	Quantity Permitted
Ice cream (the fruit therein)	acidulant	such quantity as seasons the finished product and meets the standards for ice cream
Margarine	preservative	ascorbyl palmitate and/or ascorbyl stearate 0.02%
Nonfruit water ices	acidulant	such quantity as seasons the finished product
Tomato juice	nutrient	amount to provide 10 mg/fl oz (total vitamin C)
Water ices (the fruit therein)	acidulant	such quantity as seasons the finished product

Foods for which standards are established and in which nonspecified preservatives may be optional ingredients are:

dry whole milk

dry cream

breads, rolls, buns	dough conditioners not referred to in standard if the total quantities are not more than 0.5 part for each 100 parts by weight of flour used
frozen raw breaded shrimp	antioxidant preservative—may be used to retard development of rancidity of the fat content

ᵃ Compiled by D. M. Pinkert. Consult regulations for current status and interpretation.

very specific. It would take a number of pages to detail such information for each food product for each country having regulations. For example, in considering ascorbic acid as a flour improver, the level of permissible addition ranges from 50 mg to 10 g/kg of flour (Table XXIX). Certain countries such as Australia, Canada, Chile, Holland, Japan, Kenya, New Zealand, Sweden, United States, Uruguay, and Zambia permit both L-ascorbic acid and bromate as flour improver while a number of other countries only allow L-ascorbic acid. In the ECC countries permissible L-ascorbic acid levels for technical application to food vary from 100 mg/kg to 2 g/kg of food product.

THE JOINT FAO/WHO CODEX ALIMENTARIUS COMMISSION. The Joint FAO/WHO Codex Alimentarius Commission (the Commission) was established to implement the Joint FAO/WHO Food Standards Program. Membership of the Commission comprises those Member Nations and Associate Members of FAO and/or WHO that have notified

Table XXVI. U.S. Regulations on Ascorbic Acid Addition to Meat

Food	Purpose	Quantity Permitted
Ascorbic acid in: cured pork and beef cuts, cured comminuted meat food product	to accelerate color fixing	70 oz per 100 gal pickle at 10% pump level; 0.75 oz per 100 lb meat or meat byproduct; 10% solution to surfaces of cured cuts prior to packaging (the use of such solution shall not result in the addition of a significant amount of moisture to the product)
Sodium ascorbate in: cured pork and beef cuts, cured comminuted meat food product	to accelerate color fixing	87.5 oz per 100 gal pickle at 10% pump level; 0.88 oz per 100 lb meat or meat byproduct; 10% solution to surfaces of cured cuts prior to packaging (the use of such solution shall not result in the addition of a significant amount of moisture to the product)

Table XXVII. U.S. Regulations on Ascorbic Acid Addition to Alcoholic Beverages

Alcohol and Tobacco Tax Div., U.S. Dept. of Treasury Regulations

Food	Purpose of Ascorbic Acid	Quantity Permitted
Wine	to prevent darkening of color and deterioration of flavor, and over-oxidation	within limitations which do not alter the class or type of the wine (use need not be declared on the label)
Beer	antioxidant and bio-logical stabilization	to be used only by agreement between U.S. Dept. of Treasury and the brewer

the Organizations of their wish to be considered as Members. By February 1979, 117 countries had become Members of the Commission. Other countries participating in the work of the Commission or its subsidiary bodies in an observer capacity are expected to become Members in the near future.

The purpose of the Joint FAO/WHO Food Standards Program is to elaborate international standards for foods aimed at protecting the health of the consumer, to ensure fair practices in the food trade, and to facilitate international trade. In addition to compositional criteria and labeling, food standards incorporate provisions in respect to food hygiene,

**Table XXVIII. Armed Forces Regulations on
Ascorbic Acid Addition to Food**[a]

Food	Purpose of Ascorbic Acid	Quantity Permitted
Beverage base powders prepared from dehydrated fruit juices (Type II)	nutrient	20–30 mg/12 fl oz of reconstituted powder
Cocoa beverage powder	nutrient	Not less than 25 mg/oz by weight
Coffee, instant, Type I	nutrient	Not less than 15 mg/2.5 g
Dehydrated white potatoes	nutrient	Not less than 50 mg/oz of dehydrated product
Milk, non-fat dry (Type II, Style B)	nutrient	20 mg/oz
Peanut butter, vitamin fortified	nutrient	37.5 mg/1.5 oz of product

[a] Compiled by N. E. Harris.

food additives, pesticide residues, other contaminants, and methods of analysis and sampling.

L-Ascorbic acid and certain derivatives (Table XXX) have been designated toxicologically as category A (1) in the release designated CAC/FAL 5-1979. Category A (1) additives are those that have been fully cleared by the Joint FAO/WHO Expert Committee on Food Additives and either have been given an "acceptable daily intake" (ADI) or have not been limited toxicologically. Approved uses of L-ascorbic acid have been indicated, maximum levels (ML) have been shown, and good manufacturing practice (GMP) has been established. ADI is expressed as milligrams per kilogram body weight; ML is expressed as weight per kilogram of product. GMP refers to the limitation of food additive in specified foods. It means that the additive in question is self-limiting in food for technological, organoleptic, or other reasons and that, therefore, the additive need not be subject to legal maximum limits. It also means that the food additive must be used according to good manufacturing practice, and in accordance with the General Principles for the Use of Food Additives.

Industrial Applications

An extensive list of patents and scientific papers exists on proposed uses of ascorbic acid in various industries; however, the amount of com-

Table XXIX.   Legal Status of L-Ascorbic
Acid as a Flour Improver

Country	Maximum Level Permitted
Australia	GMP[a]
Austria	200 mg/kg
Belgium	50 mg/kg
Brazil	2 g/kg
Canada	200 mg/kg
Chile	20–50 mg/kg
Cyprus	75 mg/kg
Denmark	200 mg/kg
England	GMP[a]
Finland	200 mg/kg
France	500 mg/kg[b]
Germany	GMP[a]
Greece	GMP[a]
Holland	50 mg/kg
Italy	200 mg/kg
Japan	GMP[a]
Kenya	200 mg/kg
New Zealand	GMP[a]
Norway	GMP[a]
Portugal	8–10 g/kg
South Africa	200 mg/kg
Spain	200 mg/kg
Sweden	GMP[a]
Switzerland	GMP[a]
Uruguay	20 mg/kg
United States	200 mg/kg
Zambia	200 mg/kg

[a] GMP = Good Manufacturing Practice.
[b] May only be added by the baker.

pound used in the industrial applications is small relative to pharmaceutical and food applications. While ascorbic acid may be declared
to be functional with meritorious advantages, there is a strong preference
to find and use more economical chemical aids, even though they may not
be quite as effective. The greatest activity in pursuing uses appears to
be for polymerization reactions in the plastics industry, for uses in printing inks, in photoprocessing, in metal technology, and in miscellaneous
areas, including cosmetics, tobacco, fibers, analytical assays, preservation
of blood, preservation of cut plants, and cleaning agents.

Polymerization Reactions. Polymerization reactions take place
under high and low temperatures. Where an aqueous phase exists such
as in emulsions, or if a polar solvent is involved, ascorbic acid is solubilized and may have merit, because of its reducing power, in facilitating
the polymerization with a temperature advantage, a rate of reaction,
better control, or a superior end product.

Table XXX.   Antioxidants and Antioxidant Synergists

Number	List	Additive	Evaluation and Maximum Limit
.230	A(1)	ascorbic acid (Syn: L-ascorbic acid)	ADI: 0–15 mg/kg body weight, sum of ascorbic acid and ascorbates from all sources (Ref.: Tox. 29, 30, 32; Spec. 47 Techn. Eff. 28) Codex Specification: ALINORM 76/41
.231	A(1)	ascorbate, potassium	ADI: 0–15 mg/kg body weight, sum of ascorbic acid and ascorbates from all sources (Ref.: Tox. 29, 30, 32; Spec. 1; Techn. Eff. 28)
.232	A(1)	ascorbate, sodium	ADI: 0–15 mg/kg body weight, sum of ascorbic acid and ascorbates from all sources (Ref.: Tox. 29, 30, 32; Spec. 47 Techn. Eff. 28) Codex Specification: ALINORM 76/41

Approved Uses of .230 in:	Evaluation and Maximum Limit
Canned tropical fruit salad	ML: 700 mg/kg
Canned peaches	ML: 550 mg/kg
Canned applesauce	ML: 150 mg/kg
Edible fungi and fungus products	ML: limited by GMP
Apricot, peach and pear nectars[a]	ML: limited by GMP
Apple juice[a]	ML: limited by GMP
Quick frozen strawberries	ML: limited by GMP
Canned mushrooms	ML: limited by GMP
Canned asparagus	ML: limited by GMP
Concentrated apple juice[a]	ML: limited by GMP
Table olives	ML: 200 mg/kg
Quick frozen peaches	ML: 750 mg/kg
Canned fruit cocktail	ML: limited by GMP
Jams and jellies	ML: 500 mg/kg
Black currant jam	ML: 750 mg/kg
Citrus marmalade	ML: 500 mg/kg
Grape juice[a]	ML: 400 mg/kg
Concentrated grape juice[a]	ML: 400 mg/kg
Sweetened concentrated Labrusca type grape juice[a]	ML: 400 mg/kg
Quick frozen shrimps and prawns	ML: limited by GMP

Approved Uses of .230 and .232 in:	
Canned corned beef	ML: 500 mg/kg, expressed as the acid
Luncheon meat	ML: 500 mg/kg, singly or in combination with isoascorbic acid, isoascorbate, expressed as ascorbic acid
Cooked cured chopped meat	
Cooked cured pork shoulder	
Cooked cured ham	
Canned baby foods	ML: limited by GMP
Cereal-based processed foods for infants and children	ML: limited by GMP

Continued on next page.

Table XXX.   Continued

Approved uses of .231 and .232 in:

Quick frozen lobsters	ML: 1 g/kg, expressed as the acid
Quick frozen fillets of ocean perch	ML: 1 g/kg, expressed as the acid
Quick frozen fillets of cod and haddock	ML: 1 g/kg, expressed as the acid
Quick frozen fillets of flat fish	ML: 1 g/kg, expressed as the acid
Quick frozen fillets of hake	ML: 1 g/kg, expressed as the acid

Number	List	Additive	Evaluation and Maximum Limit
.236	A (1)	ascorbyl palmitate	ADI: 0–1.25 mg/kg body weight, singly or in combination (Ref.: Tox. 29, 30; Spec. 47; Techn. Eff. 28) Codex Specification: ALINORM 76/41
.237	A (1)	ascorbyl stearate	

Approved Uses of .236 in:

Infant formula	ML: limited by GMP
Canned baby foods	ML: limited by GMP
Cereal-based processed foods for infants and children	ML: limited by GMP

Approved Uses of .236 and .237 in:

Edible fats and oils	ML: 200 mg/kg, singly or in combination
Margarine	ML: 200 mg/kg, singly or in combination

ᵃ Preserved exclusively by physical means.
ᵇ In products intended for vending machines only.

In vinyl compound polymerization of vinyl acetate, alcohol, bromide, chloride, or carbonate, ascorbic acid can be a component of the polymerization mixture (733–749). Activators for the polymerization have been acriflavine (734), other photosensitive dye compounds (737, 738), hydrogen peroxides (740, 741, 742), potassium peroxydisulfate (743), ferrous sulfate, and acyl sulfonyl peroxides (747). Nagabhooshanam and Santappa (748) reported on dye sensitized photopolymerization of vinyl monomers in the presence of ascorbic acid–sodium hydrogen orthophosphate complex. Another combination is vinyl chloride with cyclohexanesulfonyl acetyl peroxide with ascorbic acid, iron sulfate, and an alcohol (749). Use of low temperature conditions in emulsion polymerization, with ascorbic acid, is mentioned (750, 751). Clarity of color is important and impact-resistant, clear, moldable polyvinyl chloride can be prepared with ascorbic acid as an acid catalyst (752) in the formulation.

Similar reports have appeared in the technology of polymerizing acrylic monomers such as acrylonitrile (753–759) or acrylamide (760–763). Korolev et al. (764) have used ascorbic acid as a reducing agent in the mixture to increase the polymerization rate. The kinetics of polymerization in the presence of oxygen has been studied in systems containing ascorbic acid (765). Recent patents (766, 767) have been issued with ascorbic acid in the dispersion of acrylic aqueous resins.

A third type of polymers is polymerized methyl methacrylate or methacrylamide (768–773). Strubell (768) has carried out polymerization of methyl methacrylate with an ascorbic acid–benzoyl peroxide system. In an aqueous polymerization of methyl methacrylate, Misra and Gupta (770) used the redox system of potassium peroxydisulfate and ascorbic acid. A similar system was reported by Pattnaik et al. (773).

Ascorbic acid is declared to function as an antioxidant for polyethylene (774), for light-sensitive polymer mass (775), for clear thermoplastics (776), and for colorless synthetic rubber (777). It is listed as an accelerator for curing anaerobic resins (778) and for hardening processes of unsaturated polyester resins (779–783). Ascorbic acid is an additive with synergistic effect upon other compounds in stabilized premixes for polyurethane foam (784) and as a stabilizer for polyesters to be used as an lubricant additives or plasticizers (785). Ascorbic acid triggers polymerizing resin-forming materials used in well bore holes as drilling fluids (786) and in fire-resistant polymer compositions (787). Ferrocene-containing polymers and their photooxidation–reduction reaction (788, 789), and synthesis and reactions of porphyrin and metalloporphyrin polymers (790) are other systems for utility of ascorbic acid.

In plastics and polymerization reactions there appears to be much art within the systems—what may work in one case or what may be a plus feature in one may be undesirable in another. Trials must be run to substantiate where and how much of the more expensive ascorbic acid has merit over economical inorganic and organic substitutes. Ascorbic acid may have a better opportunity where color, odor, or safety are important in the end product.

Photographic Developing and Printing. The association of ascorbic acid and derivatives with the photographic industry is not a new relationship; it goes back over 45 years when ascorbic acid was first produced commercially by chemical synthesis. During this four-decade period many patents have been issued around the world. Some will be mentioned in this review. Basically, in the technology of photographic material development, ascorbic acid has been considered a component of film emulsions and in film developers both in color and black and white photography. It has been studied as an investigational material, and while merit may be shown for its image quality or for functional qualities in the developing solution, its instability, rapidity of exhaustion in action, or higher cost are disadvantageous considerations that keep its usage in this industrial application at a lower level than its potential.

Ascorbic acid has been declared as a useful optional ingredient in developer compositions (791–799). Ascorbic acid can be used without sulfite addition and it has no solvent effect on silver halides (793). Its addition increases the activity of certain developer components (800) and may stabilize the image (801–804) or intensify it (805). In a Belgian patent (806) both L-ascorbic acid and a 2,3-diphenyl-L-ascorbic acid are cited as additives. For developers functioning at an alkaline pH, ascorbic acid borate (807) was declared to be stable while acting as a reducing agent. Ascorbic acid is useful in bleaching processes (808, 809, 810): in the bleaching of photographs obtained by the silver salt diffusion process (808), in bleach–fix bath desilvering (809), and as a color photography bleaching agent (810). The kinetics of development and silver formation have been investigated by Willis et al. (811) and Pontius et al. (812).

Applications for ascorbic acid have been considered in color photography where it may be a component of the developer for special purpose such as to reduce froth (813, 814), or in image stabilization in color photographic material (815, 816). Ascorbic acid may be involved in image transfer processes (817, 818), direct positive photographic emulsions (819), one-step diffusion processes (820) in a photographic product incorporating a developer yielding images by simple treatment with water (821), or as a binder for photographic materials (822).

In the preparation of lithographic materials and in the lithographic process, ascorbic acid may be useful. The production of lithographic masters is improved by inclusion of ascorbic acid in the hardener and receiving sheet (823) and, in general, in processing silver halide lithographic materials (824). Ascorbic acid has been considered in several investigations (825–828) as a component of the developers used in lithography. In offset printing plates by colloid transfer (829), ascorbic acid and 1-phenyl-3-pyrazolidinone are used as nonhardening agents. Ink with high power to absorb light (830) is benefited by ascorbic acid addition. Other applications involve light-sensitive copy material (831), heat-developable imaging systems (832, 833), powderless etching (834), and various recording and print-out papers (835–838).

There is a metal aspect of photography where ascorbic acid may be involved. Several patents claim ascorbic acid useful as a sequestering or chelating agent (839, 840), or, to prevent iron spotting of photographic material (841, 842). It is included in a two-stage copper development of a silver latent image in semiconductor photographic layers (843), and in a study of silver-free physical development process by electrochemical methods, ascorbic acid acts as a physical developer in the form of cupriascorbic acid (*844*). Chromate dermatitis (hand lesions) is an occupational health problem in the printing and lithographic industries. A preventive regimen (*845*) involving use of a 10% ascorbic acid solution is beneficial in preventing or controlling the occurrence.

Metal Technology. The patent and scientific literature reveals some potential uses for ascorbic acid in metallic reductions, coating compositions, electroplating processes, and oxidation control. Metal ion and metal complex catalyzed reactions (*846*) and the structure of ascorbate complexes of metals (*847*) have been investigated. The kinetics and mechanism of the reduction of platinum (*848*), vanadium (*849*), cerium (*850*), molybdenum (*851*), gold (*852*), and silver (*853, 854*) by ascorbic acid have been examined. Other topics of ascorbic acid involvement are providing resistance to metal surfaces (*855, 856*), metallizing nonmetallic substrates (*857*), oxidation-resistant coating for copper and copper alloys (*858*), copper plating (*859*), nickel plating (*860, 861*), electrodeposition of nickel alloy films (*862–865*), of zinc alloys (*866, 867*), of tin alloys (*868*), electrodeposition of aluminum (*869, 870*), and activation of zinc phosphate compositions for steel (*871*). Rust remover composition (*872*) for steels, rust inhibiting uses (*873, 874*), and rustproofing agents (*875*) for ferrous and nonferrous metals and alloys are other cited applications.

Miscellaneous Applications

Ascorbic acid and derivatives are cited as potential ingredients in cosmetic formulations (*876–879*). Specific uses involve cosmetic compositions for thermal dispensing (*880*), dentifrice tablets (*881*), bath preparations (*882*), deodorants and mouthwashes (*883–886*), skin preparations such as skin lightening preparations (*887*) or protective creams (*888–890*). The more active areas have been hair and scalp preparations (*891, 892*), hair setting compositions (*893*), hair bleaching programs (*894, 895*), and hair dyeing preparations (*896, 897, 898*).

Ascorbic acid has been declared useful in intravaginal contraceptives in reducing sperm motility (*899, 900*). The preservation of human blood by the addition of sodium ascorbate (*901*) has been found to have some merit. The usefulness of ascorbic acid in the treatment of industrial chemical toxicity (*902, 903*), in the preservation of cut-blooms in water (*904, 905*), in water treatment of the ferruginous type (*906*), in inhibiting corrosion (*907*), in treatment for the production of durable creases in cloth (*908*), and in brightened yarns with high light fastness (*909*) is mentioned. Adhesive compositions (*910*) and special cleansers (*911, 912*) are other potential applications.

The purging of nitrogen oxides from exhaust gases (913) and treatment of smoking materials (914) with ascorbates are of interest, particularly the latter, wherein a lower production of potentially carcinogenic nitrosated compounds may result if the application were to be put into effect.

An extensive literature exists on the use of ascorbic acid in chemical analytical assays.

Literature Cited

1. Szent-Györgyi, A. *Biochem. J.* 1928, 22, 1387.
2. Ibid., 1931, 90, 385.
3. Waugh, W. A.; King, C. G. *Science* 1932, 76, 630.
4. Waugh, W. A.; King, C. G. *J. Biol. Chem.* 1932, 97, 325.
5. Svirbely, J. L.; Szent-Györgyi, A. *Nature* 1932, 129, 576.
6. Svirbely, J. L.; Szent-Györgyi, A. *Biochem. J.* 1932, 26, 865.
7. Svirbely, J. L.; Szent-Györgyi, A. *Nature* 1932, 129, 690.
8. Svirbely, J. L.; Szent-Györgyi, A. *Biochem. J.* 1933, 27, 279.
9. Haworth, W. N.; Hirst, E. L.; Herbert, R. W.; Percival, E. G. V.; Reynolds, R. J. W.; Smith, F. *J. Soc. Chem. Ind.* 1933, 52, 221.
10. Karrer, P.; Schoepp, K.; Zehnder, F. *Helv. Chim. Acta* 1933, 16, 1161.
11. Michael, F.; Kraft, K. *Z. Physiol. Chem.* 1933, 222, 235.
12. von Euler, E.; Klussman, E. *Arkiv. Kemi, Mineral. Geol.* 1933, 7.
13. Reichstein, T.; Gruessner, A.; Oppenauer, R. *Helv. Chim. Acta* 1933, 16, 1019.
14. Ault, R. G.; Baird, D. K.; Carrington, H. C.; Haworth, W. N.; Herbert, R.; Hirst, E. L.; Percival, E. G. V.; Smith, F.; Stacey, M. *J. Chem. Soc.* 1933, 1419.
15. "U.S. Pharmacopoeia"; 20th revision, U.S. Pharmacopoeia: Rockville, MD, 1979.
16. "Food Chemical Codex"; NAS–Natl. Res. Council: Wash., D.C., 1976.
17. Hoffman, F. S.; Nowosad, F. S.; Cody, W. J. *Can. J. Bot.* 1967, 45, 1859.
18. Rosenfield, H. J.; Meldinger, *Fra Nor. Landbrukshogskole* 1978, 57(5), 28.
19. Vardjan, M. *Biol. Vestn.* 1977, 25(1), 19.
20. Viswanath, D. P.; Sastry, K. S. K.; Rao, B. V. V. *Mysore J. Agric. Sci.* 1972, 6, 24.
21. Saxena, O. P.; Abraham, P. G.; Pandya, R. B.; Dave, I. C. *Vidya* 1969, 12(1), 189.
22. Yadava, R. B. R.; Singh, A.; Tripathi, M. *Indian Grassland Seed Res.* 1976, 4(1), 120.
23. Chinoy, J. J.; Abraham, P. G.; Pandya, R. B.; Saxena, O. P.; Dave, I. C. *Indian J. Plant Physiol.* 1970, 13(1), 40.
24. Singh, C.; Bhan, A. K.; Kaul, B. L. *Seed Sci. Technol.* 1974, 2(4), 421.
25. Vyas, L. N.; Garual, S. *Phyton (Buenos Aires)* 1971, 28(1), 1.
26. Kanchan, S. D.; Jayachandra, Y. *Curr. Sci.* 1974, 43(16), 520.
27. Severi, A.; Laudi, G. L. *G. Bot. Ital.* 1976, 110(3), 231.
28. Maity, S. C.; Maity, S. K.; Sen, P. F. *Indian Agric.* 1972, 16(2), 201.
29. Mazumder, B. C.; Chatterjee, S. K. *Bull. Bot. Soc. Bengal* 1971, 25(1–2), 71.
30. Yadava, R. B. R.; Sreenath, P. R. *Indian J. Plant Physiol.* 1975, 18(2), 135.
31. Zhukora, P. S. *Vestsi Akad. Navuk, B. SSR., Ser. Sel'skagaspad. Navuk* 1975, (1), 48.

32. Srivastava, G. C.; Sirohi, G. S. *Indian J. Exp. Biol.* **1973,** *11*(5), 470.
33. Mehta, D. H. *Vidya, B* **1977,** *20*(1), 7.
34. Singh, G.; Sareen, K. *Indian Sugar* **1976,** *25*(12), 911.
35. Huang, M-C. *Proc. Natl. Sci. Counc. Part 2* **1974,** 7, 333.
36. Garg, O. P.; Kapoor, V. *J. Exp. Bot.* **1972,** *23*(76), 699.
37. Bharti, S.; Garg, O. P. *Plant Cell Physiol.* **1970,** *11*(4), 657.
38. Singh, G.; Singh, T. H. *J. Res., Punjab Agric. Univ.* **1975,** *12*(4), 329.
39. Saimbhi, M. S. *J. Res., Punjab Agric. Univ.* **1974,** *11*(4), 369.
40. Johnnykulty, A. T.; Khudairi, A. K. *Physiol. Plant.* **1972,** *26*(3), 285.
41. Pyasyatskene, A. A. *Liet. TSR Mokslu Akad. Darb., Ser. B* **1974,** *1*(65), 55; *2*(66), 65; *4*(68), 35; **1975,** 3(71), 41.
42. Pastena, B. *Riv. Vitic. Enol.* **1974,** 27(5), 197.
43. Subbotovich, A. S.; Perstnev, N. D.; Foksha, M. G. *Tr. Kishinev. S-kh. Inst.* **1973,** *118,* 8.
44. Swaraj, K.; Garg, O. P. *Physiol. Plant.* **1970,** 23(5), 889.
45. Sinha, N. B.; Naudi, P.; Belgrami, K. S. *"Today Tomorrow's";* Printers Publ.: New Delhi, 1977; p. 191–197.
46. Sharma, V. K.; Singh, R. P.; Dua, K. L. *India Sci. Cult.* **1975,** *41*(8), 383.
47. Freebairn, H. T. *Science* **1957,** *126,* 303.
48. Middleton, J. T.; Kendrick, J. B. Jr.; Darley, E. F. *Proc. Natl. Air Pollut. Symp., 3rd* **1955.**
49. Erickson, L. C.; Wedding, R. T. *Physiol. Plant.* **1956,** 9, 421.
50. Freebairn, H. T. *Calif. Citrogr.* **1957,** Feb., 137.
51. Freebairn, H. T.; Davidson, J., Univ. Calif. News Release, Dec. 11, 1957.
52. Freebairn, H. T. *Farm Management* **1958,** June.
53. Freebairn, H. T. *J. Air Pollut. Control Assoc.* **1960,** *10*(4), 314.
54. Freebairn, H. T.; Taylor, O. C. *HortScience* **1960,** 76, 693.
55. Weaver, G. M.; Aylesworth, J. W.; Dass, H. C. *Can. Agric.* **1968,** *13*(4), 24.
56. Hanson, G. P.; Jativa, C. D. *Lasca Leaves* **1970,** *20,* 6.
57. Cathey, H. M.; Heggestad, H. E. *J. Am. Soc. Hort. Sci.* **1972,** 97(6), 695.
58. Miyake, Y. *Utsunomiya Tab. Shinkenjo Hokoku* **1973,** *12,* 55.
59. Ordin, L.; Taylor, O. C.; Probst, B. E.; Cardiff, E. A. *Int. J. Air Water Pollut.* **1962,** *6,* 223.
60. Mehta, K. G.; Mehta, D. H.; Chinoy, J. J. *Indian J. Plant Physiol.* **1976,** *19*(2), 244.
61. Saimbhi, M. S.; Arora, S. K.; Padda, D. *Plant Sci.* **1970,** *2,* 123.
62. Gonzalez, J. *Proc. Tropical Region, J. Amer. Soc. Hort. Sci.* **1973,** *17,* 285.
63. Wang, C. Y.; Mellenthin, W. M. *HortScience* **1973,** *8*(4), 321.
64. Cooper, W. C.; Rasmussen, G. K.; Smoot, J. J. *Citrus Ind.* **1968,** *49*(10), 25.
65. Cooper, W. C.; Rasmussen, G. K.; Smoot, J. *Agric. Res. Washington* **1969,** *17*(8), 11.
66. Tomer, N. S.; Kumar, H. *Indian J. Hort.* **1977,** 34(1), 30.
67. Schilling, G. *Wiss. Z., Martin-Luther-Univ., Halle-Wittenburg, Math.-Naturwiss. Reihe* **1974,** 23(2), 15.
68. Cooper, W. C.; Henry, W. H. *Citrus Ind.* **1967,** *48*(6), 5.
69. Cooper, W. C.; Henry, W. H. *Proc. Fl. State Hortic. Soc.* **1968,** *80,* 7.
70. Ibid., **1969,** *81,* 62.
71. Wilson, W. C. *Proc. Fl. State Hortic. Soc.* **1969,** *82,* 72.
72. Wilson, W. C.; Coppock, G. E. *Proc. Int. Citrus Symp., 1st,* **1969,** *3,* 1125.
73. Wilson, W. C.; Coppock, G. E. *Proc. Fl. State Hortic. Soc.* **1969,** *81,* 39.
74. Ben. Yehoshua, S.; Eaks, I. L. *J. Am. Soc. Hort. Sci.* **1969,** *94*(3), 292.
75. Ben. Yehoshua, S. *J. Am. Soc. Hortic. Sci.* **1973,** 98(3), 265.
76. El-Zeftawi, B. M. *J. Aust. Inst. Agric. Sci.* **1970,** *36,* 139.

77. Palmer, R. L.; Hield, H. Z.; Lewis, L. N. *Proc. Int. Citrus Symp., 1st* **1969,** *3,* 1135.
78. Rasmussen, G. K.; Cooper, W. C. *J. Am. Soc. Hortic. Sci.* **1968,** *93,* 191.
79. Rasmussen, G. K.; Jones, J. W. *Proc. Fl. State Hortic. Soc.* **1969,** *81,* 36.
80. Rasmussen, G. K.; Jones, J. W. *HortScience* **1969,** *4,* 60.
81. Edgerton, L. J. *HortScience* **1971,** *6*(4), 378.
82. Mazumdar, B. C.; Chatterjee, S. K. *Indian J. Plant Physiol.* **1968,** *11*(2), 188.
83. Hartmann, H. T.; Fadl, M.; Whisler, J. *Calif. Agric.* **1967,** *21*(7), 5.
84. Edgerton, L. J.; Hatch, A. N. *Proc. N.Y. State Hortic. Sci.* **1969,** *114,* 109.
85. Knight, J. N. *Acta Hortic.* **1976,** (60), 99.
86. Chatterjee, S.; Chatterjee, S. K. *Indian J. Exp. Biol.* **1971,** *9*(4), 485.
87. Varma, S. K. *Indian J. Agric. Chem.* **1976,** *9*(1–2), 159.
88. Varma, S. K. *Indian J. Exp. Biol.* **1976,** *14*(3), 305.
89. Varma, S. K. *Indian J. Plant Physiol.* **1977,** *20*(1), 85.
90. Ohta, Y.; Nakayama, M.; Yokota, K., *Japan Kokei,* 738, 2033, 11/2/73.
91. Leonard, C. D. *Plant. Dis. Rep.* **1974,** *58*(10), 918.
92. Glushchenko, I. E.; Khor'kov, E. I.; Resh, F. M. *Dokl. Vses., Akad. Skh. Nauk* **1973,** *8,* 2.
93. Glushchenko, I. E.; Khor'kov, E. I.; Resh, F. M. *Nauchn. Tr., Vses. Sel.-Genet. Inst.* **1974,** *11,* 122.
94. Bode, H. R. *Planta.* **1961,** *57,* 138.
95. Arrigoni, O. In "Root-Knot Nematodes: Meloidogyne Species: Systematics, Biology, and Control"; Lamberti, F.; Taylor, C. E., Eds.; Academic: London, 1979; pp. 457–467.
96. Arrigoni, O.; Zacheo, G.; Arrigoni-Liso, R.; Bleve-Zacheo, T.; Lamberti, F. In "Root-Knot Nematodes: Meloidogyne Species: Systematics, and Biological Control"; Lamberti, F.; Taylor, S. E., Eds.; Academic: London, 1979; pp. 469–470.
97. Arrigoni, O.; Zacheo, G.; Arrigoni-Liso, R.; Bleve-Zacheo, T.; Lamberti, F. *Phytopathology* **1979,** *69*(6), 574.
98. Markov, I. L.; *Nauk. Pr., Ukr. Sil's'kogospod. Akad.* **1975,** *171,* 79.
99. Van Lelyveld, L. J. *Agroplantae* **1975,** *7*(3), 45.
100. Plakhova, T. M. *Tr. Vses. Nauchno-Issled. Inst. Efirnomaslichn. Kul't.* **1973,** *6,* 173.
101. Plakhova, T. M. *Byul. VNII Rastenievodstva* **1975,** *47,* 86.
102. Anderson, R. A.; Linney, T. L. *Chem. Biol. Interact.* **1977,** *19*(3), 317.
103. Bocion, P. F.; DeSilva, W. H.; Hueppi, G. A.; Szkrybalo, W. *Nature* **1975,** *258*(5531), 142.
104. Sachs, R. M.; Hield, H.; Debie, J. *HortScience* **1975,** *10,* 367.
105. Heursal, J.; *Med. Fac. Landbouw. Ryks-Univ. Gent (Belgium)* **1975,** *48,* 849.
106. DeSilva, W. H.; Bocion, P. F.; Walter, H. R. *Science* **1976,** *11*(6), 569.
107. Sanderson, K. C.; Martin, W. C., Jr. *HortScience* **1977,** *12,* 337.
108. Larson, R. A. *J. Hortic. Sci.* **1978,** *53,* 57.
109. Orson, P.; Kofranek, A. M. *J. Am. Hortic. Soc.* **1978,** *103*(6), 801.
110. Breece, J. R.; Furuta, T.; Hield, H. Z. *Calif. Agric.* **1978,** May 23.
111. Cohen, M. A. *Sci. Horticult.* **1978,** *8,* 163.
112. Worley, R. E. *HortScience* **1980,** *15*(2), 180.
113. Lumis, G. P.; Johnson, A. G. *Can. J. Plant Sci.* **1979,** *59,* 1161.
114. Hield, H.; Sachs, R. M.; Hemstreet, S. *HortScience* **1978,** *13,* 440.
115. Johnson, A. G.; Lumis, G. P. *HortScience* **1979,** *14,* 626.
116. Chatterjee, I. B.; Majumder, A. K.; Naudi, B. K.; Subramanian, N. *Ann. N.Y. Acad. Sci.* **1975,** *258,* 24; *Science* **1973,** *182,* 127.
117. McCay, C. M.; Tunison, A. V. "Cortland Hatchery Rept. for 1933," State of N.Y. Conservation Dept., Albany, N.Y., 1934.
118. Kitamura, S.; Ohara, S.; Suwa, T.; Nakagawa, K. *Bull. Jap. Soc. Sci. Fish.* **1965,** *31,* 818.

119. Nakagawa, K.; *Kagaku To Seibutsu* **1967**, *3*, 19.
120. Poston, H. A. *N.Y. St. Cons. Dept. Fish. Res. Bull.* **1967**, *30*, 46.
121. John, T. M.; George, J. C.; Hilton, J. W.; Slinger, S. J. *Int. J. Vitam. Res.* **1979**, *49*, 400.
122. Halver, J. E. *Bull. Jap. Soc. Sci. Fish.* **1972**, *38*(1), 79.
123. Hilton, J. W.; *Diss. Abstr. Int. B* **1979**, *39*(11), 5322.
124. Magarelli, P. C., Jr.; Hunter B.; Lightner, D. V.; Covin, L. B. *Comp. Biochem. Physiol.* **1979**, *63A*(1), 103.
125. Lovell, R. T. *J. Nutr.* **1973**, *103*(1), 134.
126. Wilson, R. P.; Poe, W. E. *J. Nutr.* **1973**, *103*(9), 1359.
127. Andrews, J. W.; Murai, T. *J. Nutr.* **1975**, *105*(5), 557.
128. Lim, C.; Lovell, R. T. *J. Nutr.* **1978**, *108*(7), 1137.
129. Lovell, R. T.; Lim, C. *Trans. Amer. Fish. Soc.* **1976**, *107*(2), 321.
130. Halver, J. E.; Ashley, L. M.; Smith, R. R. *Trans. Amer. Fish. Soc.* **1969**, *98*(4), 762.
131. Halver, J. E.; Smith, R. R.; Baker, E. M.; Tolbert, B. M. *Abstr. FASEB Meeting 1974, April 7–12*, Atlantic City.
132. Ashley, L. M.; Halver, J. E.; Smith, R. R. "The Pathology of Fishes"; Ribelin, W. E.; Migaki, G., Eds.; Univ. Wisc. Press: Madison, Wisc., 1975; pp. 769–786.
133. Ikeda, S.; Sato, M. *Bull. Jap. Soc. Sci. Fish.* **1964**, *30*, 365.
134. Arai, S.; Nose, T.; Hashimoto, Y. *Tansuiku Suisan Kenkyusho Kenkyu Hokoku* **1972**, *22*, 69.
135. Quadri, S. F.; Seib, P. A.; DeYoe, C. W. *Carbohydr. Res.* **1973**, *29*, 259.
136. Halver, J. E.; Smith, R. R.; Tolbert, B. M.; Baker, E. M. *Ann. N.Y. Acad. Sci.* **1975**, *258*, 81.
137. Murai, T.; Andrews, J. W.; Bauernfeind, J. C.; *J. Nutr.* **1978**, *108*, 1761.
138. Kuenzig, W.; Avenia, R.; Kamm, J. J. *J. Nutr.* **1974**, *104*, 952.
139. Machlin, L. J.; Garcia, F.; Guenzig, W.; Richter, C. B.; Spiegel, H. E.; Brin, M. *Am. J. Clin. Nutr.* **1976**, *29*, 825.
140. Mehrle, P. M.; Mayer, F. L. *J. Fish Res. Board Can.* **1975**, *32*(5), 593.
141. Mayer, F. L.; Mehrle, P. M.; *Toxicol. Appl. Pharmacol.* **1976**, *37*(1), 168.
142. Mayer, F. L.; Mehrle, P. M.; Schoettger, R. A. "EPA-600/3-77-085, US-EPA," U.S. Environ. Prot. Agency, Off. Res. Dev., Duluth, Minn. 1977, pp. 1–24.
143. Mayer, F. L.; Mehrle, P. M.; Crutcher, L. P. *Trans. Am. Fish. Soc.* **1978**, *107*(2), 326.
144. Briggs, G. M.; Luckey, T. D.; Elvehjem, C. A.; Hart, E. B. *Proc. Soc. Exp. Biol. Med.* **1944**, *55*, 130.
145. Dietrich, L. S.; Monson, W. J.; Elvehjem, C. A. *J. Biol. Chem.* **1949**, *181*, 915.
146. March, B.; Biely, J. *Poult. Sci.* **1953**, *32*, 768.
147. Baldissera-Nordio, C. B. *Riv. Zootec.* **1957**, *30*, 64.
148. Bzowska, B., Dissertation, Univ. of Zurich, Switzerland, 1965, p. 86.
149. Gogus, K. A.; Griminger, P. *Poult. Sci.* **1959**, *38*, 533.
150. Dietrich, L. S.; Monson, W. J.; Elvehjem, C. A. *Proc. Soc. Exp. Biol. Med.* **1950**, *75*, 130.
151. Luckey, T. D.; Moore, P. R.; Elvehjem, C. A.; Hart, E. P. *Science* **1936**, *103*, 682.
152. Lepp, A.; Moore, P. R.; Elvehjem, C. A.; Hart, E. B. *Poult. Sci.* **1947**, *26*, 594.
153. Lyle, G. R.; Moreng, R. E. *Poult. Sci.* **1968**, *47*, 410.
154. Brant, A. W.; Otee, A. W.; Chin, C. *U.S. Dep. Agric., Tech. Bull.* **1953**, 1066.
155. Perek, M. *Wiss. Veroeff. Dsch. Ges. Ernaehr.* **1965**, *14*, 81.
156. Sung, Y-Y.; Chiang, I-N; Tai, G. *Iippon Chikusan Gakkai Ho* **1979**, *50*(7), 507.
157. Thorton, P. A.; Deeb, S. S. *Poult. Sci.* **1961**, *40*, 1063.

158. Nestor, K. E.; Touchburn, S. P.; Treiber, M. *Poult. Sci.* **1972**, *51*, 1676.
159. Perek, M.; Kendler, J. *Poult. Sci.* **1962**, *41*, 677.
160. Perek, M.; Kendler, J. *Br. Poult. Sci.* **1963**, *4*, 191.
161. Ahmad, M. M.; Moreng, R. E.; Muller, H. D. *Poult. Sci.* **1967**, *46*(1), 6.
162. Pasual, V. C.; Angel, R. S., Jr. *Philipp. J. Vet. Med.* **1967**, *6*(1/2), 124.
163. Oluyemi, J. A.; Adetowun, A. *Poult. Sci.* **1979**, *58*(4), 767.
164. Thorton, P. A. *Poult. Sci.* **1960**, *39*, 1072.
165. Ibid., **1962**, *41*, 1832.
166. Thorton, P. A.; Moreng, R. E. *Poult. Sci.* **1958**, *37*(3), 691.
167. Ibid., **1959**, *38*(3), 594.
168. El-Boushy, A. R. *Meded. Landbouwhogesch. Wageningen* **1966**, *7*, 79.
169. Mather, F. B. *Poult. Sci.* **1962**, *41*, 963.
170. Sullivan, T. W.; Gehle, M. H. *Poult. Sci.* **1962**, *41*, 1016.
171. Sullivan, T. W.; Kingam, J. R. *Poult. Sci.* **1962**, *41*, 1596.
172. El-Boushy, A. R. P.; Simons, P. C. M.; Wiertz, G. *Poult. Sci.* **1968**, *47*, 456.
173. El-Boushy, A. R.; Van Albada, M. *J. Agric. Sci.* **1970**, *18*(1), 62.
174. Kivimäe, A. K. *Lantbrukshögoko. Statens Lantbruks för, Statens Husdjursför, Särtr Förhandsmedd* **1962**, *154*.
175. Heywang, B. W.; Kemmerer, A. R. *Poult. Sci.* **1955**, *34*, 1032.
176. Heywang, B. W.; Reid, B. L.; Kemmerer, A. R. *Poult. Sci.* **1964**, *43*, 625.
177. Hunt, J. R.; Sitkin, J. R. *Poult. Sci.* **1962**, *41*, 219.
178. Harms, R. H.; Waldroup, P. W. *Poult. Sci.* **1961**, *40*, 1345.
179. Wilkinson, W. S. *Poult. Sci.* **1961**, *40*, 1470.
180. Pepper, W. F.; Winget, C. M.; Slinger, S. J. *Poult. Sci.* **1961**, *40*, 657.
181. Arscott, G. H.; Rachapaetayakom, P.; Bernier, P. E.; Adams, F. W. *Poult. Sci.* **1962**, *41*, 485.
182. Hartung, T. E.; Moreng, R. E. *Feedstuffs* **1964**, *36*, 30.
183. Ahmad, M. M.; Moreng, R. E. *Poult. Sci.* **1964**, *43*, 1298.
184. Dorr, P. E.; Nockels, C. F. *Poult. Sci.* **1971**, *50*, 1375.
185. Kechik, I. T.; Sykes, A. H. *Br. Poult. Sci.* **1974**, *15*, 449.
186. Mostert, G. C. *Farming S. Afr.* **1960**, *36*, 53.
187. Herrick, R. B.; Nockels, C. F. *Poult. Sci.* **1969**, *48*, 1512.
188. Chen, A. A-T.; Nockels, C. F. *Poult. Sci.* **1973**, *52*, 1862.
189. Rauch, W., *Arch. Gefluegelkd.* **1964**, *28*, 437.
190. Wawrzyniak, M. *Penn. Univ. Marie Curie-Skladovska* **1956**, *2*, 1.
191. Zanelli, C. *Quad. Nutr.* **1958**, *18*, 171.
192. Perek, M.; Snapir, N. *Br. Poult. Sci.* **1963**, *4*, 19.
193. Polster, J., *Mh. Veterinaermedizin* **1963**, *18*, 34.
194. Tagwerker, F. *Arch. Gefluegelkd.* **1960**, *2*, 160.
195. Barber, R. S.; Braude, R.; Cooke, P. *Proc. Nutr. Soc.* **1962**, *21*, 27.
196. Bowland, J. P. *Proc. 45th Annu. Feeders Day Report, Univ. Alberta, Edmonton, Canada* **1966**, 12.
197. Travnicek, J.; Simek, L.; Mandel, L. *Sb. Cesk. Akad. Zemed. Ved. Zivocisna Vyroba* **1961**, *6*, 421.
198. Cromwell, G. L.; Hayes, V. W.; Overfield, J. R. *J. Anim. Sci.* **1970**, *31*, 63.
199. Dvorak, M., Thesis, Vet. Fak. Vys. Skola Zemedel, Brno, **1968**, p. 1–130.
200. Brown, R. G.; Young, L. G.; Sharma, V. D.; Buchanan-Smith, J. G. *Proc. Univ. Quelph Nutr. Conf. Feed Manuf.*, March 9–10, 1971.
201. Burnside, J. E. *Proc. S. Illinois Univ. Beef-Swine Nutrition Seminar* 1969.
202. Valdmauis, A. *Zinatr. Akad. Vestis* **1953**, *5*, 721.
203. Andresen, H. U. T., Thesis, Tieraeztl. Hochschullehrb., Hanover, 1963.
204. Faller, H. *Dsch. Gefluegelwirtschaft u. Schweinefutter* **1973**, *25*(6), 142.
205. Ivos, J.; Dopliher, C.; Muhaxhiri, G. *Vet. Arch.* **1971**, *41*(7–8), 202.
206. Dvorak, M.; *Zentrabl. Veterinaermed. Reihe* **1967**, *14*, 216.

207. Gipp, W. F.; Pond, W. G.; Kallfelz, F. A.; Tasker, J. B.; Van Campen, D. R.; Krook, L.; Visek, W. J. *J. Nutr.* **1974**, *104*, 532.
208. Lundquist, N. S.; Phillips, P. H. *J. Dairy Sci.* **1943**, *26*, 1023.
209. Phillips, P. H. *Feedstuffs* **1944**, June 9, 24.
210. Phillips, P. H. *J. Vet. Med. Assoc.* **1947**, *111*(846), 218.
211. Norton, C. L.; Eaton, H. D.; Loosli, J. K.; Spielmann, A. A. *J. Dairy Sci.* **1946**, *29*, 231.
212. Nevins, W. B.; Kendol, K. A. *J. Dairy Sci.* **1947**, *30*, 175.
213. Cole, C. L.; Rasmussen, R. A.; Thorp, F., Jr. *Vet. Med. (Kansas City, Mo.)* **1944**, *39*(5), 204.
214. McPherson, E. A.; Beattie, I. S.; Young, G. B., III *Intern. Tagung Rinderkrankheiten* **1964**, *2*(3–4), 533.
215. Olson, H. E.; Tammeus, J. *J. Amer. Vet. Med. Assoc.* **1967**, *150*(11), 1299.
216. Duncan, C. W.; Huffman, C. F.; Mitchell, R. L., Jr.; Reid, J. T., unpublished data.
217. Phillips, P. H.; Lardy, H. A.; Heizer, E. E.; Rupel, I. W. *J. Dairy Sci.* **1940**, *23*, 873.
218. Phillips, P. H.; Lardy, H. A.; Boyer, P. D.; Werner, G. M. *J. Dairy Sci.* **1941**, *24*, 153.
219. Elliott, J. G.; LaChance, P. A. *J. Nutr.* **1980**, *110*, 1488.
220. Jungeblut, C. W.; Zwemer, R. L. *Proc. Soc. Exp. Biol. Med.* **1935**, *52*, 1229.
221. Jungeblut, C. W. *J. Exp. Med.* **1939**, *70*, 315.
222. McCorkle, F.; Taylor, R.; Stinson, R.; Day, E. J.; Glick, B. *Poult. Sci.* **1980**, *59*(6), 1324.
223. Bissel, M. J.; Hatie, C.; Farson, D. A.; Schwarz, R. I.; Soo, W-J. *Proc. Natl. Acad. Sci. U.S.A.* **1980**, *77*, 2711.
224. McCormick, W. J. *Arch. Pediatr.* **1951**, *68*, 1.
225. Ibid., **1952**, *69*, 151.
226. Klenner, F. R. *Proc. Tri-State Med. Assoc. Carolinas and Virginia, Columbia Feb. 19–20, 1951.* So. Med. Surg. **1951**, *113*, 101.
227. Murata, A. *Proc. Intersect. Congr. Internat. Assoc. Microbiol. Soc.* **1970**, *3*, 432.
228. Hill, C. H.; Garren, H. W. *Ann. N.Y. Acad. Sci.* **1955**, *63*, 186.
229. Salo, R.; Cliver, D. O. *Appl. and Environmental Microbiol.* **1978**, *36*, 68.
230. Luberoff, B. J. *Chem Technol.* **1978**, Feb., 76.
231. Nungester, W. J.; Ames, A. M. *J. Infect. Dis.* **1948**, *83*, 50.
232. DeChatelet, L. R.; Cooper, M. R.; McCall, C. E. *J. Clin. Invest.* **1971**, *50*, 24a.
233. Belfield, W. O. *Vet. Med.* **1967**, *62*(4), 345.
234. Edwards, W. C. *Vet. Med.* **1968**, *63*(7), 696.
235. Brandt, M. E. *Vet. Med.* **1967**, *62*(7), 616.
236. Leveque, J. I. *Vet. Med.* **1969**, *64*(11), 997.
237. Ward, D. E. *Vet. Med.* **1967**, *62*(7), 617.
238. Kalokerinos, J. *Med. J. Aust.* **1974**, *1*(12), 457.
239. Andrews, J. W.; Davis, J. M. *Feedstuffs* **1979**, Jan. 15, 33.
240. Hill, C. H. *Fed. Proc. Fed. Am. Soc. Exp. Biol.* **1980**, *39*, 396.
241. Berg, L. R.; Lawrence, W. W. *Poult. Sci.* **1971**, *50*, 1399.
242. Chatterjee, G. C.; Banerjee, S. K.; Pal, D. R. *Int. J. Vitam. Nutr. Res.* **1973**, *43*, 370.
243. Spivey Fox, M. R.; Fry, B. E., Jr. *Science* **1970**, *169*(3949), 989.
244. Spivey Fox, M. R.; Fry, B. E., Jr.; Harland, B. F.; Schertel, M. E.; Weeks C. E. *J. Nutr.* **1971**, *101*, 1295.
245. Matkovics, B.; Barabas, K.; Szabo, L.; Berencsi, C. *Gen. Pharmacol.* **1980**, *11*(5), 455.

246. Kallistratos, G.; Fasske, E. *J. Cancer, Res. Clin. Oncol.* **1980**, 97(1), 91–96.
247. Kratzing, C. C.; Willis, R. J. *Chem. Biol. Interact.* **1980**, 30(1), 53.
248. Free, V.; Sanders, P. *J. Psychedelic Drugs* **1979**, 11(3), 217.
249. Hamdy, M. K.; May, K. N.; Powers, J. J.; Pratt, D. E. *Proc. Soc. Exp. Biol. Med.* **1961**, 108, 189.
250. Szepesy, A.; Keseru, P. *Acta Pharm. Hung.* **1966**, 36, 264.
251. Maly, J.; Starho, L. *Cesk. Farm.* **1967**, 16, 345.
252. Kedvessy, G.; Keresztes, A.; Selmeczi, B. *Zentralblat. Pharm. Pharmakother. Laboratoriumsdiagn* **1971**, 110, 3.
253. Abbott Laboratories British Patent 1 270 781, 1972.
254. Asker, A. F.; Saied, K. M.; Abdel-Khalck, M. M. *Pharmazie* **1975**, 30, 463.
255. Abd-Elbary, A.; Kandil, F. *Bull. Fac. Pharm., Cairo Univ.* **1975**, 12(1), 1.
256. Chalabala, M. *Acta Fac. Pharm. Univ. Comenianae* **1975**, 27(5), 7.
257. Nürnberg, E.; Bleimüller, G. *Dsch. Apoth. Ztg.* **1977**, 117, 460.
258. Seth, S. K.; Mital, H. C. *Indian J. Pharm.* **1965**, 27, 119.
259. Lee, S.; Dekay, G. H.; Banker, G. S. *J. Pharm. Sci.* **1965**, 54, 1153.
260. Wortz, R. B. *J. Pharm. Sci.* **1967**, 56, 1169.
261. Sabri, M. I.; Rao, V. K. M. *Indian J. Technol.* **1966**, 4, 191.
262. Trivedi, B M..; Patel, N. J. *Indian J. Pharm.* **1971**, 33, 15.
263. Pelletier, O. *Can. J. Pharm. Sci.* **1973**, 8, 103.
264. Anantha-Narayana, D. B.; Khare, R. L. *Indian J. Pharm.* **1975**, 37, 46.
265. Shah, D. H.; Arambule, A. S. *Drug. Dev. Commun.* **1975**, 1, 495.
266. Faguet, J. R.; Duchene, E.; Puisieux, F. *Pharm. Acta. Helv.* **1975**, 50, 251.
267. Khana, S.; Sharma, S. N. *Indian J. Hosp. Pharm.* **1974**, 11, 111.
268. Ibid., 138.
269. Kassem, A.; Said, S.; El-Bassouni, S. *Manuf. Chem. Aerosol News* **1975**, 46, 53.
270. Chapman, D. G.; Crisafio, R.; Campbell, J. A. *J. Am. Pharm. Assoc., Sci. Ed.* **1954**, 43, 297.
271. Morrison, A. B.; Chapman, D. G.; Campbell, J. A. *J. Am. Pharm. Assoc., Sci. Ed.* **1954**, 48, 634.
272. Middleton, E. J.; Davies, J.; Morrison, A. B. *J. Pharm. Sci.* **1965**, 54, 1.
273. Ida, T.; Takahashi, S.; Noda, K.; Kishi, S.; Nakagami, S.; Utsumi, I. *J. Pharm. Sci.* **1963**, 52, 472.
274. Allen, E. S. *Curr. Ther. Res., Clin. Exp.* **1969**, 11, 745.
275. DeRitter, E.; Magid, L.; Osadca, M.; Rubin, S. H. *J. Pharm. Sci.* **1970**, 59, 229.
276. Rubin, S. H.; DeRitter, E.; Johnson, J. B. *J. Pharm. Sci.* **1976**, 65(7), 963.
277. Blaug, S. M.; Hajratwala, B. *J. Pharm. Sci.* **1972**, 61(4), 556.
278. Rogers, A. R.; Yacomeni, J. A. *J. Pharm. Pharmacol.* **1971**, 23, Suppl. 218S.
279. Finholt, P.; Paulssen, R. B.; Higuchi, T. *J. Pharm. Sci.* **1963**, 52(10), 948.
280. Finholt, P.; Kristiansen, H.; Krowczynski, L.; Higuchi, T. *J. Pharm. Sci.* **1966**, 55(12), 1435.
281. Bielski, B. H. J.; Comstock, D. A.; Bowen, R. A. *J. Am. Chem. Soc.* **1971**, 93(22), 5624.
282. Kirino, Y.; Kuan, T. *Chem. Pharm. Bull.* **1971**, 19(4), 718, 831; **1972**, 20(12), 2651.
283. Schoeneshoefer, M. *Z. Naturforsch. Teil B* **1972**, 27(6), 649.
284. Bielski, B. H. J.; Allen, A. O. *J. Am. Chem. Soc.* **1970**, 92, 3793.
285. Laroff, G. P.; Fessenden, R. W.; Schuler, R. H. *J. Am. Chem. Soc.* **1972**, 94, 26.

286. Bielski, B. H. J.; Richter, H. W. *Ann. N.Y. Acad. Sci.* **1975**, *258*, 231.
287. Katz, M.; Westley, J. *J. Biol. Chem.* **1979**, *254*(18), 9142.
288. Hand, D. B.; Guthrie, E. S.; Sharp, P. F. *Science* **1938**, *87*, 439.
289. Guttman, D. E.; Brooke, D. *J. Am. Pharm. Assoc. Sci. Ed.* **1963**, *52*, 941.
290. Newmark, H. L., U.S. Patent 2 823 167, 1958.
291. Delgado, J. N.; Lofgren, F. V.; Burlage, H. M. *Drug Stand.* **1958**, *26*, 51.
292. Jager, H. *Pharmazie* **1948**, *3*, 536.
293. Kassem, M. A.; Kassem, A. A.; Ammar, H. O. *Pharm. Acta Helv.* **1972**, *47*, 89.
294. Scheindlin, S. *Drug and Cosmetic Ind.* **1958**, *83*, 46.
295. Porikh, B. D.; Lofgren, F. V. *Drug Stand.* **1958**, *26*, 56.
296. Kato, Y., *Yakuzaigaku* **1965**, *25*, 131.
297. Baudelin, F. J.; Tuschhoff, J. V. *J. Am. Pharm. Assoc., Sci. Ed.* **1955**, *44*, 241.
298. Poust, R. I.; Colaizzi, J. L. *J. Pharm. Sci.* **1968**, *57*, 2119.
299. Fabrizi, G.; Galloni, M.; Lotti, B.; Vezzosi, O. *Boll. Chim. Farm.* **1971**, *110*, 726.
300. Nixon, J. R.; Chawla, B. P. S. *J. Pharm. Pharmacol.* **1965**, 558.
301. Tanaka, I.; Otani, S. *Yakuzaigaku* **1962**, *22*, 150.
302. Otani, S. *Yakuzaigaku* **1963**, *23*, 138.
303. Ibid., **1964**, *24*, 59.
304. Paker, E. A.; Boomer, R. J.; Bell, S. C. *Bull. Parenteral Drug Assoc.* **1967**, *21*, 197.
305. Saikovska, Y. R.; Gnidets, I. R.; Pruts, V. M. *Farm. Zh.* **1967**, *22*, 42.
306. Kassem, M. A.; Kassem, A. A.; Ammar, H. O. *Pharm. Acta Helv.* **1969**, *44*(10), 611.
307. Akers, M. J.; Lach, J. L. *J. Pharm. Sci.* **1976**, *65*, 216.
308. West, K. R.; Sansom, L. N.; Cosh, D. G.; Thomas, M. P. *Pharm. Acta. Helv.* **1976**, *51*, 19.
309. Gupta, V. D. *Am. J. Hosp. Pharm.* **1977**, *34*, 446.
310. Bauernfeind, J. C. *Proc., SOS/70, Int. Congr. Food Sci. Technol., 3rd* **1970**, 217.
311. Bauernfeind, J. C. *Adv. Food Res.* **1953**, *4*, 359.
312. Bauernfeind, J. C.; Pinkert, D. M. *Adv. Food Res.* **1970**, *18*, 219.
313. Napier, C. E. *Austr. Chem. Inst. J. Proc.* **1946**, *13*, 19.
314. Klaeui, H. In "Vitamin C: Recent Aspects of Its Physiological and Technological Importance" Birch, G. G.; Parker, K. J., Eds., John Wiley & Sons: N.Y. 1974; pp. 16–30.
315. Ammon, R. *Wiss. Veroeff. Dsch. Ges. Ernaehr.* **1965**, *14*, 206.
316. Klaeui, H. *Symp. Rancidity in Fatty Foods, Univ. Technology, Loughborough IFST, Proc.* **1973**, *6*, 195.
317. Klaeui, H. *Proc. Int. Congr. Food Sci. Technol. 4th,* **1974**, *1*, 740.
318. Bauernfeind, J. C. *Symp. Fruchtsaft-Konzentrate, Bristol, England* **1958**, 159–185.
319. Birch, G. G.; Bointon, B. M.; Rolfe, E. J.; Selman, J. D. In "Vitamin C: Recent Aspects of Its Physiological and Technological Importance"; Birch, G. G.; Parker, K. J., Eds.; John Wiley & Sons: N.Y., 1974; pp. 161–166.
320. Szotyari-Lindnerne, K., *Elelmez Ipar.* **1973**, *27*, 161.
321. Klaeui, H., *Proc. Univ. Nottingham Resid. Semin. on Vitam.* **1971**, 110–143.
322. Gresswell, D. M. In "Vitamin C: Recent Aspects of Its Physiological and Technological Importance"; Birch, G. G.; Parker, K. J., Eds.; John Wiley & Sons: N.Y., 1974; pp. 136–149.
323. Henshall, J. D. In "Vitamin C: Recent Aspects of Its Physiological and Technological Importance"; Birch, G. G., Parker, K. J., Eds.; John Wiley & Sons: N.Y., 1974; pp. 104–120.

324. Rankin, M. D. In "Vitamin C: Recent Aspects of Its Physiological and Technological Importance"; Birch, G. G.; Parker, K. J., Eds.; John Wiley & Sons: N.Y., 1974; pp. 121–135.
325. Thewlis, B. H. In "Vitamin C: Recent Aspects of Its Physiological and Technological Importance"; Birch, G. G.; Parker, K. J., Eds.; John Wiley & Sons: N.Y., 1974; pp. 150–160.
326. Newmark, H. L.; Mergens, W. J. *Proc. IUFOST Symposium, Einsiedeln, Switzerland 1979* (in press).
327. Watts, B. M. *Food Res.* **1954**, *5*, 1.
328. Lueck, E. *Food Process. Indust.* **1969**, *38*(459), 53.
329. Klaeui, H. *Int. Flavours Food Addit.* **1976**, *7*(4), 165.
330. Bauernfeind, J. C.; Pinkert, D. M. In "Encyclopedia of Food Technology"; Johnson, A. H.; Peterson, M. S., Eds.; AVI: Westport, CT, 1974; pp. 67–75.
331. Webb, G. K. *Flavour Ind.* **1972**. Aug., 401.
332. Diemar, W.; Postel, W. *Wiss. Veroeffent. Dsch. Ges. Ernaehr.* **1965**, *14*, 248.
333. Bodannes, R. S.; Chan, P. C. *FEBS Lett.* **1979**, *105*(2), 195.
334. Lee, S. H.; Labuza, T. P. *J. Food Sci.* **1975**, *40*, 370.
335. Tatum, J. H.; Shaw, P. E.; Berry, R. E. *J. Agric. Food Chem.* **1969**, *17*(1), 38.
336. Kamiya, S. *Nippon Nogei Kagaku Kaishi* **1959**, *33*, 398.
337. Thompson, L. U.; Fennema, O. *J. Agric. Food Chem.* **1971**, *19*(1), 2.
338. Timberlake, C. F. *J. Food Sci.* **1960**, *11*(5), 258.
339. Singh, R. P.; Heldman, D. R.; Kirk, J. R. *J. Food Sci.* **1976**, *41*, 304.
340. Mizrahi, S.; Karel, M. *J. Food Sci.* **1977**, *42*, 958, and 1575; **1978**, *43*, 753.
341. Lee, Y. C.; Kirk, J. R.; Bedford, C. L.; Heldman, D. R. *J. Food Sci.* **1977**, *42*(3), 640.
342. Kirk, J. R.; Dennison, D.; Kokoczka, P., Heldmann, D. R. *J. Food Sci.* **1977**, *42*(5), 1274.
343. Dennison, D. B.; Kirk, J. R. *J. Food Sci.* **1978**, *43*, 609.
344. Report of the Committee on International Dietary Allowances of the International Union of Nutritional Sciences, *Nutrition Abstracts and Reviews.* **1975**, *45*(2), 89.
345. Del Monte Food Eng. **1975**, Nov., 31.
346. Flinn, G. L. *Diss. Abstr. Int. B* **1975**, *34*(5), 2080.
347. Pope, G. G.; Gould, W. A. *Food Prod./Mngt.* **1973**, *96*(5), 14.
348. Guy, E. J.; Vettel, H. E. *J. Dairy Sci.* **1975**, *58*, 432.
349. Dellamonica, E. S.; McDowell, P. E.; Campbell, R. B. *J. Dairy Sci.* **1979**, *62*, 499.
350. Anon. *Bios. (Madison, N.J.)* **1977**, *8*(10), 51.
351. Mrozewski, S. *Prezm. Ferment. Rolny* **1966**, *2*, 72.
352. Bright, R. A.; Potter, H. N. *Food Prod. Dev.* **1979**, *13*(4), 34–37.
353. Peter, A. *Fruchtsaft Ind.* **1966**, 11.
354. Fetter, F.; Stehlik, G.; Kovacs, J.; Weiss, S. *Mitte. Hoeheren Bundeslehr Versuchsanst. Weir-Obstbau, Klosterneuburg* **1969**, *19*(2), 140.
355. Kyzlink, V.; Hostasova, B. *Sb. Vys. Sk. Chem.-Technol. Praze, Anal. Chem.* **1970**, *28*, 131.
356. Beston, G. H.; Henderson, G. A. *Can. Inst. Food Sci. Technol. J.* **1974**, *7*(3), 183.
357. Robertson, J. M.; Sibley, J. A. *Food Technol. N. Z.* **1974**, *9*(10), 13.
358. Mahmoud, M. I. *Diss. Abstr. Internat. B* **1976**, *37*(5), 2142.
359. Svorkova, L. *Lebensm-Indust.* **1977**, *24*(4), 169.
360. Brin, M.; Bauernfeind, J. C. *Postgrad. Med.* **1978**, *63*(3), 155.
361. Gage, J. W. *Food Prod. Dev.* **1972**, *6*(7), 40.

362. Cancel, L. E.; deHernandez, E. R.; Rivera-Ortiz, J. M. *J. Agric. Univ. P. R.* **1976**, *60*(4), 478.
363. Pederson, C. S. *Adv. Food Res.* **1960**, *10*, 233.
364. Leverton, R. M. *Nutr. Rev.* **1964**, *22*, 321.
365. Remmers, P. A. J. F.; Booij, M. H.; Bergervoet, M. E. M. *Internat. Z. Vitamin Forschung* **1968**, *38*, 292.
366. Meyers, P. W.; Roehm, G. H. *J. Am. Diet. Assoc.* **1963**, *42*, 325.
367. Cording, J., Eskew, R. K.; Salinard, G. J.; Sullivan, J. F. *Food Technol.* **1961**, *15*, 279.
368. Bring, S. V.; Grassl, C.; Hofstrand, J. T.; Willard, M. J. *J. Am. Diet. Assoc.* **1963**, *42*(4), 321.
369. Bring, S. V.; Raab, F. P. *J. Am. Diet. Assoc.* **1964**, *45*, 149.
370. Bring, S. V. *J. Am. Diet. Assoc.* **1966**, *48*(2), 112.
371. Maga, J. A.; Sizer, C. E. *Lebensm.-Wiss. Technol.* **1978**, *11*(4), 192.
372. Ibid., 195.
373. Voirol, F. *Food Trade Rev.* **1974**, *44*(9), 7.
374. Somogyi, J. C.; Schiele, K. *Inter. Z. Vitaminforsch.* **1966**, *36*, 337.
375. Sweeney, J. P.; Hepner, P. H.; Libeck, S. T. *Am. Potato J.* **1969**, *46*, 463.
376. Peterson, D. C. Presented at the Meeting Inst. Food Technol., May, 1972.
377. Augustin, J.; McMaster, G. M.; Painter, C. G.; Sparks, W. C. *J. Food Sci.* **1975**, *40*, 415.
378. Franke, W. *Ernaehr. Umsch.* **1972**, *19*, 118.
379. Hawkins, W. W.; Leonard, V. G.; Armstrong, J. E. *Food Technol.* **1961**, *15*, 410.
380. Austin, J. E. "Report of Harvard Univ. to U.S. Agency for International Development, Office of Nutrition," 1977.
381. Anon. *Food Process.* **1975**, *36*(3), 54.
382. CoHon, R. H.; Allgauer, A. J.; Nelson, A. W.; Koedding, D. W.; Baldwin, R. R. *Cereal Sci. Today* **1971**, *16*(6), 188.
383. Seib, P. A.; Hoseney, R. C. *Baker's Dig.* **1974**, *48*(5), 46.
384. Quadri, S. F.; Liang, Y. T.; Seib, P. A.; Deyoe, C. W.; Hoseney, R. C. *J. Food Sci.* **1975**, *40*(4), 837.
385. Vojnovich, C.; Pfeifer, V. F. *Cereal Sci. Today* **1970**, *15*(9), 317.
386. Linko, P. *Suomen Kemistil. B* **1971**, *44*(2), 183.
387. Steele, C. J. *Cereal Foods World* **1976**, *21*(10), 538.
388. Gravani, R. B. *Cereal Foods World* **1976**, *21*(10), 528.
389. Quaker Oats British Patent 1 328 608, 1973.
390. Anderson, R. H.; Maxwell, D. L.; Mulley, A. E.; Fritsch, C. W. *Food Technol.* **1976**, *30*(5), 110.
391. Gage, J. *Snack Food* **1971**, *60*(80), 60.
392. Finch, C. A. *Hrana Ishrana* **1977**, 3–4, 12.
393. Basta, S. S. *Hrana Ishrana* **1977**, 3–4, 15.
394. Hallberg, L.; Baker, S. J.; Chichester, C. O.; Cook, J. O.; DeMaeyer, E. M.; Newmark, H.; Shapiro, H. L.; Tepley, L. J. *Pharm. Technol.* **1979**, Oct.
395. Sayers, M. H.; Lynch, S. R.; Jacob, P.; Charlton, R. W.; Bothwell, T. H.; Walker, R. B.; Mayet, F. *Br. J. Haematol.* **1973**, *24*, 209.
396. Sayers, M. H.; Lynch, S. P.; Charlton, R. W.; Bothwell, T. H.; Walker, R. B.; Mayet, F. *Br. J. Nutr.* **1974**, *31*, 367.
397. Sayers, M. H.; Lynch, S. P.; Charlton, R. W.; Bothwell, T. H.; Walker, R. B.; Mayet, F. *Br. J. Haematol.* **1974**, *28*, 483.
398. Derman, D.; Sayers, M.; Lynch, S. R.; Charlton, R. W.; Bothwell, T. H.; Mayet, F. *Br. J. Nutr.* **1977**, *38*, 261.
399. Disler, P. B.; Lynch, S. R.; Charlton, R. W.; Bothwell, T. H.; Walter, R. B.; Mayet, F. *Br. J. Nutr.* **1975**, *34*, 141.
400. Bjorn-Rasmussen, E.; Hallberg, L. *Nutr. Metab.* **1974**, *16*(2), 94.

401. Hegenauer, J.; Saltman, P.; Ludwig, D. *J. Dairy Sci.* **1979**, *62*, 1037.
402. Kiran, R.; Amma, M. K.; Sareen, K. N. *Indian J. Nutr. Diet.* **1977**, *14*, 260.
403. Stekel, A.; Olivares, M.; Amar, M.; Chadud, P.; Pizarro, F.; Lopez, I. *Symp. US-AMA Dept. Food and Nutr., Univ. Chile* **1978**, 416.
404. Stekel, A.; Olivares, M.; Lopez, I.; Pizarro, F.; Amar, M.; Chadud, F.; Llaguno, S. *Pediatr. Res.* **1980**, *14*, 74.
405. Johnson, P. E.; Evans, G. W. *Nutr. Rep. Int.* **1977**, *16*, 89.
406. Klug, S. L.; Patrizzio, F. J.; Einstman, W. J. U.S. Patent 4 006 263, 1973.
407. Layrisse, M.; Martinez-Torres, C. *Am. J. Clin. Nutr.* **1977**, *30*, 1166.
408. Viteri, F. E.; Garcia-Ibanez, R.; Torun, B. *Amer. J. Clin. Nutr.* **1978**, *31*, 1961.
409. Lee, S. *Tea Coffee Trade J.* **1974**, *146* (6), 6.
410. Morse, L. D.; Hammes, P. A. U.S. Patent 3 958 017, 1976.
411. Pelletier, O.; Morrison, A. B. *Can. Med. Assoc. J.* **1965**, *92*, 1089.
412. Phillips, M. B.; Wardlow, J. M. *Can. Med. Assoc. J.* **1967**, *97*, 1384.
413. Bullock, D. H.; Singh, S.; Pearson, A. M. *J. Dairy Sci.* **1968**, *51* (6), 921.
414. Anon. INACG Report "Guidelines for the Eradication of Iron Deficiency Anemia," Nutrition Foundation, New York, 1977.
415. Head, M. K.; Hansen, A. P. *J. Dairy Sci.* **1979**, *62*, 352.
416. Weinstein, B.; Lowenstein, M.; Olson, H. C. *Milk Plant Mon.* 37 (10), 116.
417. Anderson, H. C.; Thomas, H. C.; Thomas, E. I. "Abstracts of Papers," Dairy Sci. Assoc. Meet., June 23–26, 1974.
418. Cameron, D. J. *Food Chem.* **1978**, *3*, 103.
419. Joslyn, M. A.; Ponting, J. D. *Adv. Food Res.* **1950**, *3*, 1.
420. Bauernfeind, J. C.; Jahns, F. W.; Smith, E. G.; Siemers, G. F. *Fruit Prod. J. Am. Food Manuf.* **1946**, *25*, 324.
421. Bauernfeind, J. C.; Smith, E. G.; Siemers, G. F. *Fruit Prod. J. Am. Food Manuf.* **1947**, *27*, 68.
422. Reeve, R. M. *Food Res.* **1953**, *18*, 604.
423. Ponting, J. D.; Jackson, R.; Watters, G. *J. Food Sci.* **1972**, *37* (3), 434.
424. Luther, H. G.; Cragwell, G. O. *Food Ind.* **1946**, *18*, 690.
425. Ponting, J. D.; Jackson, R. *J. Food Sci.* **1972**, *37* (6), 812.
426. Ulrich, R.; Delaporte, N. *Ann. Nutr. Aliment.* **1970**, *24* (3), B287.
427. Heaton, E. K.; Boggess, T. S.; Li, K. C. *Food Technol.* **1969**, *23* (7), 956.
428. Senina, E. P. *Intensif. Sadovod.* **1974**, 182.
429. Nicotra, A.; Fideghelli, C.; Crivelli, G. *Ann. Inst. Sper. Vallorizzazione Technol. Prod. Agric.* **1971**, *2*, 147.
430. Pech, J. C.; Fallot, J. *Ann. Technol. Agric.* **1972**, *21* (1), 81.
431. Rouet-Mayer, M. A.; Philippon, J. *Proc., Int. Congr. Food Sci. Technol., 4th* **1974**, *1b*, 89.
432. Eid, K.; Holfelder, E. *Erwerbsobstbau* **1973**, *15* (4), 55.
433. Kats, Z. A.; Rysin, A. B.; Shetsova, E. A. *Konser. Ovoshch. Prom.* **1971**, *7*, 15.
434. Sanchez-Nieva, F.; Hernandez, I. *J. Agric. Univ. P. R.* **1977**, *61* (3), 354.
435. Bates, R. P. *Proc. Fl. State Hort. Soc.* **1968**, *81*, 230.
436. Halim, D. H.; Montgomery, M. W. *J. Food Sci.* **1978**, *43* (2), 603.
437. Hudson, M. A.; Holgate, M. E.; Gregory, M. E.; Pickford, E. *J. Food Technol.* **1975**, *10* (6), 689.
438. Sarhan, M. A. I.; ElWakeil, F. A.; Morsi, M. K. S.; Sudan, J. *Food Sci. Technol.* **1971**, *3*, 41.
439. Tressler, D. K.; Joslyn, M. A. "Fruit and Vegetable Processing"; AVI: Westport, CT, 1961.
440. Bauernfeind, J. C.; Batcher, O. M.; Shaw, P. *Glass Packer* **1947**, *26* (4), 268; *26* (5), 358.
441. Hope, G. W. *Food Technol.* **1961**, *15*, 548.

442. Montgomery, M. W.; Petropakis, H. J. *J. Food Sci.* **1980**, *45*, 1090.
443. Payumo, E. M.; Pilac, L. M.; Maiquis, P. L. *Philipp. J. Sci.* **1968**, *97*(2), 127.
444. Kelly, S. H.; Finkle, B. J. *Am. J. Enol. Viti.* **1969**, *20*(4), 221.
445. Anon. *Quick Frozen Foods* **1971**, *33*(9), 109.
446. Choi, K. S.; Han, P. J.; Suh, K. B.; Yun, J. H. *Nongsa Sihom Yongu Pogo* **1969**, *12*(6), 55.
447. Berezovskaya, N. N.; Brumshtein, V. D.; Tishko, G. M. *Tr. Vses. Nauchno-Issled Inst. Konservn. Ovoshchesush. Prom.* **1974**, *21*, 6.
448. Pilnik, W.; Piek-Faddegon, M. *Schweiz. Z Obst Weinbau* **1970**, *106*(6), 133.
449. Huelin, F. E.; Coggiola, I. M.; Sidhu, G. S.; Kennett, B. H. *J. Sci. Food Agric.* **1971**, *22*, 540.
450. Anon., *Rev. Conserve Alim. Moderne* **1962**, 1.
451. Yourga, F. J. *Food Ind.* **1948**, *20*, 47.
452. U.S. Patent 3 894 157, 1975.
453. Bano, Z.; Singh, N. S. *J. Food Sci. Technol.* **1972**, *9*(1), 13.
454. Ueno, S.; Ohmura Y. Japanese Patent 7 310 223, 1973.
455. Varoquaux, P.; Sarris, J. *Lebensm. Wiss. Technol.* **1979**, *12*(6), 318.
456. Chandler, B. V. *J. Sci. Food Agric.* **1964**, *16*, 11.
457. Gstirner, F.; Saad, S. N. I. *Z. Lebensm.-Unter.-Forschung* **1959**, *110*, 9.
458. Mori, H. *Eiyo To Shokuryo* **1956**, *9*, 41.
459. Chen, L. M.; Peng, A. C. *J. Food Sci.* **1980**, *45*(6), 1556.
460. Tarr, H. L. A. *Fish. Res. Board Can. Prog. Rep. Pac. Coast Stn.* **1946**, *66*, 17.
461. Tarr, H. L. A.; Southcott, B. A.; Bissett, H. M. *Fish. Res. Board Can. Prog. Rep. Pac. Coast Stn.* **1951**, *88*, 67.
462. Andersson, K.; Danielson, C. E. *Food Technol.* **1961**, *15*, 55.
463. Jadhav, M. G.; Magar, N. G. *Fish. Technol.* **1970**, *7*(2), 146.
464. Japanese Patent 16941, 1971.
465. Menillo, J. J. French Patent 2 142 881, 1973.
466. Moody, M. W.; Novak, A. F. *Diss. Abstr. Int. B* **1974**, *35*(2), 880.
467. Alsina, L. U.S. Patent 3 859 450, 1975.
468. Tozawa, H.; Sato, K. *Bull. Jpn. Soc. Sci. Fish.* **1974**, *40*(4), 425.
469. Yoshinaka, R.; Shiraishi, M.; Ikeda, S. *Bull. Jpn. Soc. Sci. Fish.* **1972**, *38*(5), 511.
470. Moledina, K. N.; Regenstein, J. M.; Baker, R. C.; Steinkraus, K. H. *J. Food Sci.* **1977**, *42*(3), 759.
471. Baldrati, G.; Guidi, G.; Pirazzoli, P.; Vicini, E. *Ind. Conserve* **1974**, *49*(1), 10.
472. Deng, J. C. *J. Food Sci.* **1978**, *43*, 337.
473. Deng, J. C.; Matthews, R. F.; Watson, C. M. *J. Food Sci.* **1977**, *42*(2), 344.
474. Deng, J. C.; Watson, C. M.; Bates, R. F.; Schroeder, E. *J. Food Sci.* **1978**, *43*(2), 457.
475. Watts, B. W.; Lehmann, B. T. *Food Technol.* **1952**, *6*, 194.
476. Watts, B. W.; Lehmann, B. T. *Food Res.* **1952**, *17*, 100.
477. Brockmann, M. C.; Morse, R. E. *Proc. 5th Amer. Meat Inst. Res. Conf.*, *Univ. Chicago* 1953, 111–112.
478. Hollenbeck, C. M.; Monahan, R. *Proc. 5th Amer. Meat Inst. Res. Conf.*, *Univ. Chicago* 1953, 106–110.
479. Grau, R. *Wiss. Veroeffent. Dsch. Ges. Ernaehr.* **1965**, *14*, 262.
480. Grau, R. *Proc. Inst. Food Technol.* **1969**, *2*(2), 43.
481. Moehler, K. *Z. Lebesm.-Unters.-Forschung* **1970**, *142*, 169.
482. Ibid., **1972**, *147*, 123.
483. Frati, G. *Indust. Conserve* **1972**, *47*, 200.
484. Greenberg, R. A. *Proc. Int. Sym. Nitrite Meat Prod.*, *Zeist, Netherlands* **1973**, 179–188.

485. Gilmour, R. H. *IFST Proc.* **1973**, *6*(3), 163.
486. Giddings, G. G. *CRC Crit. Rev. Food Sci. Nutr.* **1977**, *9*(1), 81.
487. Gallert, H. *Fleischerei* **1971**, *22*(9), 43.
488. Koermandy, L.; Viragh, A. *Husipar* **1972**, *21*(4), 175.
489. Gallert, H. *Fleischerei* **1970**, *21*(7), 18.
490. Anon. *Fleischwirtschaft* **1978**, *58*(2), 230.
491. Luks, D.; Lenges, J.; Jacqmain, D. *Ind. Aliment. Agricol.* **1973**, *90*(5), 599.
492. Sharma, N.; Mahadevan, T. D. *Indian Food Packer* **1973**, *27*(6), 25.
493. Palmin, V. V.; Prizenko, V. K. *Izv. Vyssh. Uchebn. Zavend.* **1974**, *3*, 51.
494. Polymenidis, A. *Fleischwirtschaft* **1978**, *58*(4), 585.
495. Parolari, G.; Baldini, P.; Pezzani, G.; Farina, G. *Ind. Conserve* **1978**, *53*(2), 81.
496. Wirth, F.; Boehm, H.; Schmidt, M. *Fleischwirtschaft* **1973**, *53*, 363.
497. Brown, C. L.; Hedrick, H. B.; Bailey, M. E. *J. Food Sci.* **1974**, *39*(5), 977.
498. Olsman, W. J. *Proc. Int. Sym. Nitrite Meat Prod. Conf. Publ.* ISBN 90–220–0463–5, 1974, p. 129–137.
499. Frouin, A. *Ind. Aliment. Agricol.* **1978**, *95*(4), 285.
500. Mathey, R. *Fleischwirtschaft* **1979**, *59*(11), 1639.
501. Borenstein, B. B.; Smith, E. G. U.S. Patent 3 386 836, 1968.
502. Borenstein, B. *J. Food Sci.* **1976**, *41*, 1054.
503. Brendl, J.; Kyzlink, V.; Klein, S.; Davidek, J. *Sb. Vys. Sk. Chem.-Technol. Praze* **1971**, *32*, 173.
504. Ando, N. *Proc. Int. Sym. Nitrite Meat Prod., Zeist, Netherlands,* **1973**, 149–160.
505. Mori, K.; Akahane, Y.; Nakao, K.; Kawano, K. *Bull. Jpn. Soc. Sci. Fish.* **1973**, *39*(12), 1285.
506. Fox, J. B., Jr.; Nicholas, R. A. *J. Agric. Food Chem.* **1974**, *22*(2), 302.
507. Baird-Parker, A. C.; Baille, N. A. *Proc. Int. Sym. Nitrite Meat Prod., Zeist, Netherlands,* 1973, pp. 77–90.
508. Christiansen, L. N.; Johnston, R. W.; Kautter, D. A.; Howard, J. W.; Aunan, W. J. *Appl. Microbiol.* **1973**, *25*, 357.
509. Bowen, V. G.; Deibel, R. N. *Proc. Meat Inst. Res. Conf. AMIF, Chicago, IL, 1974; Abstr. Annu. Meet. Am. Soc. Microbiol.* **1974**, *74*, 13.
510. Bowen, V. G.; Cerveny, J. G.; Deibel, R. N. *Appl. Microbiol.* **1974**, *27*(3), 605.
511. Crowther, J. S.; Holbrook, R.; Baird-Parker, A. C.; Austin, B. L. *Proc. Int. Sym. Nitrite Meat Prod., 2nd, Unilever Res., Bedford, UK,* **1977**, 13–20.
512. Baldini, P.; Ambanelli, G.; Casolari, A. *Ind. Conserve* **1974**, *49*(3), 155.
513. Liu, H. P.; Watts, B. M. *J. Food Sci.* **1970**, *35*(5), 596.
514. Greene, B. E.; Hsin, I. M.; Zipser, M. W. *J. Food Sci.* **1971**, *36*(6), 940.
515. Unglaub, W. *Fleischwirtschaft* **1979**, *59*, 43–45, 72.
516. Harbers, C. A. Z.; Harrison, D. L.; Kropf, D. H. *J. Food Sci.* **1981**, *46*, 7.
517. Hopkins, E. W.; Sato, K. U.S. Patent 3 597 236, 1971.
518. Korschgen, B. M.; Baldwin, R. E. *J. Food Sci.* **1971**, *36*(5), 756.
519. Kwoh, T. L. *J. Am. Oil Chem. Soc.* **1971**, *48*(10), 550.
520. Hood, D. E. *J. Sci. Food Agric.* **1975**, *26*(1), 85.
521. Hood, D. E. *Ohio Farm Home Res.* **1975**, *6*(1), 9.
522. Hood, D. E. U.S. Patent 4 016 292, 1977.
523. Taluntais, A. F. British Patent 1 465 116, 1977.
524. Potthast, K.; Reise, K. H.; Reuter, H. *Feinkostwirtschafte* **1972**, *9*(9), 254.
525. Dawson, L. E.; Uebersax, M. A.; Uebersax, K. L. *Proc. World's Poultry Congr., 16th,* **1978**, *12*, 2009.
526. Kilgore, L. T.; Watson, K.; Kren, N.; Rogers, R. W.; Windham, F. *J. Am. Diet. Assoc.* **1977**, *71*(2), 135.

527. Magee, P. N.; Barnes, J. M. *Br. J. Cancer* **1956**, *10*, 114.
528. Sen, N. P.; Smith, D. C.; Schwinghamer, L.; Marldau, J. *J. Assoc. Off. Anal. Chem.* **1969**, *52*(1), 47.
529. Sen, N. P.; Smith, D. C.; Schwinghamer, L.; Howsan, B. *Can. Inst. Food Tech. J.* **1970**, *3*(2), 66.
530. Williams, A. A.; Timberlake, C. F.; Tucknott, O. E.; Patterson, L. S. *J. Sci. Food Agric.* **1971**, *22*, 431.
531. Telling, G. M.; Bryce, T. A.; Althorpe, J. *J. Agric. Food Chem.* **1971**, *19*(5), 937.
532. Fazio, T.; Damico, J. N.; Howard, J. W.; White, R. H.; Watts, J. O. *J. Agric. Food Chem.* **1971**, *19*(2), 250.
533. Ender, F.; Ceh, L. *Z. Lebensm. Unters. Forsch.* **1971**, *145*(3), 133.
534. Fiddler, W.; Doerr, R. C.; Ertel, J. R.; Wasserman, A. E. *J. Am. Off. Anal. Chem.* **1971**, *54*(5), 1160.
535. Singer, G. M.; Lijinsky, W. *J. Agric. Food Chem.* **1976**, *24*, 550.
536. White, J. W., Jr. *J. Agric. Food Chem.* **1975**, *23*(5), 887.
537. Mirvish, S. S. *J. Toxicol. and Environ. Health* **1977**, *2*, 1267.
538. Anon. *J. Am. Med. Assoc.* **1977**, *238*(1), 19.
539. Ibid., *216*(7), 1106.
540. Swann, P. F. *J. Sci. Food Agric.* **1975**, *26*, 1761.
541. Maga, J. A. *Crit. Rev. Food Sci. & Nutr.* **1978**, *19*(4), 373.
542. Scanlan, R. C. *Crit. Rev. Food Technol.* **1975**, *5*(4), 357.
543. Walter, C.; Manning, K. *Z. Lebensm.-Unters.-Forsch.* **1977**, *1965*, 21.
544. Mergens, W. J.; Vane, F. M.; Tannenbaum, S. R.; Green, L.; Skipper, P. L. *J. Pharm. Sci.* **1979**, *68*(7), 827.
545. Anon. *Chem. Week.* **1977**, Oct. 26, 16.
546. Mergens, W. J. *J. Am. Oil Chem. Soc.* **1980**, *57*, Abstr. 213.
547. Mergens, W. M.; DeRitter, E. *Cosmet. Technol.* **1980**, *2*(1), 34.
548. Mirvish, S. S.; Walcave, L.; Egan, M.; Shubik, P. *Science* **1972**, *177*, 65.
549. Greenblatt, M. *J. Natl. Cancer Inst.* **1973**, *50*, 1055.
550. Kamm, J. J.; Dashman, T.; Conney, A. H.; Burns, J. J. *Proc. Natl. Acad. Sci. U.S.A.* **1973**, *70*(3), 747.
551. Dashman, T.; Kamm, J. J.; Conney, A. H.; Burns, J. J. *Pharmacologist* **1973**, *15*, 261.
552. Kamm, J. J.; Dashman, T.; Conney, A. H.; Burns, J. J. *Proc. 3rd Meet. N-Nitroso Compds. Environ., Lyons* **1974**, 200–204.
553. Kamm, J. J.; Dashman, T.; Conney, A. H.; Burns, J. J. *Ann. N.Y. Acad. Sci.* **1975**, *258*, 169.
554. Kamm, J. J.; Dashman, T.; Newmark, H. L.; Mergens, W. J. *Toxicol. Appl. Pharmacol.* **1977**, *41*, 575.
555. Mergens, W. J.; Kamm, J. J.; Newmark, H. L.; Fiddler, W.; Pensabene, J. *Proc. 5th Mtg. N-Nitroso Compds. Environ., Lyons* **1978**, 199–212.
556. Fiddler, W.; Pensabene, J. W.; Piotrowski, E. G.; Phillips, J. G.; Keating, J.; Mergens, W. J.; Newmark, H. L. *J. Agric. Food Chem.* **1978**, *26*(3), 653.
557. Johnson, F. C. *Crit. Rev. Food Sci. & Nutr.* **1979**, *11*(3), 210.
558. Packer, J. E.; Slater, T. F.; Willson, R. L. *Nature* **1979**, *278*(5706), 737.
559. Jaeger, A. *Fleischerei* **1977**, *28*(9), 64.
560. Cassens, R. G.; Greaser, M. L.; Ito, T.; Lee, M. *Food Technol.* **1979**, *33*(7), 46.
561. Sebranek, J. G. *Food Technol.* **1979**, *33*(7), 58.
562. Herring, H. K. *Proc. Meat Ind. Res. Conf. Chicago* **1973**, 47–60.
563. Herring, H. K. *Proc. XIX Meet. Meat. Res. Workers, Paris* **1973**, *4*, 1517.
564. Mottram, D. S.; Patterson, L. S.; Rhodes, D. N.; Gough, T. A. *J. Sci. Food Agric.* **1975**, *26*, 47.
565. Greenberg, R. A. *Proc. Int. Sym. Nitrite Meat Prod., Conf. Publ.* ISBN 90–220–0463–5, **1974**, 179–185.
566. Walters, C. L.; Edwards, M. W.; Elsey, T. S.; Martin, M. *Z. Lebensm.-Unters.-Forsch.* **1976**, *162*, 377.

567. Mottram, D. S.; Patterson, R. L. S. *J. Sci. Food Agric.* **1977**, *28*, 352.
568. Woolford, G.; Cassem, R. G. *J. Food Sci.* **1977**, *42*(3), 586.
569. Ranieri, S. *Food Prod. Dev.* **1979**, *13*(10), 28.
570. Pensabene, J. W.; Fiddler, W.; Feinberg, J.; Wasserman, A. E. *J. Food Sci.* **1976**, *41*, 199.
571. Newmark, H. L.; Osadca, M.; Araujo, M.; Gerenz, C. N.; DeRitter, E. *Food Technol.* **1974**, *28*(5), 28.
572. Mergens, W. J.; Keating, J. F.; Osadca, M.; Araujo, M.; DeRitter, E. *Food Technol.* **1978**, *32*(11), 40.
573. Fiddler, W. J.; Pensabene, J. W.; Kushnir, I.; Piotrowsky, E. G. *J. Food Sci.* **1973**, *38*, 714.
574. Sen, N. P.; Donaldson, B.; Charbonneau, C.; Miles, W. F. *J. Agric. Food Chem.* **1974**, *22*(6), 1125.
575. Kasper, W. *Rev. Conserv Aliment. Moderne* **1977**, *51*, 43.
576. Mirna, A.; Spiegelhalder, B.; Eisenbrand, G. *Fleischwirtschaft* **1979**, *59*(4), 553.
577. Walters, C. L. In "Vitamin C: Recent Aspects of Its Physiological and Technological Importance"; Birch, G. G.; Parker, K. J., Eds.; John Wiley & Sons: N.Y., 1974; pp. 78–90.
578. Jorgensen, H. *Muehlenlaboratorium* **1935**, *5*, 114.
579. Anon. *Agrisearch Notes* **1976**, *24*(8), 15.
580. Elkassabany, M.; Hoseney, R. C.; Seib, P. A. *Cereal Chem.* **1980**, *57*(2), 85.
581. Maltha, P. *Getreide Mehl* **1953**, *3*, 65.
582. Grosch, W.; Weber; Mair, G. *Getreide, Mehl, Brot* **1978**, *32*(7), 175.
583. Boeck, D.; Grosch, W. *Z. Lebensm-Unters. Forsch.* **1976**, *162*(3), 243.
584. Mair, G.; Grosch, W. *J. Sci. Food Agric.* **1979**, *30*(9), 914.
585. Lillard, D. L.; Seib, P. A.; Hoseney, R. C., unpublished data.
586. Mann, D. L.; Morrison, W. R. *J. Sci. Food Agric.* **1975**, *24*, 493.
587. Grant, D. R.; Soot, V. K. *Cereal Chem.* **1980**, *57*(3), 231.
588. Tagliabo, G. *Tech. Molitoria* **1970**, *21*(24), 709.
589. Alexander, J. *Milling* **1971**, *153*(5), 48; *153*(6), 32; *153*(7), 33; *153*(8), 30.
590. Johannson, H.; Cooke, A. *Baker's Dig.* **1971**, *45*(3), 30.
591. Trenery, R. D. *Food Technol. N.Z.* **1971**, *6*(6), 31.
592. Ikezoe, K.; Tipples, K. H. *Cereal Sci. Today* **1968**, *13*(9), 327.
593. Johnston, W. A.; Mauseth, R. E. Canadian Patent 808590, 1969.
594. Dahle, L. K.; Murthy, P. R. *Cereal Chem.* **1970**, *47*(3), 296.
595. Coppo, V.; Genotti, G. *Ind. Aliment. (Pinerolo, Italy)* **1971**, *10*(11), 108.
596. Thewlis, B. H. *Ber. Getreidechem.-Tag., Detmold* **1972**, *7*(146), 23.
597. Schafer, W. *Bull. Anc. Eleves Ec. Fr. Meun.* **1972**, *252*, 271.
598. Cavel, R. *Bull. Anc. Eleves Ec. Fr. Meun.* **1974**, *263*, 250.
599. Ibid., 245.
600. Anon. *Muehle Mischfuttertechnik* **1974**, *111*(8), 109.
601. Chumachenko, N. A.; Markianova, L. M.; Demchuk, A. P.; Roister, I. M. *Khlebopek. Konditer. Prom.* **1974**, *5*, 17.
602. Bolling, H.; ElBaya, A. W.; Zwingelberg, H. *Getreide, Mehl, Brot* **1975**, *29*(3), 62.
603. Lehmann, G. *Gordian* **1976**, *76*(2), 36.
604. Westermarck-Rosendahl, C.; Junnila, L.; Koivistoinen, P. *Rev. Ferment. Ind. Aliment.* **1979**, *12*(6), 321.
605. Zentner, H. *J. Sci. Food Agric.* **1968**, *19*(8), 464.
606. Grant, D. R. *Cereal Chem.* **1974**, *51*(5), 684.
607. Morse, L. D.; Hammes, P. A. U.S. Patent 3 701 668, 1972.
608. Johnston, W. R.; Mauseth, R. E. *Baker's Dig.* **1972**, *46*(2), 20.
609. Palla, J-C.; Verrier, J. *Ann. Technol. Agric.* **1974**, *23*(2), 151.
610. Grosch, W. *Getreide, Mehl, Brot*, **1975**, *29*(11), 273.
611. Elkassabany, M.; Hoseney, R. C. *Cereal Chem.* **1980**, *57*(2), 88.

612. Giacanelli, E. *Ind. Aliment. (Pinerolo, Italy)* 1972, *11*(5), 93.
613. Moss, R. *Cereal Sci. Today* 1974, *19*(12), 557.
614. Moss, R. *Cereal Food World* 1975, *29*(6), 289.
615. Schuler, P. *Lebensm.-Wiss. Technologie* 1979, *12*(3), 13.
616. Grandvoinnet, P.; Berger, M. *Ind. Aliment. Agric.* 1979, *96*(9), 941.
617. Berger, M.; Grandvoinnet, P. *Ann. Technol. Agric.* 1979, *28*(3), 273.
618. Maureth, R. E.; Johnston, W. R. *Baker's Dig.* 1968, *42*(5), 58.
619. Jelaca, S.; Dodds, N. J. H. *J. Sci. Food Agric.* 1969, *20*(9), 540.
620. Prihoda, J.; Hampl, J.; Holas, J. *Cereal Chem.* 1971, *48*(1), 68.
621. Marston, P. E. *Baker's Dig.* 1971, *45*(6), 16.
622. Popadich, K. A.; Kashcheeva, G. M.; Lipyuk, F. A.; Maslova, L. G. *Khlebopek. Konditer. Prom.* 1972, *16*(8), 10.
623. Roiter, I. M. *Kharchova Prom.* 1971, *1*, 29.
624. Tanka, Y.; Koyanagi, Y.; Kawaguchi, M. *Shokukir Kenkyusho Kenkyu Hokuku* 1975, *30*, 28.
625. Kamenetskaya, A. M. *Dokl TSK* 1971, 62.
626. Marston, P. E. *Cereal Sci.* 1966, *11*(12), 530.
627. Thewlis, B. H. *J. Sci. Food Agric.* 1971, *22*, 1.
628. Fowler, A. A. *Food Ind. S. Afr.* 1972, *24*(12), 3.
629. Tolley, Jr., J. H. *Baker's Dig.* 1971, April, 51.
630. Leach, P. *Baker's Rev.* 1976, *5*, 10.
631. Magoffin, C. D.; Finney, P. L.; Finney, K. F. *Cereal Chem.* 1977, *54*(4), 760.
632. Powell, A. G. *Food Eng.* 1977, *49*(5), 88.
633. Stenvert, N. L.; Moss, R.; Bond, E. E. *Getreide, Mehl, Brot* 1979, *33*(11), 302.
634. Kilborn, R. H.; Tipples, K. H. *Cereal Chem.* 1979, *56*(5), 407.
635. Hoseney, R. D.; Seib, P. A.; Deyoe, C. W. *Cereal Chem.* 1977, *54*(5), 1062.
636. Cantroll, S. L., Thesis, Univ. of Tennessee, 1979.
637. Abrol, Y. P.; Uprety, D. C.; Sinha, S. K. *J. Food Sci. Technol.* 1970, *7*(3), 159.
638. Dahle, L. K. U.S. Patent 3 503 753, 1970.
639. Walsch, D. E.; Youngs, V. L.; Gillen, K. A. *Cereal Chem.* 1970, *47*(2), 49.
640. Lingnert, H. *SIK Rapport* 1972, *319*, 1–58.
641. Pongracz, G. *Int. J. Vitam. Nutr. Res.* 1973, *43*(4), 517.
642. Cort, W. M. *J. Am. Oil Chem. Soc.* 1974, *51*, 321.
643. Kawashima, K.; Itoh, H.; Chibata, I. *Agric. Biol. Chem.* 1979, *43*(4), 827.
644. Ayano, Y.; Furuhashi, T.; Watanabe, Y. *Nippon Shokuhin Kogyo Gakkai-Shi* 1977, *24*(7), 372.
645. Japanese Patent 37 543, 1972.
646. Kim, H-L.; Kim, D-H. *Hanguk Sikp'um KwahaKhoe Chi* 1972, *4*(4), 245.
647. Bauernfeind, J. C. *Crit. Rev. Food Sci. Nutr.* 1977, *8*(4), 337.
648. Wilson, H. K.; Herreid, E. O. *J. Dairy Sci.* 1969, *52*(8), 1229.
649. Iveleva, E. A.; Kaurtseva, I. E.; Nikitina, K. A.; Pugach, G. O. *Tr. Vses. Nauch.-Issled. Inst. Konservervn. Ovoshchesush. Prom.* 1970, *136*, 210.
650. Sokolov, F. *Sb. Dokl. Mezhvuz. Konf. Moloch. Delu* 1971, 377.
651. Portmann, A. *Rev. Gen. Froid* 1971, *62*(11), 1043.
652. El-Hagarawy, I. S.; Tahoon, M. K. *Alexandria J. Agric. Res.* 1972, *20*(1), 97.
653. Hsu, H.; Hadziyev, D.; Wood, F. W. *Can. Inst. Food Sci. Technol. J.* 1972, *54*(4), 191.
654. Spurgeon, K. R.; Seas, S. W.; Gudeikis, A. E. *Food Prod. Dev.* 1973, *7*(5), 104.
655. Jha, Y. K.; Singh, S. *Indian J. Dairy Sci.* 1977, *30*(1), 1.

656. Stone, I.; Gray, P. P. *Wallerstein Lab. Comm.* **1956,** *19,* 287.
657. Napier, C. E. *Wallerstein Lab. Comm.* **1956,** *19,* 193.
658. Knorr, F. *Wiss Veroeffent. Dsch. Ges Ernaehr.* **1965,** *14,* 271.
659. van Ghelurve, J. E. A.; Williams, R. S.; Besko, O.; Brenner, M. M.; Canales, D. M.; Dono, J. M.; Feeley, R.; Garza, A. C.; Hoover, D.; Stone, I.; Skocic, G. P.; West, D. B.; Grants, C. S. *Proc. Am. Soc. Brew. Chem.* **1969,** 156.
660. van Ghelurve, J. E. A.; Valyi, Z.; Dadie, M. *Brew. Dig.* **1970,** *45*(11), 70.
661. Anon. *Int. Brew. J.* **1970,** *106*(1254), 39.
662. Scriban, R.; Stienne, M. *Eur. Brew. Conv. Proc. Congr.* **1971,** *13,* 393.
663. Mitsuda, H. *Memo. Coll. Agric., Kyoto Univ.* **1971,** *100,* 1.
664. Postel, W. *Brauwissenschaft* **1972,** *25*(7), 196.
665. Cerutti, G.; Zappavigna, R.; Semenza, F. *Sci. Technol. Aliment.* **1973,** *3*(2), 111.
666. Baetsle, G. *Voedingsmiddelentechnologie* **1974,** *7*(38), 6.
667. Komornicka, W. *Przem. Ferment. Rolny* **1974,** *18*(8), 5.
668. Baetsle, G. *Fermentatio* **1974,** *70*(1), 23; *70*(2), 83.
669. Mastor, S.; Surminski, J.; Glowinski, B. *Przlm. Ferment. Rolny* **1975,** *19*(2), 4.
670. Franzy, M. *Ann. Technol. Agric.* **1959,** *8,* 285.
671. Kielhoefer, E.; Wuerdig, G. *Weinberg Keller* **1958,** *5,* 644.
672. Peynaud, E. *C.R. Acad. Agric. Fr.* **1961,** *47,* 67.
673. Tanner, H. *Wiss. Veroefft. Dsch. Ges. Ernaehr.* **1965,** *14,* 229.
674. Brun, P.; Mainguy, P. *Riv. Viti. Enol.* **1964,** *17*(2), 73.
675. Orechkina, A. E. *Bull. OIV* **1971,** *44*(481), 240.
676. Vieira, M. *Bull. OIV* **1971,** *44*(488), 926.
677. Lupadatu, Y. *Bull. OIV* **1971,** *44*(488), 928.
678. Wuerdig, G. *Bull. OIV* **1971,** *44*(488), 932.
679. Peynaud, E. *Vini Ital.* **1969,** *11*(61), 283.
680. Merzhanian, A. A.; Tagunkov, Yu. D. *Izv. Vyssh. Uchebn. Zaved. Pishch. Tekhnol.* **1969,** *6,* 77.
681. Hermandaz, M. R. *Semana Vitivinicola* **1973,** *28*(1380), 167.
682. Ferenczi, S.; Kerenyi, Z. *Borgazdasag* **1973,** *21*(2), 65.
683. Ivanova, I. P.; Belova, V. K.; Bastannaya, I. I. *Sadovod. Vinograd. Vinodel. Mold.* **1974,** *29,* 31.
684. Mueller, H. P. West German Patent 1 517 866, 1969.
685. Warkentin, H. U.S. Patent 3 518 089, 1970.
686. Otsuka, K.; Totsuka, A.; Ito, M.; Miyazaki, K.; Mukoyama, H.; Kawamatsu, M.; Zenibayashi, Y. *Nippon Joz. Kyokai Zasshi* **1973,** *68*(7), 535.
687. Schenk, W.; Bach, H. P.; Hoffmann, P. *Alkohol-Ind.* **1979,** *115*(1–2), 19.
688. Svejcar, V.; Kynicky, F. *Acta Univ. Agric., Brno, Fac. Agro.* **1973,** *2*(3), 569.
689. Brown, M. S. *Am. J. Enol. Viti.* **1975,** *26*(2), 103.
690. Svejcar, V. *Vinohrad* **1975,** *13*(8), 185.
691. Mueller, T. *Alkohol-Ind.* **1977,** *113*(36/37), 993.
692. Noonan, J. In "Handbook of Food Additives", 2nd ed.; Furia, T. E., Ed.; CRC: Cleveland, Ohio, 1972; pp. 587–615.
693. Banerjee, S. K.; Mathew, T. V.; Mukherjee, A. K.; Mitra, S. N. *Res. Indust.* **1970,** *15*(1), 1821.
694. Eisenbrand, J. *Dsch. Lebensm-Rundsch.* **1973,** *69*(4), 167.
695. Yasui, Y.; Tani, Y.; Seto, M. *Hyogo-ken Eisei Kenkyusho Kenkyu Hokoku* **1974,** *9,* 29.
696. Schara, A.; Tsoumanis, A. *Mineralwasserzeitung* **1963,** *16,* 610.
697. Bellanca, N.; Leonard, W. J., Jr. In "Current Aspects of Food Colorants"; Furia, T. E., Ed.; CRC: Cleveland, Ohio, 1977; pp. 49–60.
698. Beattie, H. G.; Wheeler, K. A.; Pederson, C. S. *Food Res.* **1943,** *8,* 395.

699. Habib, A. T.; Brown, H. D. *Proc. Am. Soc. Hort. Sci.* **1956,** *68,* 482.
700. Daravingas, G.; Cain, R. F. *J. Food Sci.* **1965,** *30,* 400.
701. Sistrunk, W. A.; Cash, J. N. *Food Technol.* **1970,** *24,* 473.
702. Starr, M. S.; Francis, F. J. *Food Technol.* **1968,** *22*(10), 1293.
703. Starr, M. S.; Francis, F. J. *J. Food Sci.* **1974,** *38*(6), 1043.
704. Segal, B.; Dima, G. *Ind. Aliment.* **1969,** *20*(7), 357.
705. Ikawa, F. *Aichni-ken Nogyo Shikenj Nempo* **1973,** *14,* 1.
706. Muschiolik, G.; Schmandke, H. *Nahrung* **1978,** *22*(7), 637.
707. Pasch, J. H.; von Elbe, J. H. *J. Food Sci.* **1979,** *44*(1), 72.
708. Int. Flavors and Fragr. Inc. U.S. Patent 4132-793, 1979.
709. Bauernfeind, J. C.; Osadca, M.; Bunnell, R. H. *Food Technol.* **1962,** *16,* 101.
710. Klaeui, H., Manz, U. *Beverages* **1967,** *8*(1), 16.
711. Terasaki, M.; Mima, H.; Fujita, E. *Eiyo To Shokuryo* **1964,** *17,* 115.
712. Loeblich, K-R. West German Patent 1 492 746, 1969.
713. Artem'ev, B. V.; Arkhiptsev, N. E.; Chepurnoi, I. P.; Mazunin, V. V.; Soldunova, V. M. *Konservn. Ovoshchesush. Prom.* **1972,** *27*(5), 18.
714. Co, H.; Sanderson, G. W. *J. Food Sci.* **1970,** *35*(2), 160.
715. Corsiglia, P. French Patent 2 082 421, 1971.
716. Swiechowski, C. *Przegl. Piekarski i Cukierniczy* **1975,** *23*(1), 14.
717. Vandercook, C. E.; Borden, C. M. *Food Prod. Develop.* May 1973.
718. Ninomiya, T. *Eiyogaku Zasshi* **1975,** *33*(3), 139.
719. Jaeger, A. *Zucker-Suesswaren Wirtsch.* **1976,** *1–2,* 1.
720. Ilany, J. *Gordian* **1977,** *77*(1), 19.
721. Horubalowa, A.; Sonnenberg, J.; Matyjasek, K. *Przegl. Piekarski Cukierniczy* **1978,** *26*(6), 113.
722. Nesmeyanov, A. N.; Rogozhin, S. V.; Slonimsky, G. L.; Tolstoguzov, V. B.; Ershova, V. A. U.S. Patent 3 589 910, 1971.
723. Szent-Györgyi, A. E. U.S. Patent 3 026 208, 1962.
724. Nulli, E. German Patent 1 938 735, 1970.
725. Kominato, J. Japanese Patent 7 903 358, 1979.
726. Anon. *Med. Tribune* **1977,** Mar.
727. Arafa, A. S.; Chen, T. C. *Poult. Sci.* **1978,** *57*(1), 99.
728. Svorcova, A. L. *Lebensm.-Industrie* **1979,** *26*(4), 170.
729. Baldini, P.; Ambanelli, G.; Casolari, A. *Ind. Conserve* **1974,** *49*(3), 155.
730. Reddy, S. G.; Chen, M. L.; Patel, P. J. *J. Food Sci.* **1975,** *40*(2), 314.
731. Takeda, M.; Nakazato, A. *Nippon Jozo Kyokai Zasshi* **1976,** *71*(4), 273.
732. Takeda, M.; Nakazato, A.; Tsukahara, T. *J. Agric. Sci.* **1977,** *21*(1), 55.
733. Kobunski Chemical Industry Co. Japanese Patent 8340, 1959.
734. Takayama, G. *Kobunshi Kagaku* **1960,** *17,* 644.
735. Kurema Chemical Industry Co. Japanese Patent 16 591, 1960.
736. Kurema Chemical Works. British Patent 895 153, 1962.
737. Sheriff, A. I.; Santappa, M. *J. Polymer Sci. Part A* **1965,** *3,* 3131.
738. Buning, R.; Diessel, K. H.; Bier, G. British Patent 1 180 363, 1970.
739. Hayashi, S.; Iwase, K.; Hojo, N. *Polym. J.* **1972,** *3*(2), 226.
740. Tsuchida, E. Japanese Patent 7 320 884, 1973.
741. Shinohara, I.; Aoyagi, J. Japanese Patent 73 102 881, 1973.
742. Roll, H.; Wergau, J.; Dockhorn, W. German Patent 2 208 422, 1973.
743. Mehta, P.; Nair, G. P. Indian Patent 131 842, 1974.
744. Fischer, N.; Kemp, T.; Boissel, J.; Eyer, H. German Patent 2 427 385, 1974.
745. Brunold, M.; Wicht, P.; Vonalnthen, C. German Patent 2 503 453, 1975.
746. Reddy, G.; Nagabhushanani, T.; Santappa, M. *Curr. Sci.* **1978,** *47*(17), 620.
747. Sanchez, I. German Patent 2 028 363, 1970.
748. Nagabhooshanam, T.; Santappa, M. *J. Polym. Sci., Polym. Chem. Ed.* **1972,** *10*(5), 1511.
749. Dynamit-Nobel, A. G. Netherlands Patent 6 408 790, 1965.

750. Japan Syn. Chem. Ind. Co. Japanese Patent 10 593, 1962.
751. Kurema Chemical Industry Co. Japanese Patent 7493, 1960.
752. Sengoku, T.; Shinke, S.; Okuyama, S.; Naganuma, K. Japanese Patent 7 138 344, 1971.
753. Lueck, H. East German Patent 18 905, 1960.
754. Csuros, Z.; Gara, M.; Gyurkovics, I. *Acta Chim. Acad. Sci. Hung.* **1961,** *29,* 207.
755. Societe des Usines Chimiques Rhone-Poulenc. French Patent 1 486 471, 1967.
756. Imamura, T.; Koseki, T.; Ito, I.; Kitagawa, H.; Sakai, H. Japanese Patent 7 225 241, 1972.
757. Suzuki, Z.; Nakahama, F.; Ito, I.; Kitagawa, H.; Sakai, H. Japanese Patent 7 414 870, 1974.
758. Koseki, T. Japanese Patent 7 334 985, 1973.
759. Nayak, P. L.; Samai, R. K.; Nayak, M. C.; Dhal, A. K. *J. Macromol. Sci. Chem.* **1979,** *13*(2), 261.
760. Delzenne, G.; Toppet, S.; Smets, G. *Bull. Soc. Chim. Belg.* **1962,** *71,* 857.
761. Gezy, I.; Nasr, H. I. *Kolor. Ert.* **1970,** *12*(7–8), 138.
762. Sierocka, M.; Tomaszewska, H.; Baczynska, E. *Pr. Wydz. Nauk. Tech., Bydgoskie Tow. Nauk. Ser. A* **1971,** *2*(6), 77.
763. Shukla, J. S.; Misra, D. C. *J. Polym. Sci. Polym. Chem. Ed.* **1973,** *11*(4), 751.
764. Korolev, G. V.; Kondratieva, A. G.; Berlin, A. A. Russian Patent 173 941, 1965.
765. Delzenne, G.; Dewinter, W.; Toppet, S.; Smets, G. *J. Polymer Sci. Part A* **1964,** *2,* 1069.
766. Ishino, H.; Fujii, S. Japanese Patent 7 906 089, 1979.
767. Tahara, S.; Hashimoto, S. Japanese Patent 7 988 985, 1979.
768. Strubell, H. *Acta Chim. Acad. Sci. Hung.* **1959,** *21,* 467.
769. Kudaba, J.; Ciziunaite, E.; Alishauskiene, T. *Polim. Mater. Ikh. Issled. Mater. Resp. Nauchno-Tekh. Konf. 13th* **1973,** *13,* 303.
770. Misra, G. S.; Gupta, C. V. *India Makromol. Chem.* **1973,** *165,* 205.
771. Nakahira, T.; Shinomiya, E.; Fukumoto, T.; Iwabucchi, S.; Kojima, K. *Eur. Polym. J.* **1978,** *14*(4), 317.
772. Kudaba, J.; Ciziunaite, E.; Levina, N. *Chem. Chem. Technol.* **1978,** 1967.
773. Pattnaik, S.; Roy, A. K.; Baral, N.; Nayak, P. L. *J. Macromol. Sci., Chem.* **1979,** *13*(6), 797.
774. Yoshikawa, T.; Sakamoto, N.; Nagamori, T. Japanese Patent 7 462 533, 1974.
775. Akama, T.; Sakai, K. German Patent 2 749 639, 1978.
776. Ichikura, Y.; Maki, H. Japanese Patent 7 375 691, 1973.
777. Bunawerke Huels G.m.b.h. Belgian Patent 618 500, 1962.
778. Suzuki, O. Japanese Patent 7 318 181, 1973.
779. Gavurina, R. K.; Mitrofanova, A. V.; Dmitrieva, N. S. *Zh. Prikl. Khim.* **1958,** *31,* 1227.
780. Takeda Chemical Industries. Japanese Patent 15 393, 1961.
781. Suzuki, O. Japanese Patent 7 406 072, 1974.
782. Atobe, D.; Makino, N.; Imai, M. Japanese Patent 7 532 284, 1975.
783. Akaoka, T.; Watanabe, K. Japanese Patent 7 405 215, 1974.
784. Ayre, J. E.; Willeboorose, F. G. U.S. Patent 3 280 049, 1966.
785. Leach, G. M. U.S. Patent 2 894 979, 1959.
786. Boyd, J. L.; Perry, R. D. U.S. Patent 3 199 589, 1965.
787. Kaneta, T.; Funai, H.; Suzuki, H. Japanese Patent 7 417 434, 1974.
788. Kojima, K.; Iwabuchi, S.; Nakahira, T.; Uchiyama, T.; Koshiyama, Y. *J. Polym. Sci., Polym. Lett. Ed.* **1976,** *14*(3), 143.
789. Nakahira, T.; Minami, C.; Iwabuchi, S.; Kojima, K. *Makromol. Chem.* **1978,** *179*(6), 1593.
790. Kamogawa, H. *J. Polym. Sci., Polym. Chem. Ed.* **1974,** *12*(10), 2317.

791. Maurer, K.; Zapf, G. *Photogr. Ind.* **1935**, *33*, 90.
792. Bills, C. E. *Science* **1935**, *81*, 257.
793. Itek, Corp. Netherland Patent 6 604 424, 1966.
794. Williams, L. A.; Lee, W. E. U.S. Patent 896 022, 1970.
795. Eastman Kodak Co. German Patent 2 145 414, 1972.
796. Fisch, R. S.; Newman, N.; Bexell, J. L. U.S. Patent 3 721 563, 1973.
797. Jacobs, J. H.; Corrigan, R. A.; Gaynor, J. U.S. Patent 3 826 653, 1974.
798. Nagae, T.; Iwano, H.; Shimamura, I. German Patent 1 772 378, 1975.
799. Katz, J. U.S. Patent 3 865 591, 1975.
800. Stjaenrukvist, O. N. British Patent 875 453, 1959.
801. Glasset, J. W.; Sutton, F. S. British Patent 875 878, 1958.
802. Societe Lumiere S.A. French Patent 1 258 356, 1960.
803. Kodak-Pathe French Patent 1 324 814, 1963.
804. Land, E. H.; Bloom, S. M.; Farney, L. C. German Patent 2 224 330, 1972.
805. Williams, J.; Gilman, P. U.S. Patent 3 730 721, 1973.
806. Kodak Soc., Anon. Belgian Patent 646 505, 1964.
807. Willems, J. F.; VanHoof, A. E. U.S. Patent 2 967 772, 1961.
808. Weyde, E. German Patent 946 327, 1956.
809. Fisch, R.; Newman, N. U.S. Patent 4 038 080, 1977.
810. Schellenberg, M.; Marthaler, M. German Patent 1 924 723, 1970.
811. Willis, R. G.; Pontius, R. B.; Ford, F. E. *Photogr. Sci. Eng.* **1970**, *14*(6), 384.
812. Pontius, R. B.; Willis, R. G.; Newmiller, R. J. *Photogr. Sci. Eng.* **1972**, *16*(6), 406.
813. Mason, L. F. A. German Patent 1 057 875, 1959.
814. Cohen, D. L.; McCauley, A. British Patent 1 131 096, 1968.
815. Yost, R. A.; Heidke, R. L. French Patent 2 005 772, 1969.
816. Tsubota, M.; Kato, K.; Yoshida, Y.; Yoshida, T. *Japanese Patent* 76 142 327, 1976.
817. Land, E. H.; Morse, M. M.; Farney, L. D. French Patent 1 579 011, 1969.
818. Lumoprint-Zindler, K. G. French Patent 1 510 383, 1968.
819. Branitskii, G. A.; Rakhmanov, S. K.; Ragoisha, G. A.; Sviridov, V. V. *Zh. Nauchn. Prikl. Fotogr. Kinematogr.* **1977**, *22*(6), 455.
820. Petrov, B. I.; Veidenbakh, V. A. *Zh. Nauchn. Prikl. Fotogr. Kimematogr.* **1972**, *19*(4), 264.
821. Bayol, R. M. A.; Knuz, P. M.; Pfaff, M. E. French Patent 2 109 249, 1972.
822. Brunold, M.; Vonlanthen, C.; Wicht, P. German Patent 2 421 859, 1975.
823. Ritzerfeld, W.; Ritzerfeld, G. German Patent 1 164 427, 1964.
824. Okutsu, E.; Iwano, H.; Nakanishi, I. German Patent 2 235 714, 1973.
825. Ebato, S.; Ito, N.; Uemura, S.; Oka, S. Japanese Patent 7 622 438, 1976.
826. Ijima, Y.; Shimamura, I.; Iwano, H. German Patent 2 113 587, 1971.
827. Prchal, G. L.; Kulus, R. W. British Patent 1 266 533, 1972.
828. Kobotera, K.; Ikenoue, S.; Mizuki, E.; Fujiuara, T. German Patent 2 250 308, 1973.
829. Leone, J. T. Belgian Patent 633 206, 1965.
830. Ozalid Group Holdings Ltd. French Patent 2 315 528, 1977.
831. Van den Heuval, W. A.; Vanhalst, J. E.; Brinckman, E. W. German Patent 1 956 513, 1970.
832. Okubo, K.; Masuda, T.; Noguchi, J. French Patent 1 542 505, 1968.
833. Shuman, D. C.; James, T. H. U.S. Patent 869 012, 1969.
834. Borth, P. F.; McKeone, J. French Patent 1 494 622, 1967.
835. Cole, D. H. British Patent 1 133 577, 1968.
836. Cole, D. H. British Patent 1 133 576, 1968.
837. Berman, J. R.; Lieblich, I. U.S. Patent 3 402 109, 1968.
838. O'Neill, A. D.; Sutherns, E. A. British Patent 1 285 696, 1972.
839. Luckey, B. W.; Rasch, A. A. British Patent 984 157, 1965.

840. Newman, N.; Fisch, R. S. U.S. Patent 3 942 985, 1976.
841. Cassio Photographic Paper Co. Belgian Patent 619 110, 1962.
842. Ilford Ltd. Netherlands Patent 6 407 905, 1965.
843. Sviridov, V. V.; Kondrat'ev, V. A.; Ivanovskaya, M. I.; Gaevskaya, T. V.;
     Bezuevskaya, V. N. *Zh. Nauchn. Prikl. Fotogr. Kinematogr.* **1976,**
     21(5), 223.
844. Gol'dshtein, M. D.; Kondrat'ev, V. A.; Bagdasar'yan, Kh. S. *Zh. Nauchn.
     Prikl. Fotogr. Kinematogr.* **1979,** *24*(2), 122.
845. Samitz, M. H.; Shraga, J. *Arch. Dermatol.* **1966,** *94*(3), 307.
846. Hanaki, A. *Kagaku No Ryoki, Zokan* **1976,** *113,* 53.
847. Kriss, E. E., *Zh. Neorg. Khim.* **1978,** *23*(7), 1825.
848. Ripan, R.; Pop, Gh.; Pop, I. *Rev. Roum. Chim.* **1974,** *19*(10), 1593.
849. Kusten, K.; Toppen, D. L. *Inorg. Chem.* **1973,** *12*(6), 1404.
850. Bhatt, K.; Nand, K. C. *Z. Phys. Chem.* **1979,** *260*(5), 849.
851. Rudenko, V. K. *Khim. Kinet. Kataliz.* **1979,** 109.
852. Ripan, R.; Pop, G.; Pop, I.; Nascu, C. *Rev. Roum. Chim.* **1977,** *22*(3),
     361.
853. Mushan, S.; Agraual, M. C.; Mehrotra, R. M.; Sanehi, R. *J. Chem. Soc.
     Dalton Trans.* **1974,** *14,* 1460.
854. Perman, C. A. *Talanta* **1979,** *26*(7), 603.
855. Castellucci, N. T. U.S. Patent 4 120 996, 1978.
856. Manning, John A. U.S. Patent 3 349 043, 1967.
857. Ceson, L. A. U.S. Patent 3 492 151, 1970.
858. Kobayashi, T.; Nakano, T.; Kishni, I. Japanese Patent 7 657 731, 1976.
859. Ogato, M. *Kinzoku Hyomen Gijutsu* **1974,** *25*(1), 20.
860. Kamiya, N.; Shinohaara, T.; Funada, K.; Imai, H. German Patent
     1 960 964, 1970.
861. Funada, K.; Shinohara, T.; Imai, H. Japanese Patent 7 317 384, 1973.
862. Lyubimora, M. K.; Savenkova, G. A.; Konevichev, B. N.; Girgori'eva,
     E. V. Russian Patent 206 265, 1967.
863. Khamaev, V. A.; Krivtsov, A. K. *Izv. Vyssh. Ucheb. Zaved., Khim.
     Khim. Tekhnol.* **1968,** *11*(3), 309.
864. Singh, V. B.; Tikoo, P. K. *J. Appl. Electrochem.* **1978,** *8*(1), 41.
865. Bielinski, J.; Przyluski, J. *Surf. Technol.* **1979,** *9*(1), 65.
866. Revyakin, V. P.; Katanaev, A. G.; Shefer, V. V.; Bastiani, E. E. Russian
     Patent 374 383, 1973.
867. Takasaki, H.; Sasaki, T.; Matsumoto, T.; Igarashi, T. Japanese Patent
     75 131 628, 1975.
868. Khamaer, V. A. Prom Obratztsy, Tovarnye Znaki Russian Patent 467 145,
     1975.
869. Tsuru, T.; Shimokawa, W.; Kobayashi, S.; Inui, T. *Kinzoku Hyomen
     Gijutsu* **1977,** *28*(5), 272.
870. Tsuru, T.; Ohba, K.; Kobayashi, S.; Inui, T. *Kyushu Sangyo Daigaku
     Kogakubu Kenkyu Hokoku* **1977,** *14,* 24.
871. Ziemba, V. F. U.S. Patent 3 923 554, 1975.
872. Miyosawa, Y. Japanese Patent 7 403 832, 1974.
873. Anon. *Europ. Chem. News* **1978,** Sept. 29, 24.
874. Castellucci, N. T. *Frankfurter Allgemeine* **1928,** *24,* 288.
875. Aizawa, Y.; Kashiwagi, H.; Takamura, S. Japanese Patent 7 593 241,
     1975.
876. Takeda Chemical Industries, Ltd. French Patent 1 489 249, 1967.
877. Hasunuma, K. Japanese Patent 7 486 554, 1974.
878. Kumiai, M.; Takahashi, Y.; Sato, H. Japanese Patent 75 117 945, 1975.
879. Ando, Y.; Tsuchiya, N. Japanese Patent 7 695 140, 1976.
880. Shubert, W. R.; Marshall, J. R. U.S. Patent 3 819 524, 1974.
881. Evers, H. C. A.; Fischler, M. Swedish Patent 367 319, 1974.
882. Iwao, S.; Tsuchiva, S. Japanese Patent 75 129 733, 1975.
883. Meisel, U.; Schiller, F. East German Patent 130 307, 1978.

884. Evers, H. C. A.; Fischler, M. German Patent 2 331 681, 1974.
885. Kraus, A.; Kraus, H. German Patent 1 142 676, 1963.
886. Keyes, P. H.; McCabe, R. M. *J. Am. Dent. Assoc.* **1973,** *86*(2), 396.
887. Curray, K. V. South African Patent 7007699, 1972.
888. Gati, T. Hungarian Patent 154 674, 1968.
889. Ozaki, Y.; Goi, H. Japanese Patent 7 028 918, 1970.
890. Selisskii, G. D.; Somov, B. A.; Ado, V. A.; Goryachkina, L. A. Russian Patent 552 083, 1977.
891. Aslan, A.; Polovrageanu, E. Romanian Patent 50 627, 1968.
892. Kop, M. H.; Quist, J. Netherlands Patent 7 314 699, 1975.
893. Cosmital Fribourg, S. A. German Patent 2 213 671, 1973.
894. Wolfram, L. J.; Hall, K. E. German Patent 2 021 099, 1970.
895. Takeda, I. Japanese Patent 75 119 781, 1974.
896. Interpal, S. A. German Patent 1 149 497, 1963.
897. Clairol International British Patent 995 948, 1965.
898. Chemitril, Inc. French Patent 1 498 572, 1967.
899. Sillo-Seidl, G. *Zentr. Gynaekol.* **1962,** *84*, 1662.
900. Ivanyuta, L. I. *Akush. Ginekol.* **1964,** *40*, 119.
901. Beutler, F. *Hered. Disord. Erythrocyte Metab., Proc. Symp.* Report 1, 1972.
902. Singh, G. B. *Indian J. Med. Sci.* **1974,** *28*(45), 219
903. Samitz, M. W. *Acta Derm. Venereol.* **1970,** *50*(1), 59.
904. Parups, E. V.; Chan, A. P. U.S. Patent 3 865 569, 1975.
905. Parups, E. V.; Chan, A. P. British Patent 1 383 272, 1975.
906. Belen-kü, S. M.; Leonova, V. G.; Klyachko, Yu. A.; Sergreeva, L. A. Russian Patent 501 978, 1976.
907. Saruwatari, Y.; Fukuda, M. Japanese Patent 77 111 846, 1977.
908. Davidson, A. N.; Howitt, F. O. *J. Text. Inst. Proc.* **1962,** *53*, 862.
909. Imai, S.; Hanyu, T. Japanese Patent 75 155 783, 1975.
910. Nakano, T.; Kato, T. Japanese Patent 76 116 835, 1976.
911. Haruta, Y.; Inoue, S. Japanese Patent 77 140 508, 1977.
912. Nakai, S. Japanese Patent 7 908 482, 1979.
913. Okada, H.; Takeuchi, M.; Mori, T.; Kamo, T.; Yamashita, T.; Kumagai, T.; Nakajima, F. Japanese Patent 78 146 284, 1978.
914. Mergens, W. J.; Newmrk, H. L. German Patent 2 506 100, 1975.
915. Burns, J. J. In "The Pharmeceutical Basis of Therapeutics", 4th ed.; Goodman; Gilman, Eds.; MacMillan: New York, 1970; pp. 1665–1671.
916. Libby, A. F.; Stone, I. *J. Orthomolecular Psych.* **1977,** *6*(4), 300.
917. Hauser, E.; Heiz, G. T. *Arch. Lebensmittelhyg.* **1980,** *31*(2), 43.
918. Chatterjee, J. B. *Science* **1973,** *182*, 1271.
919. DeChaletet, L. R.; Cooper, M. R.; McCall, C. E.; Shirley, P. S. *Proc. Soc. Exp. Biol. Med.* **1974,** *145*, 1170.
920. Free, V.; Sanders, P. *J. Orthomolecular Psych.* **1978,** *7*(4), 264.
921. Peynaud, E. *Wines Vines* **1961,** Nov.

RECEIVED for review April 16, 1981. ACCEPTED June 27, 1981.

Harvesting, Processing, and Cooking Influences on Vitamin C in Foods

JOHN W. ERDMAN, JR.
Department of Food Science, University of Illinois, Urbana, IL 61801

BARBARA P. KLEIN
Department of Foods and Nutrition, Bevier Hall, University of Illinois, Urbana, IL 61801

Vitamin C is considered the most labile of the vitamins in our food supply. Reduced ascorbic acid (RAA), which is the predominant form found in foods of plant origin, can be reversibly oxidized to dehydroascorbic acid (DHA). Further irreversible oxidation of RAA or DHA to diketogulonic acid or other products results in loss of biological activity. Oxidation can occur in the presence of metal catalysts, or plant oxidase enzymes, particularly following cell damage, or as a result of heat during food processing. Vitamin C is easily leached from foods during processing and is discarded with washing, soaking, or cooking water. Ascorbic acid losses begin with harvesting and continue through handling, industrial or home preparation, cooking, and storage of plant foods.

Vitamin C is widely distributed in the plant kingdom, particularly in fruits such as citrus, guava, tomatoes, strawberries, and black currants and in most vegetables, especially the green leafy vegetables. For a listing of the vitamin C contents of some selected fresh fruits and vegetables, *see* Table I.

The vitamin C activity of L-ascorbic acid or reduced ascorbic acid (RAA) and its oxidized form, dehydroascorbic acid (DHA) is essentially the same, while D-ascorbic acid (isoascorbic acid or erythroascorbic acid) has little of the vitamin's biological potency (*1*). The readiness with which RAA is reversibly oxidized to DHA is the basis of its physiological activity, and of its use as an antioxidant in food systems.

The aerobic oxidation of RAA (Figure 1) occurs rapidly when metal catalysts, particularly copper or iron, or enzymes such as ascorbic acid oxidase, polyphenol oxidase, peroxidase, and cytochrome oxidase are present. The anaerobic destruction of ascorbic acid may proceed by a variety of mechanisms that have been postulated (2,3) but not verified.

DHA can be reduced to RAA by chemical agents, such as hydrogen sulfide or enzymatically, by dehydroascorbic acid reductase. The conversion of DHA to diketogulonic acid (DKG) is irreversible and occurs both aerobically and anaerobically, particularly during heating. This reaction results in loss of biological activity. The total oxidation of RAA may result in the formation of furfural by decarboxylation and dehydration. With subsequent polymerization, the formation of dark-colored pigments results. These compounds affect the color and flavor of certain foods, such as citrus juices, and decrease nutritive value.

Because vitamin C is the most labile vitamin in our food supply, it is important to define those conditions that are particularly detrimental to maintaining optimal ascorbic acid content in foods. In this chapter we review the effects of genetic variation, environmental factors during growth, as well as harvesting, preparation, cooking, and storage practices upon the retention of vitamin C in foods "as consumed." Emphasis will be placed on those practices that adversely affect ascorbic acid retention in foods. No effort will be made to completely review the literature on the subject. However, review articles will be cited along with selected research papers. Sections are also included on assay methodology and kinetics of destruction of the vitamin.

Table I. Concentration of Ascorbic Acid in Selected Fresh Vegetables and Fruits

Fruit or Vegetable	Ascorbic Acid (mg/100 g)	Fruit or Vegetable	Ascorbic Acid (mg/100 g)
Kale	186	Kohlrabi	66
Collard	152	Strawberry	59
Turnip green	139	Spinach	51
Green pepper	128	Orange	50
Broccoli	113	Cabbage	47
Brussel sprout	109	Rutabaga	43
Mustard green	97	Apricot, peach, plum,	10 or less
Watercress	79	grape, apple, pear,	
Cauliflower	78	banana, carrot, lettuce, celery	

Source: Compiled by Salunkhe et al. (97) from various nutrition handbooks.

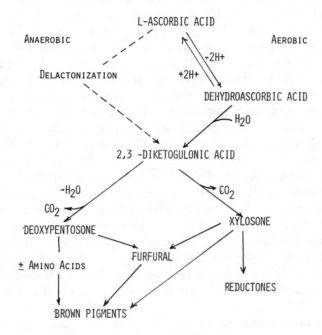

Figure 1.   Degradation of ascorbic acid.

Methodology for Determining Ascorbic Acid

The determination of ascorbic acid in foods is based, in part, on its ability to be oxidized or to act as a reducing agent. The most common method for determination of vitamin C in foods is the visual titration of the reduced form with 2,6-dichloroindophenol (DCIP) (4–7). Variations in this procedure include the use of a potentiometric titration (6), or a photometric adaptation (8) to reduce the difficulty of visually determining the endpoint in a colored extract. The major criticisms of this technique are that only the reduced vitamin, and not the total vitamin C content of the food, is measured, and that there can be interference from other reducing agents, such as sulfhydryl compounds, reductones, and reduced metals (Fe, Sn, Cu), often present in foods. The DCIP assay can be modified to minimize the effects of the interfering basic substances, but the measurement is still only of the reduced form. Egberg et al. (9) adapted the photometric DCIP assay to an automated procedure for continuous analysis of vitamin C in food extracts.

In most plant foods, the predominant form of ascorbic acid present is the reduced compound. Thus, the error introduced by the use of DCIP assay is considered negligible by some investigators (10). However, others have reported that during heat processing or storage, the amount of DHA increases substantially as percent of total ascorbic acid (TAA), and these workers suggest that DHA should not be neglected (11, 12). Brecht et al. (13) reported that ripe tomatoes contained negligible quantities of DHA, but green mature tomatoes had higher amounts. These factors should be considered in selection of assay method.

Determination of TAA can be performed by several methods. The official Association of Official Analytical Chemists (AOAC) method (7) is the microfluorometric assay developed by Deutsch and Weeks (14). In this procedure, RAA is oxidized to DHA using activated charcoal (Norit). The oxidized ascorbic acid is reacted with o-phenylenediamine (OPDA) forming a condensation product that fluoresces at 430 nm, following excitation at 350 nm. One of the disadvantages of the OPDA method is the development of fluorescing compounds from OPDA in the presence of light. Therefore, the procedure must be performed under reduced light conditions. Another complication may be the interference from DKG formed in the food prior to the assay as a result of processing and storage (15).

Several modifications of the OPDA procedure have been reported for automated analysis. Kirk and Ting (16) described a continuous flow analysis in which DCIP was substituted for Norit in the oxidation step. TAA and DHA can be determined directly; RAA is calculated as the difference between TAA and DHA. Good agreement between the manual and automated procedures was achieved, with a considerable decrease in analytical time for the automated assay. Kirk and coworkers (17–19) have used the continuous flow analysis for studies of the kinetics of ascorbic acid degradation in model systems.

Roy et al. (20) developed an automated procedure for fluorometric determination of TAA, DHA, and RAA in which N-bromosuccinimide was used for the oxidation step. This mild oxidizing agent selectively oxidizes RAA before other interfering reducing compounds. Also, N-bromosuccinimide does not react with reductones present in fruits and vegetables.

Egberg et al. (21) used Norit as the oxidant in a semiautomated total vitamin C determination, using a simultaneous oxidation and extraction step. DHA could be determined by omitting Norit in the extraction. The procedure was successfully used on a variety of foods; correlation with manual procedures was excellent.

The automated procedures, which enable the the operator to analyze many samples accurately, precisely, and rapidly, are particularly important in laboratories responsible for obtaining data for nutritional labeling. Dunmire et al. (*22*) compared the methods of Egberg et al. (*21*) and Roy et al. (*20*) with the manual AOAC visual titration and microfluorometric techniques. Forty products, including cereals, fruits, vegetables, baby foods, juices, and pet foods, were included in the study. For those samples exhibiting color interference, the titration method was not used. The results of this study indicated that for laboratories doing automated analysis of a wide spectrum of products, the procedure described by Egberg et al. (*21*) is the most widely applicable.

In the method of Roe and Kuether (*23*) suggested for total vitamin C determination (*6*), ascorbic acid is oxidized and reacted with 2,4-dinitrophenylhydrazine (DNPH). The osazone formed is extracted in sulfuric acid yielding a red solution whose intensity is proportional to the ascorbic acid concentration. Reductones and DKG may also form osazones, thus causing spuriously high vitamin C values (*24, 25*). The presence of DKG is believed to interfere to some extent with the OPDA method as well (*25*), although Egberg et al. (*21*) did not observe this. In addition Roe (*24*) noted that high concentrations of sugar can interfere with this analysis, but the sugar osazones decompose in the sulfuric acid if the preparation is allowed to stand. The interference by sugar can be compensated for by the addition of constant amounts of fructose and glucose to the standards (*11*). Pelletier and Brassard (*11*) suggested the use of a modified manual or automated DNPH procedure, based on a method designed for biological materials (*26*). Although the proposed automated assay is less tedious than Roe's manual assay (*24*) and as accurate, the long reaction times needed still make the DNPH procedure more time-consuming than the titration or fluorometric analysis.

A different method for determination of RAA, DHA, and DKG, based on the work of Roe et al. (*27*), has been used by some investigators (*12, 13, 28*). Total AA is determined by the DNPH method previously described, where the RAA is oxidized with Norit or bromine to DHA. DHA and DKG react with the DNPH to form the red osazones. To determine DHA and DKG, the extract is not oxidized, but is reacted directly with the DNPH. The RAA is determined by difference. Total DKG is measured by reducing the DHA in the extract to RAA, prior to osazone formation. In cases where it is suspected that a relatively large proportion of the RAA has been oxidized, either to DHA or DKG, as in the case of frozen fruits and vegetables (*12, 29*), the differential assay may be of use. However, for routine assays, the DCIP or microfluorometric assays, or a combination of the two will yield adequate information.

The use of high performance liquid chromatography (HPLC) has been proposed (*30–32*) but not widely applied. The interference of reductones, nonenzymatic browning compounds, and condensation products formed during processing and cooking of foods would be eliminated by an analytical technique, such as HPLC, specific for the various forms of ascorbic acid.

At this time, the selection of the method for determining ascorbic acid content requires some knowledge of the forms of vitamin C likely to be present in a given food product, the number of assays to be performed, and the spectrum of foods being assayed. In addition, the presence of interfering substances must be assessed.

Genetic and Environmental Factors

The ascorbic acid content of fruits and vegetables is markedly affected by variety, and to a lesser degree by maturity and climate. Increased exposure to sunlight and ripening on the plant generally enhances the vitamin C content of the edible portion. Ascorbic acid concentration within a fruit or vegetable often varies largely from part to part.

The variability of the naturally occurring nutrients, such as ascorbic acid, in fruits and vegetables has been a genuine concern to fruit and vegetable processors who have elected to participate in voluntary nutritional labeling programs (33). The large variation of vitamin C content due to genetic and environmental factors makes it necessary to reduce label claims to avoid over labeling.

Genetic Variation. The concentration of many individual nutrients in foods of plant origin is under genetic control. Baker (34) reviewed some examples of genetic manipulation that improved the quantity of β-carotene in tomatoes, methionine in beans, and lysine in corn. Variations of ascorbic acid content of different varieties of raw vegetables and fruits is notoriously high (35). Twofold variation in vitamin C concentration in different strains of a vegetable or a fruit is common and a fivefold variation can be found. Differences in ascorbic acid contents (35- to 300-fold) of different strains of a fruit were reported prior to 1950 (36). These reports have not been substantiated.

Stage of Maturity. In general, ascorbic acid concentration, but not necessarily total vitamin C content, decreases with maturity. Immature cabbage (37), citrus fruit (38), tomatoes (39, 40), and potatoes (41, 42) were reported to contain higher concentrations (mg/100 g of tissue) of ascorbic acid than when mature. However, there may be some varietal variation. For example, the H-1783 variety of tomatoes had higher vitamin C content when fully ripe than when green (Table II) (43). Although concentration decreased during ripening, the total content of vitamin C per citrus fruit tended to increase because of

**Table II.   Environmental Factors Affecting the Vitamin C
Content of the H-1783 Variety of Tomatoes**

Environmental Factor	Total Ascorbic Acid Concentration (mg/100 g)
Fully ripe, light foliage	23
Not fully ripe[a], light foliage	17
Fully ripe, heavy foliage	18
Fully ripe, heavy foliage, high nitrogen fertilization[b]	10

Source: Reference *43*.
[a] One week prior to fully ripe.
[b] Twice the amount for other treatments: 100 lbs/acre.

increased volume of juice and size of fruit (*38*). However, total vitamin C content of Russet Burbank potatoes gradually decreased after early harvest ($\sim$ 110 d) (*41, 44*).

Brecht et al. (*13*) harvested eight cultivars of mature-green and table-ripe tomatoes on the same day and found no differences in TAA concentrations. However, table ripe fruits were considerably higher in RAA than the mature-green fruits. Negligible quantities of DHA were found in ripe fruits.

Watada et al. (*45*) reported that RAA content was not significantly different in ripe or mature-green tomatoes. Ethylene-treated tomatoes were higher in ascorbic acid than untreated fruit but the differences could not be directly attributed to ethylene. The differences between cultivars were greater than those between maturity stages.

Betancourt et al. (*46*) found that in two varieties of tomatoes, plant-ripened fruit accumulated more (22%) RAA than did fruit ripened off the plant. Unfortunately, these researchers did not measure the total ascorbic acid content of tomatoes in their study. Pantos and Markakis (*47*) found that two cultivars of tomatoes contained 25–33% more total vitamin C when they were ripened on the vine rather than artificially. Conversely, Matthews et al. (*48*) reported that RAA of Walter tomatoes harvested at the green-mature stage and ripened off the plant was essentially the same as in those ripened on the plant. Thus, there may be varietal differences in this regard.

Most commercially grown fresh market tomatoes are harvested at the mature-green or partially ripe ("breaker") stages and are ripened off the plant. Further research should clarify the effect of stage of ripeness at picking on vitamin C content. Nearly all canned tomato products are prepared from field-ripened tomatoes so varietal variation, but not stage of ripeness, determines the vitamin C in processed products.

Climate. Climatic factors, principally temperature and amount of sunlight, have a strong influence on the composition of fruits and vegetables, especially ascorbic acid. Turnip greens, tomatoes (Table II), and strawberries (36) all had increased vitamin C concentration when grown with greater light exposure. Tests with nine varieties of apples showed that the side exposed to the sun was higher in ascorbic acid than the more shaded side (49). Sites and Reitz (50) removed all the oranges from a single Valencia tree and divided and assayed portions of each orange on the basis of their relation to the direction of sunlight exposure and the amount of light or shade (outside, canopy, inside) that was received. The authors found that ascorbic acid concentration was directly related to exposure of that portion of the fruit to sunlight.

Sunlight is not necessary for the synthesis of ascorbic acid in plants but is needed to produce optimal vitamin C concentrations. Photosynthesis produces the precursor hexoses needed for ascorbic acid synthesis (38, 51).

The temperature optimum for the most rapid rate of growth of a species of edible plant is not usually optimal for the synthesis and storage of nutrients in its tissue. In fact, the optimal temperature necessary to produce and store one nutrient will often be different for greatest storage of another nutrient (36).

Although more research needs to be conducted, it appears that citrus fruit grown in tropical or desert climates accumulated less ascorbic acid than fruits grown in a more moderate climate (38). Augustin et al. (44) could find no statistical effect of location (i.e., California vs. Maine), per se, upon ascorbic acid content of potatoes. Burge et al. (43) reported that tomatoes of the same variety, grown in different areas of the United States, may have vitamin C concentrations that deviate as much as 17% from the average value for that variety. However, some varieties had higher values grown in California, while others were higher in other areas.

Soil Fertility. In general, the principal effect of improvement of soils is to increase the yield rather than to enhance the concentration of nutrients in plants grown on these soils (36, 52). Increased nitrogen fertilization has been reported to decrease vitamin C concentration in potatoes (42), grapefruit (53), and several other citrus fruits (38). Harris (36) noted that some early researchers reported that increased nitrogen fertilization resulted in increased ascorbic acid in cabbage, collards, spinach, and Swiss chard. More recently, Burge et al. (43) showed that application of 100 lbs of nitrogen/acre produced tomato plants with heavy foliage and tomatoes with low vitamin C (Table II). Fertilization with 50 lbs/acre increased vitamin C in tomato fruit by 80%. Shekhar et al. (42) also found that high nitrogen fertilization resulted in lowered ascorbic acid content in potato tubers. The effects of phosphorus and potassium fertilization on vitamin C are inconclusive.

Once minimal mineral content of soil for optimal growth of a particular crop is achieved, no increased concentration of vitamin C is found with more fertilization. In the case of nitrogen, increased fertilization may decrease ascorbic acid concentration.

Variation Among Vegetable or Fruit Parts. Fruit juices are widely recognized for their high concentrations of ascorbic acid. Other portions of citrus fruits are often higher in concentration of the vitamin. Nagy (*38*), in his review of ascorbic acid in citrus products, pointed out that only about 25% of the vitamin C content of citrus fruit is found in the juice (Table III). For four varieties of orange, the peel contained 52%, while the pulp and rag contained 21%, of the total vitamin C in the oranges (*54*).

Table III. Vitamin C Contents of Component Parts of Citrus Fruit

Fruit	Peel		Pulp	Rag	Juice
	Flavedo	*Albedo*			
Orange, pineapple	377	206	—	68	68
Grapefruit	239	148	—	47	36
Lemon	144	—	49	—	34

Source: Compiled by Nagy (*38*).
Note: Data presented as milligrams of vitamin C per 100 g of fresh weight.

The apical portions of potato tubers are higher in ascorbic acid than the basal portions (*42*). The locular (soft, gelatin-like and seed-containing inner material) tissues of four varieties of tomatoes averaged about 25% higher in ascorbic acid concentrations than the pericarp (outer wall tissues) (*13*) although with greater amounts of sunlight, wall tissue may be equal or greater than placental (inner core) tissue in reduced ascorbic acid (*55*).

Ascorbic acid concentration in peaches and apples is highest just under the skin (*36*). The outer green leaves of cabbage, which are generally trimmed off, and the inner core are higher in ascorbic acid than the edible portion (*37*). This is consistent with the notion that when trimming foods of plant origin, the nutrient losses generally exceed the weight losses, because nutrient concentration is usually higher in the outer layers of vegetables, seeds, tubers, and fruits (*56, 57*).

Effect of Season. The observation that nutrient compositions of edible portions of plants produced from the same variety are different from one season to another probably results from differences in temperature, length of day, light intensity, and light spectrum, as well as from other minor factors (36). The literature shows inconsistent fluctuation in ascorbic acid content of vegetables and fruits produced over the four seasons.

Effect of Harvesting and Storage of Fresh Fruits and Vegetables

The procedures utilized during harvesting and the ensuing handling and storage period prior to commercial or at-home processing can dramatically affect both nutritional value and sensory quality of fruits and vegetables. Ascorbic acid is particularly sensitive to both enzymatic and nonenzymatic oxidation during this period.

Harvesting. Mechanical harvesting of some vegetable and fruit crops has increased markedly in the last decade. Over 95% of the California tomato crop is machine harvested (43). The mechanical shaker harvester used for some tree fruits can cause severe bruising of the fruit. Injury can be reduced by harvesting in the cool hours of the night, quick application of precooling, rapid and careful transportation, and immediate processing (58). Generally, fruits and vegetables will reach the food processor within hours but take much longer to get from the field to the retail fresh market. For this reason the mechanical harvesting method has not been satisfactory for the fresh fruit market for oranges, pears, plums, apples, or apricots (58, 59).

New varieties are being developed to withstand better mechanical harvesting. Burge et al. (43) reported that the ascorbic acid content of tomato varieties developed for this purpose contain as much ascorbic acid as do conventional varieties.

Intact plant tissue ascorbic acid is protected from oxidation by cellular compartmentation. However, when tissues are disrupted after bruising, wilting, rotting, or during advanced stages of senescence, oxidation of the vitamin can easily take place. In plants at least four enzymes— ascorbic acid oxidase, polyphenol oxidase, cytochrome oxidase, and peroxidase—are thought to oxidize vitamin C in damaged or overripe tissue (35, 58, 60). It has also been suggested that plant tissues contain reductase systems that can regenerate ascorbic acid when it is oxidized in situ. When the cellular integrity is damaged (e.g., after bruising), these reductase systems are inactivated and ascorbic acid oxidation continues without control (35).

The maximum activity of ascorbic acid oxidase is at 40°C, but it is almost completely inactivated at 65°C. Therefore, blanching of vegetables or fruits prior to further processing (freezing or canning) is ideal for protection of vitamin C from enzymatic oxidation, although some regeneration of heat-inactivated peroxidases may occur after blanching (35).

Storage of Newly Harvested Crops. Enzymatic destruction of ascorbic acid can begin as soon as a crop is harvested. Kale can lose 1.5% of its vitamin C per hour and about one-third in 24 h. Storage in cool conditions and increased humidity, factors that reduce wilting, reduce losses of ascorbic acid during storage. Wilting (moisture loss) is particularly prevalent with the fresh, green, leafy vegetables with large surface areas. Ezell and Wilcox (*61*) observed that ascorbic acid destruction in kale was accelerated by room temperature storage, particularly if the humidity was low. Fresh raw spinach stored overnight at 4°C in a walk-in cooler lost as much as 40% of its initial ascorbic acid. The degree of loss depended on the condition of the leaves at the time of storage (*62*). Control of temperature and humidity is essential for preservation of vitamin C in these products.

Green beans, which have less surface area than the leafy vegetables, stored at 10°C for 24 h, lost only 10% of their ascorbic acid concentrations, but when stored at room temperature for the same time, lost 24% of their ascorbic acid concentration (*35,63*). Only minor losses of ascorbic acid are found after 1 or 2 months storage of fresh citrus fruit, which have very low surface areas and a protective peel, if they are stored in cool temperatures (3.3–5.6°C) (*38*).

Eheart (*64*) found that the ascorbic acid content of broccoli held at 3°C increased during storage. In a follow-up study, Eheart and Odland (*65*) found no significant losses of ascorbic acid during a 1-week storage period, and in fact, a 36% increase was noted for one variety. This was attributed to ascorbic acid synthesis from monosaccharides during the storage period. Green beans, on the other hand, lost significant amounts of ascorbic acid (up to 88%) after 1 week at the same temperature, although decreases were small in the first 48 h.

Refrigeration (0–10°C) of fresh fruits and vegetables is commonly used to retard deterioration in eating qualities (flavor, texture, appearance, and color) and nutritive value. Reduction of temperature slows respiratory activity in plant products, reduces moisture loss, and decreases the rate of decay due to microorganisms. In the home, fresh produce is generally stored refrigerated for a relatively short period of time. Once fruit is ripened, it should be refrigerated promptly to prevent undesirable softening and subsequent bruising, which increases losses of ascorbic acid due to enzymatic action and oxidation. Vegetables, particularly leafy ones, should be stored in plastic bags or in a vegetable crisper, to minimize moisture loss that accelerates ascorbic acid degradation (*61, 66*).

Some vegetables are subject to chilling injury at refrigeration temperatures. This includes failure to ripen normally (mature-green tomatoes, immature bananas, and eggplants), susceptibility to decay (sweet potatoes), undesirable increases in sugars (potatoes), as well as an increase in lesions (pitting, internal and external discoloration). Membrane damage during chilling increases the possibility of enzyme release in the plant tissue, resulting in further softening and oxidative reactions. These effects decrease the eating quality and acceptability of the produce, reducing its consumption. The nutritive value of chill-injured foods has not received much attention, because the visible deterioration is more important economically. In general, chilling has little effect on the ascorbic acid content of fresh fruits and vegetables under reasonable conditions of distribution, storage, and marketing (58). The effect of controlled atmosphere storage on ascorbic acid content of fruits and vegetables stored under those conditions has not been well investigated.

Temperature of storage is important in maintaining the ascorbic acid content of potatoes. In general, potatoes are stored at relatively high temperatures (40–50°F), which results in better ascorbic acid retention as well as better quality (67).

A major factor contributing to the variability in vitamin C content of potatoes is the storage time. Augustin et al. (44) reported a sharp decrease in the vitamin during the first 4 months of storage of potatoes at about 7°C and 95% relative humidity. Over the next 4 months there was either a complete leveling out or a less pronounced decrease. After 8-months storage all varieties appeared to contain about the same concentration of vitamin C (40–50 mg/100 g DWB).

Kinetics of Ascorbic Acid Destruction During Processing and Storage

An interest in quantitative approaches to changes in food quality has been stimulated in part by government regulation of nutritional labeling (68). The relative instability of ascorbic acid under usual conditions of food storage and processing is well documented (69, 70). However, the prediction of vitamin C losses is complicated by lack of information about the mechanisms of degradation and the factors that influence them. The loss of ascorbic acid is dependent on the presence or absence of oxygen, the rate of oxygen transfer, pH, and water content and activity of the food (17, 71–74).

To predict nutrient deterioration, knowledge of the reaction rate as a function of temperature of storage or processing is needed. The kinetics of ascorbic acid destruction have been examined most extensively in model systems, with particular attention being given to intermediate moisture foods (17, 71, 78, 79). Most of the data available for vitamin C losses in actual food systems are insufficient to calculate the kinetic parameters needed to predict losses during heat treatment or storage.

Lund (*80*) and Labuza (*71, 76*) have reexamined the data in the literature to derive some of the values. However, in many cases, the information presented in the reviewed studies is inadequate to establish the
conditions that were used for processing or storage. The interpretation
of data was sometimes based on erroneous assumption of reaction orders,
leading to inaccurate predictions of nutrient losses (*76*).

According to Lenz and Lund (*72*), kinetic models for destruction
of food components are needed to improve products by minimizing
quality changes for new product development and to predict shelf life
during storage. Numerous reports and reviews of the kinetics of ascorbic
acid destruction can be found in the literature (*68–88*). A brief overview
is presented here to indicate the need for further research in this area.

Nutrient destruction is usually described in terms of time and
temperature effects using the reaction rate and the dependence of the
reaction rate on temperature. The parameters most frequently used by
physical chemists and in engineering applications are the reaction rate
constant (k), at a given temperature (T), and the Arrhenius activation
energy (E_a). In the food industry, the time to reduce the concentration
of a component to 10% of the initial value (D), at a given temperature
(usually 121°C), and the change in degrees Fahrenheit required for a
ten-fold change in D (z), are used to describe the reaction rates. The
Q_{10} value, which is the ratio of the reaction rate (k) at $T(°C) + 10$, to
the reaction rate at T, is often used in biological descriptions of kinetics.

For ascorbic acid, losses are generally considered to follow first-order
kinetics as described by:

$$\frac{-dC}{dt} = kC \tag{1}$$

where C = the concentration of the nutrient, t = time, and k = the rate
constant (time^{-1}). If $C = C_o$ at time zero, integration of Equation 1
yields:

$$C = C_o \exp(-kt) \tag{2}$$

For the first-order reaction, a plot of $\log C$ vs. t will yield a straight line,
and the rate constant (k), can be derived from the slope. It is possible
to plot the log of the ratios of concentrations at two times, or the log of
the percent nutrient remaining, vs. time to obtain the rate constant at
a particular temperature (*71, 77*). The half-life (time required for
destruction of 50% of the initial vitamin present) at a given temperature
can also be used to calculate k since the half-life is independent of the
initial concentration.

If the destruction of a component is presumed to be zero-order, a plot of C vs. t should give a straight line. Certain losses of vitamin C, particularly in frozen foods, are presumed to follow first-order kinetics (89). Labuza (76) observed that zero-order reaction rates for quality losses may be assumed in some fluctuating temperature studies, but this may lead to a miscalculation of predicted changes. Therefore, from a theoretical standpoint, it is important that the proper order be used for predictions. In general, ascorbic acid destruction is assumed to be first-order, or pseudo first-order (17, 27) except under specific conditions of heat and moisture (79).

The temperature dependence of the reaction is usually described by the Arrhenius equation:

$$k = k_o \exp \ (-E_a/RT) \tag{3}$$

where $k =$ the first-order rate constant, $k_o =$ pre-exponential constant or frequency factor or Arrhenius constant (time^{-1}), $R =$ gas constant (1.987 cal/K-mol), and $T =$ absolute temperature (K). The activation energy (E_a) is equivalent to $-2.303R$ times the slope of a plot of log k vs. $1/T$.

The energy of activation for most vitamins is considered to be 20–30 kcal/mol (69), but the value can be affected by a number of factors. The E_as for destruction of enzymes or microorganisms used as indicators of adequacy of thermal processing are generally much higher. Because an increase in temperature has a greater effect on the reaction rate when the E_a is higher, if k_os are comparable, more rapid destruction of enzymes and microorganisms than vitamins may result at the elevated temperatures used for thermal processing. Therefore, it has been assumed that vitamins are more stable than other food components. However, relatively little data are available to support this.

Some information regarding the E_a for ascorbic acid in food systems can be found in the literature. Kirk et al. (17) determined that the vitamin C destruction in a model dehydrated food system could be described by the first-order function. Rates of destruction were influenced by a_w, moisture, and temperature of storage. Activation energies for TAA destruction at a_ws above 0.24 were approximately 18 kcal/mol, similar to those reported for RAA by Lee and Labuza (78). Lower E_as were reported at a_ws less than 0.24, suggesting a different mechanism for ascorbic acid destruction, perhaps by an anaerobic pathway. Rate constants were also influenced by the packaging used for the model food system, which may be attributed to the amount of dissolved oxygen present.

Lee et al. (81) reported that the E_a for the anaerobic destruction of added ascorbic acid in tomato juice at pH 4.0 during storage was 3.3

kcal/mol, which is lower than the values for ascorbic acid destruction in buffered solutions reported by Blaug and Hajratwala (82). The anaerobic destruction of ascorbic acid is generally believed to proceed at a slower rate than aerobic degradation. In canned foods, the absence of oxygen alters the mechanism of destruction, and thus the reaction rate (72, 75).

Lathrop and Leung (75) reported that the E_a for ascorbic acid degradation in canned peas during processing at 110–132°C was 41 kcal/mol. This was higher than the E_as reported for other nutrients, although in a similar range (83, 84). Contrary to other studies, these investigators suggested that ascorbic acid destruction in canned peas was much more heat sensitive than that in model systems. Rao et al. (90), in a similar investigation with canned peas, reported an E_a of 13.1 kcal/mol, significantly lower than that found by Lathrop and Leung (75). Differences in the destruction mechanism (aerobic vs. anaerobic), oxygen concentration, and actual temperature in the center of the food might account for some of the variation.

Nagy (38) reported that for stored citrus juices, the loss of vitamin C was not necessarily a first-order reaction. For grapefruit juice, the E_a was 18.2 kcal/mol, and the reaction was first-order. For orange juice, two E_as were determined: 12.8 kcal/mol in the temperature range 4–28°C, and 24.5 kcal/mol in the range 28–50°C. The change in reaction kinetics was attributed to different destruction mechanisms, although no explanation was offered.

The lack of data for actual food systems, and the discrepancies cited above, indicate the difficulty in predicting ascorbic acid losses that might occur during processing and storage of foods. With the advent of nutritional labeling, the processor must be able to provide foods containing at least the amount of a nutrient listed at the time of purchase. Therefore, the determination of losses as outlined by Labuza et al. (85) or Lenz and Lund (72) should be part of the quality control program in a food company. The development of computer simulation models for prediction of quality losses, including nutrients, will become increasingly important (85–88).

Ascorbic Acid Losses During Industrial Processing

Because of vitamin C's lability to heat-induced oxidation and its high solubility in water, major losses of the vitamin can occur during food processing techniques that utilize long heat treatments or that involve large quantities of soaking, rinsing, or cooking water (35, 91, 92). This section reviews the effects of different food preservation processes on the retention of vitamin C in commercial food products.

Blanching. Hot water, microwave, or steam blanching is used prior to freezing, canning, or drying operations primarily to inactivate enzymes that cause deterioration during storage of frozen foods. Blanching is also used to clean and reduce the microbial population on the vegetable or fruit, to soften bulky vegetables and reduce volume prior to packaging, to expel gasses that can create excessive pressure in the can, and to maintain or "fix" color (35).

Hot water blanch and subsequent water-cooling is undesirable because of leaching of various water-soluble nutrients, especially ascorbic acid. Losses of ascorbic acid are especially high when the surface area per mass of the food is large (small pieces), when there is a large water to food ratio, when the contact time is long, and when the product is extensively stirred in water. When blanch conditions are favorable, loss of ascorbic acid can be less than 10%, but the loss can be 50% or more under severe conditions. The wide range of ascorbic acid retention in canned fruits and vegetables may reflect the varying conditions of blanching, although in some cases high losses result from the use of copper salts as color stabilizers (93).

Lathrop and Leung (94) collected pea samples at various points along a commercial canning line in Washington State (Table IV). They found a total 8% loss of ascorbic acid concentration during soaking, cleaning, and sizing operations due to leaching (no heat applied). Hot water blanching (3 min at 82–88°C) caused a further 19% reduction

Table IV. Vitamin C Losses Due to Specific Operations in Commercial Thermal Pea Processing

	Vitamin C		
Process	*Content*[a] *(mg/100 g of Peas)*	*Loss After Each Operation (%)*	*Cumulative Losses (%)*
Receiving	24.9 ± 0.9	0	0
Soaking	24.3 ± 1.5	2.4	2.4
Washing and sizing	22.9 ± 2.9	5.8	8.0
Blanching	18.5 ± 1.1	19.2	25.7
Hot filling			
still	10.4 ± 0.1	43.8	58.2
continuous	10.3 ± 1.4	44.3	58.6
Thermal processing			
still	8.2 ± 1.1	21.2	67.1
continuous	8.0 ± 0.9	22.3	67.9

Source: Lathrop and Leung (94).
[a] Mean ± sd for five or more samples.

in vitamin C. The same authors further studied the effect of blanch time on the ascorbic acid content of 20–40-g quantities of peas blanched in a pilot-scale steam blancher at 100°C or in distilled water (4:1, water:peas) at 85°C. After 3 min the retention was 78.5% after steam and 71.9% after water blanching. About one-third or one-half of the vitamin C lost from hot-water-blanched peas was leached into the blanch water.

Selman, in his review of vitamin C losses during processing of peas (*95*), observed that there was a large variation among varieties for both the vitamin C content and retention during processing steps such as blanching. The losses were not related to the initial ascorbic acid content of the variety. The work of Morrison (*96*) shows a threefold variation of vitamin C loss from six cultivars of peas blanched in water for 1 min at 97°C.

In general, steam blanching appears to result in lower loss of ascorbic acid although some studies have shown no difference between steam and hot water. Leaching loss is less with steam but increased oxidation may occur because of longer blanch times (*35*). Microwave blanching has been shown in some cases to be superior to steam blanching for vitamin C retention (*80, 97*) probably because of less leaching loss. The hot gas and superheated steam blanching procedures have yet to be adequately tested for their effects on ascorbic acid retention in a variety of products.

Pasteurization and Commercial Sterilization (Canning). Along with blanching, pasteurization and sterilization are the common thermal preservation procedures in industrial processing. The objective of pasteurization is to inactivate vegetative cells of pathogenic or spoilage organisms. Other than milk, most pasteurized products have a low pH to reduce the rate of microbial growth. Many orange and other fruit juices and drinks are pasteurized. Pasteurization is usually followed by other special treatments such as refrigeration or fermentation.

The commercial sterilization procedure uses sufficient heat to inactivate spores of pathogenic or spoilage organisms. Sterilization usually is used in conjunction with anaerobic storage conditions (*68, 80*).

Pasteurization requires considerably less thermal input than does sterilization. Therefore, the thermal losses during pasteurization processing are quite low. However, oxidative losses can be high if care is not taken to deaerate and if high-temperature–short-time (HTST) conditions are not used (*80*).

Thompson (*98*) investigated the loss of nutrients from milk after pasteurization and sterilization. A portion of his results are found in Table V. HTST (72°C for 15 s) pasteurization of the fluid milk prior

Table V. Loss of Nutrients in Milk During Processing

| | Pasteurized | | Sterilized | |
| | HTST | Holder | UHT | In Bottle |
Nutrient	(%)	(%)	(%)	(%)
Thiamine	10	10	10	35
Vitamin C	10	20	10	50
Folic acid	0	0	10	50
Vitamin B_{12}	0	10	20	30

Source: Thompson (98) as noted by Lund (80).

to bottling is superior to pasteurization of the previously bottled milk. Ultrahigh temperature (144°C for a few seconds) is far superior to sterilizing in the bottle for retention of four measured vitamins.

Commercial sterilization of peas in a retort resulted in a 33% retention of the initial ascorbic acid in one study (Table V) (94) and 38–60% retention in another study (99). The latter study reported considerably lower vitamin C loss during the blanching operation and thus higher total retention. Final retention of vitamin C in other vegetables after canning was 40% for corn and 23% for beets (99). The low total retention of vitamin C for beets was largely because of blanching and peeling operations. Large blanching losses for wax beans and green beans were also reported (99).

Moisture Removal (Drying). Ascorbic acid is the most difficult of the vitamins to preserve during the dehydration of foods. Losses of 20% have been reported in spray-dried milk and 30% in roller-dried milk (93). Those drying procedures that require shorter drying times will improve vitamin C retention (35). Retention can also be improved by application of vacuum or by use of nitrogen atmosphere during drying (97), or by the addition of sulfur dioxide to fruits and vegetables prior to drying (93). Sulfur dioxide must be used with caution, however, as it destroys thiamine.

The rate of ascorbic acid destruction and the activation energy are very sensitive to water activity. The reaction rate constant varies over three orders of magnitude for the entire water activity range (100). At high water activities, ascorbic acid is rapidly destroyed, but it is quite stable at low water activity. The sensitivity of ascorbic acid to temperature at high water activity suggests that vitamin C retention is dependent on the wet bulb temperature at the beginning of drying and on the temperature of evaporation. Control of drying rate and conditions is essential for retention of vitamin C, and is particularly important for drying of fruit slices or halves.

Concentration of fruit juices should not result in marked loss of ascorbic acid if the pressed juice is deaerated and and evaporated at low temperatures (*100*). Ascorbic acid retentions in excess of 90% have been reported for concentration and freezing processes (*38, 101*) and can be expected for freeze concentration processes (*100*).

Gee (*102*) dried slices of carrots and tomatoes and whole spinach leaves at 47°C for 16–24 h in a forced-draft oven to a water activity of 0.33. No pre-blanch chemical treatment was used. During dehydration no loss in total ascorbic acid was detected for carrots and less than 20% loss was noted for tomatoes. Ascorbic acid loss for spinach was 62%. Ascorbic acid content remained rather stable in carrots and tomatoes for about 1 month stored in air, but losses accelerated rapidly thereafter. No benefit of nitrogen or vacuum packaging on vitamin C retention during storage was noted. These are surprising results. The high retention of vitamin C under drying conditions should be verified.

Dehydration of potatoes can result in highly variable ascorbic acid retention depending upon the process techniques used. Jadhav et al. (*103*) found a maximum loss of 78% of RAA in an add back, air-drying process and a maximum loss of only 30% in a freeze–thaw process for producing dehydrated mashed potatoes. Maga and Sizer (*104*) studied vitamin C and thiamin retention in extrusion processed potato snack-like flakes. At high extrusion temperatures, the best ascorbic acid retention occurred in the low moisture potato meal (25% water). However, thiamine retention at high extrusion temperatures was generally best from high-moisture meal (59% water) and poor from low-moisture meal.

Low Temperature Treatment.   Many commercial frozen food products are high in ascorbic acid. Refrigeration is used for various fresh fruit juices and for holding many fruits and vegetables prior to retail sale or further processing.

Freezing, if properly conducted, is considered the best long-term food preservation technique for both optimal sensory quality and nutrient retention (*35, 57, 105, 106*). The average retention of reduced ascorbic acid in different vegetables that were blanched, frozen, or stored for 6–12 months at −18°C and thawed was about 50% (*106*). Losses during the entire process are largely attributed to blanching and to the prolonged frozen storage. Losses differ markedly among products and within varieties of a cultivar.

Under proper processing conditions, fruits lose less than 30% of their original vitamin C content through the entire freezing and frozen storage period (*106*). Frozen concentrated fruit juices can retain over 90% of their ascorbic acid (*38, 106*). Packing in syrup is generally protective of ascorbic acid.

The temperature of frozen storage is critical for optimal nutrient retention. The International Institute of Refrigeration (*107*) recommends that for good retention of nutrients and quality of foods the maximum freezing storage temperature should be −18°C (0°F). At this temperature there is a slow but acceptable deterioration of food quality (*35*).

Ascorbic acid loss in frozen foods is highly temperature dependent. For example, when peaches, boysenberries, or strawberries are stored at −7°C instead of −18°C, the rate of ascorbic acid degradation increases by a factor of 30–70 (*105, 106*).

Kramer et al. (*108*) measured ascorbic acid retention at constant (±1°C) and fluctuating (±5°C each 20 min) temperatures in salisbury steaks stored for 3 or 6 months (Table VI). They found good retention of vitamin C stored at constant −20°C or lower for 3 months. At higher temperatures, or at fluctuating temperatures, there was substantial reduction of vitamin C within 3-months storage. No other studies of vitamin C retention under both constant and fluctuating temperature were found.

Proper storage of canned and bottled single-strength fruit juices is essential for maximal vitamin C retention. Nagy, in his review of the literature (*38*), concludes that storage at 21°C (the temperature that may be close to the average year-round nonrefrigerated commercial storage conditions) for upwards of a year results in vitamin C retentions of greater than 75%. However, storage temperatures in excess of 28°C cause marked ascorbic acid destruction, and at 38°C little vitamin C was retained. Refrigeration storage (4–10°C) resulted in excellent (90% or more) retention of the vitamin, after 1 year.

Table VI. Effect of Constant and Fluctuating Temperatures Upon the Ascorbic Acid and Thiamine Contents of Salisbury Steak

Storage Conditions	Ascorbic Acid Content		Thiamine Content	
	Constant Temperature	Fluctuating Temperature	Constant Temperature	Fluctuating Temperature
Initial	3.6		3.0	
3 Months				
−10°C	1.8	1.0	2.8	1.8
−20°C	2.8	2.0	2.9	2.1
−30°C	2.8	2.5	3.2	2.6
6 Months				
−10°C	1.2	1.1	1.9	1.8
−20°C	1.6	1.1	2.7	1.7
−30°C	1.3	1.1	2.7	2.6

Source: Reference *108*.
Note: Data presented as milligram of vitamin specified per 100 g.

Squires and Hanna (*109*) collected samples of seventeen brands of commercial reconstituted orange juices in plastic-coated cardboard containers and stored them under refrigeration at 4°C. They reported that the average reduction in RAA was about 2%/d.

Fermentation. Selective fermentation of foodstuffs for preservation, enhancement of nutritive value, improvement of flavor, or preparation of alcoholic beverages has been practiced probably since prehistoric times by peoples of nearly every civilization (*110*). During fermentation of foods, one often can find a net increase in content of certain B vitamins, such as riboflavin and niacin, because of microbial synthesis. However, depending upon other processing steps, the fermented food may or may not retain the newly synthesized nutrients.

Separation of milk into the curd and whey fractions prior to cheese manufacture causes a partition of water-soluble substances (whey) from the curd. More than 80% of the vitamin C and thiamine is removed with the whey fraction (*111*). Desalting of the brine during pickle manufacture results in a 100% vitamin C loss. When desalting is not practiced, losses of ascorbic acid are about 40–50% (*110*).

It was reported in 1939 (*112*) that during the active fermentation period of sauerkraut production, the vitamin C content was equal to that of the original cabbage. Then, during vat storage, a slow, progressive loss of vitamin C occurred. Further destruction (25–35%) occurred during preheating and canning operations. Marked loss of vitamin C was found in canned kraut stored at elevated temperatures (*113*). In a recent report Ro et al. (*114*) investigated the vitamin B_{12} and ascorbic acid content of Kimchi, a chinese cabbage fermented with *Propionibacterium freundenreichii ss. shermanii*. Although vitamin B_{12} content increased, vitamin C content decreased (when compared with fresh unfermented Kimchi) during the first 5 weeks of fermentation.

From these and other studies one must conclude that most fermented foods are not good sources of vitamin C. Exceptions would be fresh cabbage and other fermented vegetables that have not been desalted.

Irradiation. Ionizing radiation for use in food systems can come from electrons, x-rays, or gamma rays from cobalt-60 or cesium-137. There is little rise in the temperature within the foodstuff, so heat destruction of nutrients is minimized. However, free radicals and peroxides are formed within the food. In the United States, irradiation is classified as a food additive and its use in the food industry has been severely restricted to such areas as prevention of potato sprouting and wheat infestation.

As is noted in Chapter 3 in this book, ascorbic acid reacts very rapidly with free radicals formed from water. The end products of this reaction could be DHA or other nonbiologically active forms of the vitamin. Vitamin C in irradiated food systems can be considered to act as a free radical scavenger, but as such its overall content in irradiated food would be reduced.

Josephson et al. (115) conclude from their review of the effects of ionizing radiation treatment of foods that nutrient destruction, such as to vitamin C, in irradiated foods is no greater than that occurring when food is preserved by more conventional means. In addition, if irradiation is performed on frozen foods, the losses of vitamin C are reduced.

Storage of Preserved Foods. Proper storage conditions for preserved foods will extend their shelf life. Extended storage at high temperatures, or at high humidity with inadequate packaging will lead to deterioration of the food products' sensory quality and nutrient content. An example of the effects of poor packaging and poor storage conditions for cranberry sauce is illustrated in Table VII.

Table VII.   Effects of Packaging Upon Quality of Cranberry Sauce (pH = 2.7)

		After Storage for 5 Weeks at 37°C at 80% RH in Packages Made of:			
Test	Prior to Storage	No. 2 Lined Tin Can	Aluminum Laminated Film	Polyester Film (2 layers)	Polyester Film (1 layer)
Moisture (%)	56.1	55.9	56.0	54.5	53.5
Acceptability (hedonic scale)	7.3	6.7	7.2	6.3	5.3
Ascorbic acid (mg/100 g)	89.2	73.4	71.7	0.4	0.0

Source: Reference 149.

Ascorbic Acid Losses During Food Preparation

It has been suggested that, during preparation of food for the table either in or out of the home, losses of nutrients occur that surpass those incurred during processing (116). An extensive review of the literature done in 1960 (117), which was updated in 1975 (92), revealed that few new data have been reported in the intervening years. Erdman (57) suggested that more information, particularly on the effects of cooking procedures on nutrient retention, was necessary.

We do not intend to provide comprehensive coverage of the early work on ascorbic acid retention in home prepared foods in this section, but to indicate the critical points where losses may occur. The increased consumption of food away from home, in a food service facility, such as school and business cafeterias, restaurants, and fast food stands, will influence the nutrients available to the consumer. Nutrient data collected in the 1940s have become less useful because of changes in raw materials, food processing, technology, and equipment (118). Therefore, one must view the information available about the influence of various processes and procedures on vitamin C content of foods as indicative, rather than absolute.

In most studies of vitamin C content of prepared food, the variety of fruit or vegetable is rarely reported or known. The consumer, unless she/he is the gardener as well, has little control over the variety of fruit or vegetable purchased or available. In commercial retailing of fruits and vegetables, the decisions regarding variety are influenced by season, growing area, and quality characteristics of the product other than nutritive value.

Preparation for Cooking. During preparation for cooking, most plant materials require some peeling and trimming. In addition, subdivision of large whole vegetables is often done to speed cooking times and to provide more uniform size pieces. Trimming losses vary considerably depending on the type of food, its condition and freshness, and the method of cooking to be used. A handbook of food yields (119) provides extensive information about losses and gains in weight of food during different stages of preparation.

The extent of trimming for most fruits and vegetables will influence the total initial nutrient content. Since ascorbic acid is usually concentrated in the outer leaves or layers of the fruit or vegetables, removal of these portions may result in a considerable loss (37, 67, 120, 121).

Losses in ascorbic acid content owing to advance preparation (cutting and shredding) do occur (122–125), but the amount is unpredictable and inconsistent. The losses are influenced by the degree of subdivision, soaking in water, material of the cutting instrument, time of standing, and temperature of storage during standing. Destruction of ascorbic acid in cut cabbage has been reported to be as low as 3% (121) and as high as 40% (122). According to Van Duyne et al. (122) retention of reduced ascorbic acid in cabbage that was shredded and allowed to stand for 1 h in air, 1 h in water, or 3 h in water was over 87% in all cases. Similarly, peeled potatoes, quartered or whole, did not lose significant amounts of ascorbic acid during a 1–3-h soaking period (126). Based on the sparse data, it appears that the soaking of vegetables in water for short periods of time prior to cooking results in small losses of ascorbic acid. If a vegetable is shredded or cut, the losses will be increased.

Cooking of Vegetables. In the 1940s, many of the studies of ascorbic acid retention were concerned with processes of blanching and freezing; in the next decade, studies of cooking methods including pressure cooking, "waterless" cooking, and steaming were more common. The development of electronic cooking also stimulated research in the early 1960s. Since that time, there have been relatively few new reports on vitamin retention in cooked foods.

In assessing the cooking studies, caution must be used in interpreting results. Clearly, the amount of water and the time of heating must be specified. Difficulty in determining the degree of "doneness" may influence the observations. The amount of subdivision of the vegetables must also be considered. It should be pointed out that in almost all of the investigations cited only one cooking time, an "optimum", was used. Although there are recommendations for cooking times and amounts of water to be used in home cooking, it is likely that the average food preparer deviates substantially from the recommendations because of personal preferences, inexperience, or other factors. It would be interesting to determine what cooking methods are actually used, and to determine the effects of a range of heating times and temperatures on ascorbic acid retention in vegetables.

BAKING, STEAMING, AND PRESSURE COOKING. The most common method of cooking vegetables is by boiling in water. The proportion of water to vegetable used can vary greatly from a 0:1 (waterless cooking) to a 5:1 ratio (water to cover). Usual recommendations for vegetable cookery are to use a "minimum amount" of water, which can range from a ratio of 0.25:1 to 1:1 depending on the food. In making recommendations for the amount of water to be used, palatability as well as nutrient retention are considered.

Examples of the effects of different ratios of water to vegetable used in various cooking methods on ascorbic acid retention are shown in Table VIII. The water to vegetable ratio used in the cooking procedure is important because losses of ascorbic acid are primarily caused by leaching of the vitamin. Cooking methods that reduce exposure to large quantities of water, such as pressure cooking, steaming, and microwave cooking, would be expected to result in higher total ascorbic acid retention (10, 127–132). When the same or similar ratio of water to vegetable is used in any of the cooking methods, ascorbic acid losses are approximately the same, if cooking times are comparable (131–135). In almost all vegetables cooked in a minimum amount of water, ascorbic acid retention in the vegetables was over 70%, regardless of the cooking method used. Eheart and Gott (136) noted that when no water or very small amounts were used, ascorbic acid retention was about the same. However, if large quantities of water (5:1 ratio) were used for boiling

Table VIII. Effects of Some Common Cooking Methods on Ascorbic Acid Retention in Vegetables

Vegetable and Cooking Method	Water: Vegetable Ratio	Cooking Time (min)	Percent Retention	References
Broccoli				
microwave	2:1	3	72	*150*
saucepan (boiling)	2:1	10	59	*150*
microwave	0.4:1	5	87	*130*
saucepan (boiling)	5.5:1	6.5	45	*130*
saucepan	0.5:1	10	88	*132*
waterless cooking	0.2:1	8	82	*132*
Cabbage				
microwave	0:1	5	93	*150*
microwave	3.5:1	4	85	*150*
saucepan (boiling)	4:1	25	20	*150*
pressure cooker	1.25:1	3	50	*150*
microwave	0.25:1	4	80	*130*
saucepan (boiling)	5:1	6.5	38	*130*
microwave	0.5:1	12	72	*134*
saucepan (boiling)	0.5:1	14	69	*134*
Spinach				
microwave	0:1	7	56	*134*
saucepan	0:1	7	61	*134*
microwave	0.25:1	6.5	47	*135*
saucepan	0.25:1	7	50	*135*

vegetables, as was done by Gordon and Noble (*130*), ascorbic acid retention was much lower in conventionally cooked than in microwave cooked vegetables, even though cooking times were similar.

Studies in which the ascorbic acid retention and content of the cooking liquid were determined (*130, 133, 134*) showed that total ascorbic acid retention was generally about 90% after cooking. Sweeney et al. (*137*) reported that total percent retention in broccoli solids plus cooking liquid did not decrease greatly with time. Therefore, ascorbic acid appeared to be relatively heat stable although it was easily leached into the cooking water. When larger proportions of water were used (*130*), a higher percentage of ascorbic acid was found in the cooking liquid, which emphasizes the importance of using minimum amounts of water in vegetable cookery.

It is frequently stated that steaming vegetables is most beneficial in retaining ascorbic acid in the food. An examination of the sparse data (*56*) in the literature does not support this theory, however. In many cases, the lengthened cooking time necessary to soften the vegetables can result in destruction of vitamin C by heat and oxidation. If vegetables are extensively subdivided prior to cooking (e.g., shredded or thinly sliced), then steaming methods are satisfactory for palatable, nutritious vegetables. For larger pieces or whole vegetables, the use of small amounts of water and conventional or microwave cooking methods will be quicker and more effective in retaining ascorbic acid. It should be pointed out that the data for steamed and boiled vegetables from the same sources are not readily available. Thus, the recommendations regarding steaming are inferred rather than known.

MICROWAVE COOKING. When sales of microwave ovens increased in the 1970s, the nutritional benefits were advertised. Recent studies have confirmed the early findings (134, 136) that microwave cooking results in good retention of ascorbic acid, presumably because of the low water to vegetable ratios and short cooking times used. In a review of microwave effects on nutrient retention, Klein (138) pointed out that the amount of water used in cooking, and to a lesser extent, the cooking time, affect ascorbic acid losses more than the source of energy or the type of cooking. If short cooking times and small amounts of water are used, more ascorbic acid will be retained in any cooking method.

Mabesa and Baldwin (139) found that frozen peas, cooked with or without water in microwave ovens or conventionally, varied in ascorbic acid content. When the same ratio of water to vegetable (1:4) was used in the microwave and conventional methods, ascorbic acid retentions were similar (70%), but lower than when no water was used in the microwave oven (retention >96%).

In a study of ascorbic acid retention in frozen cauliflower (Table IX) (140), the ascorbic acid content and retention in the vegetables cooked with no water was significantly higher ($p < 0.05$) than those cooked with increasing proportions of water (0.25:1, 0.5:1, 1:1). However, the cauliflower cooked without water was not as palatable.

Table IX.   Ascorbic Acid Retention in Frozen Cauliflower Cooked with Various Ratios of Water to Vegetable

	Water: Vegetable Ratio	Cooking Time (min)	Ascorbic Acid[a] (mg/100 g)	Percent Retention[a]
Uncooked cauliflower			51.4 ± 3.9	100
Cooked cauliflower	0:1	5.5	52.2 ± 8.1	99.8 ± 7.7
	0.25:1	5.5	45.5 ± 2.5	88.0 ± 4.9
	0.5:1	5	43.1 ± 1.5	82.9 ± 2.8
	1:1	5	42.3 ± 0.7	81.1 ± 1.6

[a] Mean ± sd for four samples.

Klein et al. (*135*) found that approximately one-half of the initial ascorbic acid in fresh raw spinach was retained in the cooked vegetable. The amount of water and vegetable (1:4) used in each method was constant, and cooking times were similar. No significant differences in ascorbic acid content between conventionally and microwave cooked spinach were found.

In most frozen vegetables, sufficient ice clings to the product to provide adequate moisture for cooking in the microwave oven. When fresh vegetables are prepared by this method, some water is generally added to prevent scorching or undesirable palatability characteristics. The microwave method can be considered essentially a waterless method, since it is unnecessary to add large quantities of water to the vegetable.

FRYING. The deep fat frying technique is used for relatively few vegetables with the notable exception of potatoes. Domas et al. (*141*) reported that retention of ascorbic acid was over 75% in fried potatoes, while Pelletier et al. (*142*) noted about 60% retention. Augustin et al. (*143*) observed that with deep fat fried potato products, ascorbic acid retentions were unrealistically high. These investigators suggested that this result was caused by interference with the commonly used assay methods by browning compounds formed during cooking. Thus, no conclusions can be drawn from the available studies. Augustin et al. (*32*) suggested that the high performance liquid chromatographic method of determining ascorbic acid should be of use in separating the browning compounds and ascorbic acid.

There has been some interest in the oriental method of stir-frying because this is essentially a waterless method of cooking, usually with very short cooking times. Theoretically, this would provide maximum vitamin C retention. Eheart and Gott (*136*) found that when broccoli was cooked by a stir-frying method, ascorbic acid retention was higher than when it was cooked by microwaves or in large amounts of water. Using a low ratio of water to vegetable (0.5:1) in conventional cooking resulted in less loss of ascorbic acid than did the microwave cooking method used (0.9:1). In green beans, conventional cooking in the lowest water to vegetable ratio (0.5:1) resulted in higher ascorbic acid retention than microwave or stir-frying.

Bowman et al. (*144*) studied the effect of stir-frying on ascorbic acid retention in green peppers and spinach. Cooking times for the stir-fried vegetables were considerably shorter than those used for conventional cooking methods, and ascorbic acid retention was higher. These investigators noted that ascorbic acid retention was slightly higher in microwave than conventionally boiled vegetables, but the differences were significant in only three of the sixteen vegetables tested.

Chapman (*145*) compared ascorbic acid content and retention in three vegetables (broccoli, cabbage, and cauliflower) cooked by stir-frying, microwave cooking, and conventional cooking. With the times and methods used (Table X) ascorbic acid retention was highest in conventionally cooked vegetables, followed by microwave and stir-fried. At least two factors could be responsible for low values associated with stir-frying; size of pieces, length and temperature of cooking. To ensure more uniform heating of stir-fried vegetables, the food was cut in smaller pieces, and the time was increased to provide a product with texture comparable with conventional and microwave cooked products. The higher heat used in stir-frying together with long exposure could result in low ascorbic acid retention.

Table X. Percent Retention of Ascorbic Acid in Vegetables Cooked by Three Methods

Method of Preparation	Water: Vegetable Ratio	Cooking Time (min)	Percent Retention		
			Vegetables	Liquid	Total
Broccoli					
conventional	0.9:1	11	81	12	93
microwave	0.9:1	11	76	14	90
stir-fry	no water	15	72	—	72
Cabbage					
conventional	0.5:1	6	83	10	93
microwave	0.5:1	8	78	8	86
stir-fry	no water	6	81	—	81
Cauliflower					
conventional	0.5:1	8	84	6	90
microwave	0.5:1	8	84	5	88
stir-fry	no water	14	79	—	79

Source: Reference *145*.

BAKING. Potatoes are among the most commonly baked vegetables. Most of the studies indicate that there is good retention of ascorbic acid in baked potatoes (*143, 146*). Pelletier et al. (*142*) reported that potatoes baked in the skin retained 78% of the ascorbic acid, as compared with boiled in the skin, 81%; peeled and boiled, 73%; and fried 72%. Augustin et al. (*143*) reported 91% retention in baked potatoes.

Holding and Reheating of Cooked Foods. Recent work by Augustin et al. (*44, 143*) on home and institutional preparation of potatoes emphasizes the points at which ascorbic acid losses can occur. The increased use of precooked foods in households and institutions suggests the need for further investigation. Very few studies of the effects of cooking, holding, and reheating procedures appear in the literature.

Crosby et al. (*147*) reviewed the effects of institutional food service methods on ascorbic acid losses in vegetables held hot, and showed that considerable losses of vitamin C can be expected during holding. In 1975, Ang et al. (*148*) indicated that ascorbic acid in mashed potatoes prepared and reheated and held by conventional food service methods was extremely unstable, with losses of over 75% reported in some cases.

Augustin et al. (*143*) reported that the ascorbic acid content of cooked, chilled, and reheated baked potatoes decreased during refrigeration and microwave reheating, resulting in a net loss of approximately 30% of the ascorbic acid (dry weight basis). Similar results were noted for ascorbic acid fortified, rehydrated mashed potatoes, such as those commonly used in school lunch programs, although the losses were not as high as with baked potatoes.

A study done by Charles and Van Duyne (*132*) is widely cited as evidence of losses of ascorbic acid during home refrigerator storage and reheating of cooked vegetables. In seven of the nine vegetables examined, the concentrations of ascorbic acid were significantly reduced by holding in the refrigerator for 1 d (Table XI). After 1 d of refrigeration and reheating, the losses were significant in all products and ranged from 34 to 68%. Further holding for 2 or 3 d prior to reheating resulted in further significant decreases in ascorbic acid content. Therefore, the practice of refrigerating and warming leftover vegetables is not recommended from the standpoint of ascorbic acid retention.

Table XI. Effect of Holding and Reheating Cooked
Vegetables on Ascorbic Acid Retention

Vegetable	Ascorbic Acid Retention		
	Freshly Cooked	Refrigerated 1 d	Refrigerated 1 d, Reheated
Asparagus	86	82	66[b]
Broccoli	88	68[a]	60[a]
Cabbage, shredded	73	44[b]	33[b]
Peas	88	52[b]	43[b]
Snap beans	83	41[a]	29[b]
Spinach	52	48	32[a]

Source: Reference *132*.
[a] Significantly lower ($p > 0.05$) than corresponding mean for freshly cooked sample.
[b] Significantly lower ($p > 0.01$).

Conclusions

Ascorbic acid stability during harvesting, handling, storage, or processing of foods is often quite poor unless steps are taken to prevent vitamin C destruction. The major routes of vitamin C loss from foods are through thermal destruction, water leaching and enzymatic oxidation. One can minimize enzymatic destruction by avoiding bruising of fruit and vegetables and through proper storage conditions. Water leaching can also be reduced during soaking, washing, blanching, and cooking by use of minimal water, and in the case of blanching and cooking, the use of steam or microwave processing.

Some thermal destruction of the vitamin is inevitable in blanching, drying, canning, and cooking operations. However, some types of thermal processing, such as high temperature, short-time cooking, will usually result in optimal amounts of vitamin C in the food "as consumed".

Lund (69) has published a table containing the D_{121} values for destruction of constituents in foods. From Table XII it is evident that vitamins are more thermally resistant than are vegetative cells, spores, or destructive enzymes. In fact, most vitamins are more thermally resistant than are the organoleptic qualities of color, flavor, and texture. As a general rule, one can process a food for optimal sensory quality and be relatively sure of optimal thermal stability of the vitamins contained in the foods.

Table XII. Thermal Resistance of Constituents in Foods

Constituents	$D_{121}{}^a$ *(min)*
Vitamins	100–1,000
Color, texture, flavor	5–500
Enzymes	1–10
Spores	0.1–5.0
Vegetative cells	0.002–0.02

Source: Reference *69*.
^{a} Time at 121°C to decrease concentration by 90%.

Unfortunately, the thermal resistance of ascorbic acid falls in the low end of the scale (around 100, depending on a_w, pH, and other factors) in Table XII. Therefore, a final food product could display acceptable sensory qualities but still have lost a significant amount of vitamin C. If one is concerned with the vitamin C retention in foods, then great care must be taken in all facets of handling, storage, and processing of that food.

Literature Cited

1. Berk, Z. "Introduction to the Biochemistry of Foods"; Elsevier: Amsterdam, 1976; p. 92.
2. Bauernfeind, J. C.; Pinkert, D. M. *Adv. Food Res.* **1970**, *18*, 219.
3. Tannenbaum, S. R. In "Principles of Food Science, Part I"; Fennema, O., Ed.; Dekker: New York, 1976.
4. Bessey, O. A.; King, C. G. *J. Biol. Chem.* **1933**, *103*, 687.
5. Bessey, O. A. *J. Biol. Chem.* **1938**, *126*, 771.
6. Association of Vitamin Chemists, "Methods of Vitamin Assay," 3rd ed.; Interscience: New York, 1966; p. 287.
7. Association of Official Analytical Chemists, "Official Methods of Analysis," 12th ed.; Freed, M. Ed.; AOAC: Washington, D. C., 1975.
8. Loeffler, H. J.; Ponting, J. D. *Ind. Eng. Chem., Anal. Ed.* **1942**, *14*, 846.
9. Egberg, D.; Larson, P.; Honold, G. *J. Sci. Food Agric.* **1973**, *24*, 789.
10. Noble, I.; Hanig, M. M. D. *Food Res.* **1948**, *13*, 461.
11. Pelletier, O.; Brassard, R. *J. Food Sci.* **1977**, *42*, 1471.
12. Matthews, R. F.; Hall, J. W. *J. Food Sci.* **1978**, *43*, 532.
13. Brecht, P. E.; Keng, L.; Bisogni, C. A.; Muager, H. M. *J. Food Sci.* **1976**, *41*, 945.
14. Deutsch, M. J.; Weeks, C. E. *J. Assoc. Off. Agric. Chem.* **1965**, *48*, 1248.
15. Mills, M. B.; Damron, D. M.; Roe, J. H. *Anal. Chem.* **1949**, *21*, 707.
16. Kirk, J. R.; Ting, N. *J. Food Sci.* **1975**, *40*, 463.
17. Kirk, J.; Dennison, D.; Kokoczka, P.; Heldman, D. *J. Food Sci.* **1977**, *42*, 1274.
18. Dennison, D. B.; Kirk, J. R. *J. Food Sci.* **1978**, *43*, 609.
19. Singh, R. P.; Heldman, D. R.; Kirk, J. R. *J. Food Sci.* **1976**, *41*, 304.
20. Roy, R. R.; Conetta, A.; Salpeter, J. *J. Assoc. Off. Anal. Chem.* **1976**, *59*, 1244.
21. Egberg, D. C.; Potter, R. H.; Heroff, J. C. *J. Assoc. Off. Anal. Chem.* **1977**, *60*, 126.
22. Dunmire, D. L.; Reese, J. D.; Bryan, R.; Seegers, M. *J. Assoc. Off. Anal. Chem.* **1979**, *62*, 648.
23. Roe, J. H.; Kuether, C. A. *J. Biol. Chem.* **1943**, *147*, 339.
24. Roe, J. H. "Methods of Biochemical Analysis"; Interscience: New York, 1954; Vol. 1, p. 115.
25. Bourgeois, C. F.; Mainguy, P. R. *Int. J. Vitam. Res.* **1975**, *44*, 70.
26. Pelletier, O. *J. Lab. Clin. Med.* **1968**, *72*, 674.
27. Roe, J. H.; Mills, M. B.; Oesterling, M. J.; Dameron, C. M. *J. Biol. Chem.* **1948**, *174*, 201.
28. Smoot, J. M.; Nagy, S. *J. Agric. Food Chem.* **1980**, *28*, 417.
29. Guadagni, D. G.; Nimmo, C. C.; Jansen, E. F. *Food Technol.* **1957**, *11*, 389.
30. Sood, S. P.; Saitori, L. E.; Wittmer, D. P.; Haney, W. G. *Anal. Chem.* **1976**, *48*, 796.
31. Pachla, L. A.; Kissinger, P. T. *Anal. Chem.* **1976**, *48*, 364.
32. Augustin, J.; Beck, C.; Morousek, G. I. *Food Sci.* **1981**, *46*, 312.
33. Farrow, R. P.; Kemper, K.; Chin, H. B. *Food Technol.* **1979**, *33*(2), 52.
34. Baker, L. R. In "Nutritional Evaluation of Food Processing"; Harris, R. S.; Karmas, E., Eds.; Avi: Westport, CT, 1975; p. 19.
35. Bender, A. E. "Food Processing and Nutrition"; Academic: New York, 1978.
36. Harris, R. S. In "Nutritional Evaluation of Food Processing"; Harris, R. S.; Karmas, E., Eds.; Avi: Westport, CT, 1975; p. 33.
37. Patton, M. B.; Green, M. E. *Ohio Agric. Exp. Stn., Res. Bull.* **1954**, 742.

38. Nagy, S. *J. Agric. Food Chem.* **1980,** *28,* 8.
39. Liu, Y. K.; Luh, B. S. *J. Food Sci.* **1979,** *44,* 425.
40. Malewski, W.; Markakis, P. *J. Food Sci.* **1971,** *36,* 537.
41. Augustin, J.; McDole, R. E.; McMuster, G. M.; Painter, C. G.; Sparks, W. C. *J. Food Sci.* **1975,** *40,* 415,
42. Shekhar, V. C.; Iritani, W. M.; Arteca, R. *Am. Potato J.* **1978,** *55,* 663.
43. Burge, J.; Mickelsen, O.; Nicklow, C.; Marsh, G. L. *Ecol. Food Nutr.* **1975,** *4,* 27.
44. Augustin, J.; Johnson, S. R.; Tertzel, C.; Toma, R. B.; Shaw, R. L.; True, R. H.; Hogan, J. M.; Deutsch, R. M. *J. Food Sci.* **1978,** *43,* 1566.
45. Watada, A. E.; Aulenbach, B. B.; Worthington, J. T. *J. Food Sci.* **1976,** *41,* 856.
46. Betancourt, L. A.; Stevens, M. A.; Kader, A. A. *J. Am. Soc. Hortic. Sci.* **1977,** *102,* 721.
47. Pantos, C. E.; Markakis, P. *J. Food Sci.* **1973,** *38,* 550.
48. Matthews, R. F.; Crill, P.; Locascio, S. J. *Proc. Fla. State Hortic. Soc.* **1974,** *87,* 214.
49. Murphy, E. F. *Proc. Am. Soc. Hortic. Sci.* **1939,** *36,* 498.
50. Sites, J. W.; Reitz, H. J. *Proc. Am. Soc. Hortic. Sci.* **1951,** *56,* 103.
51. Isherwood, F. A.; Mapson, K. W. *Annu. Rev. Plant Physiol.* **1962,** *13,* 329.
52. Anonymous *Food Technol.* **1974,** *28* (1), 71.
53. Smith, P. F. *Proc. Int. Citrus Symp., 1st* **1969,** 1559.
54. Atkins, C. D.; Wiedenhold, E.; Moore, E. L. *Fruit Prod. J.* **1945,** *24,* 260.
55. McCollum, J. P. *Proc. Am. Soc. Hortic. Sci.* **1944,** *45,* 382.
56. Lachance, P. A. In "Nutritional Evaluation of Food Processing," 2nd ed.; Harris, R. S.; Karmas, E., Eds.; Avi: Westport, CT, 1975; p. 463.
57. Erdman, J. W., Jr. *Food Technol.* **1979,** *33* (2), 38.
58. Krochta, J. M.; Feinberg, B. In "Nutritional Evaluation of Food Processing"; Harris, R. S.; Karmas, E., Eds.; Avi: Westport, CT, 1975; p. 98.
59. O'Brien, M.; Kasmire, R. F. *Trans. ASAE* **1972,** *15,* 566.
60. Mapson, L. W. In "The Biochemistry of Fruits and Their Products"; Hulme, A. C., Ed.; Academic: New York; Vol. 1, 1970.
61. Ezell, B. D.; Wilcox, M. S. *J. Agric. Food Chem.* **1959,** *7,* 507.
62. Klein, B. P., unpublished data.
63. Zepplin, M.; Elvehjem, C. A. *Food Res.* **1944,** *9,* 100.
64. Eheart, M. S. *Food Technol.* **1970,** *24,* 1009.
65. Eheart, M. S.; Odland, D. *J. Am. Diet. Assoc.* **1972,** *60,* 402.
66. Curran, J.; Erdman, J. W., Jr. *Prof. Nutr.* **1980,** *12* (3), 7.
67. Smith, O. "Potatoes: Production, Storing, Processing," 2nd ed.; Avi: Westport, CT, 1977.
68. Saguy, I.; Karel, M. *J. Food Technol.* **1980,** *34* (2), 78.
69. Lund, D. B. *Food Technol.* **1977,** *31* (2), 78.
70. Ibid., **1979,** *33* (2), 28.
71. Labuza, T. P. *CRC Crit. Rev. Food Technol.* **1972,** *3,* 217.
72. Lenz, M. K.; Lund, D. B. *Food Technol.* **1980,** *34* (2), 51.
73. Villota, R.; Karel, M. *J. Food Process. Preserv.* **1980,** *4,* 141.
74. Mohr, D. H., Jr. *J. Food Sci.* **1980,** *45,* 1432.
75. Lathrop, P. J.; Leung, H. K. *J. Food Sci.* **1980,** *45,* 152.
76. Labuza, T. P. *J. Food Sci.* **1979,** *44,* 1162.
77. Wanninger, L. A. *Food Technol.* **1972,** *26,* 42.
78. Lee, S. H.; Labuza, T. P. *J. Food Sci.* **1975,** *40,* 370.
79. Laing, B. M.; Schlueter, D. L.; Labuza, T. P. *J. Food Sci.* **1978,** *43,* 1440.
80. Lund, D. B. In "Nutritional Evaluation of Food Processing"; Harris, R. S.; Karmas, E., Eds.; Avi: Westport, CT, 1975; p. 205.
81. Lee, Y. C.; Kirk, J. R.; Bedford, C. L.; Heldman, D. R. *J. Food Sci.* **1977,** *42,* 640.
82. Blaug, S. M.; Hajratwala, B. *J. Pharm. Sci.* **1972,** *61* (4), 556.

83. Mulley, E. A.; Stumbo, C. R.; Hunting, W. M. *J. Food Sci.* **1975**, *40*, 985.
84. Hamm, D.; Lund, D. B. *J. Food Sci.* **1978**, *43*, 631.
85. Labuza, T. P.; Shapero, M.; Kamman, J. *J. Food Process. Preserv.* **1979**, *2*, 91.
86. Purwadaria, H. K.; Heldman, D. R.; Kirk, J. R. *J. Food Process. Eng.* **1979**, *3*, 7.
87. Saguy, I.; Mizrahi, S.; Villota, R.; Karel, M. *J. Food Sci.* **1978**, *43*, 1861.
88. Riemer, J.; Karel, M. *J. Food Process. Preserv.* **1978**, *1*, 293.
89. Van Arsdel, W. B.; Guadagni, D. G. *Food Technol.* **1959**, *13*, 14.
90. Rao, M. A.; Lee, C. Y.; Katz, J.; Cooley, H. J. *J. Food Sci.* **1981**, *46*, 636.
91. Priestley, R. J. "Effects of Heating on Food Stuffs"; Appl. Sci.: London, 1979.
92. Harris, R. S.; Karmas, E. "Nutritional Evaluation of Food Processing," 2nd ed.; Avi: Westport, CT, 1975.
93. Benterud, A. In "Physical Chemical and Biological Changes in Food Caused by Thermal Processing"; Hoyem, T.; Kvale, O., Eds.; Appl. Sci.: London, 1977; p. 185.
94. Lathrop, P. J.; Leung, H. K. *J. Food Sci.* **1980**, *45*, 995.
95. Selman, J. D. *Food Chem.* **1978**, *3*, 189.
96. Morrison, M. H. *J. Food Technol.* **1974**, *9*(4), 491.
97. Salunkhe, D. K.; Pao, S. K.; Dull, G. G. *CRC Crit. Rev. Food Technol.* **1973**, *4*(1), 1.
98. Thompson, S. Y. "Ultra-high Temperature Processing of Dairy Products"; Soc. Dairy Technologists: London, 1969.
99. Lee, C. Y.; Downing, D. L.; Iredale, H. D.; Chapman, J. A. *Food Chem.* **1976**, *1*, 15.
100. Bluestein, P. M.; Labuza, T. P. In "Nutritional Evaluation of Food Processing," 2nd ed.; Harris, R. S.; Karmas, E., Eds.; Avi: Westport, CT, 1975; p. 289.
101. Henshall, J. D. *Proc. Nutr. Soc.* **1973**, *32*, 17.
102. Gee, M. *Lebensm.-Wiss. Technol.* **1979**, *12*, 147.
103. Jadhav, S.; Steele, L.; Hadziyev, D. *Lebensm.-Wiss. Technol.* **1975**, *8*, 225.
104. Maga, J. A.; Sizer, C. E. *Lebensm.-Wiss. Technol.* **1978**, *11*, 192.
105. Fennema, O. In "Nutritional Evaluation of Food Processing," 2nd ed.; Harris, R. S.; Karmas, E., Eds.; Avi: Westport, CT, 1975; p. 244.
106. Fennema, O. *Food Technol.* **1977**, *31*(12), 32.
107. "Recommendations for the Processing and Handling of Frozen Foods," 2nd ed.; International Institute of Refrigeration: Paris, 1972; p. 144.
108. Kramer, A.; King, R. L.; Westhoff, D. C. *Food Technol.* **1976**, *30*(1), 56.
109. Squires, S. R.; Hanna, J. G. *J. Agric. Food Chem.* **1979**, *27*, 639.
110. Jones, I. D. In "Nutritional Evaluation of Food Processing," 2nd ed.; Harris, R. S.; Karmas, E., Eds.; Avi: Westport, CT, 1975; p. 324.
111. Kon, S. K. *FAO Nutr. Stud.* **1959**, *17*.
112. Pederson, C. S.; Mack, G. L.; Athawes, W. L. *Food Res.* **1939**, *4*, 31.
113. Pederson, C. S.; Whitcombe, J.; Robinson, W. B. *Food Technol.* **1956**, *10*, 365.
114. Ro, S. L.; Woodburn, M.; Sandine, W. E. *J. Food Sci.* **1979**, *44*, 873.
115. Josephson, E. S.; Thomas, M. H.; Calhoun, W. K. In "Nutritional Evaluation of Food Processing," 2nd ed.; Harris, R. S.; Karmas, E., Eds.; Avi: Westport, CT, 1975; p. 393.
116. Anonymous. *Food Technol.* **1974**, *28*, 77.
117. "Nutritional Evaluation of Food Processing"; Harris, R. S.; Von Loesecke, H., Eds.; John Wiley & Sons: New York, 1960.
118. Watt, B. K.; Murphy, E. W. *Food Technol.* **1970**, *24*, 50.

119. Matthews, R. H.; Garrison, Y. J. "Food Yields Summarized by Different Stages of Preparation," *USDA* **1975**, *102*.
120. Schroder, G. M.; Satterfield, G. H.; Holmes, A. D. *J. Nutr.* **1943**, *25*, 503.
121. Kirk, M. M.; Tressler, D. K. *Food Res.* **1941**, *6*, 395.
122. Van Duyne, F. O.; Chase, J. T.; Simpson, J. I. *Food Res.* **1944**, *9*, 164.
123. Munsell, H. E.; Streightoff, F.; Bender, B.; Orr, M. L.; Ezekiel, S. R.; Leonard, M. H.; Richardson, M. E.; Koch, F. G. *J. Am. Diet. Assoc.* **1949**, *25*, 420.
124. Walker, A. R. P.; Arvidsson, U. B. *S. Afr. J. Med. Sci.* **1952**, *17*, 143.
125. Millross, J.; Speht, A.; Holdsworth, K.; Glew, G. "The Utilization of the Cook-Freeze Catering System for School Meals"; W. S. Maney & Son: Leeds, England, 1973.
126. Van Duyne, F. O.; Chase, J. T.; Simpson, J. I. *Food Res.* **1945**, *27*, 72.
127. Noble, I.; Waddell, E. *Food Res.* **1945**, *10*, 246.
128. Krehl, W. A.; Winters, R. W. *J. Am. Diet. Assoc.* **1950**, *26*, 1966.
129. Fisher, K. H.; Dods, M. L. *J. Am. Diet. Assoc.* **1952**, *28*, 726.
130. Gordon, J.; Noble, I. *J. Am. Diet. Assoc.* **1959**, *35*, 241.
131. Van Duyne, F. O.; Owen, R. F.; Wolfe, J. C.; Charles, V. R. *J. Am. Diet. Assoc.* **1951**, *27*, 1059.
132. Charles, V.; Van Duyne, F. O. *J. Home Econ.* **1954**, *46*, 659.
133. Thomas, M. H.; Brenner, S.; Eaton, A.; Craig, V. *J. Am. Diet. Assoc.* **1949**, *25*, 39.
134. Kylen, A. M.; Charles, V. R.; McGrath, B. H.; Schleter, J. M.; West, L. C.; Van Duyne, F. O. *J. Am. Diet. Assoc.* **1961**, *39*, 321.
135. Klein, B. P.; Kuo, C. H. Y.; Boyd, G. *J. Food Sci.* **1981**, *46*, 640.
136. Eheart, M. S.; Gott, C. *Food Technol.* **1964**, *19*, 867.
137. Sweeney, J. P.; Gilpin, G. L.; Staley, M. G.; Martin, M. E. *J. Am. Diet. Assoc.* **1959**, *35*, 354.
138. Klein, B. P. *CRC Handb. Nutr. Foods*, in press.
139. Mabesa, L. B.; Baldwin, R. E. *J. Food Sci.* **1979**, *44*, 932.
140. Klein, B. P., Reich, L., unpublished data.
141. Domas, A. A. M. B.; Davidek, J.; Velisek, J. Z. *Lebensm.-Unters. Forsch.* **1974**, *154*, 270.
142. Pelletier, O.; Nantel, C.; Leduc, R.; Tremblay, L.; Brassard, R. *Can. Inst. Food Sci. Technol. J.* **1977**, *10*, 138.
143. Augustin, J.; Marousek, G. I.; Tholen, L. A.; Bertelli, B. *J. Food Sci.* **1980**, *45*, 814.
144. Bowman, F.; Berg, E. P.; Chuang, A. L.; Gunther, M. W.; Trump, D. C.; Lorenz, K. *Microwave Energy Applications Newsletter* **1975**, *8*(3), 3.
145. Chapman, J. L., M.S. Thesis, Univ. Illinois, Urbana, 1978.
146. Kahn, R. M.; Halliday, E. G. *J. Am. Diet. Assoc.* **1944**, *20*, 220.
147. Crosby, M. W.; Fickle, B. E.; Andreassen, E. G.; Fenton, F.; Harris, K. W.; Burgain, A. M. *N. Y. Agric. Exp. St.*, Cornell, *Bull.* **1953**, *1891*.
148. Ang, C. Y. W.; Chang, C. M.; Frey, A. E.; Livingston, G. E. *J. Food Sci.* **1975**, *40*, 997.
149. Heidelbaugh, N. D.; Karel, M. *Mod. Packag.* **1970**, *43*(11), 80.
150. Campbell, C. L.; Lin, T. Y.; Proctor, B. E. *J. Am. Diet. Assoc.* **1958**, *34*, 365.

RECEIVED for review January 22, 1981. ACCEPTED July 20, 1981.

Antioxidant Properties of Ascorbic Acid in Foods

WINIFRED M. CORT

Hoffmann-LaRoche, Inc., Kingsland Road, Nutley, NJ 07110

Ascorbic acid and its esters function as antioxidants with some substrates by protecting double bonds and scavenging oxygen. Activity of ascorbates has been shown on vegetable oils, animal fats, vitamin A, carotenoids, citrus oils, and in fat-containing foods such as fish, margarine, and milk. Ascorbates also scavenge oxygen out of aqueous solutions and out of certain oxygen-containing compounds. This oxygen scavenging ability has resulted in ascorbic acid addition to beer, wine, meat, and bread. Ascorbic acid also lowers the oxidation state of many metals and valence may thus affect oxidation catalysis. The efficiency of ascorbates as antioxidants is dependent upon the substrate and the compounds to be protected. Because the 2- and 3-positions of ascorbic acid must be unsubstituted, the two free radicals formed at these positions may be intermediates in scavenging oxygen and inhibiting radical formation at double bonds.

A ntioxidants are listed in the Code of Federal Regulations (CFR) under food and chemical preservatives (1, 2). The listing includes phenolics such as butylated hydroxyanisole (BHA) indexed in Chemical Abstracts as [phenol, (1,1-dimethylethyl)-4-methoxy-25013-16-5] and butylated hydroxytoluene (BHT) [phenol, 2,6-bis(1,1-dimethylethyl)-4-methyl 128-37-0] as well as tetrabutylated hydroxyquinone (TBHQ) [(1,4-benzenediol, 2-(1,1-dimethylethyl 1948-33-0)], the thiodipropionates, tocopherols, bisulfites, and ascorbates. Only the latter two scavenge oxygen out of solution. The rest of the antioxidants have been used predominantly in fats and oils, and in most cases, with the exception of tocopherols and ascorbyl palmitate (AP) (**I**) [1-ascorbic ester 6-hexadecanoate 137-66-6], at the legal limit of 0.02% of the fat. Propyl gallate

(PG) [benzoic acid, 3,4,5-trihydroxypropyl ester 121-79-9], although listed with the other antioxidants in 1973, is now listed in 184.1660 as an antioxidant with a maximum level of 0.015% in food. Ethoxyquin (EMQ) [quinoline, 6-ethoxy-1,2-dihydro-2,2,4-trimethyl 91-53-2] has been used in animal feeds and the carry-over in animals is limited to 5 ppm. EMQ is allowed in paprika and chili powder at 100 ppm. Nordihydroguaiaretic acid (NDGA), allowed prior to 1968, is now illegal and foods containing it are deemed adulterated.

The use of ascorbic acid (II), as with other antioxidants, involves the specific substrate into which they are incorporated. In certain circumstances, additives that are present in foods and beverages inactivated a given antioxidant when used in the same formulation. In other cases, certain antioxidants reacted chemically with the materials they were intended to stabilize.

L-ascorbyl palmitate

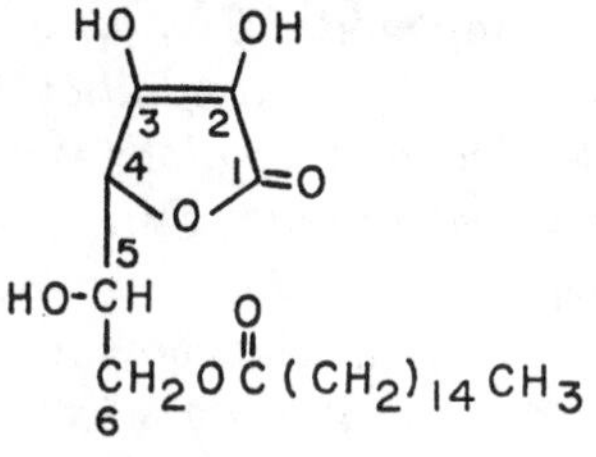

L-ascorbic acid

I

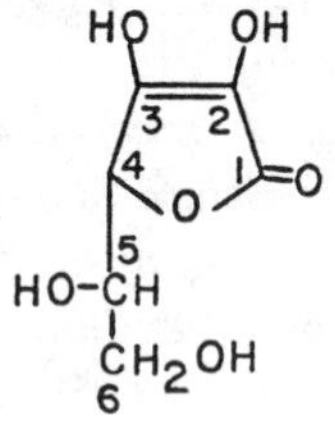

II

Ascorbic acid was studied in fats many years ago and reviewed by Chipault (3) who reported some activity, alone and with other antioxidants, in lard, cottonseed oil, meats, fish, mayonnaise, vegetable fats, baked and fried foods, milk powders, and irradiated foods. In these systems he reports that ascorbic acid doubles the stability of lard in the presence of either tocopherol or NDGA.

Ascorbic acid was used to prevent the oxidation of olive oil, milk, arachis nut oil, lard, ethyl ester of lard, cottonseed oil, pork, and beef fat (4); data showing activity alone and as a synergist are reviewed. Ascorbyl laurate, myristate, palmitate, and stearate were similarly active, although only AP is listed as a preservative in CFR. Ascorbic acid synergy with tocopherol was also reviewed.

Tappel (5) showed that ascorbic acid acts synergistically with food antioxidants and because of the great increase in effectiveness resulting from a small amount of ascorbic acid, he suggested mixtures would be effective in preventing oxidative rancidity in meats, poultry, and fish.

Ingold (6) did not review ascorbic acid per se, but did present a chapter on metal catalysis including the metal content of vegetable oils and the effect of valence state of the metals on oxidation of fats and oils. He reports cobalt, manganese, copper, iron, and zinc at the higher valences acted catalytically to oxidize many substrates. The author discussed the antioxidant activity of ascorbic acid in radiation-induced free radicals, fats in emulsions, fluid milk, and frozen fish. He also discussed the quandary of metal reactions vs. valence state.

Uri (7) has previously noted that Fe^{2+} reacts with peroxides:

$$Fe^{2+} + ROOH \rightarrow Fe^{3+} + OH^- + RO\cdot$$

thus, the organic peroxides such as linoleic hydroperoxides are decomposed to chain-initiating alkoxy radicals. When ferrous phthalocyanine is added to a saturated solution of quercetin in ethyl benzoate treated with methyl linoleate hydroperoxide, a deep red color forms that is attributed to the formation of an o-quinone at the $3' + 4'$-position of the flavone. Also, bleaching of β-carotene in ethyl benzoate by methyl linoleate hydroperoxide does not take place until ferrous ions are added and then this bleaching is completed within 10 min. The formation of the alkoxy radical in this reaction is the basis of the oxidizing power, which Uri refers to as "reductive activation." In his outline of activity of different metal catalysts he lists Co^{2+}, Mn^{2+}, and Ce^{3+} as most active. However, he shows reaction of all the lower oxidation states of the metals with peroxide. On the other hand, all the metals in the lower oxidation state, that is, Co^{2+}, Fe^{2+}, V^{2+}, Cr^{2+} Cu^+, Mn^{2+}, reacted with oxygen to form the higher valence state.

In certain systems ascorbic acid was so effective in lowering the valence state of metals that it was used in analytical chemistry (8). Ascorbic acid was used with gold, lead, bismuth, tellurium, copper, phosphorus, uranium, halogens, mercury, and cobalt.

In addition to the reports on the ascorbic acid effect on fats and metals, there are numerous reports that in certain media ascorbic acid may remove oxygen from solution; phenolic antioxidants are not effective in scavenging.

Experimental

Studies reported here use standard assay methods for antioxidants such as thin layer tests (Schaal oven) and the active oxygen method (AOM) (9) assayed by measuring peroxide formed, and an emulsion system using hemoglobin peroxidation of safflower oil measuring removal of oxygen from solution (10). Experiments on oxygen scavenging were performed in all glass equipment and in glass bottles with metal closures with a measured volume of headspace air. Experiments on additional substances, vitamin A, carotenoids, and citrus oil also were performed in thin layer tests measuring the loss of vitamin A at 325 nm and apocarotenal at 460 nm. Experiments with water solutions and sodium nitrite were also included. Ascorbic acid derivatives including ascorbic acid 2-sulfate (**III**), ascorbyl palmitate and laurate, sodium ascorbate, 2,3-di-*O*-methylascorbic acid (**IV**), benzoylascorbic acid, isopropylideneascorbic acid (**V**), and 3-*O*-[(dimorpholino)phosphinate]-5,6-*O*-isopropylidene L-ascorbate (**VI**) were also studied in the test systems. All figures reported here were collected in duplicate and were within a 10% variation.

L-ascorbic acid-2-sulfate
(potassium salt)

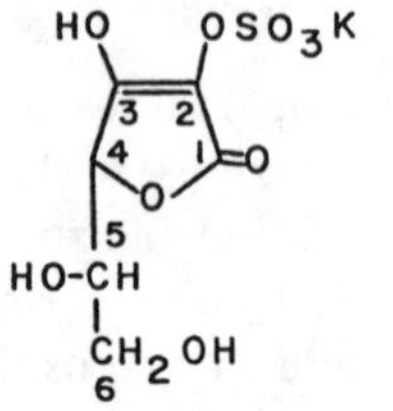

2,3-di-*O*-methylascorbate

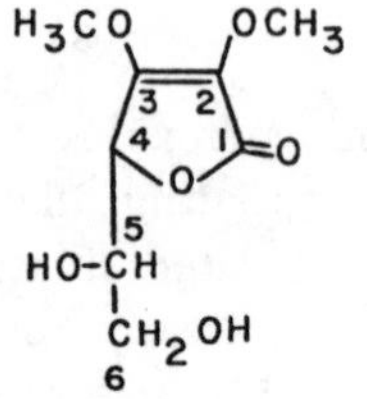

III

IV

5,6-isopropylidene
L-ascorbic acid

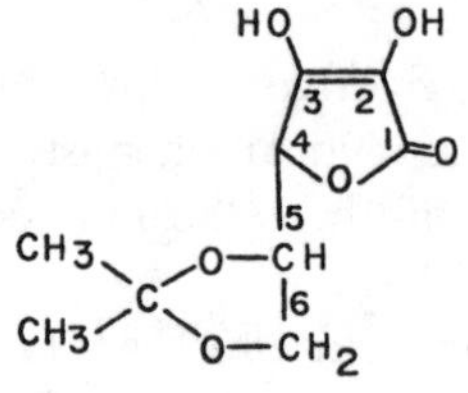

3-*O*-[(dimorpholino)phosphinate]-5,6-*O*-isopropylidene-L-ascorbate

V

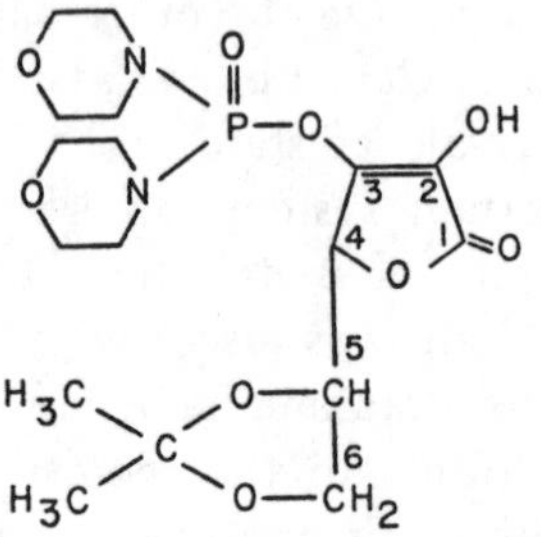

VI

Results

A series of antioxidant experiments illustrating comparative anti-oxidant activity in the specific systems tested is presented in Tables I–IX. Because many of the food-grade antioxidants except ascorbates and tocopherols are limited in the United States to 0.02% of the fat or oil, Table I compares the activity in soybean oil at that level. Although ascorbic acid and AP are more active than BHT and BHA, they are not as active as PG and TBHQ. Table II compares the activity of various ascorbates. Substitution in the 2- or 3-position of ascorbic acid makes it no longer active as an antioxidant, whereas compounds substituted in the 6- or 5,6-positions are active antioxidants. In Table III, antioxidant activities of ascorbic acid and AP are greater than BHT and BHA in safflower, sunflower, peanut, and corn oil. On pork and chicken fat, which are low in tocopherols, the ascorbates are less effective than BHT and BHA (Table IV); ascorbates are synergistic with tocopherols (*11*).

Wheat germ oil was studied in similar experiments, and it rapidly forms peroxides (Table V). Ascorbic acid and AP were more efficient antioxidants here than was BHT. To investigate the effect on wheat, whole berries were added to water and mixed with 0.1 g of antioxidants/ 100 g of berries and then dried at 60°C overnight. The dried mass was pulverized in a Waring blender and 10 g was added to petri dishes and titrated daily for peroxide after extraction into chloroform–acetic acid.

Table I. Comparative Antioxidant Activity in Soybean Oil

Antioxidant (0.02%)	*Days to Reach PV[a] 70*
None	5
BHT	8
BHA	7
PG	15
TBHQ	25
Ascorbic acid	10
AP	14

Note: α-Tocopherol content 10 mg %, total tocopherols 95%, thin layers, 45°C.
[a] PV is peroxide value (milliequivalents per kilogram).

Table II. Comparative Antioxidant Activity of Ascorbic Acid Derivatives in Soybean Oil

Antioxidant (0.05%)	*Days to Reach PV 70*
None	5
L-Ascorbic acid	17
D-Isoascorbic acid (erythorbic)	17
L-Ascorbyl palmitate	21
L-Ascorbyl laurate	21
D-Isoascorbyl laurate	21
L-Ascorbic acid 2-sulfate	5
2,3-Di-O-methyl-1-ascorbic acid	5
3-Benzoyl-L-ascorbic acid	5
5,6-Isopropylidene-L-ascorbic acid	23
2,3:4,6-Di-O-isopropylidene-2-keto-L-gulonate	5
3-O-[(Dimorpholino)phosphinate]-5,6-O-isopropylidene-L-ascorbate	5

Note: Thin layers, 45°C.

Table III.   Comparative Antioxidant Activity in Vegetable Oil

| | Substrate Oil | | | |
Antioxidant	Safflower	Sunflower	Peanut	Corn
None	6	6	15	12
BHT (0.02%)	10	9	15	13
BHA (0.02%)	8	8	15	15
AP (0.01%)	11	10	26	21
Ascorbic acid (0.02%)	10	10	NR[a]	NR[a]

Note: Thin layers, 45°C. Data given as days to reach PV 70.
[a] NR = not run.

Table IV.   Comparative Antioxidant Activity in Animal Fats

Antioxidant (0.02%)	Pork Lard	Chicken Fat
None	3	5
BHT	18	15
BHA	26	20
Ascorbic acid	8	10
AP	9	10
α-Tocopherol	15	13
α-Tocopherol and AP	28	28

Note: Thin layers, 45°C. Data given as days to reach PV 20.

Table V.   Comparative Antioxidant Activity in Wheat Germ Oil

| | Day | | | | |
Antioxidant	1	2	3	4	11
None	10	35	86	102	NR[a]
BHT (0.02%)	8	29	76	110	NR[a]
AP (0.2%)	0	18	50	98	NR[a]
AP (0.06%)	0	0	NR[a]	0	70
Ascorbic acid (0.06%)	0	0	NR[a]	0	12
BHT (0.06%)	0	0	NR[a]	70	NR[a]

Note: Thin layers, 45°C, data given as peroxide values.
[a] NR = not run.

Untreated controls reached peroxide value (PV) 70 in 11 d; those with BHT treatment lasted 20 d, with TBHQ 24 d, and with AP 31 d.

Results on comparative antioxidant efficiency on crude palm oil (Table VI) again show ascorbic acid to be very active.

Studies made on human fat were performed simply because of curiosity (Table VII). Oxidation was not very rapid, but the fat contained 14 mg % tocopherols (8.5 mg % gamma and 5.5 mg % alpha). AP had activity on this fat that may or may not be caused by synergism

Table VI.   Comparative Antioxidant Activity in Crude Palm Oil

Antioxidants	Days to Reach 70 PV
None	33
BHT (0.02%)	44
BHA (0.02%)	45
PG (0.02%)	60
TBHQ (0.02%)	45
Ascorbic acid (0.02%)	60
Ascorbic acid (0.1%)	100

Note: Thin layers, 45°C.

Table VII.   Compartive Antioxidant Activity in Human Fat

	PV on Days Shown					Days to
Antioxidant	7	16	21	39	64	Reach 20 PV
None	5	19	24	52	425	21
BHT (0.02%)	0	0	0	12	42	45
BHA (0.02%)	2	18	23	55	270	21
PG (0.02%)	0	0	0	4	18	78
TBHQ (0.02%)	0	0	0	0	0	ND[a]
α-Tocopherol (0.02%)	3	19	26	60	426	21
AP (0.02%)	0	0	13	43	317	28
AP (0.1%)	0	0	0	0	63	64
AP (1.0%)	0	0	0	0	0	ND[a]

Note: Thin layers, 45°C, human fat obtained from new cadaver rendered in autoclave. Fat filtered through cheesecloth and Whatman No. 2 paper.
[a] ND = not detected in 64 d.

of the tocopherols, a phenomenon to be discussed later. The unusual result is the dramatic effects of TBHQ.

The AOM test, in which air is bubbled at a constant rate at 98°C, shows ascorbic acid and AP to be active (Table VIII). The unexpected result here is the very large activity of ascorbic acid. However, Berner et al. (*12*) reported an AOM value of 8.3 for BHA, which on the addition of ascorbic acid at 0.03% became 44.2; this value was their highest AOM value. In a recent review, Porter (*13*) noticed this anomaly and included it in his theory of lipophilic, amphiphilic classification of antioxidants.

To determine quickly if a compound had any activity as an antioxidant, a hemoglobin-catalyzed emulsion test (*10*) was developed and at the same time a similar test was developed by Berner et al. (*12*). In the system (*10*) the antioxidants were added at 100 μg and compared to BHT at the same concentration. Ascorbic acid and AP are weak in this system but they exhibit some activity, whereas ascorbates substituted

Table VIII. Comparative Antioxidant Activity

Antioxidant	Soybean Oil	Crude Palm Oil
None	5	11
BHT (0.02%)	11	31
BHA (0.02%)	9	30
PG (0.02%)	14	50
AP (0.02%)	13	NR[a]
TBHQ (0.02%)	26	17
Ascorbic acid (0.02%)	43	NR[a]
Citric acid (0.1%)	NR[a]	51
Ascorbic acid (0.1%)	150	95

Note: AOM, 98°C, data given as hours to reach PV 70.
[a] NR = not run.

Table IX. Antioxidant Activity

Antioxidant[a]	Activity (% BHT)[a]	PV Formed in 10 min
None	0	30
BHT	100	28
BHA	200	10
PG	108	22
TBHQ	100	25
AP	64	14
Ascorbic acid	5	14
2,3-Di-O-methylascorbic acid	0	30
Ascorbic acid 2-sulfate	0	30

Note: Emulsion test, hemoglobin peroxidation.
[a] 100 μg added to 20 mL 10% stripped safflower oil emulsion.

in the 2- and 3-positions have no activity. The data presented here corroborate Porter's theory because the oil-soluble antioxidants are more active in the emulsion system and the more water-soluble compounds, such as ascorbic acid and citric acid, are more active in the all oil systems.

Tocopherol was effective and ascorbic acid ineffective in the protection of citrus oils evaluated by aroma (13). In a typical study, 5 g of orange oil was oxidized in 75-mL open brown bottles at 45°C and was evaluated by a panel after 6 d, at which time it was ranked as off-odor, "terpeney." The peroxide value of the initial oil was zero; the oxidized material had a PV of 100. As a result, days to reach 100 PV was used as an endpoint. Comparative antioxidant effects on a number of citrus oils and on D-limonene [cyclohexene, 1-methyl-4-(1-methylethenyl)-(R)-5989-27-5] are presented in Table X. BHA is the most active while AP has no activity alone but does synergize with tocopherol.

Vitamin A with its five conjugated double bonds oxidizes to 5,8-epoxides (*15*) with subsequent loss of UV absorption at 325 nm. Thus, vitamin A was studied with the addition of various antioxidants (Table XI) in open bottles in thin layers. Although EMQ was the best, it is limited to use in vitamin A for animal feeds. AP activity was not great, but when added to a mixture of tocopherol, BHT, and diethanolamide, AP gave excellent protection. Klaui (*16*) has shown stability of vitamin A palmitate with tocopherol, AP, and an amine equal to 1300 h, compared to a control equal to 100 h. However, the antioxidants in the dry market form (beadlets) protect the vitamin A in the beadlets as well as the end use of the product. For example, spray-dried vitamin A can be pro-

Table X.   Citrus Oils Antioxidant Activity

Antioxidants[a]	Orange (Fla.)	Orange (Calif.)	Lemon	Grape-fruit	Lime	D-Limo-nene
None	6	4	9	3	9	5
BHT	35	32	24	27	9	> 56
BHA	44	49	91	34	15	> 56
PG	18	36	17	20	9	> 56
dl-α-Tocopherol	15	10	9	7	15	15
AP	6	4	9	3	9	5
Tocopherol and AP	21	16	19	7	15	30

Note: Data given as days to reach 100 PV, 45°C.
[a] Antioxidants at 0.02% ; sample size, 5 g in 75-mL open bottles.

Table XI.   Comparative Activity on Antioxidants on Crystalline Vitamin A Acetate

Antioxidant[a]	Days				
	2	5	8	12	15
None	62	27	15	10	7
BHT	89	79	73	59	52
BHA	57	30	19	12	9
PG	57	28	15	10	7
TBHQ	88	82	80	71	70
dl-α-Tocopherol	89	70	57	42	33
AP	70	40	23	18	10
EMQ	98	91	89	84	75
BHT (at 1.2 g)	87	81	74	59	56
BHT, Tocopherol, AP, diethanolamine	98	93	88	85	75
Tocol mix[b]	95	89	81	81	79
BHT and either ethanolamine diethanolamine Tween 60 or 80	100	89	85	67	60

Note: Sample size, 5 g in 100-mL open brown bottles, 45°C. Data given as percent retention.
[a] At 100 mg/bottle unless noted.
[b] Mix = α-tocopherol 230, diethanolamine 460, Tween 80, 1151 mg.

duced with only tocopherol for protection, and the vitamin is stable for several years. However, if the vitamin is mixed in flour with the moisture encountered at the mills (12–13%), it must have BHT to survive (17).

Carotenoids such as β-apo-8'-carotenal with its nine conjugated double bonds also form epoxides and lose all their color on oxidation. Thus, experiments using color loss at 460 nm were performed to study antioxidant activity. Table XII shows that γ-tocopherol followed by BHA and α-tocopherol are the best antioxidants for apocarotenal, and if AP is added, both tocopherols are the very best. Ascorbic acid and AP both have some antioxidant activity for apocarotenal without tocopherol.

Oxygen scavenging experiments were performed on compounds dissolved in oxygenated distilled water in brown bottles with 2 cm³ of headspace, testing all the compounds at 20 mg/bottle. The bottles were shaken in a rotary shaker at 150 rpm for 19 h at room temperature. Immediately after opening, oxygen in solution was read on the Orion Electrode (Orion Research) (Table XIII). Additional experiments, read within 5 min, showed that the inorganics reacted immediately; however, after bubbling in air for 5 min, only the sodium sulfite continued to keep oxygen in solution at zero. Ascorbic acid and cysteine took

Table XII. Comparative Activity of Antioxidants on Apo-8'-carotenal

Antioxidant[a]	Day (45°C)							Day (room temperature)
	4	6	8	12	16	20	28	28
None	72	59	40	16	6	2	>1	80
BHT	100	92	88	70	40	25	7	91
BHA	100	100	98	88	72	59	40	95
PG	95	95	92	85	65	52	36	93
Ascorbic acid	80	78	52	29	7	3	1	87
AP	96	88	78	46	16	5	1	91
dl-α-Tocopherol	100	100	95	92	72	48	28	95
dl-α-Tocopherol and AP	100	100	98	92	75	65	42	100
dl-α-Tocopherol and ascorbic acid	100	100	100	95	78	62	43	96
dl-γ-Tocopherol	100	100	100	100	82	72	48	96
dl-γ-Tocopherol and AP	100	100	100	92	78	72	56	96
dl-γ-Tocopherol and ascorbic acid	100	100	100	92	75	70	55	96

Note: 200 μg/g in coconut oil. Data given as percent ret ention. 3.3 g Petri plate 150 × 15 mm.
[a] Antioxidants at 200 μg/g.

**Table XIII. Oxygen Scavenging Experiment Effect of
Compounds on Residual Oxygen in Solution**

Compounds Added[a]	Oxygen (ppm)	Odor
None	8	OK
$Na_2S_2O_4$	0–1	SO_2-like
$Na_2S_2O_5$	0–1	SO_2-like
Na_2SO_3	0	OK
L-Ascorbic acid	0	OK
Sodium-L-ascorbate	0	OK
2,3-Di-O-methylascorbic acid	8	OK
3-Benzoyl ascorbate	8	OK
5,6-Isopropylidene-L-ascorbic acid	0	OK
3-O-[(Dimorpholino)phosphinate]-5,6-O-isopropylidene-L-ascorbate	8	OK
Potassium-L-ascorbate 2-sulfate	8	OK
Cysteine HCl	5	+ odor
Cysteine free base	0	+ odor
D-Isoascorbic acid	0	OK
Dehydro-L-ascorbic acid	8	OK

Note: 50-mL brown bottles, closed metal lids, 2 cm³ of headspace air, shaken
150 rpm for 19 h, room temperature.
[a] 20 mg/bottle.

17–24 h of shaking in closed bottles to come to completion. As previously shown, in fat oxidation the 2- and 3-positions of ascorbic acid have to be unsubstituted to allow oxygen scavenging. Measurement of UV absorption showed an optical density at 290 nm of 1.0 and at 260 nm of 1.4 for the sodium ascorbate; these readings might indicate formation of the free radical in the 2-position, which reportedly absorbs at 290 nm (*18*).

Ascorbyl palmitate, laurate, and stearate were tested in this system. However, their water solubilities were so low that they did not function as oxygen scavengers until the pH was adjusted to 9 to solubilize all three esters. Subsequently they removed all of the oxygen from solution at 20 mg/bottle with 2 cm³ of headspace air.

Theoretically 3.3 mg of ascorbic acid will consume the oxygen in 1 cm³ of headspace air (*19*). Additional experiments were performed with measured amount of headspace air and ascorbic acid (Table XIV). These experiments were performed in 37-mL bottles with metal lids in a shaker at 150 rpm for 19 h. Six milligrams of ascorbic acid removed oxygen in the bottles with 1 cm³ of headspace and reduced the oxygen in the bottles with 2 cm³ of headspace. Ascorbic acid assays measured by absorption at 260 nm indicate a lack of material balance. Therefore, additional studies were performed in all glass bottles (Table XV). In this experiment 3.4–3.6 mg of ascorbic acid was required for each cubic centimeter of headspace, which is close to the theoretical value. In additional experiments not included in this table, metal caps were inserted into the all glass equipment; less time was required to remove the oxygen from the solutions and more ascorbic acid per cubic centimeter of headspace was required.

Water solutions of ascorbic acid measured in the UV required gassing with nitrogen to slow down the destruction of ascorbic acid. Nitrogen-gassed ascorbic acid solutions at 10 μg/mL were scanned spectrophotometrically at 360–200 nm for 24 h with no change in optical density (peak, 260 nm). By comparison, 10-μg/mL solutions of ascorbic acid, containing 8 ppm oxygen in all glass equipment with 10 cm^3 of headspace air, were scanned hourly also. Within 6 h the UV peak was reduced, no new peaks were formed, and more than 90% of the ascorbic acid was gone.

Anaerobic degradation of ascorbic acid in grapefruit juice is a zero-order reaction (20), but degradation of fish is either first or zero order depending on the type of fish (21). Ascorbic acid degradation in peas is

Table XIV. Residual Oxygen in Solution

	Ascorbic Acid Content (mg)		
Headspace (cc)	3	6	9
0	0.0	0.0	0.0
1	1.2	0.0	0.0
2	2.2	0.2	0.0
3	3.6	2.8	0.3
5	4.7	5.1	1.4
7	7.0	6.0	5.0
10	8.0	7.0	6.0

Note: Closed bottles, metal lids, shaken 19 h at room temperature. Data given as parts per million.

Table XV. Oxygen Scavenging by Ascorbic Acid with Reduced Metal Contamination

Ascorbic Acid	Oxygen (ppm)	Residue Ascorbic Acid (mg)	Ascorbic Acid Consumed (mg)
none	8.0	0.0	0.0
3 mg	0.4	1.3	1.7
6 mg	0.0	4.2	1.8
9 mg	0.0	7.2	1.8

Note: 0.5 cm^3 of headspace, glass flasks and stopper; shaken 24 h at room temperature.

a first-order degradation (22, 23). First-order degradation of ascorbic acid was shown in limited oxygen, but oxygen had a profound effect on the rate (24); these findings agree with our data. Studies on ascorbic acid in relation to water activity indicate that the lack of water in the AOM probably prevents ascorbic acid from breaking down, allowing it to remain active.

Further studies on the ability of ascorbic acid to scavenge oxygen by reacting with nitrogen have been of interest. Ascorbic acid added to sodium nitrite solutions immediately produces bubbles, with the release of nitric oxide. Mergens (26) studied the addition of all of the precursors of ascorbic acid synthesis as well as the 6- and 5,6-derivatives discussed here. His system is similar to that reported previously (27). The loss of nitrite was measured within 1 min from a 7 mM solution of sodium nitrite. Ascorbic derivatives in the 6- and 5,6-positions were active, and all precursors were inactive, in nitrite decomposition. More recently Mergens found that III and VI are inactive. Thus, reaction with nitrite parallels the requirement for oxygen scavenging and antioxidant in fats, namely that the 2- and 3-positions of ascorbic acid must be unsubstituted and remain as the enediol or enediol anion to be active.

Table XVI   Oxygen Scavenging from Nitrogen Dioxide by Ascorbates

Active	Inactive
L-Ascorbic acid	Ascorbic acid precursors glucose, sorbose, 2-ketogulonic, etc.
AP	
5,6-Isopropylidene-L-ascorbic acid	L-Ascorbic acid 2-sulfate
d-Isoascorbic acid (erythorbic)	3-O-[(Dimorpholino)phosphinate]-5,6-O-isopropylideneascorbic acid

Discussion

Metal Effects and Prooxidant Action. Ascorbic acid is prooxidant in some situations. Kanner et al. (28) showed that Cu^{2+} increased the oxidation of linoleate using loss of β-carotene as an indicator. However, when sufficient ascorbic acid was added to his system, copper catalysis was reversed. Furthermore, when Fe^{3+} was added, the addition of ascorbic acid increased the prooxidant effect. Previous publications (29) have discussed the deactivation of copper catalysis by ascorbic acid, but in iron-catalyzed oxidation, Fe^{2+} initiates oxidation of lipid (2). Fe^{2+} *is* formed from Fe^{3+} by ascorbic acid. Many foods contain metals, and the addition of ascorbic acid will lower their valence. These lower valence metals may cause problems.

The role of ascorbic acid in enzyme systems has been known for a long time. The ascorbic acid requirement was reviewed along with α-ketoglutaric acid, oxygen, and Fe^{2+} in propyl and lysyl hydroxylases and the possibility that ascorbic acid's function is to keep to iron as Fe^{2+} (30). More recently researchers claim that ascorbic acid does not participate in the hydroxylation reaction but is specifically required to keep the enzyme Fe^{2+} in the reduced form (31). The peptide-bound proline is transformed to hydroxyproline and α-ketoglutarate to succinate and carbon dioxide. Ascorbic acid as a cofactor functions to keep iron as Fe^{2+} in not only propyl hydroxylase but also lysyl hydroxylase, p-hydroxyphenyl pyruvate hydroxylase, indoleamine-2,3-dioxygenase, and α-ketoglutarate and 5-hydroxymethyluracil dioxygenases.

One of the most interesting papers on ascorbic acid–Cu^{2+} reactions showed that ascorbic acid–Cu^{2+} catalyzes the formation of ethylene from several precursors. The interest in ethylene was as an abscission agent in plants. All alcohols, aldehydes, acids, ethers, and epoxides formed ethylene when mixed with Cu^{2+} and ascorbic acid in 5-mL closed bottles at 30°C for 1 h. Methional was the most active, followed by propanal, propanol, propyl ether, ethyl ether, and ethanol. This reaction may be part of the oxygen scavenging system because Cu^{2+} increases ascorbic acid's ability to scavenge oxygen. The authors claim this reaction cannot be attributed to copper in its lower valence state.

Either Fenton reagent or a mixture of ascorbic acid, Fe^{3+}, and ethylenediaminetetraacetic acid catalyzed the production of acetyldehyde from ethanol, ethylene from methional derivative, and methane from dimethyl sulfoxide (34). The authors claimed that both hydroxy radicals and singlet oxygen were found as intermediates, and, indeed, ascorbic acid scavenged both hydroxyl radical and singlet oxygen.

Ascorbic Acid and Tocopherol. In certain foods and beverages ascorbic acid and AP synergized other antioxidants and tocopherols, and some of this data was reviewed (5, 35). Both α- and γ-tocopherol, similar to ascorbic acid, react with Cu^{2+} and Fe^{3+}, and as a result ascorbic acid may sacrificially stabilize tocopherols (36). However, ascorbic acid transforms α-tocopheroxide to α-tocopherol and the dimeric keto ether to "bi-α-tocopheryl," thus regenerating the two antioxidant species from oxidized tocopherols (37). Packer et al. (38) mixed trichloromethylperoxy radical with α-tocopherol under pulse radiolysis to form tocopherol radical (absorbs at 425 nm). When ascorbic acid was added, ascorbic radical formed, absorbing at 360 nm; the 425-nm absorption was lost. The rapid interaction may recycle tocopherol at the expense of ascorbic acid.

Biological Systems. In biological systems, oxidation may proceed through superoxide radical O_2^-, which forms from molecular oxygen by addition of a single electron (*39*). Superoxide dismutase (SOD) acts on O_2^- to yield hydrogen peroxide and oxygen, which reacts with another O_2^- to produce hydroxy radical. This latter reaction is catalyzed by Fe^{3+}; the hydroxy radicals are considered most toxic. Superoxide radical is produced by respiration and a number of enzymes, including xanthine oxidase, aldehyde oxidase, dihydro-orotic acid dehydrogenase, galactose oxidase, indoleamine and 2-nitropropane dioxygenases, diamine oxidase, and ribulose-1,5-diphosphate carboxylase. Oxidation of many compounds, including hydroquinone, flavins, thiols, catecholamines, dialuric acid, herbicides, paraquat, and carbon tetrachloride, produce O_2^-. Polluted air from burning gasoline, paper, and tobacco and ozone-contaminated air contains O_2^-.

Ascorbic acid reacts with O_2^- generated from the xanthine oxidase system and may play a role against O_2^- mediated toxicity. Ascorbic acid quenches the hydroxyl radical (*40*). Ascorbic acid may protect against free radicals in the lung because ascorbic acid is found in the fluid (*39*). The toxicity of ozone and oxygen may also be reduced by ascorbic acid (*39*). Carbon tetrachloride mortality in rats is lowered by ascorbic acid. Autoxidation of ascorbic acid did not generate O_2^-. Reduced glutathione reacts with dehydroascorbic acid (**VII**) and recycles ascorbic acid.

dehydroascorbic acid

VII

Review of Ascorbic Acid Mechanisms of Action. Ascorbic acid and AP have antioxidant activity in fats, oils, vitamin A, and carotenoids. In these systems AP is a better antioxidant than are the phenolic antioxidants BHT and BHA, both from these data and others (*29, 35*). Ascorbic acid protects against oxidation of flavor compounds in wine, beer, fruits, artichokes, and cauliflower (*29*) presumably by oxygen scavenging. The well-known formation of nitric oxide from nitrites by ascorbic acid is used not only for inhibition of nitrosamine formation, but also to promote the formation of nitrosometmyoglobin and nitrosomyoglobin to keep meat red.

Ascorbic acid, acting as an antioxidant in certain systems, scavenges oxygen out of solution at a ratio of 3.4–3.6 mg/cm^3 of headspace air, which is close to the theoretical value.

In all of the ascorbic acid reactions substitution in the 5- and 5,6-positions does not interfere with its activity. Substitution in either the 2- or 3-position or both makes ascorbic acid no longer active as an oxygen scavenger or as an antioxidant.

Olcott and Lin (41) attempted to learn the mechanism of action of certain antioxidants by studying stable free radical nitroxides. They measured the electron paramagnetic resonance (EPR) signal and as long as the nitroxide signal was obtained, oxidation was inhibited. When that signal was no longer detected, oxidation proceeded. Later (42) EMQ nitroxide prevented the oxidation of squalene and when the EPR nitroxide signal was no longer detected, oxidation proceeded. They contended that the free radical of the antioxidant keeps the the alkyl free radical in the lipid from forming; therefore, peroxides cannot form. This explanation is not universally acceptable, although the formation of a radical prior to peroxide formation of fats and oils has been accepted for many years.

Orr (43) used dimethyl sulfoxide as a free radical sink to inhibit the effect of Cu^{2+} and ascorbic acid on catalase and β-glucuronidase as well as the degradation of hyaluronic acid. The formation of a radical from ascorbic acid and Cu^{2+} in water was detected by EPR (44). Based on an EPR spectroscopic study of ascorbic acid during oxidation of methyl-arachidonate-enriched liposomes, ascorbic acid may be important in preventing free radical damage in the central nervous system (45).

Formation of the free radical of ascorbic acid (measured at 360 nm) accompanied reduction of tocopherol free radicals (38). Bielski et al. (18, 46) showed that the ascorbic acid free radical in the 3-position absorbs at 360 nm and that in the 2-position absorbs at 290 nm; also, ascorbic acid reacts with superoxide.

In certain systems ascorbic acid free radical on the 2- and 3-positions may be an intermediate in the antioxidant function, but it is a short-lived intermediate (18). An electron spin resonance flow system was used to study scavenging of a nitrosating agent by ascorbic acid, and a total spin free radical, which is the same as that produced by radiolytic oxidation (48), was determined (47).

The evidence in this chapter is that the 2- and 3-positions of ascorbic acid must be unsubstituted and available for ascorbic acid to act as an oxygen scavenger or an antioxidant.

Acknowledgments

Thanks are given to Jane Jernow and E. Oliveto for providing the ascorbic acid derivatives and to M. Mergens for experimental data.

Literature Cited

1. *Code of Federal Regulations* Title 21 121.101, 1973.
2. *Code of Federal Regulations* Title 21 172.110–172.190, 182.3013–182.3890, 1980.
3. Chipault, J. R. In "Autoxidation and Antioxidants"; Lundberg, W. O., Ed.; John Wiley & Sons: New York, 1962; Vol. 2, pp. 506–509, 523–526.
4. Emanuel, N. M.; Lyaskovskaya, Y. N. In "The Inhibition of Fat Oxidation Processes"; Pergamon Press: New York, 1967; pp. 307–315.
5. Tappel, A. L. In "Autoxidation and Antioxidants"; Lundberg, W. O., Ed.; John Wiley & Sons: New York, 1961; Vol. 1, p. 325.
6. Ingold, K. V. In "Symposium on Foods: Lipids and Their Oxidation"; Schultz, H. W.; Day, E. A.; Sinnhuber, R. O., Eds.; Avi: Westport, CN, 1962; p. 93.
7. Uri, N. In "Autoxidation and Antioxidants"; Lundberg, W. O., Ed.; John Wiley & Sons: New York, 1961; Vol. 1, pp. 55–106, 133.
8. Hay, G. W.; Lewis, B. A.; Smith, F. In "The Vitamins"; Sebrell, W. H.; Harris, R. S., Eds.; Academic: New York, 1967; Vol. 1, p. 319.
9. AOCS "Official and Tentative Methods of the Amer. Oil Chem. Soc."; AOCS: Champaign, IL, 1964; Vol. 1.
10. Cort, W. M. *Food Technol.* **1974,** *26,* 60.
11. Cort, W. M. *J. Am. Oil Chem. Soc.* **1974,** *51,* 321.
12. Berner, D. L.; Conte, J. A.; Jacobson, G. A. *J. Am. Oil Chem. Soc.* **1974,** *51,* 292.
13. Porter, W. L. In "Autoxidation in Food and Biological Systems"; Simic, M. G.; Karel, M., Eds.; Plenum: New York, London, 1980; p. 295.
14. Kesterson, J. W.; McDuff, O. R. *Am. Perfum. Essent. Oil Rev.* **1949,** *54,* 285.
15. Schweiter, U.; Isler, O. In "The Vitamins"; Sebrell, W. H.; Harris, R. S., Eds.; Academic: New York, 1967; Vol. 1.
16. Klaui, H. *Proc. Univ. Nottingham Resid. Semin. Vitam.* **1971,** 110.
17. Borenstein, B.; Cort, W. M., French Patent 2 011 564, 1970.
18. Bielski, B. H. J.; Comstock, D. A.; Bowen, R. A. *J. Am. Chem. Soc.* **1971,** *93,* 5624.
19. "The Use of Ascorbic Acid in Carbonated and Non-Carbonated Beverages," Roche Technical Service, Fine Chemical Division, 1960.
20. Smoot, J. M.; Nagy, S. *J. Agric. Food Chem.* **1980,** *28,* 417.
21. Ding, J. C.; Watson, M.; Bates, R. P.; Schroeder, E. *J. Food Sci.* **1978,** *43,* 457.
22. Lathrop, P. J.; Leung, H. K. *J. Food Sci.* **1980,** *45,* 152.
23. Blaug, S. D.; Hajratwala, B. *J. Pharm. Sci.* **1972,** *61,* 556.
24. Dennison, D. B.; Kirk, J. R. *J. Food Sci.* **1978,** *43,* 609.
25. Labuza, T. P. *Food Technol.* **1980,** *34,* 67.
26. Mergens, W.; Hoffmann-LaRoche, personal communication.
27. Raineri, R.; Weisburger, J. H. *Ann. N.Y. Acad. Sci.* **1975,** *258,* 181–189.
28. Kanner, J.; Mendel, H.; Budowski, P. *J. Food Sci.* **1977,** *42,* 60.
29. FAO-WHO "Review of the Technological Efficacy of Some Antioxidants and Synergists," *W.H.O. Tech. Rep. Ser.* **1971,** *488.*
30. Barnes, M. J. *Ann. N.Y. Acad. Sci.* **1971,** *258,* 264.

31. "The Role of Ascorbic Acid in the Hydroxylation of Peptide-Bound Pro-line," *Nutr. Rev.* **1979**, *37*, 26.
32. Hayaishi, O.; Nozaki, N.; Abbott, H. T. In "The Enzymes"; Boyer, P. D., Ed.; Academic: New York, 1974; Vol. 12, p. 119.
33. Lieberman, M.; Kunishi, A. T. *Science* **1967**, *158*, 938.
34. Cohen, G.; Cederbaum, A. I. *Arch. Biochem. Biophys.* **1980**, *199*, 438.
35. Klaui, H. In "Vitamin C: Recent Aspects of Its Physiological and Techno-logical Importance"; Birch, G.; Parker, K. J., Eds.; John Wiley & Sons: New York, 1974; pp. 16–39.
36. Cort, W. M.; Mergens, W.; Green, A. *J. Food Sci.* **1978**, *43*, 797.
37. Schuldel, P.; Mayer, H.; Isler, O. In "The Vitamins"; Sebrell, W. H.; Har-ris, R. S., Eds.; Academic: New York, 1972; pp. 168–225.
38. Packer, J. E.; Slater, T. F.; Willson, R. L. *Nature* **1979**, *278*, 737.
39. Leibovitz, B. E.; Siegel, B. V. *J. Gerontol.* **1980**, *35*, 45.
40. Fessenden, R. W.; Verma, N. C. *Biophys. J.* **1978**, *24*, 93.
41. Olcott, H. S.; Lin, J. S. "Free Radical Intermediates of Antioxidants," *66th Meet. AOCS, Dallas, TX, 1975.*
42. Lin, J. S.; Olcott, H. S. *J. Agric. Food Chem.* **1975**, *23*, 798.
43. Orr, C. W. M. *Biochemistry* **1967**, *6*, 2995.
44. Moravskii, I. *Proc. Acad. Sci. USSR Chem. Sect.* **1977**, *1*, 61; *Chem. Abstr.* **1977**, *86*, 111618C.
45. Demopoulu, S. H.; Flamm, E.; Seligman, M.; Power, R.; Pietronigro, D.; Ranschoff, J. *Oxygen Physiol. Funct., Proc. Am. Physiol. Soc. Colloq.* **1977**, 491–502; *Chem. Abstr.* **1979**, *90*, 927105.
46. Bielski, B. H. J.; Richter, H. W. *J. Am. Chem. Soc.* **1977**, *99*, 3019.
47. Kalus, W. H.; Filby, W. G. *Experientia* **1980**, *36*, 143.
48. Laroff, G. P.; Fessenden, R. W.; Schuler, R. H. *J. Am. Chem. Soc.* **1972**, *94*, 9026.
49. Jernow, J.; Blount, J.; Oliveto, E.; Perrota, A.; Rosen, P.; Toome, V. *Tetrahedron* **1979**, *35*, 1483.

RECEIVED for review January 22, 1981. ACCEPTED June 22, 1981.

Biological Interaction of Ascorbic Acid and Mineral Nutrients

NOEL W. SOLOMONS

Department of Nutrition and Food Science, Massachusetts Institute of Technology, Cambridge, MA 02139, and Division of Human Nutrition and Biology, Institute of Nutrition of Central America and Panama, Guatemala City, Guatemala, Central America, Apartado 11-88

FERNANDO E. VITERI[1]

Division of Human Nutrition and Biology, Institute of Nutrition of Central America and Panama, Guatemala City, Guatemala, Central America, Apartado 11-88

In the diet and at the tissue level, ascorbic acid can interact with mineral nutrients. In the intestine, ascorbic acid enhances the absorption of dietary iron and selenium; reduces the absorption of copper, nickel, and manganese; but apparently has little effect on zinc or cobalt. Ascorbic acid fails to affect the intestinal absorption of two toxic minerals studied, cadmium and mercury. At the tissue level, iron overload enhances the oxidative catabolism of ascorbic acid. Thus, the level of dietary vitamin C can have important nutritional consequences through a wide range of inhibitory and enhancing interactions with mineral nutrients.

The nutritional sciences have recently moved from a predominant concern with the identification and characterization of deficiency manifestations for individual nutrients to a consideration of interactions between and among nutrients. Ascorbic acid represents a vitamin that undergoes numerous interactions with other nutrients, specifically minerals; therefore, it is important and appropriate to review and update this topic. The present state of knowledge on the interaction of ascorbic acid and minerals of nutritional importance is the subject of this chapter.

[1] Current address: Division of Disease Prevention and Control, Pan American Health Organization, Washington, DC 20037.

0065-2393/82/0200-0551$06.00/0

Minerals of Nutritional Importance

Approximately fifteen minerals are considered nutrients (*calcium, chromium, cobalt, copper, iron, magnesium, manganese, molybdenum,* nickel, *phosphorus, selenium,* silicon, tin, vanadium, and *zinc*); of these minerals, those in italics are essential to mammalian nutrition. Minerals, which are important for good nutrition, are supplied in an organism's diet. However, we have recently realized that the biological availability of the minerals from their food sources is also important in nutrition (*1*). Internal metabolism, distribution, and retention are less important factors in mineral nutrition.

Nature and Scope of Ascorbic Acid–Mineral Interaction

The primary interaction of ascorbic acid with minerals occurs in the gastrointestinal tract. Significant effects on inhibiting and enhancing the uptake of minerals into the mucosa or into the body have been documented. Various investigators have postulated a number of mechanisms that alone, or in combination, would be responsible for the specific interaction of ascorbic acid with a given mineral in the gut (i.e., by affecting the pH of the intestinal environment, having an antioxidant/reducing effect, affecting intraluminal solubility, causing intraluminal complex formation, or affecting transmucosal transport). The effect of ascorbic acid on intraintestinal pH, providing a more acidic environment, has been mentioned; this would be most important in the absence of normal gastric acid production. Ascorbic acid's antioxidant or reducing effect may preserve or promote the reduced oxidation state for a given metallic ion. Depending upon the specificity of the mucosal absorption mechanism, this reducing effect can either reduce or augment uptake. Ascorbic acid, through its effects on pH and oxidation state, or by forming complexes, may promote intraluminal solubility of a mineral, preventing its olation, polymerization, precipitation, or competitive binding in the intestine. Ascorbic acid may also form complexes with minerals and be taken up into the mucosal cell as part of an ascorbic acid–mineral chelate. Finally, ascorbic acid may influence some of the transport proteins in intracellular binding systems for minerals in intestinal cells.

Within the body, ascorbic acid and minerals have two additional levels of important interaction: in the tissue storage and turnover of ascorbic acid; and in the synthesis of tissues and organs. The apparent decrease in the half-life of ascorbic acid in the presence of excess iron is an example of the former interaction, whereas the simultaneous participation of vitamin C, calcium, and phosphorus in the formation of growing bone is an example of the latter.

Ascorbic Acid–Iron Interaction

The possibility of an important interaction of ascorbic acid and iron in the human intestine was first suggested in 1940 (2). Since then, research with experimental animals and human subjects has extended and elucidated the biology of the interaction.

Animal Studies. Studies with experimental animals have demonstrated enhancement of iron absorption in the presence of ascorbic acid. Brown and Rother (3) failed to observe an enhancement of iron uptake after 30 min when 20 μg of iron-59-labeled ferrous sulfate and 100 mg of ascorbic acid were injected by stomach tube into 200-g rats, but Van Campen (4) found that 17.6 mg of ascorbic acid promoted the absorption of a 100-μg dose of iron-59-labeled ferric chloride given by stomach tube to 6-week-old rats.

Using an isolated loop technique, a twofold increase in iron-59 uptake in rat intestine in the presence of ascorbic acid was demonstrated (5), and a similar effect was noted in isolated, perfused gut segments of mice (6). Using an everted intestinal sac technique, equivalent enhancement of mucosal uptake of both ferric and ferrous ions in the presence of 8×10^{-4} mM ascorbate concentration in the buffer was shown (7). The uptake of iron-59 by everted sacs of rat intestine was linear through a 0.5–3.0 mM concentration of ascorbic acid; experiments on isolated intestinal loops of rats also have demonstrated a dose-dependent enhancement of iron absorption by ascorbic acid through an ascorbic acid:iron molar ratio of 1:1 to 4:1 (8, 9).

Ascorbic Acid and Therapeutic Doses of Iron in Humans. The potential pharmaceutical importance of an enhancement of iron absorption in the presence of ascorbic acid stimulated extensive research on the effect of ascorbic acid on therapeutic doses of iron. Two basic techniques for assessing iron absorption have been used: the change in circulating iron concentration after an oral dose of iron (ferremia method) (10–12); and the incorporation of radioiron into red cells 2 weeks following oral administration of iron-55 or iron-59 (radioiron method) (13, 15). A summary of data from various studies is shown in Tables I and II. Added ascorbic acid, in excess of 150 mg, significantly increased the absorption of iron over the control solution. The major dissenting observation is that of Grebe et al. (14) who showed that when tracer iron was ferric chloride, ascorbic acid enhanced absorption but when the tracer was ferrous sulfate, no enhancement was seen. The authors questioned the validity of using radiolabeled ferric chloride with unlabeled ferrous sulfate. Extensive subsequent experience has validated this approach, however, so that other explanation for the nonenhancement of iron absorption with the ferrous tracer must be sought.

Using a radioiron technique (15), 105 mg of iron as ferrous sulfate embedded in resin to form a tablet was better absorbed when 500 mg of ascorbic acid was incorporated into the preparation as compared with resin-embedded ferrous sulfate or an aqueous solution of ferrous sulfate. In the treatment of iron deficiency anemia, a more rapid repletion of hemoglobin was found when 500–750 mg of supplementary vitamin C was given prior to an oral dose of therapeutic metallic iron (16).

Table I. Effects of Ascorbic Acid on Absorption of Therapeutic Doses of Iron in Humans Using the Radioiron Method

Iron Dose[a] (mg of ferrous sulfate)	Dose of Ascorbic Acid (mg)	Ratio of Absorption with Ascorbic Acid/Without Ascorbic Acid[b]	Reference
30	50	0.91	(13)
30	100	1.09	(13)
30	200	1.33	(13)
30	300	1.43	(13)
30	500	1.48	(13)
60	600	1.60	(14)
60[c]	600	0.93	(14)
15	200	1.78	(15)
15	500	1.87	(15)
30	200	1.24	(15)
30	500	1.35	(15)
60	200	1.48	(15)
60	500	2.51	(15)
120[c]	200	1.00	(15)
120[c]	500	1.64	(15)

[a] $^{59}FeCl_3$ tracer.
[b] Contains 10 mg of ascorbic acid.
[c] $^{59}FeSO_4$ tracer.

Table II. Effects of Ascorbic Acid on Absorption of Therapeutic Doses of Iron in Humans Using the Ferremia Method

Iron Dose (mg of ferrous sulfate)	Dose of Ascorbic Acid (mg)	Ratio of Absorption With Ascorbic Acid/Without Ascorbic Acid	Reference
300	250	1.66	(10)
200	50	1.00	(11)
200	1000	1.41	(11)
4[a]	500	1.44	(12)

[a] In children, mg/kg.

In Achlorhydria and Postgastrectomy. The question of whether ascorbic acid would influence iron absorption in subjects whose normal acid secretory capacity had been severely compromised by achlorhydria or gastrectomy has been addressed. In an experimental animal model (*17*), addition of 10 mg of ascorbic acid to the radioiron dose increased iron absorption in anemic gastrectomized rats but not in iron-loaded gastrectomized animals. Human patients who had undergone partial gastrectomy and who were anemic at the time of study absorbed less radioiron from a meal than comparably anemic individuals with normal acid secretion (*18*). Addition of oranges (containing ascorbic acid) to the meal increased iron absorption. Similarly, iron-deficient patients with normal gastrointestinal tracts absorbed iron-59 from bread meals better than did either postgastrectomy patients or spontaneously achlorhydric patients (*19*). Addition of 1 g of ascorbic acid increased iron absorption in all groups in this study, but the added ascorbic acid had its greatest effect in the patients with apparently normal acid secretion. In studies with 105-mg doses of ferrous sulfate or slow-release iron capsules, on the other hand, addition of 500 mg of ascorbic acid potentiated iron absorption to a greater extent in anemic post-gastrectomy patients than in patients who were simply anemic (*20*). The number of observations are limited and the findings somewhat inconsistent. Thus, no simple statement about the role of acid secretion or the role of ascorbic acid as an acidifying agent can be made on the basis of these studies on achlorhydria and gastrectomy.

Ascorbic Acid and Dietary Iron Absorption in Humans. It is well known that iron occurs in two forms in the diet: as part of the heme moiety of myoglobin and hemoglobin in red meats and blood (heme iron); and in an "inorganic" form in ferritin and in all forms of plant-derived foods (nonheme iron). Phytates, oxalates, carbonates, and inorganic phosphates are among the dietary constituents that reduce the biological availability of nonheme iron (*21, 22*). Ascorbic acid has no important effect on the intraintestinal metabolism of heme iron, but a wide variety of investigations have demonstrated enhancement of the absorption of nonheme iron from dietary sources. Using intrinsically radioiron-labeled eggs, mustard greens, and spinach, the absorption of iron was increased by simultaneous consumption of 85 mg of ascorbic acid, either as 200 mL of orange juice or as crystalline ascorbate (*23*). Iron balance studies conducted on eight Indian subjects consuming their customary diets showed an increased apparent absorption of iron after their diet was supplemented with 100 mg of ascorbic acid (*24*). In studies involving extrinsic labeling of various diets with radioiron, doses of ascorbic acid ranging from 50 to 1000 mg have increased iron absorption from mixed diets (*25*), bread (*26*), eggs (*27*), wheat (*28*), soy (*28*), and maize porridge (28, 29). The inhibitory effects of the tannins in tea can be partially overcome by adding large amounts of ascorbic acid (250–500 mg) to meals (30, 31). The absorption of fortification iron as ferrous sulfate or as ferric phosphate, provided in a table salt vehicle, is increased by about threefold with the addition of 50 mg of ascorbic acid (32, 33). With a ferrous-sulfate-containing table salt mixed into a meal of cooked rice, 60 mg of ascorbic acid added during cooking produced a similar threefold increase in iron availability (34).

The uptake of iron by the human intestine is governed not only by its dietary form and companion consituents, but also by the iron condition of the individual. Iron-depleted subjects absorb all forms of iron with greater avidity than do iron-replete individuals. In human dietetics, therefore, the ascorbic content of a diet can be included in the equation for describing the bioavailability of iron from a mixed diet (35). The interaction of iron nutrition and graded intakes of ascorbic acid (< 25 mg; > 25 but < 75 mg; and > 75 mg) as a prediction of iron availability from a mixed North American diet is plotted in Figure 1.

Mechanistic Aspects of the Ascorbic Acid–Iron Interaction in the Intestine. Studies of the mechanism of the interaction of ascorbic acid and iron at the molecular and cellular levels have yielded a variety of theories. An acidic pH in the lumen of the intestine favors the absorption

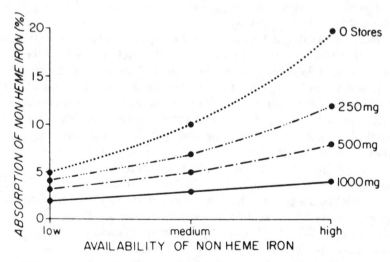

Figure 1. *The percent absorption of nonheme iron by individuals with iron body stores of 0 (· · ·), 250 (— · · · —), 500 (— · — ·), and 1000 (——) mg is shown as influenced by the availability of nonheme iron in a given metal (35). Low availability represents < 25 mg of ascorbic acid, medium availability represents 25–75 mg of ascorbic acid, and high availability represents > 75 mg of ascorbic acid.*

of iron. When the secretion of gastric acid is intact, the contribution of ingested ascorbic acid to luminal pH is probably minor. In the absence of gastric acid, the contribution of ascorbic acid to intestinal pH might be greater, but the data from the experiments in hypochlorhydric and achlorhydric animals and subjects, described above, do not allow any firm conclusions regarding pH effects of ascorbic acid. The reducing potential of ascorbic acid is important. The necessity that iron be in the divalent ferrous state has been related either to Fe^{2+} being the preferred form for transmucosal uptake or to its being less likely to polymerize or bind to other substances than the trivalent, ferric (Fe^{3+}) form. Ascorbic acid reduces ferric iron in foods such as egg yolk to ferrous iron (36). The iron in egg yolk is present as ferric hydroxide. In in vitro dialysis experiments with intrinsically labeled egg yolk (36) or in hemoglobin repletion studies in growing rats fed on egg yolk (37), only those reducing agents that also had a complexing potential could effectively reduce ferric iron in egg yolk or enhance its iron absorption into the rat. Thus, o-phenanthroline, an iron complexing agent without reducing potential, and sodium sulfite, α-tocopherol, or hydroquinone, reducing agents without complexing potential, showed no effect in these egg-yolk-related experiments. Ascorbic acid has both reducing and complexing potential.

In vitro experiments (38) showed that iron could form soluble chelates with ascorbic acid at the pH of the normal intestinal lumen. Soluble ascorbic acid–iron chelates formed at an acidic pH remained in solution even after the alkalinization of the medium (39). Intraintestinal installation of the pH-adjusted chelates into the rat enhanced the absorption of iron. The authors also suggest that the ascorbic acid normally present in mammalian bile has a physiologically important role in the absorption of nonheme iron from the diet. Whether the whole ascorbic acid–iron chelate is taken up intact into the mucosal cell under these conditions has not been established. Iron is, at the same time, more soluble, reduced, and more absorbable at intestinal pH in the presence of ascorbic acid; those factors, with or without direct mucosal uptake of ascorbic acid–iron complexes, explain the contribution of ascorbic acid to the enhancement of iron availability.

Effects of Excess Tissue Iron on Ascorbic Acid Metabolism. Epidemiological observations among the Bantu of South Africa showed an apparent association of clinical scurvy in adult males with hemosiderosis common to this group. Both plasma clearance of ascorbic acid and urinary excretion of ascorbic acid were altered in severe iron overload; plasma clearance was increased and urinary excretion was decreased in siderotic subjects (40, 41). The evidence was interpreted as a demonstration of enhanced oxidative catabolism of ascorbic acid in the presence of excess tissue iron.

Ascorbic Acid–Cobalt Interaction

Cobalt has no confirmed nutritional role in mammalian organisms aside from its participation in the corrin ring structure of cobalamins (vitamin B_{12}). Nonetheless, inorganic cobalt is absorbed by the intestine. That this absorption pathway was shared with iron was first suggested by the observation of a mineral–mineral competition (42). The use of radioisotopes of iron in diagnostic tests of absorption for characterizing iron nutrition in human subjects has been advanced (43–45). An excellent correlation between absorption of radioiron and radiocobalt has been reported (43–45).

In a series of studies conducted on human volunteers in the Division of Human Nutrition and Biology at the Institute of Nutrition of Central America and Panama, we employed the radiocobalt absorption test in the context of iron absorption tests. We used a modification of a 6-h cobalt excretion test to estimate absorption (44). Approximately 2.5 μCi of cobalt-60 mixed with 4.74 mg (20 μmol) of cobalt chloride hexahydrate was given in 100 mL of water after an overnight fast. The subjects remained fasting for 2 h postingestion and then consumed a standard breakfast. A liter or more of water was consumed during the final 4 h of the study. All urine produced during the 6 h was collected; the excreted radioactivity was measured in a well-type γ-counter.

In a group of ten urban, nonanemic adults and in nineteen rural agricultural workers with varying degrees of iron deficiency, a pair of cobalt absorption tests was performed. On one occasion, the cobalt-60 dose was given alone; on the other occasion, 1000 mg of ascorbic acid was added to the cobalt-60 dose. Table III shows the data on the ten normal

Table III. Comparison of the 6-h Excretion of Cobalt-60 When Administered Alone or with 1000 mg of Ascorbic Acid in Normal Subjects

Percent of Oral Dose Excreted in the Urine

	Without Ascorbic Acid	*With Ascorbic Acid*	Δ
	18.9	17.8	1.1
	11.5	12.5	−1.0
	22.2	24.7	−2.5
	7.6	9.9	−2.3
	15.0	11.0	4.0
	18.9	14.8	4.1
	19.0	13.2	5.8
	7.5	13.6	−6.1
	22.6	27.6	−5.0
	8.7	14.3	−5.6
mean	13.2	15.9	
se	±6.5	±5.8	

subjects. No differences of statistical significance were noted by paired Student *t*-test analysis, as was true when data from all twenty-nine subjects were grouped. The excretion of radioisotopic cobalt in 6 h as a percentage of the administered dose was 26.5 ± 13.0% with cobalt alone and 23.8 ± 12.7% with cobalt plus ascorbic acid (mean ± sd). Linear regression of the paired data revealed a correlation coefficient of $r =$ 0.768 ($p < 0.001$). Apparently, in aqueous solution, ascorbic acid has no effect—inhibiting or enhancing—on the absorption of radiocobalt. This is in contrast to the experience of workers using ferrous iron in solution, discussed earlier. We also have demonstrated a twelvefold decrease in cobalt excretion when the dose was mixed into a meal (46), but whether or not simultaneous administration of ascorbic acid would alter cobalt absorption in the presence of food has not been examined.

Ascorbic Acid–Copper Interaction

Inhibition of intestinal copper absorption by ascorbic acid was observed in experimental animals. Adding 5 g of ascorbic acid/kg of poultry ration containing 8 mg of copper exacerbated copper deficiency signs including growth retardation, anemia, and mortality from aortic rupture in chicks (47). Aortic rupture was caused by defective elastin formation, a copper-dependent function. The time to appearance of aortic rupture was also decreased by the 0.5% ascorbic-acid-containing diet. Even with a copper content of 24 mg/kg, 0.5% ascorbic acid produced anemia. Growth reduction and anemia was observed (47) in Dutch rabbits on a diet containing 3 ppm of copper by adding 1.0% ascorbic acid, although no signs of copper deficiency were evident with the 3-ppm copper ration alone (48) (Table IV). Addition of 0.1% ascorbic acid to a copper-deficient diet fed to chicks decreased growth, increased mortality, and reduced aortic elastin content (49). Essentially identical results were obtained with turkey poults (50). In guinea pigs

Table IV. Effects of Ascorbic Acid on Symptoms of Copper Deficiency in Dutch Rabbits Fed Low-Copper Diets

	Weight (%)			Hemoglobin (%)		
	6 wk	12 wk	18 wk	6 wk	12 wk	18 wk
Cu (2 ppm), AA (0%)	68	47	39	75	59	71
Cu (3 ppm), AA (0%)	96	94	—	107	93	—
Cu (3 ppm), AA (1%)	81	62	61	66	73	88

Note: Data are expressed as a percentage of value for animals consuming a control diet containing 6 ppm Cu. AA = ascorbic acid.
Source: Reference 48.

fed a ration containing 21 ppm of copper, adjusting the dietary ascorbic acid content to 1.0% caused a 39% reduction in whole blood copper concentration and a 52% reduction in liver copper content as compared with animals receiving a standard diet with 0.1% ascorbic acid (51). Addition of 2.5% ascorbic acid to the diets of minipigs consuming an adequate copper intake produced only slight retardation in weight gain (52); when the animals were placed on a copper-deficient diet, ascorbic acid provoked a sharper fall in weight and earlier death. Hepatic and serum copper levels were lower in the ascorbic-acid-supplemented animals (52).

In young swine, addition of 0.5% ascorbic acid to a diet containing a toxic amount of copper, 250 mg/kg of diet, reduced the anemia that was the toxic manifestation of copper excess, and reduced hepatic accumulation of copper (53).

Absorption of a tracer dose of copper-64 from in situ ligated segments of rat intestine in 250–350-g animals was reduced by the simultaneous administration of 2.5 mg of ascorbic acid (54). Radiocopper absorption was also reduced in chicks receiving a 0.1% ascorbic acid ration (55).

The mechanism of this effect is not known. Hill and Starcher (49) postulated that reduction of copper from its divalent (cupric) state to its monovalent (cuprous) state accounted for the impaired absorption of copper in the presence of ascorbic acid; they produced the same effect with another reducing agent, dimercaptopropanol (BAL). This explanation has been accepted by others (56), although the oxidation state of copper for maximum intestinal absorption has not been established. An intramucosal competition of ascorbic acid for sulfhydryl sites on metallothioneins was demonstrated (57). If this ligand has any regulatory role in copper uptake, this alternative mechanism of ascorbic acid–copper interaction could explain the mechanism. Experimental confirmation of an ascorbic-acid-induced inhibition of copper absorption in the human intestine has not been presented.

Ascorbic Acid–Zinc Interaction

Given the effects of ascorbic acid on the absorption of iron and copper, investigators have been interested in possibly significant interactions with zinc. The absorption of zinc and other divalent mineral ions was studied using an isolated, filled duodenal loop in situ in the rat (58). A 10^{-4}-M zinc solution was infused in the presence or absence of 10^{-2} M ascorbate or dehydroascorbate. A two-thirds reduction in the net absorption of zinc from the lumen was observed during a 5-h experiment. Over 90% of the zinc taken up in the aqueous solution alone remained in the mucosal cells; however, over 50% of the zinc absorbed in the presence of a 100-fold molar excess of ascorbic acid or dehydroascorbic acid was transferred to the body. Thus, the net amount of zinc reaching the internal organs of the rat in 5 h was four to six times greater with ascorbate or dehydroascorbate.

We have conducted in vivo experiments on the interaction of zinc and ascorbic acid in the human intestine (56). To assess absorption we monitored the plasma zinc concentration after an oral dose of 25 mg of elemental zinc as zinc sulfate in 100 mL of water taken in the fasting state. The plasma zinc level was measured prior to zinc administration and at hourly intervals thereafter for 4 h. The addition of graded doses of 0.5, 1.0, and 2.0 g of ascorbic acid, constituting Zn:AA molar ratios of 0.134, 0.067, and 0.034, respectively, to the 25-mg solution of zinc had no effect on the velocity of zinc absorption (Figure 2). However, because the effect of ascorbic acid in improving nonheme iron absorption was most dramatically seen in the presence of food or beverages, further studies were conducted in which the change in plasma zinc following the ingestion of 108 mg of zinc as zinc sulfate mixed with 120 g of black bean gruel, a known inhibitor of zinc absorption (59, 60) was measured. Studies were conducted both in the presence and absence of 2 g of ascorbic acid (Figure 3). Once again, no effect of added ascorbic acid was detected. At least for humans, there appears to be neither an inhibiting nor an enhancing influence of ascorbic acid on the biological availability of orally ingested zinc.

Zinc and Ascorbic Acid Metabolism and Excretion. Iron has an oxidizing effect on ascorbic acid, reducing its urinary excretion; therefore, Keltz et al. (61) questioned whether zinc would show a similar effect. Human subjects were fed a diet containing either 11.5 or 19.5 mg of zinc/d for 7-d balance periods. Daily ascorbic acid intake was 100 mg. Consistent with the findings from iron-loaded Africans, the higher zinc intake caused a significant 30% decrease in urinary ascorbate excretion. No explanation for the zinc-related reduction in ascorbic acid beyond the analogy with the iron-loaded individuals is readily available.

In a study with experimental animals (62), both ascorbic acid (2.5 mM/kg dose) and zinc as zinc sulfate (1.4 mM/kg dose) increased ethanol clearance from the blood of intoxicated, 250-g rats when sterile solutions of the respective compounds were injected intraperitoneally. The effects appeared to be independent, because neither additive nor synergistic effects on clearance were noted when the two agents were injected simultaneously.

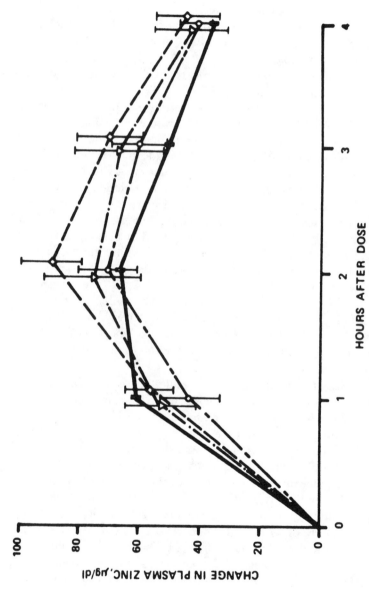

Figure 2. *The change in plasma zinc concentration (mean ± se) at 60-min intervals for 4 h after various graded doses of ascorbic acid mixed with 110 mg of $ZnSO_4 \cdot 7H_2O$ (56). Key: ◇ — ◇, 0.5 g of ascorbic acid; ▽ — · —▽, 1.0 g of ascorbic acid; and ○ — — —○, 2.0 g of ascorbic acid. Five subjects participated in each experiment. The heavy line shows the curve of zinc sulfate alone (Figure 1). No significant differences are found among any of the hourly points.*

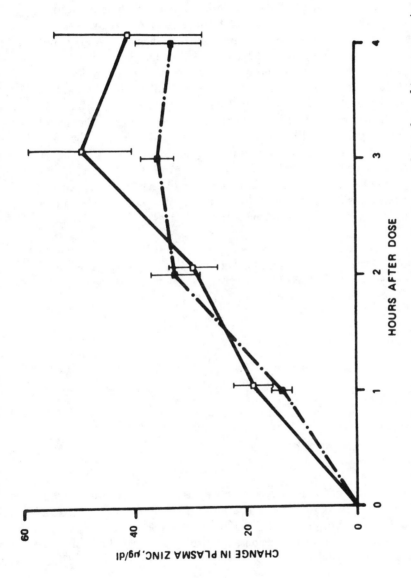

Figure 3. The change in plasma zinc concentration (mean ± se) over 4 h for five subjects consuming 475 mg of ZnSO₄ · 7H₂O (containing 108 mg of zinc) mixed into 120 g of black bean gruel (56). The mean was consumed either alone (□ —— □), or with 2.0 g of ascorbic acid (■ — · — ■), by five sub-jects. No significant differences are observed.

Ascorbic Acid–Nickel Interaction

The essentiality of nickel in various higher forms of mammals, including rats, goats, sheep, and pigs, has been demonstrated (63–66). Nickel is also homeostatically regulated in humans (66). Balance studies suggested that the absorption of nickel from normal American meals is on the order of 10% (68). Virtually nothing is known, however, about the factors affecting the bioavailability of nickel in humans.

A detectable rise in plasma nickel concentration after the oral administration of 22.4 mg of nickel sulfate was reported (69). In collaborative studies,[2] we have examined the interaction of nickel and ascorbic acid in the human intestine. Healthy volunteers received 5 mg of elemental nickel as 22.4 mg of nickel sulfate, as in the previous report. The total volume was 100 mL. This was ingested either alone or with 1 g of ascorbic acid. This constituted a Ni:AA molar ratio of 0.015. A significant depression in the rise of plasma nickel was observed when ascorbic acid was present as compared with the situation of aqueous nickel alone (see Table V). Our Ni:AA ratio of 0.015 compares with a molar ratio

Table V. Effect of Ascorbic Acid (1 g) on the Absorption of Nickel (5 mg) as Nickel Sulfate in Human Subjects

	Change in Plasma Nickel Above Fasting Levels ($\mu g/mL$)			
	1 h	*2 h*	*3 h*	*4 h*
Nickel alone	48.8 ±12.6	73.0 ±11.1	80.0 ±11.3	53.3 ±16.3
Nickel with AA	29.9 ±10.3	38.6 ±4.8	52.8 ±4.5	42.3 ±6.3
Significance	N.S.	$p < 0.05$	$p < 0.05$	N.S.

Note: Data are expressed as mean ± se.

of 0.002 that might occur in a typical meal, assuming that the United States mean nickel intake is 165 μg (55 μg in a single meal) and that a 200-mL glass of orange juice contains 100 mg of ascorbic acid.

In the same series of investigations, we also demonstrated a profound inhibition of nickel uptake in the presence of mixed meals (70). Thus,

[2] Collaborative studies with F. Nielsen and T. Shuler of the Human Nutrition Research Laboratory of the U.S. Department of Agriculture at Grand Forks, North Dakota.

in the context of a mixed diet, the nutritional implications of the inhibitory influence of ascorbic acid on nickel uptake remain to be interpreted.

Ascorbic Acid–Selenium Interaction

Selenide, the reduced form of selenium, appears to be the most usable form of the mineral (71). Moreover, vitamin E and other reducing agents tend to maintain selenium in its selenide form. In homogenated in vitro tissue, ascorbic acid is capable of reducing selenate to selenite and selenide (72). Preliminary experience with chicks suggested that ascorbic acid, acting as an antioxidant, increased the utilization of dietary selenium (73). This was confirmed (74) by the enhancement of selenium uptake from ligated duodenal loops of chicks or from dietary sources in the presence of graded doses of ascorbic acid in studies conducted with poultry.

Interaction of Ascorbic Acid and Other Mineral Nutrients

Virtually no data are available concerning the interaction of ascorbic acid and molybdenum, magnesium, vanadium, or silicon. A limited number of experiments have suggested that other minerals of nutritional importance, namely calcium and manganese, may show a physiological interaction with ascorbate. Some observations on an ascorbic acid–calcium interaction have been published. Ascorbic acid is essential to the formation of bone matrix in growing bone, but its role in skeletal mineralization was also examined. A low vitamin C intake in rhesus monkeys increased the exchangeable pool of calcium-45 and the accretion rate of calcium in the presence of sodium fluoride (75, 76). Addition of 0.3% ascorbic acid to turkey rations reduced the mineralization of poult femurs 8 weeks after hatching (77), but a 0.65% ascorbic acid content in the diet did not reduce tibial mineralization in growing chicks and Japanese quails (78). High doses of intraperitoneal ascorbic acid mobilize calcium-45 previously incorporated into skeletal bone (79–81); the same effect of ascorbic acid was shown in 5-d cultures of chick tibias labeled in ovum with calcium-45 (82). The variability in the in vivo experience and the pharmacological nature of the doses (79–82) makes any conclusions regarding a biological role of excess vitamin C intake in reducing skeletal mineralization somewhat premature.

Experiments in isolated segments of rat intestine (58) showed a reduction in net absorption of manganese from a 10^{-4}-M solution in the presence of a 10^{-2}-M solution of ascorbate. Dehydroascorbate had no effect on net manganese absorption, but it increased transfer of the manganese to the carcass.

Interaction of Ascorbic Acid with Toxic Minerals

There is evidence for an interaction between ascorbic acid and some trace minerals toxic to the vertebrate organism, although the data are not extensive. During a 5-h perfusion of intestinal segments of rats, 10^{-2} M ascorbate or dehydroascorbate did not alter the net removal from the lumen of cadmium in a 10^{-4}-M solution (58). The ratio of cadmium transported to the carcass to the total cadmium removed from the lumen was 0.14 for the cadmium alone; however, the corresponding ratios of 0.828 and 0.772 were found with 10^{-2}-M additions of ascorbate and de-hydroascorbate, respectively. Addition of ascorbic acid as 10 g/kg to the ration prevented the excess mortality, weight reduction, and anemia induced by adding 75 mg of cadmium/kg of diet (83). This dose of ascorbic acid did not reduce cadmium concentration in tissues, and it was presumed that the mechanism was not an inhibition of cadmium absorption but rather some other interaction at the level of tissue metabolism. Evans et al. (57) demonstrated decreased binding of cadmium to bovine hepatic metallothionein in vitro in the presence of ascorbic acid. This type of ascorbic acid–cadmium interaction may explain the findings of Fox and Fry (83).

Neither the uptake nor the transfer of mercury from a 10^{-4}-M solution instilled into an isolated loop of rat intestine was significantly altered by the presence of a 10^{-2}-M solution of dehydroascorbate (58). Thus, with 100-fold molar excesses of ascorbic acid the intestinal absorption of either cadmium or mercury was not affected, but at some internal location, ascorbic acid apparently counteracts the toxic activity of cadmium.

Conclusions

Studies in basic and applied physiology, primarily in experimental animals, but also in human subjects, and some research in fundamental biochemistry, are the basis of our understanding of the interaction of ascorbic acid with various minerals important to human nutrition and health. Much remains to be learned. The experiences reviewed in this chapter suggest that the level of dietary ascorbic acid intake can have important nutritional consequences for mammalian species, and possibly for humans, through a wide range of inhibiting and enhancing interactions with trace minerals at the levels of intestinal absorption. The importance of this interaction in the case of nonheme iron in the human diet is well established and provides the basis for some public health strategies to alleviate iron deficiency in some parts of the world. The public health importance of the interaction of ascorbic acid with other mineral nutrients remains to be established. At the level of internal metabolism, ascorbic

acid also interacts with certain minerals with significant biological consequences both for the respective minerals (as in the case of calcium) and
for ascorbic acid (as in the case of iron and zinc). The exciting con-
temporary trend in nutritional research is to consider nutrient–nutrient
interactions (*84*), and new and far-reaching insights into the interaction
of ascorbic acid and mineral nutrients may be forthcoming in the near
future.

Acknowledgments

N. W. Solomons is the recipient of a Clinical Investigator Award
(1 K08 AM 00715) in nutrition from the National Institutes of Health.
This is INCAP Publication #I-1131.

Literature Cited

1. "Trace Elements in Human Nutrition," *W.H.O., Tech. Rep. Ser.* **1973**, *532*.
2. Moore, C. V.; Bierman, H. Q.; Minnich, V.; Arrowsmith, W. R. *Am. Assoc. Advance Sci. Publ.* **1940**, *13*, 34.
3. Brown, E. B.; Rother, M. L.. *J. Lab. Clin. Med.* **1963**, *62*, 804.
4. Van Campen, D. R. *J. Nutr.* **1972**, *102*, 165.
5. Hopping, J. M.; Ruliffson, W. R. *Am. J. Physiol.* **1963**, *205*, 885.
6. Hamilton, D. L.; Bellamy, J. E. C.; Valberg, J. D.; Valberg, L. S. *Can. J. Physiol. Pharmacol.* **1977**, *56*, 384.
7. Pearson, W. N.; Reich, M. *J. Nutr.* **1965**, *87*, 117.
8. Hopping, J. M.; Ruliffson, W. S. *Am. J. Physiol.* **1966**, *210*, 1316.
9. Monsen, E. R.; Page, J. F. *J. Agric. Food Chem.* **1978**, *26*, 233.
10. Sörensen, E. W. *Acta Med. Scand.* **1966**, *180*, 241.
11. Lee, P. C.; Ledwich, J. R.; Smith, D. C. *Can. Med. Assoc. J.* **1967**, *97*, 181.
12. El-Hawary, M. F. S.; El-Shobaki, F. A.; Kholeif, T.; Sakr, R.; El-Bassoussy, M. *Br. J. Nutr.* **1975**, *33*, 351.
13. Brise, H.; Hallberg, L. *Acta Med. Scand.* **1962**, *171*, Suppl. 51.
14. Grebe, G.; Martinez-Torres, C.; Layrisse, M. *Curr. Ther. Res., Clin. Exp.* **1975**, *17*, 382.
15. McCurdy, P. R.; Dern, J. *Am. J. Clin. Nutr.* **1968**, *21*, 284.
16. Gorton, M. K.; Bradley, J. E. *J. Pediatr.* **1954**, *45*, 1.
17. Rieber, E. E.; Conrad, M. E.; Crosby, W. H. *Proc. Soc. Exp. Biol. Med.* **1967**, *124*, 577.
18. Turnbull, A. L. *Clin. Sci.* **1965**, *28*, 499.
19. Williams, J. *Clin. Sci.* **1959**, *18*, 521.
20. Baird, I. M.; Walter, R. L.; Sutton, D. R. *Br. Med. J.* **1974**, *4*, 505.
21. Kuhn, I. N.; Layrisse, M.; Roche, M.; Martinez, C.; Walker, R. B. *Am. J. Clin. Nutr.* **1968**, *21*, 1184.
22. Peters, T., Jr.; Apt, L.; Ross, J. F. *Gastroenterology* **1971**, *61*, 315.
23. Moore, C. V.; Dubach, R. *Trans. Assoc. Am. Physicians* **1951**, *64*, 245.
24. Apte, S. V.; Venkatachalam, P. S. *Indian J. Med. Res.* **1965**, *53*, 1084.
25. Pirizio-Biroli, G.; Bothwell, T. H.; Finch, C. A. *J. Lab. Clin. Med.* **1958**, *51*, 37.
26. Callender, S. T.; Warner, G. T. *Am. J. Clin. Nutr.* **1968**, *21*, 1170.
27. Callender, S. T.; Marney, S. R., Jr.; Warner, G. T. *Br. J. Haematol.* **1970**, *19*, 657.
28. Sayers, M. H.; Lynch, S. R.; Jacobs, P.; Charlton, R. W.; Bothwell, T. H.; Walker, R. B.; Mayet, F. *Br. J. Haematol.* **1973**, *24*, 209.

29. Björn-Rassmussen, E.; Hallberg, L. *Nutr. Metab.* **1974**, *16*, 94.
30. Derman, D.; Sayers, M.; Lynch, S. R.; Charlton, R. W.; Bothwell, T. H.; Mayet, F. *Br. J. Nutr.* **1977**, *38*, 261.
31. Disler, P. B.; Lynch, S. R.; Charlton, R. W.; Torrance, J. D.; Bothwell, T. H.; Walker, R. B.; Mayet, F. *Gut* **1974**, *16*, 1963.
32. Sayers, M. H.; Lynch, S. R.; Charlton, R. W.; Bothwell, T. H.; Walker, R. B.; Mayet, F. *Br. J. Haematol.* **1974**, *28*, 483.
33. Disler, P. B.; Lynch, S. R.; Charlton, R. W.; Bothwell, T. H.; Walker, R. B.; Mayet, F. *Br. J. Nutr.* **1975**, *34*, 141.
34. Sayers, M. H.; Lynch, S. R.; Charlton, R. W.; Bothwell, T. H.; Walker, R. B.; Mayet, F. *Br. J. Nutr.* **1974**, *31*, 367.
35. Monsen, E. R.; Hallberg, L.; Layrisse, M.; Hegsted, D. M.; Cook, J. D.; Mertz, W.; Finch, C. A. *Am. J. Clin. Nutr.* **1978**, *31*, 134.
36. Halkett, J. A.; Peters, E. T.; Ross, J. F. *J. Biol. Chem.* **1958**, *231*, 187.
37. Morris, E. R.; Greene, F. E. *J. Nutr.* **1972**, *102*, 901.
38. Anelli, J. *Acta Cient. Venez.* **1958**, *9*, 105.
39. Conrad, M. E.; Shade, S. G. *Gastroenterology* **1968**, *55*, 35.
40. Lynch, S. R.; Seftel, H. C.; Torrance, J. D.; Charlton, R. W.; Bothwell, T. H. *Am. J. Clin. Nutr.* **1967**, *20*, 641.
41. Wapnick, A.; Lynch, S.; Krawitz, P.; Seftel, H.; Charlton, R.; Bothwell, T. *Br. Med. J.* **1968**, *3*, 704.
42. Pollack, S.; George, J. N.; Reba, R. C.; Kaufman, R. N.; Crosby, W. H. *J. Clin. Invest.* **1965**, *44*, 147.
43. Sorbie, J.; Olatunbosun, D.; Corbett, W. E. N.; Valberg, L. S. *Can. Med. Assoc. J.* **1971**, *104*, 777.
44. Valberg, L. S.; Sorbie, J.; Corbett, W. E.; Ludwig, J. *Ann. Intern. Med.* **1972**, *77*, 181.
45. Wahner-Roedler, D. L.; Fairbanks, V. F.; Linman, J. W. *J. Lab. Clin. Med.* **1975**, *85*, 253.
46. Solomons, N. W.; Garcia, R.; Viteri, F. E., unpublished data.
47. Carlton, W. W.; Henderson, W. *J. Nutr.* **1965**, *85*, 67.
48. Hunt, C. E.; Carlton, W. W. *J. Nutr.* **1965**, *87*, 385.
49. Hill, C. H.; Starcher, B. *J. Nutr.* **1965**, *85*, 271.
50. Simpson, C. F.; Robbins, R. D.; Harms, R. H. *J. Nutr.* **1971**, *101*, 1359.
51. Smith, C. H.; Bidlack, W. R. *J. Nutr.* **1980**, *110*, 1398.
52. Voelker, R. W.; Carlton, W. W. *Am. J. Vet. Res.* **1969**, *30*, 1825.
53. Gipp, W. F.; Pond, W. G.; Kallfelz, F. A.; Tasker, J. B.; Van Campen, D. R.; Krook, L.; Visek, W. J. *J. Nutr.* **1974**, *104*, 532.
54. Van Campen, D. R.; Gross, E. *J. Nutr.* **1968**, *95*, 617.
55. Hill, C. H.; Starcher, B. *J. Nutr.* **1965**, *85*, 271.
56. Solomons, N. W.; Jacob, R. A.; Pineda, O.; Viteri, F. E. *Am. J. Clin. Nutr.* **1979**, *32*, 2495.
57. Evans, G. W.; Majors, P. F.; Cornatzer, W. E. *Biochem. Biophys. Res. Commun.* **1970**, *41*, 1244.
58. Sahagian, B. M.; Harding-Barlow, I.; Perry, H. M., Jr. *J. Nutr.* **1967**, *93*, 291.
59. Solomons, N. W.; Jacob, R. A.; Pineda, O.; Viteri, F. E. *J. Nutr.* **1979**, *109*, 1519.
60. Solomons, N. W.; Jacob, R. A.; Pineda, O.; Viteri, F. E. *J. Lab. Clin. Med.* **1979**, *94*, 335.
61. Keltz, F. R.; Kies, C.; Fox, H. M. *Am. J. Clin. Nutr.* **1978**, *31*, 1167.
62. Yanice, A. A.; Lindeman, R. D. *Proc. Soc. Exp. Biol. Med.* **1977**, *154*, 146.
63. Nielsen, F. H.; Myron, D. R.; Givand, S. H.; Zimmerman, T. J.; Ollerich, D. A. *J. Nutr.* **1975**, *105*, 1620.
64. Schnegg, A.; Kirchgessner, M. *Z. Tierphysiol. Tierernähr. Futtermittelkd.* **1975**, *36*, 63.
65. Schnegg, A.; Kirchgessner, M. *Nutr. Metab.* **1975**, *19*, 268.

66. Anke, M.; Hennig, A.; Grün, M.; Partschefeld, M.; Groppel, B.; Ludke, H. *Arch. Tierernähr.* **1977**, *27*, 25.
67. Sunderman, F. W., Jr.; Nomoto, S.; Nechaj, M. In "Trace Substances in Environmental Health"; Hemphill, D. D., Ed.; Univ. of Missouri Press: Columbia, 1971; Vol. 4, pp. 352–356.
68. Horak, S. E.; Sunderman, F. W., Jr. *Clin. Chem.* **1972**, *19*, 429.
69. Spruits, D.; Bongaarts, P. J. M. *Dermatologica* **1977**, *154*, 291.
70. Solomons, N. W.; Viteri, F. E.; Shuler, T.; Nielsen, F. H., unpublished data.
71. Underwood, E. J. "Trace Elements in Human and Animal Nutrition," 3rd ed.; Academic: New York, 1971.
72. Diplock, A. T.; Baum, H.; Lucy, J. A. *Biochem. J.* **1971**, *123*, 721.
73. Combs, G. F.; Scott, F. L. *J. Nutr.* **1974**, *104*, 1297.
74. Combs, G. F., Jr.; Pesti, G. M. *J. Nutr.* **1976**, *106*, 1976.
75. Reddy, G. S.; Narasinga Rao, B. S. *Metabolism* **1971**, *20*, 642.
76. Ibid. **1971**, *20*, 650.
77. Dorr, P.; Balloun, S. L. *Br. Poult. Sci.* **1976**, *17*, 581.
78. Sifri, M.; Kratzer, F. H.; Norris, L. C. *J. Nutr.* **1977**, *104*, 1484.
79. Thornton, P. A. *Proc. Soc. Exp. Biol. Med.* **1968**, *127*, 1096.
80. Thornton, P. A.; Omdahl, J. L. *Proc. Soc. Exp. Biol. Med.* **1969**, *132*, 618.
81. Thornton, P. A. *J. Nutr.* **1970**, *100*, 1979.
82. Ramp, W. A.; Thornton, P. A. *Proc. Soc. Exp. Biol. Med.* **1971**, *137*, 273.
83. Fox, M. R.; Fry, B. E., Jr. *Science* **1970**, *169*, 989.
84. Solomons, N. W.; Russell, R. M. *Am. J. Clin. Nutr.* **1980**, *33*, 2031.

RECEIVED for review January 22, 1981. ACCEPTED March 18, 1981.

Effects of Ascorbic Acid on the Nitrosation of Dialkyl Amines

YOUNG-KYUNG KIM, STEVEN R. TANNENBAUM, and JOHN S. WISHNOK

Department of Nutrition and Food Science, Massachusetts Institute of Technology, Cambridge, MA 02139

Ascorbic acid is known to inhibit the nitrosation of secondary amines. A computer model has been developed to predict the amount of nitrosamine formed under conditions that are experimentally inaccessible. The computer-calculated rates for N-nitrosomorpholine formation using rate and equilibrium constants from the literature agree well with experimental values in the absence of and presence of ascorbic acid under anaerobic conditions. In the aerobic system the inhibitory efficiency of ascorbic acid is lower, and the nature of the interactions among the various components of the mixtures is less well understood. The use of ascorbic acid for inhibition of N-nitroso compound formation both in vitro and in vivo is briefly reviewed.

Ascorbic acid, in addition to its known and potential biological properties, is an active and interesting organic chemical in its own right. Its strong reducing abilities (*1*), in particular, have stimulated interest in the possible use of ascorbic acid as an inhibitor of nitrosation reactions and, consequently, as a means of reducing human exposure to carcinogenic *N*-nitroso compounds.

Most substances containing the N—NO functionality are carcinogenic in at least one animal species (*2, 3*) and these compounds are, therefore, probably human carcinogens as well.

N-Nitroso compounds are not often found in nature, although they are occasionally detected in some industrial environments (*4, 5*). However, several *N*-nitrosoamines have been regularly detected in a wide variety of foods (*6*) and an extensive research effort has consequently been directed toward the detection and identification of these substances, the elucidation of the routes of their formation, and the evaluation of the human health hazards posed by nitrosamine exposure.

One result of these investigations has been a realization that N-nitroso compounds can form under a wide variety of conditions from reaction of nitrosatable nitrogens with any of several nitrosating species (7–13). As will be detailed later, complex equilibria among several nitrosating agents can arise from nitrite ion, NO_2^-, which is readily formed in vivo by bacterial reduction of nitrate, NO_3^- (14). Nitrosatable amines, in addition, are widely distributed in foods (15). There is, therefore, an increasing interest in the question of human exposure to endogenously formed N-nitroso compounds.

If it is found that epidemiologically significant nitrosation may occur in vivo from reactions of compounds normally present in the diet or as metabolites, then it becomes important to develop nontoxic methods for preventing these transformations.

Ascorbic acid is known to react rapidly with nitrite as well as with other nitrosating agents (16). This, along with its low toxicity and known nutritional importance, has naturally led to an evaluation of its usefulness as an inhibitor of nitrosation reactions (17). We have begun both experimental and theoretical studies of the interactions of ascorbic acid with amines, amides, and nitrosating agents. Our approaches and results are described in the following sections.

Amine Nitrosation

The nitrosation reactions of a given amine in the presence of ascorbic acid can be conceptually considered as an interacting set of several separate systems, that is, (i) a set of equilibria among various nitrogen oxides, (ii) reactions of nitrosatable nitrogen with each of the various nitrosating agents, (iii) reaction of ascorbic acid with oxygen, and (iv) reaction of ascorbic acid with the nitrosating agents.

The equilibria arising from aqueous nitrite are shown in Scheme 1, with nitrosating species italicized (18).

$$NO_2^- + H^+ \rightleftarrows HNO_2$$

$$HNO_2 + H^+ \rightleftarrows H_2NO_2^+ \rightleftarrows H_2O + NO^+$$

$$2HNO_2 \rightleftarrows N_2O_3 + H_2O$$

$$HNO_2 + HX \rightleftarrows NOX + H_2O$$

Scheme 1.

The relative importance of the various nitrosating agents is strongly dependent on the pH and, in the case of NOX, on the concentration of the halogen (e.g., Cl⁻, Br⁻) or pseudohalogen, (e.g., SCN⁻), X. A typical pH profile for the nitrosation of amines has an initial-rate maximum near pH 3.4. This behavior is the net result of an increase in the concentration of nitrosating species vs. a decrease in the concentration of nitrosatable free amine (*19*) as the pH is lowered. Although the maximum initial rate usually occurs near pH 3.4, measurable nitrosation will nonetheless occur over a wide pH range. In the presence of catalysts, for example, X = SCN⁻, the pH maximum is shifted, and the initial rates fall off more slowly as the pH decreases (Figure 1). For simple nitrosation reactions, then, the rate of nitrosation depends on the concentrations of the various nitrosating species and on the concentration of free amine, both of which are affected by pH.

Ascorbic Acid Oxidation

In anaerobic systems, ascorbic acid/ascorbate reacts with all of the nitrosating agents shown in Scheme 1. These reactions are generally faster than the reactions between amines or amides and the respective nitrosating agents, and ascorbic acid has been shown to be an effective in vitro inhibitor of amine nitrosation via competition for these agents (*17, 24*). These results have been extended to more practical areas such as the prevention of nitrosamine formation in foods and in vivo (*20, 21, 22*).

In principle, then, ascorbic acid appears to have considerable importance as an inhibitor of in vivo nitrosation of ingested or biosynthesized amines via endogenous nitrite. However, this potential is far from realized. The reaction conditions actually encountered in living organisms are complex and varied and—perhaps more importantly—the in vitro interactions among ascorbic acid, nitrite, and amines are not straightforward.

The equilibria shown in Scheme 1, for example, give rise to both polar ($H_2NO_2^+$, NO^+) and nonpolar (N_2O_3) nitrosating agents. The N_2O_3 can be intercepted by ascorbic acid to form non-nitrosating NO. In the presence of oxygen, however, N_2O_3 and N_2O_4 can be regenerated via NO and NO_2, as shown in Scheme 2 (*23, 24*).

Inhibition of nitrosation in this system, then, will be effective at best only until the ascorbate has been converted to dehydroascorbate.

The amine–nitrite reactions in physiological systems may be further obscured by carbonyl (*25*) or pseudohalogen (*19*) catalysts, by constituents of gastric juice or intestinal fluids, or by multiphasic interactions in lipid-containing micelles such as those found in the small intestine (26). Nitrosations of amines with long alkyl chains ($n \geq 6$) are enhanced by micelle formation (27). The mechanisms of these reactions are not known but, depending on whether the nitrosation occurs on the surface or in the interior of the micelles, polar and/or nonpolar nitrosating agents may be involved.

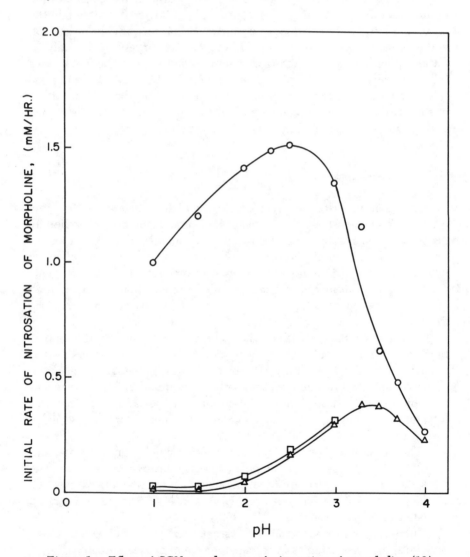

Figure 1. Effect of SCN⁻ on the rate of nitrosation of morpholine (19). Key: 5 mM nitrite, 10 mM morpholine, 2.5 mM KSCN (○); 5 mM nitrite, 10 mM morpholine, 100 mM KBr (□); 5 mM nitrite, 10 mM morpholine (△).

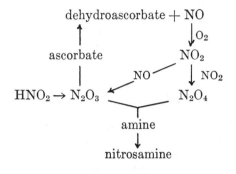

Scheme 2.

In addition to these aspects of the amine nitrosation reaction, the reactions of ascorbic acid with various components of the nitrite equilibria involve transformations that are also affected by the presence or absence of oxygen (1, 23). Some of these are shown schematically in Scheme 3. If attention is then focussed on the reactions of ascorbic acid/ascorbate rather than on the nitrosation of amines, it can be seen that the amount of ascorbic acid or ascorbate available for inhibition of nitrosation can be diminished by the presence of oxygen.

The experimental destruction of ascorbate by various combinations of nitrite, air, and nitrogen is shown in Figure 2 (24, 28). It is apparent from these experiments not only that ascorbate is sensitive to the presence of either air or nitrite but that the combination of these two reactants can completely exhaust the available ascorbate as opposed to the stoichiometric depletion observed with nitrite alone.

Variations in pH, in addition to affecting the equilibria among the nitrosating agents and the concentrations of free and protonated amines, also affect the relative concentrations of ionized (ascorbate) and nonionized forms of ascorbic acid. The reactions of ascorbic acid/ascorbate with each of the nitrosating reagents are therefore also pH-dependent, as illustrated in Figure 3 (16).

Computer Modeling

The observations above, taken together, suggest that the reactions among amines, nitrite, and ascorbic acid under physiological conditions would be expected to be extremely complex and that kinetic studies might be experimentally intractible even in vitro. A summary of the equilibria and reactions that might occur in an anaerobic model system is shown in Scheme 4. The question "How does ascorbic acid affect

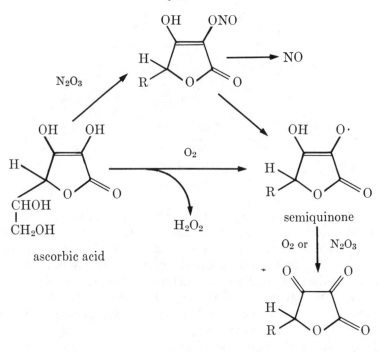

2-nitrosylascorbic acid

Scheme 3.

the rate of amine or amide nitrosation?" does not have a clearly simple answer.

Our current approach to the complexity of this problem has been to develop a computer model that can, in principle, provide guidelines for experimental designs and insight into properties of the system that may be experimentally impractical or inaccessible (29).

The rate equation for the formation of a nitrosamine from a given amine is set up as in Equation 1. Making steady state assumptions for

$$\frac{d[R_2NNO]}{dt} = k_4\,[R_2NH][N_2O_3] + k_7\,[R_2NH][NO^+] \qquad (1)$$

nitrous anhydride and nitrosonium ion allows the expression of the above equation in terms of the concentrations of various reagents and the rate and equilibrium constants in Scheme 4. The rate constants or equilibrium constants for most of the individual steps in Scheme 4 are available from

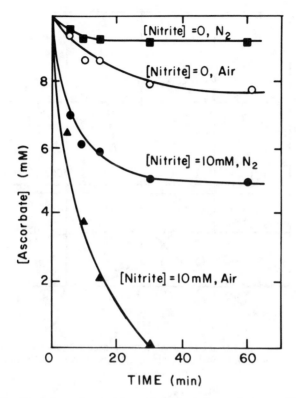

Figure 2. *Reaction of ascorbic acid with nitrite and air at pH 4 (25°C).*
(Reproduced, with permission, from Ref. 24.)

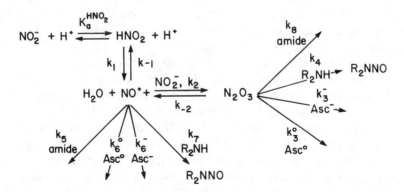

Scheme 4. *Reaction scheme for nitrosation in the presence of ascorbic acid.*

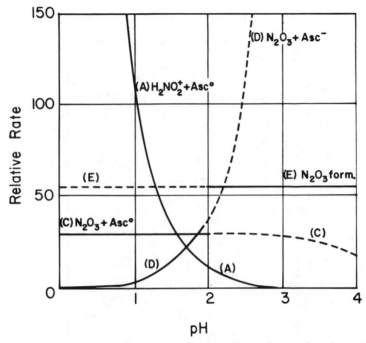

Figure 3. Effect of pH on the reactions of ascorbic acid and ascorbate anion with various nitrosating species. (Reproduced, with permission, from Ref. 16.)

the literature (*1, 16, 18, 30–34*). Arbitrary initial concentrations of the various reagents can then be entered into the computer and initial rates under that set of conditions will be calculated and printed out. Since all of the interactions among the components are considered, any perturbation of one by the other will automatically be included. If the pH is changed, for example, then the amine/ammonium-ion and ascorbic acid/ ascorbate concentrations will be appropriately adjusted.

For simple nitrosation reactions (i.e., [ascorbic acid] = 0) there is good quantitative agreement between calculated and observed initial rates as shown for morpholine → *N*-nitrosomorpholine in Figure 4.

When ascorbic acid/ascorbate is added to the system, the general behavior of the calculated initial rates is consistent with that intuitively expected, that is, the initial rates are reduced with increasing ascorbic acid, and the effect is pH dependent as shown in Table I. The versatility of the computer can also be seen in Figure 5 in which calculated pH profiles are plotted for different initial concentrations of ascorbic acid/ ascorbate. As expected, the greater the ascorbic acid/ascorbate concen-

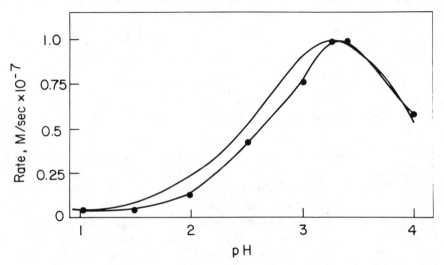

Figure 4. Calculated (———) vs. observed (●) (19) pH profile for initial rate of nitrosation of morpholine, 10 mM morpholine, 5 mM nitrite.

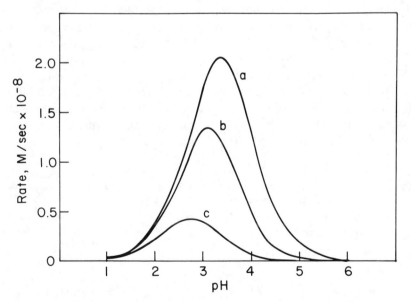

Figure 5. Initial rate profiles for the nitrosation of morpholine in the presence of various concentrations of ascorbic acid, 10 mM morpholine, 10 mM nitrite, 0°C: a, [Asc] = 0; b, [Asc] = 0.01 mM; c, [Asc] = 0.1 mM.

Table I. The Amount of Ascorbic Acid Required for 99%
Reduction in Initial Rate[a]

pH	[Asc]/[Nitrite]
2	2.9
3	0.33
4	0.05
5	0.02

[a] System: 10mM morpholine, 10mM nitrite, 0°C.

tration, the lower the initial rate of nitrosation. Additionally, however, the maximum initial rate shifts concurrently to lower pHs. This behavior, previously unreported, probably represents the decreasing concentration of ascorbate anion relative to the less active ascorbic acid.

Quantitative agreement between literature values (24) for nitrosation rates of morpholine in the presence of ascorbic acid, and those calculated by the computer model, are poor. The calculated initial rates are lower than the literature initial rates, even for a presumably degassed system (Figure 6). Recent experiments in our laboratories show that nitrosations in the presence of ascorbic acid are indeed (Schemes 2, 3, and 4) sensitive to oxygen; that is, the discrepancies beween the earlier observations (24) and the calculated initial rates may be because of incomplete degassing of the reaction mixtures. When morpholine is nitrosated at pH 4 with added ascorbic acid, the production of N-nitrosomorpholine over a 2-h period is dramatically altered by the amount of oxygen present (Figure 7). When oxygen is rigorously excluded, the observed and calculated initial rates are in good agreement as shown in Table II.

In summary, the general concept, that ascorbic acid can inhibit or prevent the nitrosation of amines, is essentially true. The specific effects, however, which can be expected in a given system, depend on a complex set of interactions among pH, the nature of the amine, the amount of

Table II. Initial Reaction Rate of N-Nitrosomorpholine Formation
in the Presence of Ascorbic Acid at pH 4

| | Initial Reaction Rate (M/s) | |
[Asc]	Measured[a]	Calculated[b]
0	1.3×10^{-8}	—
	2.0×10^{-11}	2.4×10^{-11}
3mM	3.0×10^{-11}	$(1.4–5.5)^{c} \times 10^{-11}$

[a] System: 10mM morpholine, 10mM NaNO$_2$ in pH at 0°C, kept under N$_2$ throughout the reaction.
[b] k_4 measured in this work was used for the calculation.
[c] 95% confidence interval.

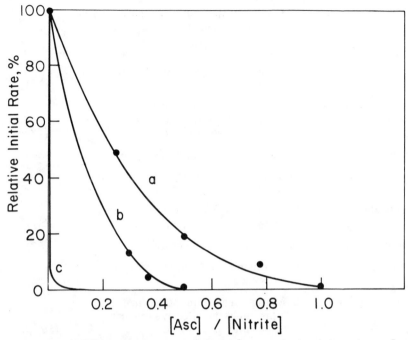

Figure 6. Effect of oxygen on the initial rates of nitrosation of morpholine in the presence of ascorbic acid, 10 mM morpholine, 10 mM nitrite, pH 4: a, air, 25°C; b, N₂ bubbling, 25°C; c, calculated anaerobic, 0°C. (Reproduced, with permission, from Ref. 24.)

oxygen present, and the presence or absence of catalysts. Although there has been both experimental and theoretical progress in this area, there is still an incomplete understanding of what might actually be anticipated for the effects of ascorbic acid on human in vivo nitrosation reactions.

Applications of Ascorbic Acid

Ascorbic acid has been shown to inhibit the formation of N-nitroso compounds both in vitro and in vivo. Although a detailed literature survey in this area is beyond the scope of this chapter, we have compiled a set of brief descriptions of a group of representative publications. Some of these have been reviewed in earlier articles (35, 50).

For convenience we have divided the studies into those that evaluate quantitative effects, that is, in vitro (Table III), and those in which inhibition of nitrosation is inferred from the absence of an expected toxic effect in intact animals (Table IV). It is remarkable that ascorbic acid is effective in systems as different as bacon fat and gastric juice.

**Table III. Inhibition of Nitrosation by
Ascorbic Acid In Vitro**

Amine or Amide	Effect	References
—	kinetics of reaction of nitrite with ascorbate	(16)
Secondary amines, methylurea	blocking of N-methylaniline not very effective compared with stronger bases and methylurea	(17)
Morpholine	blocking effective in model system	(36)
Dimethylamine	both ascorbate and erythorbate were effective in frankfurters	(22)
Dimethylamine	blocking effective in food and model systems	(37)
Piperazine	blocking effective in gastric juice	(38)
Morpholine	mechanism of blocking in presence of oxygen	(24)
Dimethylamine	blocking effective in model food systems, blocking effective in curing brines and meat slices	(39, 40)
Methylurea	blocking effective only with large excess of ascorbate in homogenized potato	(41)
Proline	formation of nitrosopyrrolidine in bacon inhibited, ascorbyl palmitate more effective than ascorbate	(42)
Piperazine, aminophenazone	blocking nitrosation in human gastric juice	(43)
Pyrrolidine	blocking in commercial bacon	(44)
Pyrrolidine	blocking in protein-based model system	(45)
Dimethylamine	blocking in seafood	(46)
Methapyrilene	blocking nitrosation under simulated gastric conditions	(47)
—	mechanism	(48)
—	inhibiting formation of a mutagen in nitrosated fish	(49)
—	review	(50)
—	review	(35)

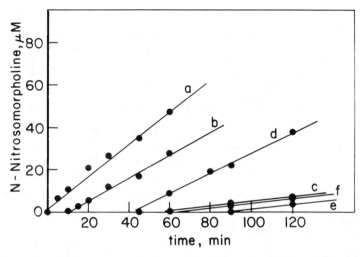

Figure 7. Time course of nitrosomorpholine formation. The reaction system was kept under N_2 unless stated otherwise, 10 mM morpholine, 10 mM nitrite, pH 4, 0°C, varying oxygen: a, without ascorbic acid; b, [Asc] = 1 mM; c,d, [Asc] = 3 mM, degassing of the solution was done by bubbling N_2 through pasteur pipet for 5 min; d,f, exposed to air 30 min after the reaction started; e,f, [Asc] = 3 mM, degassing of the solution was done by bubbling N_2 through gas dispersion tube for 1 h.

Table IV. Inhibition of Nitrosation by Ascorbic Acid In Vivo

Amine or Amide	Effect	References
Aminopyrine	inhibits hepatotoxicity	(21)
Aminopyrine	inhibits hepatotoxicity	(20, 51)
Dimethylamine	inhibits hepatotoxicity	(52)
Ethylurea	inhibits transplacental carcinogenesis	(53)
Morpholine, piperazine, methylurea	ascorbate inhibits lung adenoma formation by blocking nitrosation, some paradoxical effects when ascorbate given with preformed carcinogen	(54)
Aminopyrine	inhibits carcinogenesis	(55)
Morpholine	inhibits nitrosomorpholine formation and liver tumors, enhances fore-stomach carcinogenesis	(56)
Chlordiazepoxide	inhibits nitrosation	(57)

Literature Cited

1. Fennema, O. R. "Principles of Food Science, Part 1, Food Chemistry"; Marcel Dekker: New York, 1976; pp. 360–364.
2. Druckrey, H.; Preussmann, R.; Ivankovic, S.; Schmähl, D. *Z. Krebsforsch.* 1967, *69*, 103.
3. Magee, P. N.; Montesano, R.; Preussmann, R. In "Chemical Carcinogens," *ACS Monograph Ser.* 1976, *173*, 491–615.
4. Shapley, D. *Science* 1976, *191*, 268–270.
5. Fine, D. H.; Rounbehler, D. P.; Belcher, N. M.; Epstein, S. S. *Science* 1976, *192*, 1328–1330.
6. Scanlan, R. A. *Crit. Rev. Food Technol.* 1975, *5*, 357.
7. Wishnok, J. S. *J. Chem. Educ.* 1977, *54*, 440–442.
8. Sander, J.; Bürkle, G. *Z. Krebsforsch.* 1969, *73*, 54–66.
9. Greenblatt, M.; Mirvish, S. S.; So, B. T. *J. Natl. Cancer Inst.* 1971, *46*, 1029–1034.
10. Mysliwy, T. S.; Wick, E. L.; Archer, M. C.; Shank, R. C.; Newberne, P. M. *Br. J. Cancer* 1974, *30*, 279–283.
11. Tannenbaum, S. R.; Sinskey, A. J.; Weisman, M.; Bishop, W. W. *J. Natl. Cancer Inst.* 1974, *53*, 79–84.
12. Tannenbaum, S. R.; Archer, M. C.; Wishnok, J. S.; Bishop, W. W. *J. Natl. Cancer Inst.* 1978, *60*, 251–253.
13. Tannenbaum, S. R.; Fett, D.; Young, V. R.; Land, P. C.; Bruce, W. R. *Science* 1978, *200*, 1487–1489.
14. Tannenbaum, S. R.; Weisman, M.; Fett, D. *Food Cosmet. Toxicol.* 1976, *14*, 549.
15. Neurath, G. B.; Dünger, M.; Pein, F. G.; Ambrosius, D.; Schreiber, O. *Food Cosmet. Toxicol.* 1976, *15*, 275–282.
16. Dahn, H.; Loewe, L.; Bunton, C. A. *Helv. Chim. Acta* 1960, *43*, 320–333.
17. Mirvish, S. S.; Wallcave, L.; Eagen, M.; Shubik, P. *Science* 1972, *177*, 65–68.
18. Mirvish, S. S. *Toxicol. Appl. Pharmacol.* 1975, *31*, 325–351.
19. Fan, T. Y.; Tannenbaum, S. R. *J. Agric. Food Chem.* 1973, *21*, 237–240.
20. Kamm, J. J.; Dashman, T.; Conney, A. H.; Burns, J. J. *Proc. Natl. Acad. Sci. U.S.A.* 1972, *70*, 747–749.
21. Greenblatt, M. *J. Natl. Cancer Inst.* 1973, *50*, 1055–1056.
22. Fiddler, W.; Pensabene, J. W.; Piotrowski, E. G.; Doerr, R. C.; Wasserman, A. E. *J. Food Sci.* 1973, *38*, 1084–1085.
23. Bunton, C. A.; Dahn, H.; Loewe, L. *Nature (London)* 1959, *183*, 163–165.
24. Archer, M. C.; Tannenbaum, S. R.; Fan, T. Y.; Weisman, M. *J. Natl. Cancer Inst.* 1975, *54*(5), 1203–1205.
25. Keefer, Y. K.; Roller, P. P. *Science* 1973, *181*, 1245–1247.
26. Small, D. M. In "Molecular Association in Biological and Related Systems," *Adv. Chem. Ser.* 1968, *84*, 31.
27. Okun, J. D.; Archer, M. C. *J. Natl. Cancer Inst.* 1977, *58*, 409–411.
28. Kim, Y. K., unpublished data.
29. The computer program will be provided upon request.
30. Bayliss, N. S.; Dingle, R.; Watts, D. W.; Wilkie, R. J. *Aust. J. Chem.* 1963, *16*, 933–942.
31. Turney, T. A. *J. Chem. Soc.* 1960, 4263–4265.
32. Benton, D. J.; Moore, D. *J. Chem. Soc. A* 1970, 3179–3182.
33. Hetzer, H. B.; Bates, R. G.; Robinson, R. A. *J. Phys. Chem.* 1966, *70*, 2869–2872.
34. Ridd, J. H. *Q. Rev.* 1961, *15*, 418–441.
35. Tannenbaum, S. R.; Mergens, W. *Ann. N.Y. Acad. Sci.* 1980, *355*, 267.
36. Fan, T. Y.; Tannenbaum, S. R. *J. Food Sci.* 1974, *38*, 1067.

37. Kawabata, T.; Shazuki, H.; Ishibashi, T. *Nippon Suisan Gakkaishi* **1974**, *40*, 1251.
38. Sen, N. P.; Donaldson, B. In "N-Nitroso Compounds in the Environment"; Bogovski, P.; Walker, E. A., Eds.; IARC; Lyon, France, 1974; pp. 103–106.
39. Gray, J. I.; Dugan, L. R. *J. Food Sci.* **1975**, *40*, 981–984.
40. Mottram, D. S.; Patterson, R. L. S.; Rhodes, D. N.; Gough, T. A. *J. Sci. Food Agric.* **1975**, *26*, 47–53.
41. Raineri, R.; Weisburger, J. H. *Ann. N.Y. Acad. Sci.* **1975**, *258*, 181–189.
42. Sen, N. P.; Donaldson, B.; Seaman, S.; Iyengar, J. R.; Miles, W. F. *J. Agric. Food Chem.* **1976**, *24*, 397–401.
43. Ziebarth, D.; Scheunig, G. "Environmental N-Nitroso Compounds: Analysis and Formation"; Walker, E. A.; Bogovski, P.; Griciute, L., Eds.; IARC: Lyon, France, 1976; pp. 279–290.
44. Mergens, W. J.; Newmark, H. L. *Proc. Meat Ind. Res. Conf., Arlington, VA, Mar., 1979.*
45. Massey, R. C.; Crews, C.; Roger, D.; McWeeny, D. J. *J. Sci. Food Agric.* **1978**, *29*, 815–821.
46. Tozawa, H. *Nippon Suisan Gakkaishi* **1978**, *44*, 797.
47. Mergens, W. J.; Vane, F. M.; Tannenbaum, S. R.; Green, L.; Skipper, P. *J. Pharm. Sci.* **1979**, *68*(7), 827–832.
48. Kalus, W. H.; Filby, W. G. *Experientia* **1980**, *36*, 147.
49. Weisburger, J. H.; Marquardt, H.; Mower, H. F.; Hirota, N.; Mori, H.; Williams, G. *Prev. Med.* **1980**, *9*, 352.
50. Mirvish, S. S. *Ann. N.Y. Acad. Sci.* **1975**, *258*, 175–180.
51. Kamm, J. J.; Dashman, T.; Conney, A. H.; Burns, J. J. "N-Nitroso Compounds in the Environment"; Bogovski, P.; Walker, E. A., Eds.; IARC: Lyon, France, 1974; pp. 200–204.
52. Cardesa, A.; Mirvish, S. S.; Haven, G. T.; Shubik, P. *Proc. Soc. Exp. Biol. Med.* **1974**, *145*, 124.
53. Ivankovic, S.; Preussmann, R.; Schmähl, D.; Zeller, J. W. "N-Nitroso Compounds in the Environment"; Bogovski, P.; Walker, E. A., Eds.; IARC: Lyon, France, 1974; pp. 101–102.
54. Mirvish, S. S.; Cardesa, A.; Wallcave, L.; Shubik, P. *J. Natl. Cancer Inst.* **1975**, *55*, 633–636.
55. Fong, Y. Y.; Chan, W. C. "Environmental N-Nitroso Compounds: Analysis and Formation"; Walker, E. A.; Bogovski, P.; Griciute, L., Eds.; IARC: Lyon, France, 1976; pp. 461–464.
56. Mirvish, S. S.; Pelfrene, A. F.; Garcia, H.; Shubik, P. *Cancer Lett.* **1976**, *2*, 101–108.
57. Preda, N.; Popa, L.; Galea, V.; Simu, G. "Environmental N-Nitroso Compounds: Analysis and Formation"; Walker, E. A.; Bogovski, P.; Griciute, L., Eds.; IARC: Lyon, France, 1976; pp. 301–304.

RECEIVED for review January 22, 1981. ACCEPTED May 29, 1981.

INDEX

Copy editor: Robin Giroux
Jacket designer: Kathleen Schaner

Typesetting by Service Composition Company, Baltimore, MD.
Printing and binding by Port City Press, Washington, DC.